# High Field Brain MRI

Tommaso Scarabino • Saverio Pollice
Teresa Popolizio
Editors

# High Field Brain MRI

## Use in Clinical Practice

Second Edition

Springer

*Editors*
Tommaso Scarabino
Department of Radiology and Neuroradiology
"L. Bonomo" Hospital
Andria (BT)
Italy

Teresa Popolizio
Department of Neuroradiology
"IRCCS Casa Sollievo della Sofferenza"
San Giovanni Rotondo (FG)
Italy

Saverio Pollice
Department of Radiology and Neuroradiology
"L. Bonomo" Hospital
Andria (BT)
Italy

ISBN 978-3-319-44173-3 ISBN 978-3-319-44174-0 (eBook)
DOI 10.1007/978-3-319-44174-0

Library of Congress Control Number: 2017931059



Printed on acid-free paper

This Springer imprint is published by Springer Nature
The registered company is Springer International Publishing AG
The registered company address is: Gewerbestrasse 11, 6330 Cham, Switzerland

# Preface

The second revised and implemented edition of this text aims to provide an update on the progress achieved in the high-field MRI systems in terms of hardware, software, its use in clinical routine and in the research field.

During the last years, there has been an increase in the installation trend of MRI 3 Tesla scanner all over the world, thanks to new laws and concessions introduced by the legislative systems of different European countries and thanks to the growing interest in the experts deriving from the different utlities and diagnostic possibilities.

Through the research carried out in this area by various manufacturing companies, the 3 Tesla scanners have become more compact, powerful, and versatile. These improvements have also been accompanied by a reduction of the differences in terms of the purely economic costs compared with more widely diffused 1.5 Tesla devices.

In this text, the many benefits offered by a 3 Tesla scanner compared to 1.5 Tesla are highlighted: higher signal, higher resolution, higher sensitivity, shorter imaging times, additional more advanced study procedures and enhanced diagnostic capacity, greater accuracy in morphofunctional study of the brain.

With advances in terms of software and hardware, some of the shortcomings of the 3.0 T systems, previously put in evidence, (inhomogeneity of the field, artifacts caused by susceptibility and chemical shift, elevated SAR, high costs), are currently less relevant.

The 3.0 T MR systems currently offer morphological investigation with high spatial, temporal and contrast resolution (essential for diagnosis). They also provide physiological, metabolic and functional information, enhancing the diagnostic power of routine MR imaging in terms of sensitivity and specificity both in clinical practice and in applied research purposes.

This volume includes papers on the techniques and semeiotics of morphofunctional cerebral imaging at 3.0 Tesla (including reference to the advantages and drawbacks respect to lower field strength MR systems) and the main clinical applications in neuroradiology.

Andria (BT), Italy Tommaso Scarabino
Saverio Pollice
San Giovanni Rotondo (FG), Italy Teresa Popolizio

# Contents

# Part I

# Techniques and Semeiotics

# High-Field MRI and Safety: I. Installations

1

Alberto Maiorana and Alessandra Iannelli

High-field magnetic resonance (MR), originally developed in the framework of spectroscopy and functional neuroradiology, has become to our days an important diagnostic tool not only in research but also in advanced clinical practice.

High magnetic fields afford a better signal/noise ratio (SNR) and consequently better spatial resolution in a shorter time of acquisition, even though the diagnostic outcome is then subject to the dependence on the magnetic field of other factors that variously contribute to image quality.

The rationale for the utilization of high magnetic fields in MR diagnostic imaging is obvious: the distribution of the population into two spin levels is statistically determined.

$\frac{n_f}{n_e} = e^{\left(\frac{\Delta E}{kT}\right)}$ where $\Delta E = h \times \gamma \times B_o$ depends on the static magnetic field, $h$ and $\gamma$ are constants, $n_f$ is the spin population in the fundamental state, and $n_e$ is the population in excited state.

An increase in $B_o$ values results in an inversion of the states of the two populations and therefore in a stronger MR signal.

In fact, the signal intensity is proportional to the square of the static magnetic field, since $S \cong (N_{\text{spin}} \cdot V_{\text{spin}})$ where the number of $N_{\text{spin}}$ and $V_{\text{spin}}$ and the voltage induced by each spin both depend linearly on $B_o$ [1, 2]. However, while the signal is proportional to the square of the static field $B_o$, the noise is proportional to $B_o$, and therefore from 1.5 T to 3.0 T, the SNR doubles. This allows to obtain an acceptable image quality even with increased spatial resolution or reduced time of acquisition.

The overall MR diagnostic outcome is always a compromise between field strength and other parameter choices such as gradients used for slice selection, radio frequency, and acquisition timing.

For instance, achieving greater spatial resolution while minimizing undesired partial volume effects requires increasing gradient steepness $G_z$ and reducing the frequency bandwidth $\boldsymbol{\Delta\omega}$ in the decoding readout phase, since slice thickness is defined as $\Delta z = \frac{\Delta\omega}{\gamma G_z}$ [2].

In any case, shimming requires a very strong field homogeneity. For instance, nowadays 3 Tesla machines used routinely achieve usually field homogeneity of less than 1 1.5 ppm in a spherical volume of 45 cm and of less than 0.005 ppm in a spherical volume of 10 cm, with a peak gradient ramp of 30÷50 mT/m and slew rates of about 150÷200 T/m/s.

Another key principle is that the resonance frequency $\omega = \gamma \times B_o$ depends on the static magnetic field. It therefore is 43 MHz at 1.0 T and 128 MHz at 3.0 T, resulting in greater radio

Alberto Maiorana (✉) • Alessandra Iannelli
Health Physics Department,
"IRCCS Casa Sollievo della Sofferenza",
Viale Cappuccini, 71013,
San Giovanni Rotondo (Fg), Italy


T. Scarabino et al. (eds.), *High Field Brain MRI*, DOI 10.1007/978-3-319-44174-0_1

frequency (RF) absorption by biological tissues, whose conductivity increases with frequency. This poses problems when designing coils suitable for the greater power applied as well as for patient safety, as increased tissue temperature is one of the risks associated with RF electromagnetic fields [3, 4].

Another important note is about susceptibility. Increased susceptibility of tissues exposed to higher magnetic field can result in local inhomogeneities that cannot be corrected and eventually present as artifacts. This effect has been exploited in functional MR BOLD studies, which are based on the changes in blood oxygenation generated by magnetic susceptibility inhomogeneities [2, 4, 5].

Notwithstanding technical and cost problems, high-field MR offers very significant advantages, and several human imaging studies at 340 MHz have demonstrated that safety margins exist above 3 and 4 Tesla [6]. More recent studies exploring biological effects on vital signs and cognitive ability suggest no risk even up to 9.4 Tesla➔2010 [7].

The growing interest in 3 T and higher magnetic fields has brought the safety issues back to the forefront.

When planning the installation of a high-field MR unit, the strength of the static magnetic field is one of the major problems to be addressed by those responsible for safety and technicians alike. In fact, this is but one, albeit the most apparent, element to be considered when assessing the associated risks and benefits. Patients in the tunnel of a high-strength imager are exposed to a magnetic field many thousands of times greater than the earth's, even though no special patient or operator safety precautions are required compared with low or medium magnetic fields. However, during scanning, patients are also exposed to gradient switch-on and to RF impulses for signal decoding and spin excitation, both of which are related to the intensity of the static magnetic field and carry different though acceptable patient risk given the obviously beneficial result.

Approval of high-field MR tomographs for diagnostic purposes dates from 1997, when the US Department of Health and Human Services, Food and Drug Administration, and Center for Devices and Radiological Health (US FDA.) classified as carrying a significant risk and therefore subjected to specific authorization all MR systems having static magnetic fields exceeding 4.0 T; a specific absorption rate (SAR) exceeding 4 W/kg averaged over the whole body for any 15-min period, 3 W/kg averaged over the head for any 10-min period, 8 W/kg for any gram of body or chest tissue in any 15-min period, or 15 W/kg for any gram of tissue in the extremities in any 15-min period; field gradients sufficient to induce patient discomfort or pain; and acoustic noise reaching sound pressure levels of 99 dB (A) (with reference to the response curve of the human ear, A curve) or peak values exceeding 140 dB(A) [8]. Based on these conditions, a 3 T MR unit meeting SAR, gradient, and noise requirements is substantially equivalent to a 1.5 T unit and does not carry a significantly greater risk, hence further restrictions.

At that time, the components of the early tomographs available on the market were substantially similar to those of the 1.5 T machines from which they had been derived. They thus presented a number of drawbacks, such as poor homogeneity of the static magnetic field, insufficient gradient slew rate, inadequate coil structure in relation to the greater resonance frequency, excessive fringe field extension, noise, and weight, and were also extremely expensive. All such factors hampered the diffusion of the technique, which remained confined to specific research fields for a long time.

By contrast, last-generation units have been conceived as high-field diagnostic machines and are equipped with technical features that allow to operate with a degree of safety comparable to the conventional low- and medium-field scanners [3, 9]. The passive-shield 3 T GE prototype was bulky and heavy, and its 0.5 mT line (or 5 Gauss limit) was an ellipsoid measuring 8.5 × 6.5 m in an axial radial direction. Adequate additional shielding of the fringe field in the magnet room would have required hundreds of tons of iron. The introduction of *active shielding* has significantly reduced magnet weight. In particular, the 200 mT line, which is crucial toward meeting current operator safety regulations, is practically contained in the tomograph's volume. This feature protects staff from undue whole-body exposure even for long stays in the scan room, while also due to the presence of passive ferromagnetic barriers around the scan room perimeter, the 0.1 mT line barely exceeds the magnet room boundary of magnet room.

Due to the intrinsic weakness of the MR signal and to the high sensitivity of image reconstruction systems, the magnet room needs to be protected by a Faraday cage capable of attenuating the outside electromagnetic noise. The shielding must be able to attenuate the signals by at least 80 dB, and it obviously also works the other way around, i.e., by shielding the operators from any type of exposure to the RF electromagnetic fields generated by the coils.

In 1999, the FDA approved for sale some high-field tomographs for clinical diagnostic imaging [4].

In July 2003 it replaced its 1997 guidelines and laid down new upper static magnetic field limits for MR diagnostic units. These limits were 8.0 T for adults and 4.0 T for neonates less than 1 month old [10]. In June 2014, FDA publication about the same topic confirms field strength risk limits of 8 T for adults and 4 T for neonates and indicates 4 W/kg as SAR limit averaged over the whole body for any 15 min period and 3.2 W/kg averaged over the head for any 10 min period [21].

In Europe, particularly in Italy, the earliest reference technical regulation, CEI EN 60601-2-33/A11 of 1998 [11], was superseded by IEC 60601 1-2-33 Ed. 2.0 of 2002 [12], the consolidated current version of which is the recent CEI EN 60601-2-33/A1/A2 published in 2015 [13].

In 2004, the International Commission for Nonionizing Radiation Protection (ICNIRP) has issued patient safety guidelines for MR scanning [14] and an amendment in 2009 about patient exposure to static magnetic fields, confirming an upper limit for whole-body exposure of 4 T in normal operating mode and 8 T for controlled mode [15].

In Italy, MR units with a static field strength of or exceeding 2.0 T were not approved for clinical use [16] until the entry into force of a new law, n. 160 of 7 August 2016, that pushes the threshold for research scheme from the old limit of 2 T to the new one of 4 T, thus enabling MR units of 3 T, to be no longer restricted to documented research applications [24]. Further legislation [17, 18] lays down SAR and field gradient limits substantially in line with the indications of Comitato Elettrotecnico Italiano (CEI) [11]. Today, MR machines with static magnetic fields exceeding 4 T, can be installed only at major research institutions and are subject to ministerial authorization [24]. Such units also need to be involved in scientific or clinical research projects mandating the use of such high field strengths. The authorization of tomographs with field strength exceeding 4 T is released by the Health Ministry and is currently also subject to the prior technical opinions of the "Istituto Nazionale per l'Assicurazione contro gli Infortuni sul Lavoro e le malattie professionali" (INAIL), the "Istituto superiore di Sanità" (ISS), and the "Consiglio Superiore di Sanità" (CSS). [24]. As regards staff safety and protection, limits for *static* magnetic fields were issued by I.C.N.I.R.P. in 2009 [20]. Whereas the limits adopted in Italy [17] are substantially similar. Specifically they are named VLE (exposure limit values) and set as 2 T for sensorial effects in normal working conditions and 8 T for sanitary effects in controlled working conditions.

With high-field systems, correct dimensioning or upgrading of ventilation and helium venting pipes in relation to the type of magnet being installed and room size should be addressed at the design stage [23]. Indeed, in the event of a quench, i.e., the sudden inactivation of the magnet, the liquid helium contained in a superconducting magnet (which is more than in a high-strength unit) rapidly turns to gas and may saturate the magnet room atmosphere.

## References

1. Takahashi M, Uematsu H, Hatabu H (2003) MR imaging at high magnetic fields. Eur J Radiol 46:45–52
2. Duerk JL (1999) Principles of MR image formation and reconstruction. Magnetic Resonance Imaging Clinics of North America, Physics of MR Imaging 7(4):629–659

3. Schenck JF (1999) MR safety at high magnetic fields. Magn Reson Imaging Clin N Am MR Safety 6(4):715–730
4. Frayne R, Goodyear BG, Dickhoff P et al (2003) Magnetic resonance imaging at 3.0 Tesla: challenges and advantages in clinical neurological imaging. Invest Radiol 38(7):385–402
5. Uematsu H, Dougherty L, Takahashi M et al (2003) A direct comparison of signal behaviour between 4.0 and 1.5 T: a phantom study. Eur J Radiol 45:154–159
6. Kangarlu A, Robitaille PML (2000) Biological effects and health implications in magnetic resonance imaging. Concepts in Magnetic Resonance 12:321–359
7. Atkinson IC et al (2010) Vital signs and cognitive function are not affected by 23-sodium and 17-oxygen magnetic resonance imaging of the human brain at 9.4 T. J Magn Reson Imaging 32:82–87
8. Food and Drug Administration Center for Devices and Radiological Health (1997) Guidance for magnetic resonance diagnostic devices-criteria for significant risk investigation
9. Budinger TF (1999) MR safety, past, present and future from a historical perspective. Magn Reson Imaging Clin N Am, MR Safety 6(4):701–714
10. Food and Drug Administration Center for Devices and Radiological Health (2003) Criteria for significant risk investigations of magnetic resonance diagnostic devices
11. Comitato Elettrotecnico Italiano, Apparecchi Elettromedicali Parte 2 (1998) Prescrizioni particolari di sicurezza relative agli apparecchi a risonanza magnetica per diagnostica medica. CEI EN 60601-2-33/A11
12. International Electrotechnical Commission (2002) Medical electrical equipment Part 2-33: particular requirements for the safety of magnetic resonance equipment for medical diagnosis. IEC 60601 1-2-33 Ed. 2.0
13. International Electrotechnical Commission IEC 60601 -2-33 Ed 3.2 06-2015 Medical electrical equipment Part 2-33: particular requirements for the safety of magnetic resonance equipment for medical diagnosis. CSV
14. The International Commission on Non-Ionizing Radiation Protection [ICNIRP] (2004) Medical magnetic resonance (MR) procedures: protection of patients. Health Phys 87(2):197–216
15. Amendment to the ICNIRP "Statement on Medical Magnetic Resonance (MR) Procedures: Protection of the Patients" The International Commission on Non-Ionizing Radiation Protection (2009)
16. D.P.R 542 (1994) Regolamento recante norme per la semplificazione del procedimento di autorizzazione all'uso diagnostico di apparecchiature a risonanza magnetica nucleare sul territorio nazionale. G.U. 219
17. D.Lgs 1/8/2016, n. 159: Attuazione della Direttiva 2013/35/UE sulle disposizioni minime di sicurezza e di salute relative all'esposizione dei lavoratori ai rischi derivanti dagli agenti fisici (campi elettromagnetici) e che abroga la direttiva 2004/40/CE
18. D.M. 03/08/1993 (1993) Aggiornamento di alcune norme concernenti l'autorizzazione all'installazione ed all'uso di apparecchiature a risonanza magnetica. G.U. 187
19. Campanella F, Mattozzi M, Panebianco A S et al. (2004) Indicazioni operative e gestionali relative all'installazione ed uso di apparecchiature diagnostiche a Risonanza Magnetica. Indicazioni Operative I.S.P.E.S.L.
20. The International Commission on Non-Ionizing Radiation Protection [ICNIRP] (2009) Guidelines on limits of exposure to static magnetic fields. Health Phys 96(4):504–514
21. Criteria for Significant Risk Investigations of Magnetic Resonance Diagnostic Devices – Guidance for Industry and Food and Drug Administration Staff Document issued on: June 20, 2014
22. Indicazioni Operative dell'INAIL per la gestione della sicurezza e della qualità in Risonanza Magnetica, aa F Campanella, MA D'Avanzo, M Mattozzi, L Moretti. Edizione 2015
23. Realizzazione alla regola dell'arte degli impianti di ventilazione nelle sale di Risonanza Magnetica. Indicazioni operative, esperienze, criticità. Edizione 2012
24. Legge n. 160 del 7 Agosto 2016, del Presidente della Repubblica: *"Conversione in legge, con modificazioni, del decreto legge 24 giugno 2016, n. 113, recante misure finanziarie urgenti per gli enti territoriali e il territorio"*. (GU n.194 del 20-8-2016)

# High-Field MRI and Safety: II. Utilization

2

Alberto Maiorana and Alessandra Iannelli

The possible risks directly connected with magnetic resonance (MR) diagnostic imaging are mainly related to three components that are simultaneously active as the patient is being scanned: static magnetic field, magnetic field gradients, and radio-frequency (RF) field.

No adverse effects of static magnetic fields lower than 4.0 T have yet been demonstrated in man [1–4]; in contrast, it is well established that attempts to improve the diagnostic performance by acting on the other two elements may lead to potentially hazardous situations. Although the electric and the magnetic field are commonly conceived of as separate entities, in fact they coexist, and only rarely can they be considered separately. Several effects ascribed to variable magnetic fields are in fact due to changes in the associated electric field.

Two possible sources of indirect risk can be magnified by the intrinsic working characteristics of fast superconducting MR imagers: cryogenic gases and the noise produced by coil vibration during sequence performance.

Some of the main risks directly or indirectly connected with high magnetic fields are discussed below.

A. Maiorana (✉) • A. Iannelli
Health Physics Department,
"IRCCS Casa Sollievo della Sofferenza",
Viale Cappuccini, 71013
San Giovanni Rotondo (Fg), Italy
e-mail: a.maiorana@operapadrepio.it

## 2.1 Static Magnetic Field

The suspicion that exposure to high magnetic fields could be associated with some kind of risk dates from 1970, when MR diagnostic imaging was first introduced. However, statistical data indicate that about 150,000,000 MR diagnostic examinations have been performed in the world from 1980 to 1999 (ca. 20,000,000 a year, 50,000 a day) with very few accidents. Although the absolute accident number remains low, FDA statistics about MR officially declared that accidents occurring from 2000 to 2009 showed an increase of 523 %. [5].

The few documented cases of severe injury directly ascribable to the static magnetic field were due to magneto-mechanical effects on patient implants or devices introduced into the scan room by mistake [3, 6].

### 2.1.1 Translation and Rotation Forces

All materials that magnetize transiently have a susceptibility value $\chi_m$ other than 0; in particular, materials whose values range from −1 and 0, designated as diamagnetic, are repelled by the magnetic field. In fact, although all materials have a diamagnetic field, in some of them, the presence of ions of transition elements tends to raise the susceptibility value. Materials with positive values are attracted to the magnetic field and are called paramagnetic. Ferromagnetism is an


T. Scarabino et al. (eds.), *High Field Brain MRI*, DOI 10.1007/978-3-319-44174-0_2

extreme form of paramagnetism and characterizes some materials having high levels of susceptibility, which are strongly attracted to magnetic fields. The presence of such objects in the magnet room is extremely dangerous and must be avoided. Diamagnetic and paramagnetic materials, whose susceptibility is about 0.01, respond weakly to the magnetic field and are often considered nonmagnetic. To this group belong biological tissues, whose susceptibility is in a range of ±20 % from $-9\ 10^{-6}$, to say the susceptibility of water. For instance, when patients are slid into the tunnel, the magnet exerts a force that contrasts this movement, although it is so weak as to be negligible [6].

Magnetic flow density $B$, expressed as Tesla, represents the magnetic induction deriving from exposure to a magnetic field $H$, according to the relationship:

$B = \mu_0(1+\chi_m)H$, where the magnetic susceptibility $\chi_m = \frac{M}{H}$ is the ratio of induced magnetization to the source field and $\mu_0$ is the magnetic permeability in vacuum.

Although the distinction between source and induced magnetic field tends to be neglected in practice, in MR diagnostic imaging, it has an important role when the susceptibility has an appreciable positive value, as is the case of paramagnetic contrast agents and ferromagnetic objects.

When an object, such as the human body, a metal prosthesis, or an erythrocyte, is introduced into a MR tomograph, it is subjected to translation forces in the gradient zones and to rotation forces with respect to the direction of the static field $B$. Such forces depend on the susceptibility of the material from which the object is made, on its shape and volume, and on the intensity of the magnetic field, and in relation to them, they may be negligible or have potentially lethal effects.

The force of translation $F_{trasl} \approx \frac{\chi_m V}{\mu_0} \times B \times \frac{dB}{dz}$ depends on the volume $V$, the susceptibility value, and the magnetic field gradient, whereas the force of rotation required to oppose the object's rotation $F_{rot} \approx \frac{\chi_m^2 V}{2L\mu_0} \times B^2$ also depends on its length $L$ and volume, thus on its shape.

In general, $F_{rot} >> F_{trasl}$, thus the tissue damage induced by the rotation force generated by the field of an implanted metal object will be greater than the damage caused by the force of translation, especially in the presence of high magnetic fields, due to its quadratic dependence on $B$ [6].

In human tissue, the magneto-mechanical effects are negligible due to their weak susceptibility; for instance, the alignment of erythrocytes parallel to the magnetic field due to their ellipsoid shape is negligible because of the quadratic dependence of the torque on susceptibility. The force acting on 100 g of water in an 8 T magnetic field with a peak gradient of 7.9 T/m and a product $B \cdot \frac{dB}{dz}$, equaling 43 $T^2$/m, is negative and is ca. $-3.4 \cdot 10^{-3}$ N.

By contrast, a 100 g stainless steel wrench with susceptibility of 0.01 and a volume of 12.5 $cm^3$ will be attracted to the same field with a force of 4.3 N, an acceleration of 43 $m/s^2$, that is, more than four times of the gravitation, turning it into a bullet [3, 6]. The magnitude of the force acquired for the paramagnetic and ferromagnetic objects would be larger by a factor $10^2$ to $10^5$, posing serious hazards for workers and patients in the magnet area.

People with splinters lodged in the bodies or wearing metal prostheses are also at high risk, since these object's movements, induced by the magnetic field, may cause tissue or vessel tears.

Inside the magnet, the field gradient is zero and so is the force of translation exerted on a ferromagnetic object, which will thus remain trapped in the tunnel. Attempts to extract it forcibly in case of an accident are often vain and can impair the magnet's stability in the cryostat. Recovery of the object usually requires inactivation of the magnet. By contrast, the rotation forces, which depend solely on $B^2$, continue to be active. To prevent this type of risk, metal objects must never be introduced into the scan room. This is clearly stated in notices and is prevented from happening by taking an accurate patient history.

Since most of the data on the compatibility of several implanted devices and prostheses regard 1.5 T static magnetic fields, MR investigations of such patients at higher fields are to be avoided.

However, information on the safety and compatibility of 26 aortic aneurysm clips tested at 8.0 T and of 109 implants and devices tested at 3.0 T has been published.

Safety in this connection indicates that the objects have been shown to carry no additional patient risk save a reduction in image quality, whereas compatibility indicates demonstration of the property of not interference with image quality. The distinction between long- and short-bore magnets of equal field intensity lies in the differences in the respective position and height of gradient peaks at the tunnel aperture [7–10].

In general, patients wearing pacemakers should avoid undergoing MR imaging, especially at high magnetic field. The several effects that may derive from exposure are due to the static magnetic field (e.g., pacemaker movement, remote control switch-off, and ECG changes), to the RF field (e.g., heating, alteration of pace frequency, and device reset), and to the gradients (e.g., induction of voltage, heating, and remote control switch-off). However, these effects still present controversial aspects because, on the one hand, early compatibility studies assessed models that are no longer in use and, on the other, recent data indicate that small groups of patients underwent MR imaging for vital reasons without experiencing adverse effects [11, 12, 14–18].

In most materials, the magnetization induced is parallel to $H$; in such cases, $M$, $B$, and $H$ all point in the same direction, and the material is said to have isotropic susceptibility. If, however, the susceptibility varies within the volume of the material exposed to the magnetic field, the object becomes magnetized along directions that may not be parallel to the magnetic field; in anisotropic cell structures, this may lead to structure reorientation or distortion. In such cases, this effect, which has been documented in vitro, is stronger than the one induced by object shape [6].

Another biological effect connected with a potential risk, which in the past has been attributed to abnormal myocardial repolarization, is in fact induced by the blood flow in the large vessels within a strong magnetic field. The Lorentz force, $F$, induces on vessel walls an electric field $E = \frac{F}{q} = vBsen\theta$, where $v$ is blood velocity, $\theta$ the angle between the flow direction and the direction of the magnetic field, and $q$ the charge of the ions in the blood.

This induced electric field causes a reversible increment in T-wave amplitude in the ECG. In vivo investigation of this effect at fields greater than 8 T has demonstrated that the induced potentials are below the threshold of nerve or muscle stimulation. The migration of opposite charges to vessel walls induced by the magnetic field also causes a current in a direction perpendicular to the flow velocity in vessels and thus an additional Lorentz force in a direction opposite to the blood flow that could contrast it appreciably. However, it has been demonstrated that this effect is negligible even in the presence of magnetic fields exceeding 10 T [13].

## 2.2 Varying Electric and Magnetic Fields

During scanning, patients are also exposed to the activation of magnetic field ramps or gradients for spatial localization of the signal and to RF impulses for signal generation and decoding. Specific effects that may constitute a source of patient risk during scanning have been documented in their connection.

### 2.2.1 Magnetic Field Gradients

Many of the effects ascribed to magnetic fields that vary over time are in fact related to the associated electric field. Switching the magnetic field gradients on and off may induce electric currents capable of affecting the cell membrane potential and, if sufficiently intense, of stimulating the peripheral nervous system and the cardiac muscle. The stimulation threshold of peripheral nerves may be painful but is reversible and is used as a safety reference indicator for cardiac stimulation, which in contrast carries a risk of fibrillation. In fact, with ramp durations of less than 1 m/s, the former threshold is always lower than, and is reached before, the latter [13].

The intensity of these currents is proportional to the induced electric field and depends on the conductivity of biological tissues. The other critical factor of gradients, besides their amplitude, is their slew rate; the value of the induced electric field can be calculated using a model represented by a cylindrical object with radius $r$ as follows: $E = \frac{r}{2} \cdot \frac{\mathrm{d}B}{\mathrm{d}t}$.

For instance, if during an examination a localization ramp from 0 to 20 mT/m in 200 μs is launched from a 1 m coil, then the temporal variation of the magnetic field will be 100 T/s, and for an abdomen 0.4 m in diameter, the value of the electric field calculated using the above model will be 10 V/m, which exceeds the 6 V/m threshold of peripheral nerve stimulation [4, 20].

An ability to excite 40–50 mT/m gradients is shared by last-generation currently used MR units reaching slew-rate values of about 200 T/m/s per axis [19]; at high magnetic fields, spatial resolution can be improved by strengthening the gradients up to 80 mT/m, the highest gradient ramp clinically available. High ramp however results in an increased induced electric field that may easily exceed the safety threshold. To avoid this effect, the electric field increase could be offset by increasing gradient duration; however, an increase, for instance, from 0 to 80 mT/m in 400 μs would result in a value of $\frac{\mathrm{d}B}{\mathrm{d}t}$ of 200 T/m/s, while based on the model mentioned above, the electric field would still be 10 V/m. In addition, increasing gradient duration leads too close to the values where the thresholds of peripheral and cardiac stimulation converge, preventing peripheral nerve stimulation from being used as a safety indicator.

## 2.3 Radio-Frequency Electromagnetic Fields

The RF impulses applied in MR imaging are always accompanied by an RF electric field, which in turn induces RF electric currents in patients.

Due to the Joule effect, these currents may induce a potentially adverse heating of tissues or burns caused by conducting loops accidentally generated by the contact between the patient's limbs or by leads of auxiliary devices inadvertently left on the patient's skin [22, 23].

At 3.0 T, the resonance frequency of protons is 128 MHz, i.e., twice the value at 1.5 T, the spatial distribution of the RF field generated by the coils becomes more complex with increasing frequency, and the temperature rise may become localized, giving rise to hot spots.

At very high frequencies, the wavelength of the field is comparable to the size of the anatomical structure being scanned, a situation that may lead to generation of stationary waves that impair RF field homogeneity. In addition, as the frequency increases, so does the tissue conductivity and consequently the density of the induced current, resulting in greater power density being deposited in tissues.

Greater conductivity also involves impaired RF signal penetration, requiring greater power to obtain the same signal.

Prevention of accidental tissue heating requires a careful valuation of the energy deposited per unit of mass in unit of time or specific absorption rate (SAR), which is measured in W/kg of exposed tissue. Between 1.5 and 3.0 T, this rate increases with $B^2$, making the safety threshold more likely to be reached in the course of the same sequence performed with a 3.0 T than with a 1.5 T unit [2].

Today, FDA SAR limits are of 4 W/kg for an exposition averaged over 15 minutes for whole body and 3.2 W/kg for head exposition averaged over a time of 10 minutes [21].

## 2.4 Cryogenic Gases

With high-field systems, correct dimensioning or upgrading of ventilation and helium venting pipes in relation to the type of magnet being installed and room size should be addressed at the design stage, given that 700 l of gas are produced from 1 l of liquid helium. The cryostat of a 3.0 T superconducting magnet contains approximately 3 $m^3$ of helium, i.e., roughly three times a 1.0 T magnet. In normal boil-off, i.e., gradual, controlled evaporation conditions, the gas is channeled outside through a dedicated exhaust pipe. In case of a quench, i.e., a sudden increase in coil temperature and violent, uncontrolled evaporation of the helium in which the coils are immersed, the oxygen concentration in the scan room may drop to levels likely to cause asphyxia. In case of an emergency, the forced ventilation plant therefore needs to guarantee at least 18÷20 air changes/hour to restore safety conditions in the room as quickly as possible. In particular, the design of the ventilation plant inlet and outlet points must ensure against a short circuit of the air flow, and inlet and outlet fluxes need to be proportionate [24].

To ensure helium outflow in normal as well as emergency conditions, the quench pipe diameter must be correctly dimensioned in relation to pipe length and the number of bends. Finally, the oxygen monitor, which activates the ventilation plant in case of an emergency, needs to be placed at appropriate height in the room (since helium is lighter than air and tends to rise) and close to the likeliest point of leakage, which is the limiting pressure valve fitted on the quench pipe.

To avoid introducing cryogenic gas containers into the hospital, an insulated pipe allowing the helium to be refilled from the outside should be envisaged.

## 2.5 Acoustic Noise

In an MR unit, field gradients are the main source of acoustic noise, which is produced by the rapid current changes inside the coils. In the presence of a strong magnetic field, these currents are subject to the Lorentz force acting on the coils. Changes in gradient amplitude and steepness connected with different sequences may affect noise levels, which tend to increase with decreasing slice thickness, field of view, TR, and TE [26].

Functional MR using fast gradients involves a noise level close to 120 dB (A), which varies in relation to the sequences performed, but is consistently higher than the noise produced by a 1.5 T [25].

At present, the simplest and least expensive means to reduce noise is passive patient protection using earplugs or earphones, even though this impairs communication with the operator and may cause discomfort.

"Silent" coils made from new materials with new assembly techniques or active noise cancelation systems are being developed; moreover it should be possible to optimize the choice of the imaging parameters to obtain less noisy sequences [26–28].

## References

1. Schenck JF (1999) MR safety at high magnetic fields. Magn Reson Imaging Clin N Am MR Safety 6(4):715–730
2. Frayne R, Goodyear BG, Dickhoff P et al (2003) Magnetic resonance imaging at 3.0 Tesla: challenges and advantages in clinical neurological imaging. Invest Radiol 38(7):385–402
3. Kangarlu A, Robitaille PML (2000) Biological effects and health implications in magnetic resonance imaging. Concepts in Magnetic Resonance 12:321–359
4. Budinger TF (1999) MR safety, past, present and future from a historical perspective. Magnetic Resonance Imaging Clinics of North America, MR Safety 6(4): 701–714
5. FDA's Manufacturer and User Facility Device Experience (MAUDE) database
6. Schenck JF (2000) Safety of strong, static magnetic fields. J Magn Reson Imaging 12:2–19
7. Shellock FG (2002) Magnetic resonance safety update 2002: implants and devices. J Magn Reson Imaging 16:485–496
8. Kangarlu A, Shellock FG (2000) Aneurysm clips: evaluation of magnetic field interactions with an 8.0 T MR system. J Magn Reson Imaging 12:107–111
9. Shellock FG (2002) Biomedical implants and devices: assessment of magnetic field interactions with a 3.0 Tesla MR system. J Magn Reson Imaging 16:721–732
10. Shellock FG, Tkach JA, Ruggeri PM et al (2003) Aneurysm clips: evaluation of magnetic field interactions and translational attraction by use of "Long-Bore" and "Short Bore" 3.0-T MR imaging systems. AJNR Am J Neuroradiol 24:463–471
11. Duru F, Luechinger R, Scheidegger MB et al (2001) Pacing in magnetic resonance imaging environment: clinical and technical considerations on compatibility. Eur Heart J 22:113–124

12. Shellock FG, Tkach JA, Ruggeri PM et al (2003) Cardiac pacemakers, ICDs, and loop recorder: evaluation of translational attraction using conventional ("Long Bore") and "Short Bore" 1.5 and 3.0 Tesla MR systems. J Cardiovasc Magn Reson 5(2):387–397
13. Kangarlu A, Burgess RE, Zhu H et al (1999) Cognitive, cardiac, and physiological safety studies in ultra high field magnetic resonance imaging. Magn Reson Imaging 17(10):1407–1416
14. Baikoussis NG et al (2011) Safety of magnetic resonance imaging in patients with implanted cardiac prostheses and metallic cardiovascular electronic devices. Ann Thorac Surg 91:2006–2011
15. Buendía F et al (2010) Nuclear magnetic resonance imaging in patients with cardiac pacing devices. Rev Esp Cardiol 63:735–739
16. Calcagnini G et al (2008) In vitro investigation of pacemaker lead heating induced by magnetic resonance imaging: role of implant geometry. J Magn Reson Imaging 28:879–886
17. Colletti PM, Shinbane JS, Shellock FG (2011) "MR-conditional" pacemakers: The radiologist's role in multidisciplinary management. AJR Am J Roentgenol 197:W457–W459
18. Harden SP (2011) MRI conditional pacemakers: the start of a new era. Br J Radiol 84:773–774
19. ET T (2016) High slew-rate head-only gradient for improving distortion in echo planar imaging: preliminary experience. J Magn Reson Imaging 44:653–664
20. Schaefer DJ, Bourland JD, Nyenhuis JA (2000) Review of patient safety in time – varying gradient field. J Magn Reson Imaging 12:20–29
21. Criteria for Significant Risk Investigations of Magnetic Resonance Diagnostic Devices - Guidance for Industry and Food and Drug Administration Staff Document issued on: June 20, 2014
22. Shellock FG (2000) Radiofrequency energy-induced heating during MR procedures: a review. J Magn Reson Imaging 12:30–36
23. Dempsey MF, Condon B (2000) Thermal injuries associated with MRI. Clin Radiol 56:457–465
24. Indicazioni operative dell'Inail per la gestione della sicurezza e della qualità in Risonanza Magnetica (2015)
25. Hattori Y (2007) Measurement and evaluation of the acoustic noise of a 3 Tesla MR scanner. Nagoya J Med Sci 69(1–2):23–28
26. McJury M, Shellock FG (2000) Auditory noise associated with MR procedures: a review. J Magn Reson Imaging 12:37–45
27. Segbers M et al (2010) Shaping and timing gradient pulses to reduce MRI acoustic noise. Magn Reson Med 64:546–553
28. Lin CY, Chen JH (2012) Real-time active noise control of magnetic resonance imaging acoustic noise. J Acoust Soc Am 132:1971

# 3.0 T MRI Diagnostic Features: Comparison with Lower Magnetic Fields

**3**

Tommaso Scarabino, Giuseppe Maria Giannatempo, Saverio Pollice, Michelangelo Nasuto, Rosario Francesco Balzano, and Teresa Popolizio

3.0 T magnetic resonance (MR) units are optimized for high-resolution morphological and functional imaging, especially of the head and neck, and offer a number of advantages over lower-field systems, such as a higher signal/noise ratio (SNR) and greater spatial and temporal resolution (Fig. 3.1) [1–4]. Drawbacks include greater specific absorption rates (SAR), acoustic noise and dielectric resonance, although in the more recent imagers, these problems have largely been resolved by improvements in hardware and software.

MR scans acquired at 3.0 T and 1.5 T exhibit different diagnostic features that need to be taken into consideration when images are being interpreted and also to optimize sequence parameters. These same differences prevent transfer of 1.5 T study protocols to 3.0 T systems.

T. Scarabino (✉) • S. Pollice
Department of Radiology and Neuroradiology, PO "L. Bonomo" Hospital, Andria (BT), Italy
e-mail: tscarabino@hotmail.com

G.M. Giannatempo • M. Nasuto • R.F. Balzano
T. Popolizio
Department of Radiology and Neuroradiology, IRCCS "Casa Sollievo della Sofferenza", San Giovanni Rotondo (FG), Italy

## 3.1 Comparison of 3.0 T and 1.5 T MR Imaging

### 3.1.1 Advantages

#### 3.1.1.1 High SNR

This is undoubtedly the main advantage of high-field MR systems [5–8]. The stronger magnetic field is associated with a proportional increase in the percentage of hydrogen protons oriented parallel to the static magnetic field ($B_0$), resulting in increased macroscopic longitudinal magnetization (MLM) and thus in a better SNR. In particular, signal intensity increases with the square of $B_0$, whereas the noise is linearly proportional to it.

In principle, the linear dependence of SNR on magnetic field strength should result in its doubling from 1.5 T to 3.0 T. In practice, this is true only of some tissues such as cerebrospinal fluid (CSF). In white and grey matter and in the grey nuclei, the increase is much smaller (30–60 %) because the signal reduction induced by changes in relaxation times is associated with a greater signal loss due to susceptibility (related to the very low iron concentrations in some of these areas) and to chemical shift artefacts. Moreover, despite major advances in software and hardware directed at improving image quality and reducing imaging time, acquisition parameters can also be modified to an extent where a lower SNR can be


T. Scarabino et al. (eds.), *High Field Brain MRI*, DOI 10.1007/978-3-319-44174-0_3

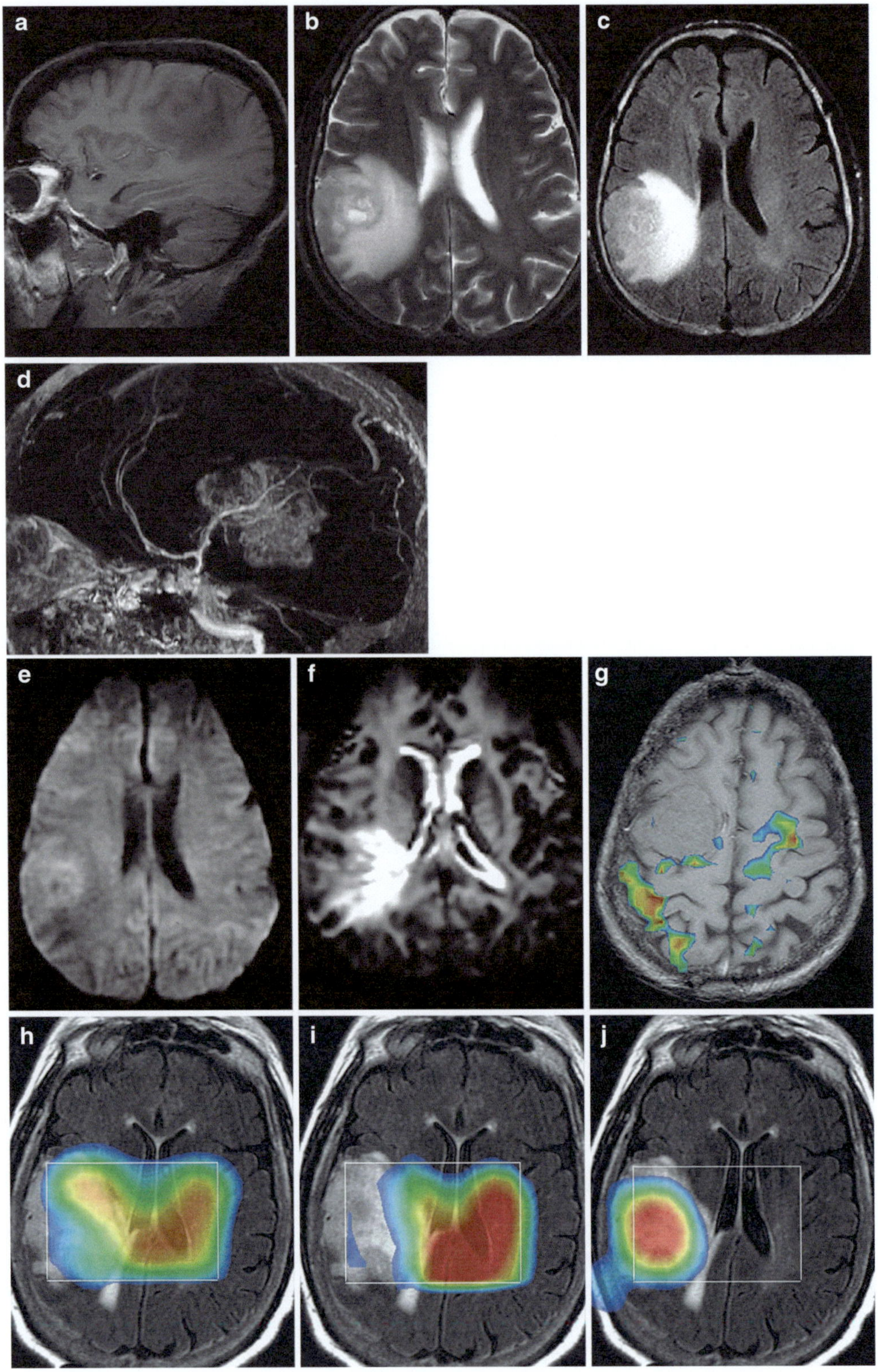


**Fig. 3.1** High-resolution morphological and functional study of cerebral glioblastoma: SE T1 (**a**), FSE T2 (**b**), FLAIR (**c**), MRA (**d**), DWI (**e**), PWI (**f**), fMRI with motor task (**g**) and spectroscopy (**h**) (Cho map; (**i**) NAA map; (**j**) Lac/Lip map)

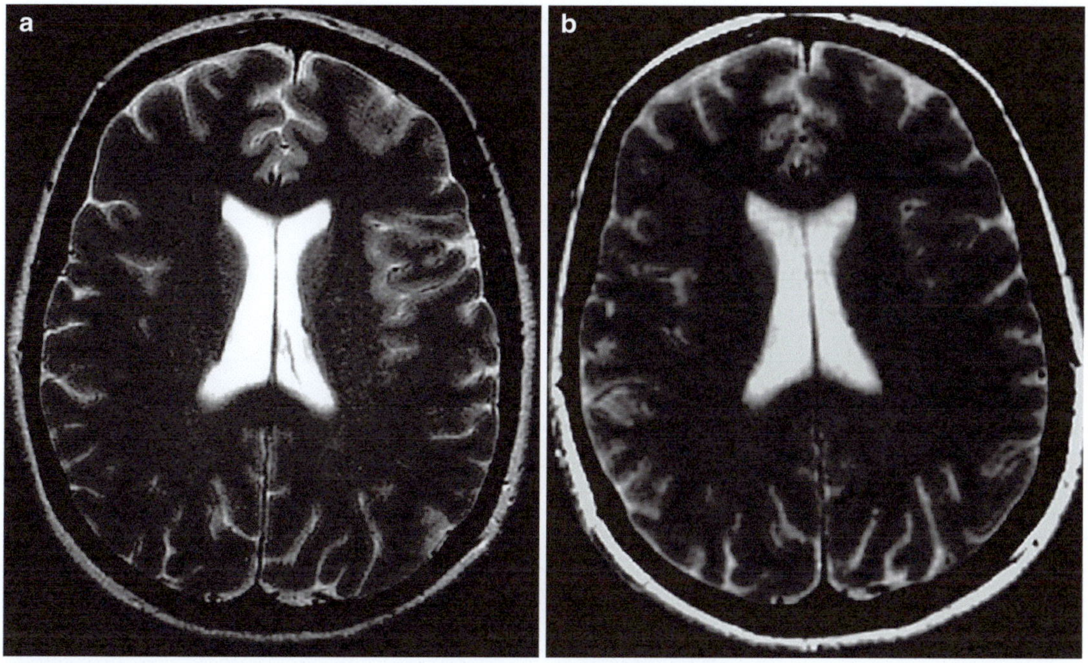


**Fig. 3.2** FSE T2 study: comparison of 3.0 T (TR/TE/ETL 4850/81/15, slice thickness 4 mm, FOV 22 cm, matrix 448×320, 2 NEX, 2:39) (**a**) with 1.5 T (TE/TE/ETL 3000/88/8, slice thickness 6 mm, FOV 24×18, 2 NEX, 256×224, 2:24) (**b**). At 3.0 T (**a**) an FSE T2 study takes a similar amount of time as at 1.5 T (**b**) but achieves greater definition (thinner and more numerous slices, broader matrices and smaller FOV)

obtained at 3.0 T than 1.5 T (Fig. 3.2). However, the use of 3.0 T systems in clinical settings requires great care to avoid compromising image quality.

#### 3.1.1.2 High Spatial Resolution

SNR is higher at 3 tesla, but the improvement varies with the category of the sequences.

The greater SNR allows increased spatial resolution to be achieved and a reduction of partial volume effects, thereby depicting structures that are difficult to visualize at 1.5 T (e.g. blood vessels measuring 200–300 μm). In addition, the resulting greater spatial resolution makes 3.0 T imaging more accurate when fine morphological detail is required, as in volumetric studies like hippocampal volumetry, which is performed to analyse the extent of hippocampal damage in patients with epilepsy and other diseases involving the brain such as Alzheimer's [9].

3 T MRI also provides accurate stereotactic data sets [10].

#### 3.1.1.3 High Temporal Resolution

Temporal resolution is also enhanced at higher field intensity due to greatly reduced acquisition time. Indeed, the fast gradients of 3.0 T units allow scanning times to be drastically shortened, resulting in a reduction of motion artefacts.

Using a 3.0 T MR system, morphological investigations of the brain, including a standard high-definition study before and after contrast administration, can be performed in 20–30 min and yield greater detail than using a 1.5 T unit. If diffusion and perfusion studies, spectroscopy and functional MR imaging (fMRI) are also performed, acquisition and processing times do not exceed 50–60 min.

Since intrinsically fast techniques like echo-planar sequences obviously involve similar acquisition times with both low and high field strengths, the greater SNR of the latter is exploited to achieve enhanced spatial resolution (Fig.3.3).

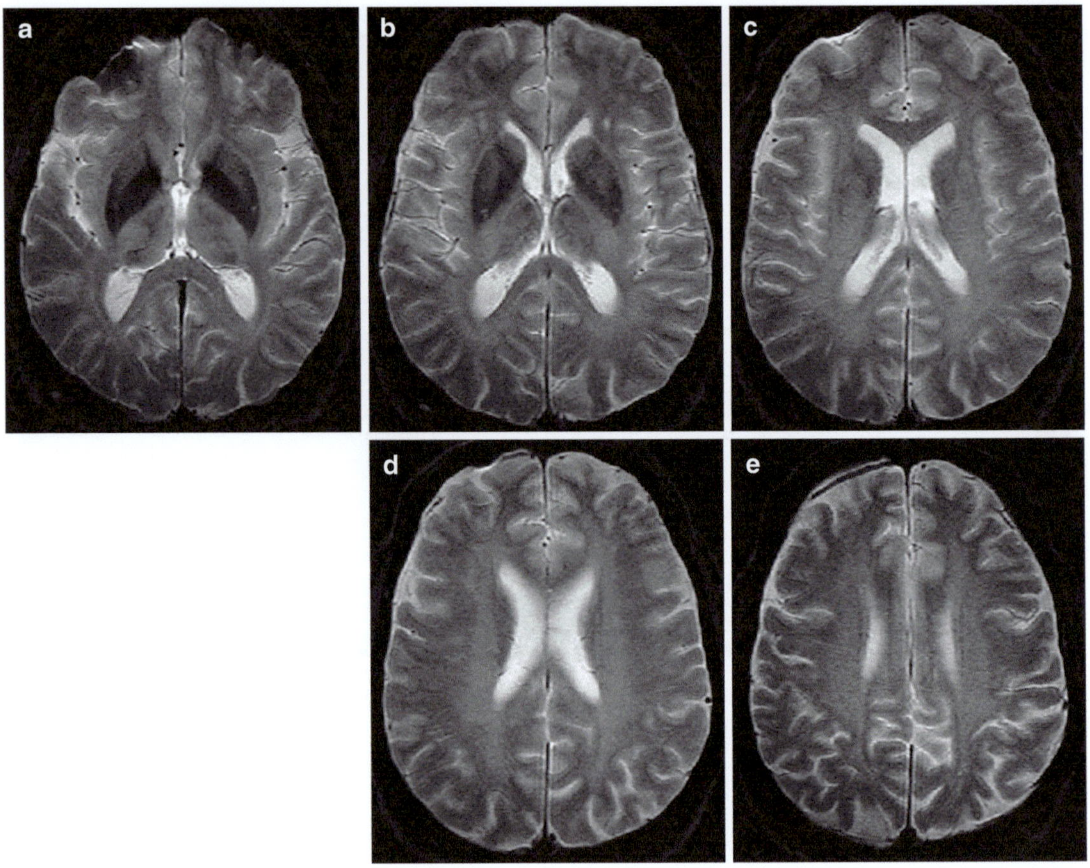


**Fig. 3.3** (**a–e**) SE-EPI (16 shots, matrix 512 × 256). The higher SNR yields greater resolution

High-strength magnetic fields are therefore indicated for fast imaging of patients in poor conditions, for long protocols (including structural, metabolic and functional imaging) and for novel applications such as continuous EEG recording and functional fMRI for the detection of seizure foci [11].

Reduced times of acquisition are also useful with uncooperative and paediatric patients. In the latter, this feature is especially valuable in the case of non-sedated children who may have difficulties in lying still or in sedated neonates in poor conditions: short examination times are thus crucial in both cases [12].

## 3.1.2 Disadvantages

### 3.1.2.1 Increased SAR

A major drawback of high magnetic fields is an increased SAR, i.e. the radiofrequency (RF) energy deposited per kilogram of tissue in unit of time. The resonance frequency of the hydrogen protons, hence the RF signal, grows proportionally with magnetic field strength, resulting in more energy being deposited in tissues. As a consequence, the SAR limits are reached sooner with 3.0 T than 1.5 T units, the SAR increasing fourfold from 1.5 T to 3.0 T [13, 14]. Because the SAR increases with the square of the field strength, RF deposition is more limiting at higher field strengths.

Moreover, as the SAR is also proportional to pulse duration and pulse and slice number, its increment at higher magnetic field strengths entails a number of drawbacks, limiting the number of slices, the use of fast spin echo (FSE) sequences, selection of the flip angle (FA) and speed of acquisition. Therefore, sequences such as FSE, which employ a large number of closely spaced RF pulses with large FA, are those most likely to cause increased energy deposition at higher fields and to be affected by SAR level limitations. Unfortunately, as FSE sequences rely on T2- rather than T2*-weighted echo trains, they are the least sensitive to susceptibility-induced image distortion and would be extremely useful at higher magnetic fields.

High magnetic field strength therefore requires a new approach to reduce the SAR, especially when using FSE. Several different strategies have been devised to do this. The most obvious one is to reduce acquisition time via an increase in echo spacing and a reduction in echo train length or by employing partial FA (e.g. 150° instead of 180°). However, these methods impair scanning efficiency (due to longer examination times or to reduced anatomical coverage) or the contrast/noise gain per unit of time. An interesting technique that is not affected by these limitations is the one using hyperechoes, which for tissues with T1>>T2 provides greater signal intensity. Using the hyperecho as the centre *k*-space line for the image, a greater SNR is achieved with respect to comparable conventional FSE sequences with a marked reduction in SAR.

With T1 sequences, the use of longer TR partially resolves the SAR problem but entails longer imaging times as well as a decrease in the T1 weighting of sequences, which is not necessarily desirable.

By contrast, in gradient echo imaging, lower FA for given TR are used to reduce the SAR. To prevent accidental heating of tissues during scanning, the SAR must always be closely monitored to avoid exceeding the limits laid down by the FDA (Food and Drug Administration) (less than 1 °C in any tissue). This threshold is rarely reached at 1.5 T even using FSE sequences.

Therefore, since sequences can be modified and still yield high-quality images, the SAR is not an insurmountable problem for brain scanning at 3.0 T with the exception of foetal imaging; high-field imagers are thus unlikely to be used for the latter applications in the foreseeable future [12].

The newer MR system designs are inherently more SAR efficient. While the earlier units were so RF intense as to require 'patient cooling' intervals between sequences in some cases, the more modern units and their protocols do not normally carry this risk. Limitations in the rate of RF energy deposition continue to place minor restrictions on the number of sections that can be acquired per TR period, thus some of the efficiency gains afforded by the potentially doubled signal intensity of 3.0 T units. The problem is much less severe with newer systems, and section reduction is currently a relatively minor concern also thanks to the increasing diffusion of parallel imaging with multichannel receiver coil arrays, which is becoming an integral part of high-field MR neuroimaging. This technique reduces the effects of SAR by means of a decreased RF exposure achieved by reducing the number of pulses required to obtain a given image with a set resolution. Although this entails an increase in dead time, it is partly offset by the greater SNR of 3.0 T systems. For this reason, high-field imaging is the ideal platform for parallel imaging because it helps to offset the low SNR of parallel imaging.

Finally, modifications in pulse sequence design by several manufacturers should in the near future lead to RF limitations and section acquisition efficiency equal to or even slightly greater than those currently available with 1.5 T units [15, 16].

#### 3.1.2.2 Increased Acoustic Noise

The acoustic noise generated by rapid gradient switching within the main magnetic field, which increases with field strength, is another considerable disadvantage of 3.0 T units. The noise is twice that generated in a 1.5 T MR system and may exceed 119 dB, especially with fast sequences like fast SE, fast gradient echo (FGE) and echoplanar imaging (EPI). However, this disadvantage can also be overcome relatively easily by using parallel imaging.

#### 3.1.2.3 Dielectric Resonance Effect

This phenomenon is connected with the distortion of the $B_1$ field by the body of the subject in the tunnel when volume coils are used at high fields. In particular, as the field strength, and therefore the Larmor frequency, increases – while the wavelength decreases – body size becomes significant with respect to the wavelength of the radiation transmitted, particularly in the presence of a high dielectric constant of the body. This results in a change in the intensity of the signal, which will often exhibit a bright centre and relatively hypointense borders [17, 18].

#### 3.1.2.4 Other Disadvantages

Other disadvantages are increased vigilance required for patient screening, increased biological effects and increased cost of equipment purchase, installation, maintenance and operation [13, 14].

## 3.2 Diagnostic Features of 3.0 T MR Imaging

The main differences compared with lower-field strength systems are (1) changes in tissue contrast, (2) increased magnetic susceptibility and (3) increased chemical shift.

### 3.2.1 Changes in Tissue Contrast

Whereas proton density is clearly a magnetic field-independent parameter, T1 and T2 relaxation times are field dependent, usually increasing and, respectively, decreasing at higher magnetic fields.

The rates at which excited protons relax are a function of magnetic field strength. In general, the longitudinal or spin-lattice relaxation rate (R1 = 1/T1) of certain tissues (e.g. semisolids) decreases with field strength, whereas the transverse relaxation rate (R2 = 1/T2) is scarcely affected [5, 19]. This leads to a 25–40 % increase in T1 relaxation time in tissues on passing from 1.5 T to 3.0 T fields. By contrast, for biological fluids (like CSF and blood), the longitudinal rate is weakly affected, so that R1 and R2 are basically equal at both field intensities. As a result, given the same TR, T1 weighting is greater at 3.0 T than at 1.5 T. Good T1 contrast can also be achieved using relatively long TR.

The increase in T1 relaxation time is a major drawback in high-field SE T1 imaging, as the reduction in T1 differences between tissues results in loss of contrast (Fig. 3.4).

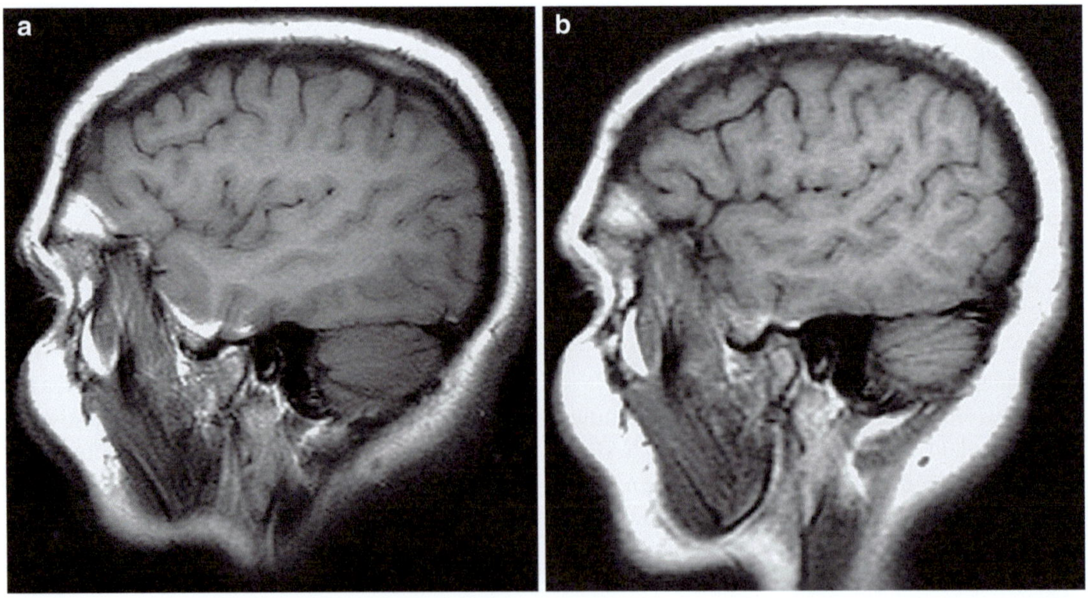


**Fig. 3.4** T1 imaging: SE T1 sequence acquired at 3.0 T (TR/TE 500/min, slice thickness 5 mm, FOV 24, matrix 320×224, 1 NEX, 2:00) (**a**) and 1.5 T (TR/TE 500/min, slice thickness 5 mm, FOV 24 cm, matrix 256×192, 1 NEX, 1:23) (**b**). The increased T1 involves reduced contrast at 3.0 T with respect to 1.5 T

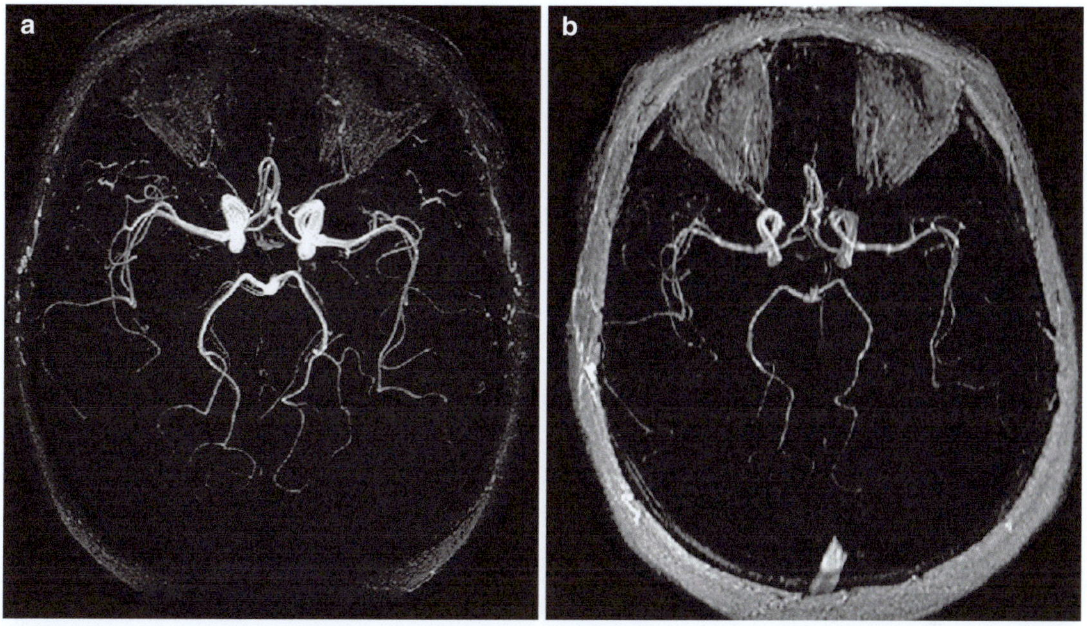


**Fig. 3.5** Normal arterial circulation: 3D TOF study at 3.0 T (**a**) and 1.5 T (**b**). Vascular conspicuity and background are greater in (**a**) (TOF SPGR TE/TE/FA 30/min/20, slice thickness 1.4 mm, matrix 512×320, ZIP 1024, ZIP 2, 1 NEX, 50 locations per slab, 6:18) than in (**b**) (TOF SPGR TE/TE/FA 45/4/20, slice thickness 1.4 mm, FOV 24×18, matrix 512×224, 1 NEX, 50 locations per slab, 6:22) resulting in greater vessel-tissue contrast

T1 lengthening with increasing magnetic field also applies to blood. Blood T1 is insensitive to the level of oxygenation and increases linearly with field strength. This is particularly valuable in MR angiography (especially in time-of-flight sequences), as it involves greater background suppression due to a lower R1 of stationary tissues and a greater flow enhancement given the broadly constant R1 of blood, thus yielding better vessel-tissue contrast (Fig. 3.5) [20, 21].

The long T1 is also useful in perfusion studies, as spin tags persist over a longer time, boosting sensitivity. As regards brain tissue T2 relaxation time, it diminishes with increasing magnetic field, albeit not linearly. In fact, T2 contrast is largely unaffected by field strength, probably due to the action of other mechanisms (like exchange and/or diffusion during gradient activation).

T2* is also shorter at 3.0 T. This may be useful when studying the deoxyhaemoglobin-containing vasculature (i.e. the venous system) and can also yield brain tissue contrast, for instance, between grey and white matter. Indeed, the shorter T2* relaxation times enhance the differences in the T2* of different tissues, resulting in greater distortion and in a larger number of artefacts due to signal loss. Indeed, changes in R2* are sensitive to changes in $B_0$ and are therefore related to differences in field susceptibility and homogeneity. Optimal $B_0$ field homogeneity, improved high-order coil shimming and broader reconstruction bandwidths are essential to improve the signal in such circumstances.

### 3.2.2 Increased Magnetic Susceptibility

Susceptibility effects increase with field strength. Increased magnetic susceptibility enhances the BOLD (blood oxygenation level dependent) effect, making clinical BOLD imaging more practical and informative as a result. BOLD contrast is the result of small magnetic susceptibility effects also responsible for the MR signal changes caused by changes in blood oxygenation under 3 %.

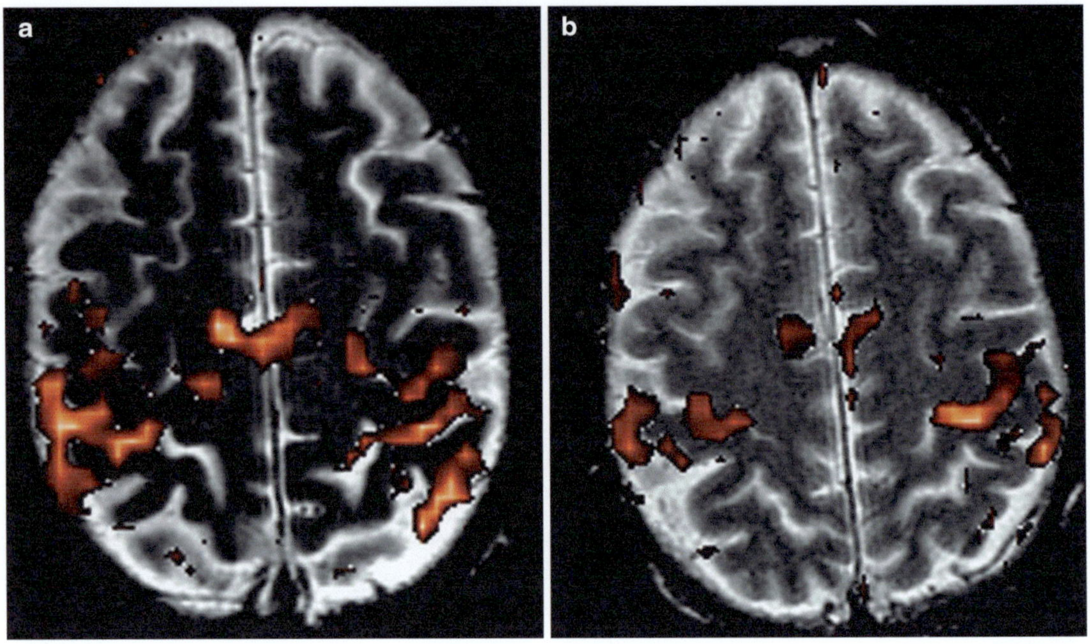


**Fig. 3.6** Motor fMRI with bilateral finger tapping: study at 3.0 T (**a**) and 1.5 T (**b**). The enhanced sensitivity to blood oxygenation and reduced background noise of the 3.0 T system (**a**) afford more reliable localization of motor areas compared with the 1.5 T imager (**b**)

3.0 T fMR images reflect greater signal changes (up to 7 %) (Figs. 3.6, 3.7 and 3.8) [22–25].

The increased static MR signal can be used to reduce the cortical volume needed for signal averaging to achieve sufficient SNR. Another potentially more important advantage of the higher $B_0$ is that as the field strength increases, the field gradient around the capillaries becomes larger and extends further into the parenchyma, thus involving a greater amount of brain tissue in producing the functional signal. In field gradients, the magnetization vectors inside voxels attain different phases and the effective transverse relaxation time T2* decreases as a result. Concurrently, the shortened T2* of blood at high $B_0$ reduces the relative contribution from the large veins. So the weighting of capillary signal contributions becomes more significant and the functional signal is more closely coupled with neuronal activity [26].

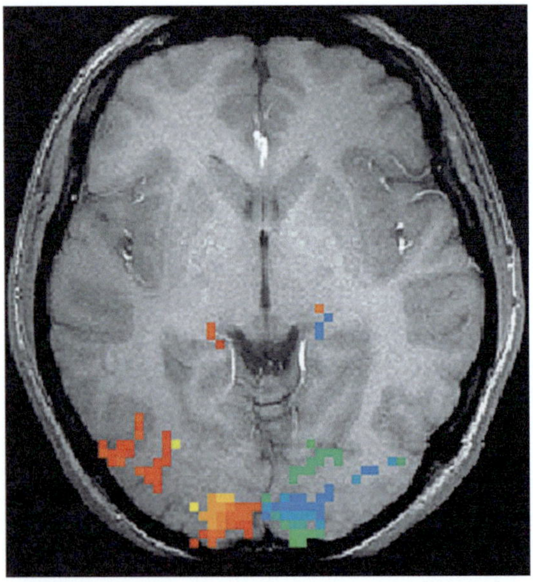

**Fig. 3.7** Visual fMRI at 3.0 T: the enhanced BOLD effect maps additional areas at the millimetre and submillimetre levels

The BOLD contrast increases as a result, becoming more sensitive to the susceptibility effects in and around the smaller vessels rather than in and around larger draining vessels. GE-EPI are usually preferred to SE-EPI sequences because they afford better discrimination of small from large vessels. SE-EPI are the sequences of choice for the study of small vessels on which the BOLD effect depends with the increase in magnetic field strength. In addition, because SE-EPI sequences are less sensitive to magnetic susceptibility effects, they are preferred for fMRI in areas where differences in susceptibility at the air-tissue interface (e.g. paranasal sinuses) are more difficult to depict at high-field strengths, resulting in marked SNR reductions.

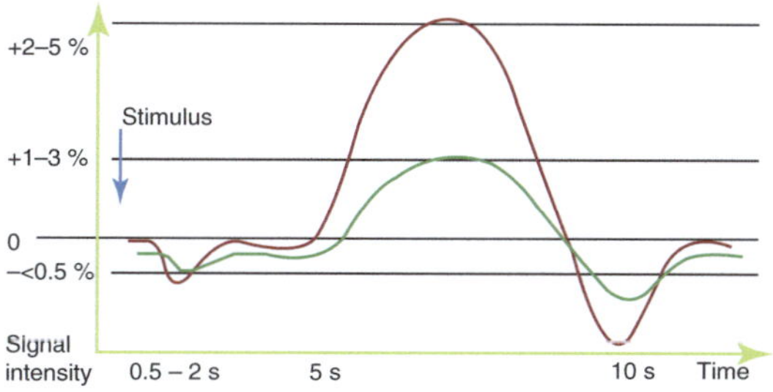


**Fig. 3.8** Visual fMRI: the signal level obtained with the 1.5 T system is 1–3 % (*green*) compared with 2–5 % with the 3.0 T system (*red*)

The greater sensitivity of high-strength magnetic fields to magnetic susceptibility can also be exploited to boost the sensitivity of contrast-enhanced perfusion studies and to improve the sensitivity of FSE sequences to haemorrhagic lesions (Figs. 3.9, 3.10 and 3.11) [19, 27, 28].

However, 3.0 T MR systems have two potential disadvantages with respect to 1.5 T scanners. Firstly, EPI sequences are usually noisier due to switching of the usually more powerful gradients, even more so when EPI sequences are acquired with GE sequences, because using SE sequence refocalization prevails over phase dispersion, thereby reducing the noise. Secondly, high-field systems are characterized by a larger number of magnetic susceptibility artefacts, especially when using GE and EPI sequences (mainly in the areas that most commonly generate artefacts, such as the temporal lobes), and from blurring when FSE sequences are performed, which often yield unsatisfactory images. In both cases, experience and use of correction systems (phase map correction) and

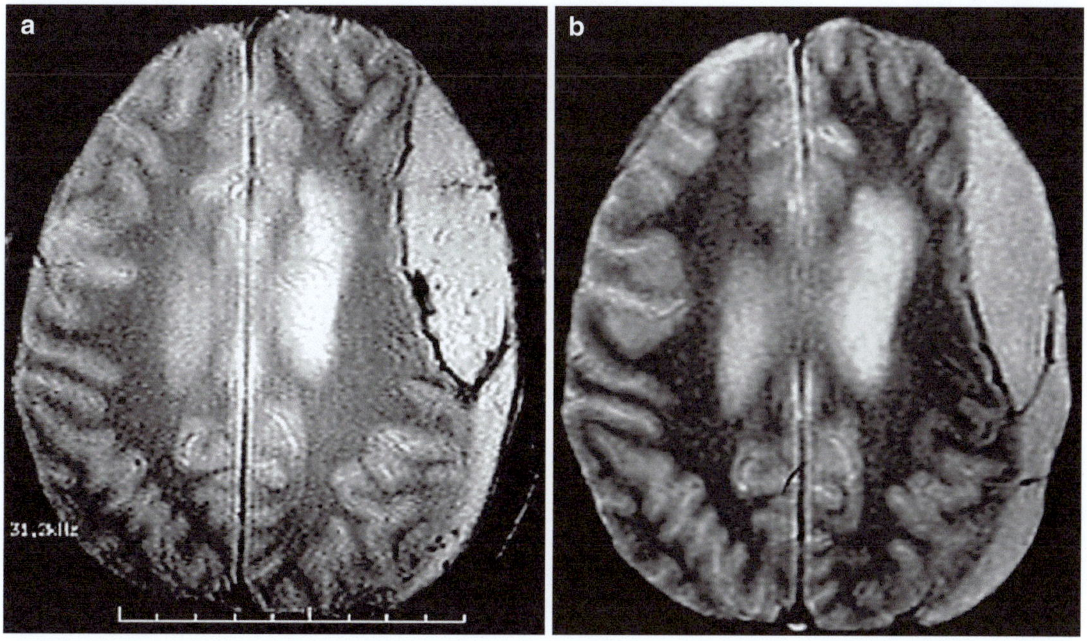


**Fig. 3.9** Arachnoid cysts complicated by haemorrhage in subacute-chronic stage after surgery. Study with GRE T2 sequences at 3.0 T (TR/TE/FA 525/9.8/20, slice thickness 5 mm, FOV 24×18, matrix 512×224, 2 NEX, 2:60) (**a**) and 1.5 T (TR/TE/FA 500/15/20, slice thickness 5 mm, FOV 24×18, matrix 320×192, 2 NEX, 2:28) (**b**). The greater sensitivity of 3.0 T MRI to the effects of magnetic susceptibility affords better depiction of haemosiderin deposits

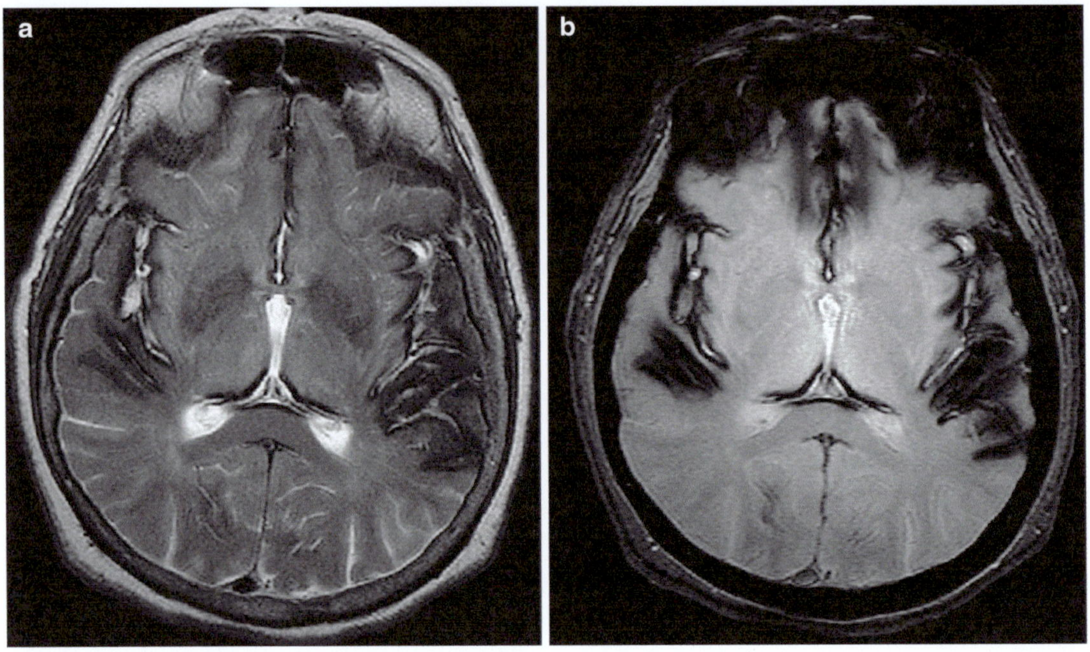


**Fig. 3.10** Leptomeningeal haemosiderosis studied with FSE (**a**) and GRE (**b**). Despite the intrinsically lower sensitivity of FSE to magnetic susceptibility, the 3.0 T imager affords excellent depiction of the low haemosiderin signal, which is visualized even more clearly in the GRE sequence

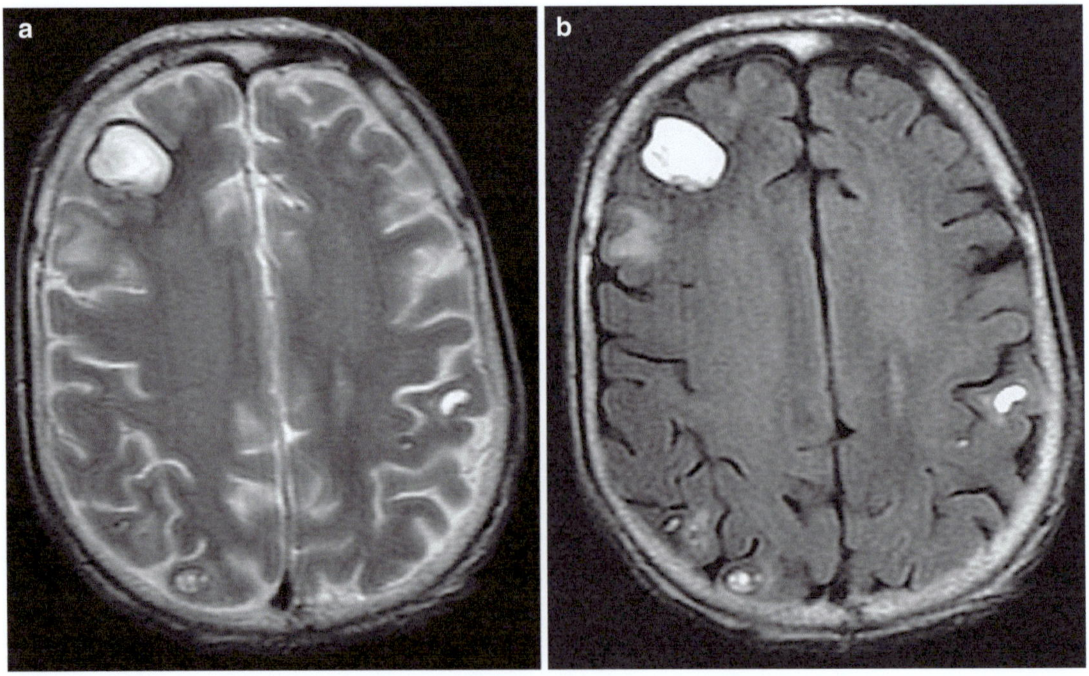


**Fig. 3.11** Multiple recent haemorrhagic foci studied with FSE (**a**) and FLAIR (**b**). Suppression of the CSF signal improves detection of the smaller lesions in the FLAIR sequence

techniques such as radial array orientation of *k*-space data and propeller CD help dispel diagnostic doubts. Finally, by reducing effective echo spacing and TE at the expense of SNR, parallel imaging allows images to be obtained with an artefact incidence comparable to that of 1.5 T units [29].

### 3.2.3 Increased Chemical Shift

Chemical shift effects also increase with magnetic field strength. The increased chemical shift enhances spectroscopic investigations via an increased chemical shift resolution, which affords wider separation of the absolute frequencies of different metabolites (Fig. 3.12) [30–32], particularly when closely located [33]. However, a larger number of artefacts are generated at the interfaces between tissues with different chemical bonds (fat/water) due to erroneous signal attribution within the reconstruction matrix, resulting in diagnostic limitations in standard anatomical imaging.

At 3.0 T, the water/fat chemical shift is around 440 Hz; this leads to the use of FSE sequences, in which more 180° pulses (greater echo train length), fewer TE and reduced slice thickness compensate for the susceptibility artefacts at the interfaces of tissues with different susceptibility constants. In addition, broader receiver bandwidths (32–125 kHz) are applied to keep the chemical shift within limits that do not impair diagnostic quality.

Indeed, to reduce these artefacts to levels seen at 1.5 T, since the chemical shift frequency between water and fat doubles at 3.0 T, the receiver bandwidth needs to be doubled too, with a consequent reduction in SNR by approximately 40 %. All other imaging parameters being equal, the images obtained at 3.0 T, which show a roughly 60 % improvement in SNR over those acquired at 1.5 T, will therefore have 20 % better SNR. Attempts to enhance spatial resolution by increasing the in-plane matrix, reducing section thickness or both will further compromise the SNR [34]. The reduced SNR associated with the receiver bandwidth is, however, partly compensated for by the higher SNR of 3.0 T systems and by last-generation multichannel coils.

One alternative to reducing chemical shift artefacts that does not entail image degradation is fat saturation, which however will further reduce the number of sections that can be acquired because it increases the SAR. Another is water

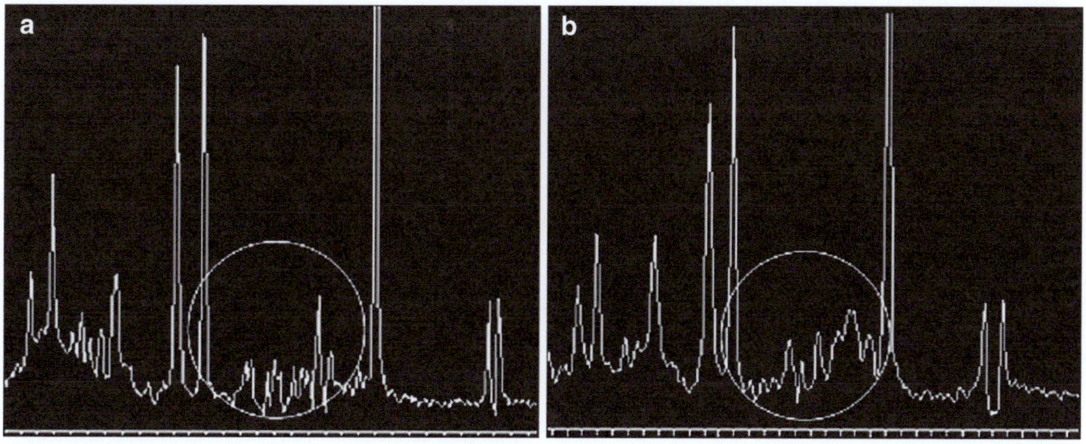


**Fig. 3.12** Single-volume spectroscopy (PRESS TR/TE 2000/30) acquired at 3.0 T (**a**) and 1.5 T (**b**). In (**a**) the increased chemical shift improves spectroscopic resolution, resulting in broader separation of the peaks of the different metabolites in the Glx

excitation, which does not increase the SAR significantly, improves image resolution and has an SNR similar to that at 1.5 T [34].

## Conclusion

High-field MR, with its intrinsically higher SNR, can be a platform for new diagnostic applications or can serve to improve existing methods. Most big improvements have been detected in research application (functional MRI and spectroscopy) and in software of automated lesion detection [35] .

However, its use is not unfettered by limitations.

In fact, the very high spatial resolution and shorter acquisition times permitted by the greater SNR result in a loss of image quality to a level below that which can be achieved with 1.5 T systems. Given the high SNR of 3.0 T MR systems, neuroradiologists can choose between imaging the brain in the same time taken with a 1.5 T unit, thus obtaining better quality images (by increasing the matrix and/or reducing slice thickness and/or FOV) and generating images of the same quality as those of a 1.5 T system in a shorter time, thus increasing patient comfort or reducing the dose of contrast medium administered.

Resolution quality tends to be privileged in clinical practice, with acquisition of a larger number of slices of reduced thickness, use of smaller FOV and broader matrices and acquisition times similar to those of 1.5 T systems (Fig. 3.3).

A compromise is generally sought between resolution and speed (e.g. by reducing the number of excitations) depending on the clinical problem and the type of patient [36].

The high SNR of high-strength magnetic fields can also be obtained with 1.5 T devices using the latest hardware (surface receiver coils used singly or in arrays, high-yield gradients to reduce TE) and software (new sequences able to optimize the contrast/noise ratio) or longer examination times. However, this cannot be done in the case of unstable or poorly cooperative patients, or it may be impossible for reasons of cost (reduced patient flow). In addition, although matrix size can be increased within 1.5 T systems, the attendant reduction in voxel size yields a more granular image.

Lastly, the higher SNR of high-field MR systems is a resource that the neuroradiologist can exploit in clinical practice, since the higher the SNR, the greater the scope for adjusting protocols.

Moreover 3-T intraoperative MRI (iMRI) is likely to become the standard of care for a wide range of neurosurgical procedures because it offers a superior visualization of soft tissue and clear delineation of any residual tumour tissue and advantages like brain activation studies and complex vascular imaging that are unavailable with low- and midfield iMRI systems [37].

## References


1. Alvarez-Linera J (2008) 3T MRI : advances in brain imaging. Eur J Radiol 67:415–426
2. Scarabino T, Nemore F, Giannatempo GM et al (2003) Risonanza Magnetica 3.0 Tesla. Riv Neuroradiol 16(Suppl):314–315
3. Scarabino T, Nemore F, Giannatempo GM et al (2004) 3.0 T imaging. Riv Neuroradiol 17:765–776
4. Scarabino T, Nemore F, Giannatempo GM et al (2003) 3.0 T magnetic resonance in neuroradiology. Eur J Radiol 48:154–164
5. Sohn CH, Sevick RJ, Frayne R, Chang HW, Kim DX (2010) Fluid attenuated inversion recovery (FLAIR) imaging of the normal brain: comparison between under conditions of 3.0 Tesla and 1.5 Tesla. Korean J Radiol 11:19–24
6. Norris DG (2003) High field human imaging. J Magn Reson Imaging 18:519–529
7. Scarabino T, Nemore F, Giannatempo GM et al (2004) Semeiological features of 3.0 T MR imaging: what changes at high magnetic field. Riv Neuroradiol 17:755–764
8. Takahashi M, Uematsu H, Hatabu H (2003) MR imaging at high magnetic fields. Eur J Radiol 46:45–52
9. Craven I, PD G, Hoggard N (2011) Magnetic resonance imaging of epilepsy at 3 Tesla. Clin Radiol 66(3):278–286
10. Azmi H, Schulder M (2003) Stereotactic accuracy of a 3 T magnetic resonance unit. Stereotact Funct Neurosurg 80(1–4):140–145
11. Briellmann RS, Syngeniotis A, Jackson GD (2001) Comparison of hippocampal volumetry at 1.5 Tesla and at 3 Tesla. Epilepsia 42(8):1021–1024

12. Rutherford M, Malamateniou C, Zeka J et al (2004) MR imaging of the neonatal brain at 3 Tesla. Eur J Paediatr Neurol 8:281–289
13. Weintraub MI, Khoury A, Cole SP (2007) Biologic effects of 3 Tesla (T) MR imaging comparing traditional 1.5 and 0.6 T in 1023 consecutive outpatients. J Neuroimaging 17:241–245
14. De Vocht F, Stevens T, van Wendel-de-Joode B, Engels H, Kromhout H (2006) Acute neurobehavioral effects of exposure to static magnetic field: analyses of exposure-response relations. J Magn Reson Imaging 23:297–297
15. Ross JS (2004) The high field strength curmudgeon. AJNR 25:168–169
16. Tanenbaum LN (2004) 3-T MR imaging: ready for clinical practice (letters). AJNR 25:1626–1627
17. Tropp J (2004) Image brightening in samples of high dielectric constant. J Magn Reson 167:12–24
18. Yang QX, Wang J, Zhang X (2002) Analysis of wave behaviour in lossy dielectric samples at high field. Magn Reson Med 47:982–989
19. Wansapura JP, Holland SK, Dunn RS et al (1999) NMR relaxation times in the human brain at 3.0 T. JMRI 9:531–538
20. Bernstein MA, Huston J 3rd, Lin C et al (2001) High-resolution intracranial and cervical MRA at 3.0 T: technical considerations and initial experience. Magn Reson Med 46:955–962
21. Reichenbach JR, Barth M, Haacke EM et al (2000) High resolution MR venography at 3.0 Tesla. J Comput Assist Tomogr 24:949–957
22. Di Salle F, Esposito F, Elefante A et al (2003) High field functional MRI. Eur J Radiol 48:138–145
23. Chen W, Ugurbil K (1999) High spatial resolution functional magnetic resonance imaging at very-high-magnetic field. Top Magn Reson Imaging 10:63–78
24. Van der Zwaag W, Francis S, Head K et al (2009) fMRI at 1.5, 3 amd 7 T: characterizing BOLD sigbal changes. Neuroimage 47:1425–1434
25. Thulborn KR, Chang SY, Shen GX et al (1997) High resolution echo-planar imaging of human cortex at 3.0 T. NMR Biomed 10:183
26. Kim D-S, Garwood M (2003) High field magnetic resonance techniques for brain research. Curr Opin Neurobiol 13:612–619
27. Sugahara T, Korogi Y, Kochi M et al (2001) Perfusion-sensitive MR imaging of glioma: comparison between gradient- echo and spin-echo echo-planar imaging techniques. AJNR 22:1306–1315
28. Wang J, Alsop DC, Li L et al (2002) Comparison of quantitative perfusion imaging using arterial spin labeling at 1.5 T and 4.0 Tesla. Magn Reson Med 48:242–254
29. Heidelmann RM, Griswold MA, Muller M et al (2004) Feasibility and limitations of high field parallel MRI. Radiologe 44(1):49–55
30. Polonara G, Scarabino T, Salvolini U (2003) Basics and new frontiers of MR spectroscopy with high Tesla. Riv Neuroradiol 16(Suppl):144–148
31. Kim JH, Chang KH, Na DG et al (2006) Comparison of 1.5 T and 3 T 1H MR spettroscopy for human brain tumor. Korean J Radiol 7:156–161
32. Di Costanzo A, Trojsi F, Giannatempo GM et al (2003) High-field proton MRS of human brain. Eur J Radiol 48:146–153
33. Wardlaw JM et al (2012) A systematic review of the utility of 1.5 versus 3 Tesla magnetic resonance brain imaging in clinical practice and research. Eur Radiol 22:2295–2303
34. Pattany PM (2004) 3 T MR imaging: the pros and cons (editorial). AJNR 25:1455–1456
35. Kim PD, Truwit CL, Hall WA (2009) Three-tesla high-field applications. Neurosurg Clin N Am 20(2):173–178
36. Shapiro MD (2004) The time for 3 T clinical imaging is now (letter). AJNR 25:1628–1629
37. Ginat DT, Swearingen B, Curry W, Cahill D, Madsen J, Schaefer PW (2014) 3 Tesla intraoperative MRI for brain tumor surgery. 3 Tesla intraoperative MRI for brain tumor surgery 39(6):1357–1365

# Standard 3.0 T MR Imaging

# 4

Tommaso Scarabino, Antonella Bacci,
Giuseppe Maria Giannatempo, Saverio Pollice,
Michelangelo Nasuto, Annamaria Pennelli,
Raffaele Agati, and Teresa Popolizio

Magnetic resonance imaging (MRI) studies of the brain can be classified into two general categories based on the type of information that is being collected: morphological or functional. Standard morphological studies are performed to depict tissue, cerebrospinal fluid (CSF) spaces, vessels and fibre bundles; functional studies include mapping of brain function (fMRI), perfusion and diffusion imaging and metabolic studies by means of spectroscopy.

Standard 3.0 T MR scanning offers better quality images than lower-strength systems, thereby providing superb detail of the brain. Its increased spatial resolution is a major advantage in investigating certain diseases, such as brain tumours, requiring tissue characterization, spatial work-up and pre-surgical planning, and difficult to identify congenital abnormalities.

T. Scarabino (✉) • S. Pollice
Department of Radiology and Neuroradiology,
PO "L. Bonomo" Hospital, Andria (BT), Italy
e-mail: tscarabino@hotmail.com

A. Bacci • R. Agati
Department of Neuroradiology, Bellaria Hospital - University of Bologna, Bologna, Italy

G.M. Giannatempo • M. Nasuto • A. Pennelli
T. Popolizio
Department of Radiology and Neuroradiology,
IRCCS "Casa Sollievo della Sofferenza",
San Giovanni Rotondo (FG), Italy

## 4.1 Pulse Sequences

Anatomical brain scanning essentially relies on proton density, differences in T1 and T2 between regions (e.g. cortex vs. subcortical nuclei) and tissue type (white matter, grey matter and CSF). Brain images can be acquired using different pulse sequences. A 3.0 T MR system implements all the pulse sequences commonly applied in clinical practice, including SE (normal, fast 2D and 3D), GE (GRASS/fast GRASS 2D and 3D, SPGR/fast SPGR 2D and 3D), EPI (single-shot/multi-shot 2D and 3D) and IR (STIR, FLAIR, normal, fast) using common imaging parameters like flow and respiratory compensation, cardiac and peripheral gating, graphic prescription, graphic saturation, fat/water saturation, variable bandwidth and asymmetric field of view.

Since the user interface and sequence parameters are the same as those employed with 1.5 T systems, at 3.0 T one should in theory obtain the same images with the advantage of high-field strength, i.e. a double signal intensity. In practice, much depends on tissue relaxation times (T1 and T2) and the specific absorption rate (SAR) [1–6]. Since relaxation times are field-dependent and affect image contrast, 1.5 T imaging sequences cannot be transferred to 3.0 T systems. In addition, the excessive RF energy that is deposited on tissues at 3.0 T needs to be



T. Scarabino et al. (eds.), *High Field Brain MRI*, DOI 10.1007/978-3-319-44174-0_4

**Table 4.1** Technical parameters of the main sequences applied with 1.5 and 3.0 T systems

| Sequence | TR (ms) | TE (ms) | Other parameters (TI, FA, ETL) | Slice thickness (mm) | No. of slices | FOV | Matrix | NEX | Examination time (min:s) |
|---|---|---|---|---|---|---|---|---|---|
| *SE* T1 / 1.5 T | 500 | Min | – | 6 | 16 | 24 | 256×192 | 1 | 1:23 |
| *SE* T1 / 3.0 T | 500 | Min | – | 5 | 18 | 24 | 320×224 | 1 | 2:00 |
| *FGE* T1 / 3.0 T | 225 | Min | FA 75 | 4 | 20 | 24 | 512×256 | 1 | 1:57 |
| *IR* T1 / 3.0 T | 2075 | 24 | TI auto | 4 | 11×2 | 24 | 256×256 | 1 | 2:49 |
| *TSE* T2 / 1.5 T | 3000 | 88 | ETL 12 | 6 | 21 | 24 | 256×224 | 2 | 2:24 |
| *TSE* T2 / 3.0 T | 4850 | 81 | ETL 15 | 4 | 25 | 22 | 448×320 | 2 | 2:39 |
| *TSE* T2 *HD* / 3.0 T | 4975 | 85 | ETL 15 | 3 | 25 | 20 | 512×320 | 4 | 7:20 |
| FLAIR / 1.5 T | 8800 | 120 | TI 2200 | 5 | 14×2 | 26 | 256×192 | 2 | 4:24 |
| FLAIR / 3.0 T | 11,000 | 130 | TI 2250 | 4 | 16×2 | 22 | 288×192 | 2 | 5:52 |

taken into account when adapting and optimizing clinical imaging protocols for use with such systems.

The technical parameters of the main sequences applied with 1.5 and 3.0 T systems are reported in Table 4.1. Higher-field systems afford greater resolution quality by allowing the acquisition of a larger number of slices (usually 25–27 vs. 18–20) of smaller thickness (4 mm vs. 5–6 mm), with narrower fields of view (20–22 vs. 24), broader matrices (512×512 vs. 256×256), and acquisition times similar to those of 1.5 T systems.

Lastly, two factors that depend on magnetic field strength need to be taken into consideration: the influence of the signal loss caused by the stronger susceptibility effects and the potentially diminished sensitivity of the radio-frequency coils at higher field intensity.

### 4.1.1 T1 Imaging

Since T1 relaxation times are longer at higher magnetic fields, entailing a reduction in the

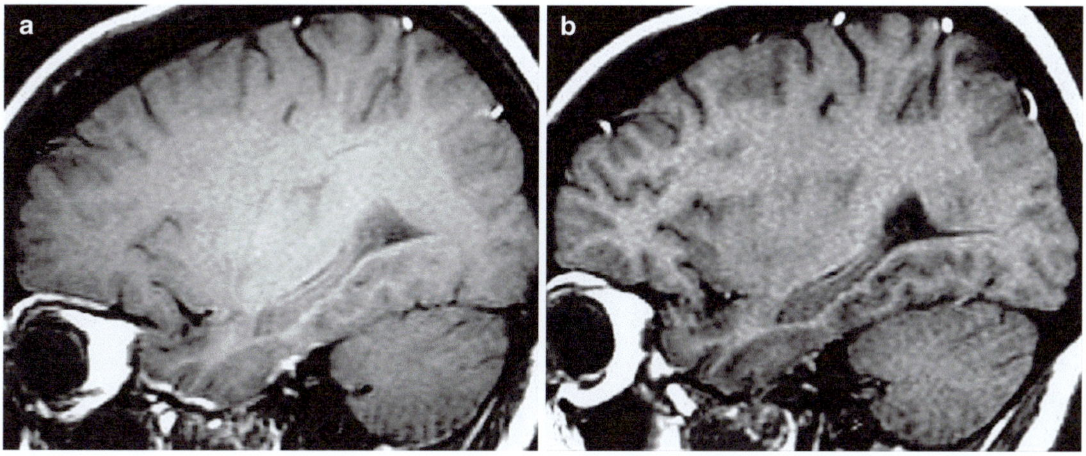


**Fig. 4.1** T1 imaging: comparison of the same SE T1 sequence (TR 500, 0.5 NEX, 1:00) acquired at 3.0 T (**a**) and 1.5 T (**b**). Note the less satisfactory white/grey matter contrast in (**a**)

relative differences among different tissue types, it is generally difficult to obtain T1-weighted images with sufficient contrast when using a 3.0 T unit [2]. In fact, not only T1 increases, but the T1 values of different tissue types actually converge, giving rise to a narrower range of distribution. For this reason, optimization of the signal-to-noise ratio (SNR) in the same sample using a higher field unit requires longer TR (and a smaller flip angle), resulting in longer scanning times. Using longer TR, the gain in signal intensity in unit of time afforded by the higher magnetic field is therefore lost. T1 saturation for a given TR is greater at 3.0 T, resulting in reduced signal gain. In other words, the SNR per unit of time would be optimized with the shortest possible TR/T1. The possibility that the SNR gain connected with the high magnetic field may substantially be offset by a longer T1 highlights the importance of optimizing the imaging parameters [3].

The increased T1 is the main problem in 3.0 T brain imaging using SE T1-weighted sequences, which afford very unsatisfactory T1 contrast (Fig. 4.1) [7–10]. Indeed, the reduction in T1 differences among different types of tissues entails a loss of contrast between white and grey matter. For T1 contrast, this has led to the application of sequences other than SE which yield high T1 contrast irrespective of field strength, i.e. fast GE T1 (spoiled gradient echo, SPGR or MP-RAGE) and fast IR or fast FLAIR T1 weighted (Figs. 4.2, 4.3 and 4.4) [7–9].

Fast SPGR allows thinner slices to be obtained in a shorter time and provides images suitable for reformatting in all three planes using a single volumetric acquisition of the whole brain, thus disclosing a larger number of lesions than can be depicted using SE T1-weighted sequences acquired in a single plane. In addition, large arterial vessels appear hyperintense on fast SPGR sequences, although this does not impair image interpretation.

In contrast, fast IR entails longer scanning times because chained acquisitions are required to image the whole brain; this can be a problem when multiple unenhanced and contrast-enhanced studies, or different views, need to be performed.

Unlike IR T1-weighted sequences, which are less satisfactory and take longer to perform, a typical FLAIR T1-weighted study of the brain coupled with parallel imaging allows higher spatial resolution protocols to be applied in a shorter acquisition time.

Greater inflow contrast and enhanced background suppression make contrast-enhanced T1 imaging a definite advantage of 3.0 T systems. For instance, when studying primary and

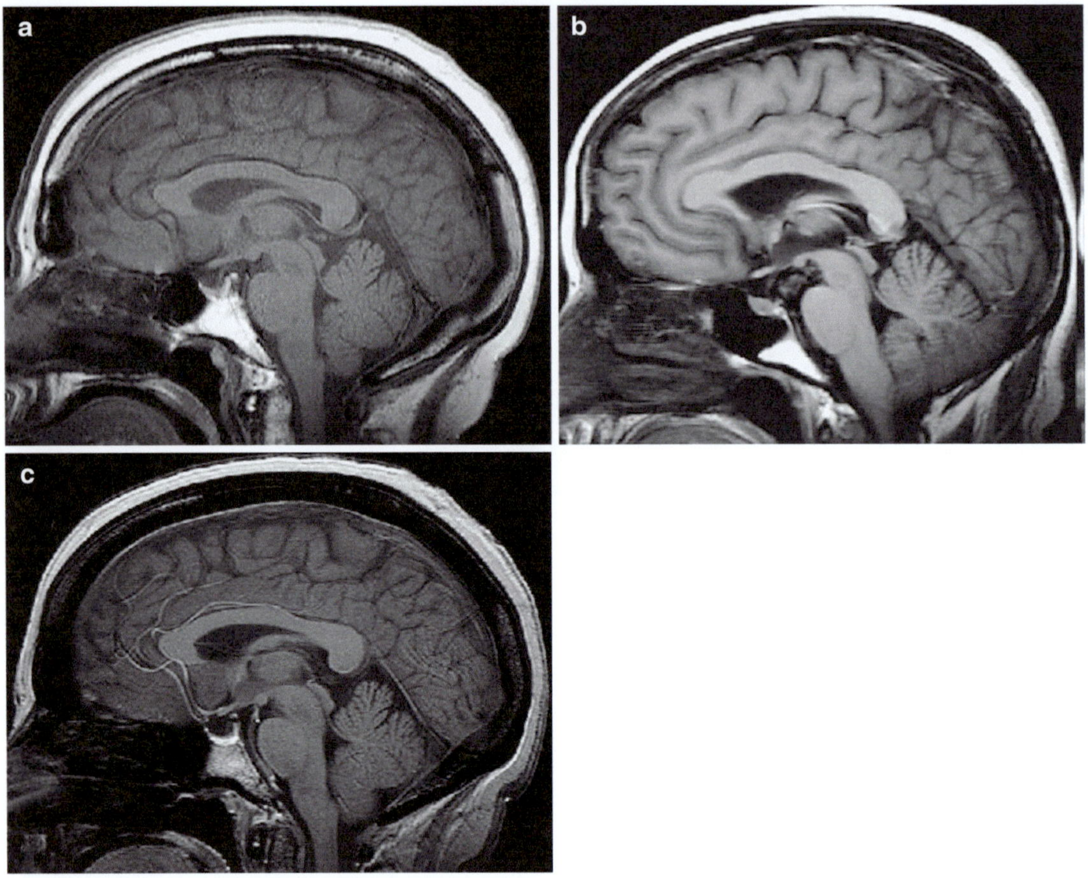

**Fig. 4.2** T1 imaging with SE T1 (**a**), FLAIR T1 (**b**) and FGRE T1 (**c**). The poor white/grey matter contrast of the SE T1 sequence (**a**) required performance of the other two high-contrast sequences. Note the typical high signal of the larger arterial vessels in (**c**) (*arrow*)

secondary brain tumours, the administration of a both single- and multiple-dose gadolinium yields greater contrast between tumour and normal brain tissue and allows the detection of more metastases and demonstrates different patterns of enhancement that may be useful to assess the degree of malignancy and to monitor response to therapy [11–13].

The greater sensitivity of 3.0 T contrast-enhanced investigations has also been demonstrated in multiple sclerosis, with a 21 %increase in the number of enhancing lesions detected, a 30 % increase in enhancing lesion volume and a 10 % increase in total lesion volume relative to scanning at 1.5 T [14].

Contrast-enhanced imaging also improves the evaluation of hypophyseal macro- and microadenomas (Figs. 4.5 and 4.6). 3.0 T MR venography is another valuable technique that provides increased spatial resolution, and thus more detailed information, in the same time of acquisition as a 1.5 T system [15].

However, contrast-enhanced T1 semeiotics requires adjustments in TR and TE and a reduction in the dose of contrast agent [3]. The usual dosage of 0.1 mmol/kg can be halved without affecting image quality. Using a standard dose, the contrast/noise ratio (CNR) is two and a half times greater than with 1.5 T systems [15]. Double or triple doses can result in meningeal contrast uptake, a common non-pathological finding, at 3.0 T which at lower field strengths may, however, mimic carcinomatosis or meningitis and should thus be avoided.

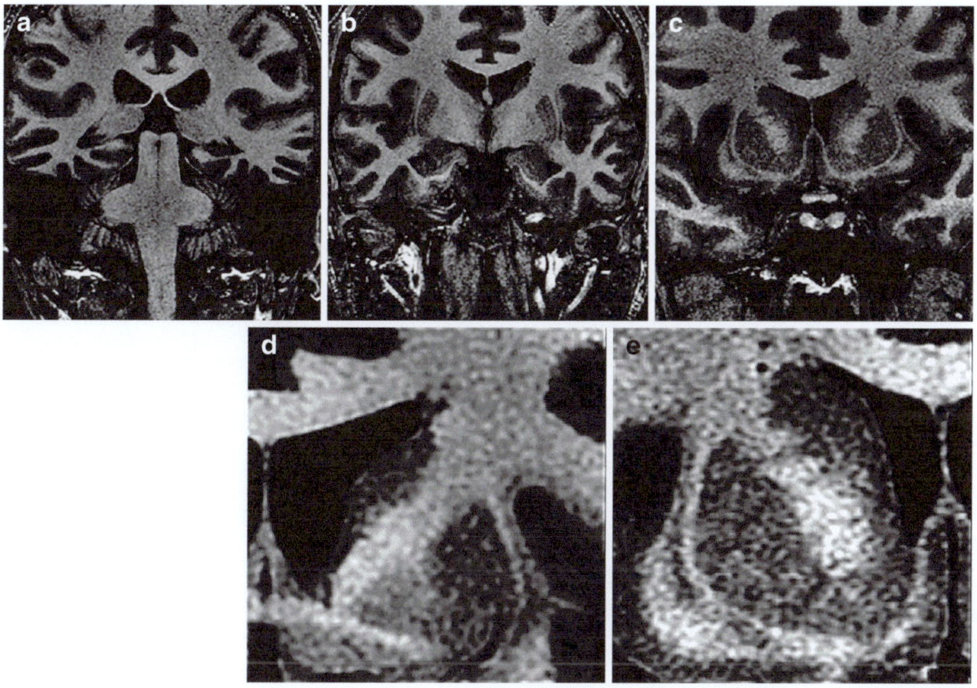

**Fig. 4.3** (**a–e**) High-definition T1 images acquired with a 3D FSPGR IR-Prep sequence (750 ms, TR 8.4, TE 3.8, BW 50 kHz, FOV 160, matrix 416×320, slice thickness 2 mm). Coronal views (**a–c**, **d**, **e**) details

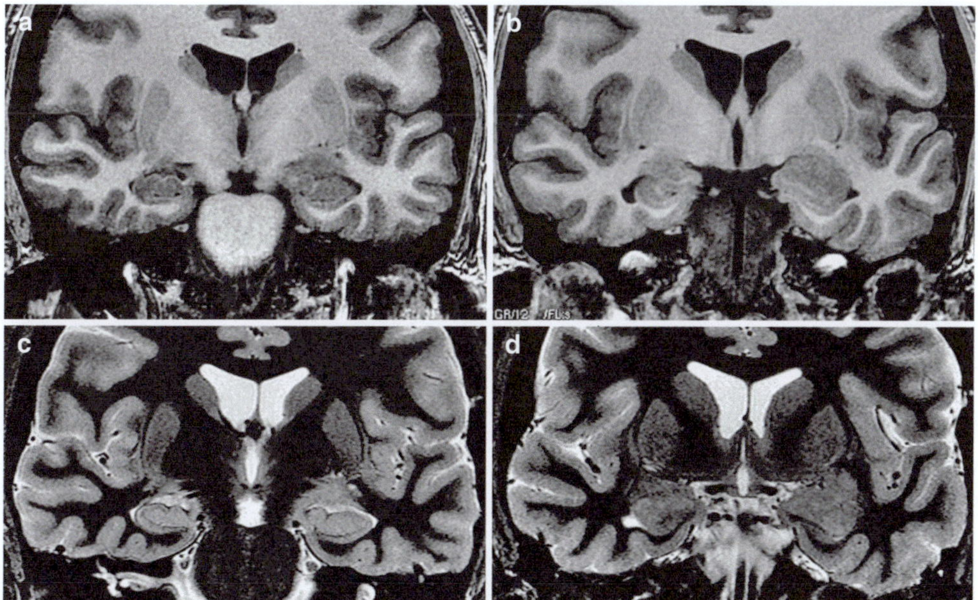

**Fig. 4.4** High-definition images: comparison of a 3D FSPGR IR-Prep sequence (**a**, **b**) (TR 9.1, TE 4.0, FOV 170, slice thickness 2 mm, matrix 320×288) with an FSE-IR sequence (**c**, **d**) (TI 250 ms, FOV 160, slice thickness 3 mm, matrix 512×256). Note the optimum anatomical depiction of the cortico-subcortical junction on both sequences

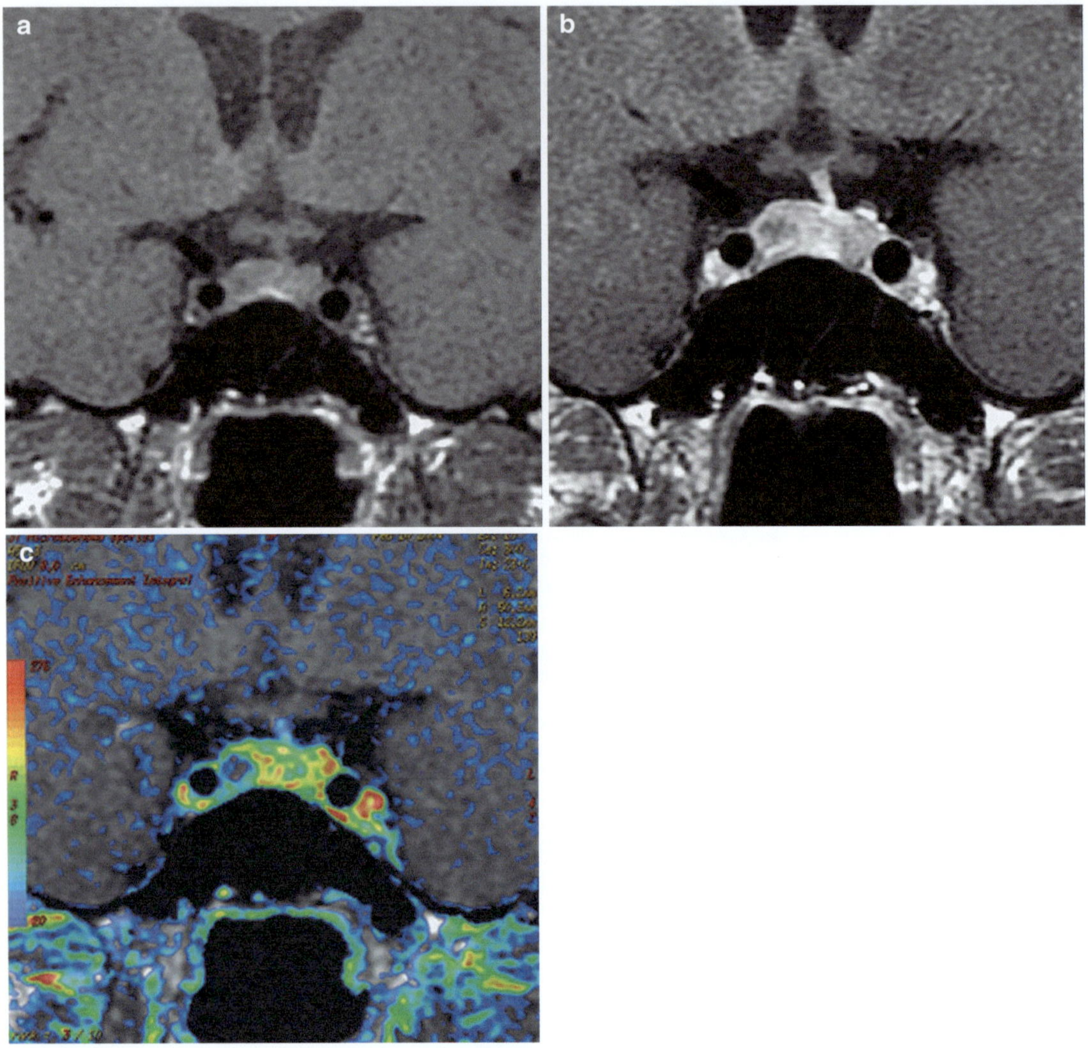

**Fig. 4.5** Unenhanced (**a**) and contrast-enhanced (**b**) hypophyseal microadenoma. PEI processing using Functool 2 (**c**)

To enhance sensitivity or highlight minimal changes in the blood-brain barrier, a double dose of contrast agent may be employed in selected investigations of brain metastases or inflammatory disease [16, 17]. In such cases, greater lesion enhancement with respect to normal brain parenchyma results in improved sensitivity and resolution.

Fast GE T1, rather than standard SE sequences, are preferred for contrast-enhanced T1 imaging, as they offer better contrast in the same acquisition time. SE T1 sequences are, however, consistently improved by contrast administration (Fig. 4.7).

### 4.1.2 T2 Imaging

In T2 contrast imaging, the advantages of high magnetic field strength are best exploited by performing fast SE sequences acquired using

**Fig. 4.6** Hypophyseal macroadenoma: (**a**) unenhanced image (**b**) dynamic contrast-enhanced image

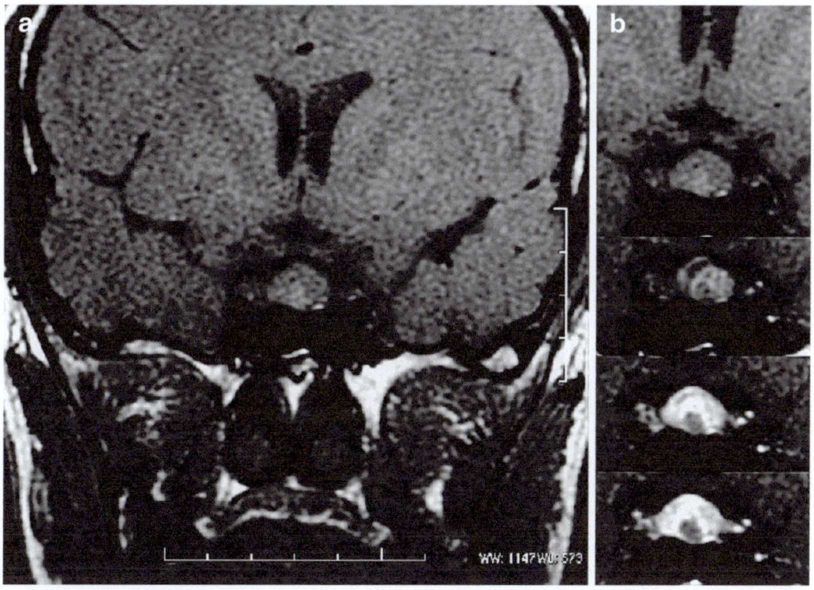

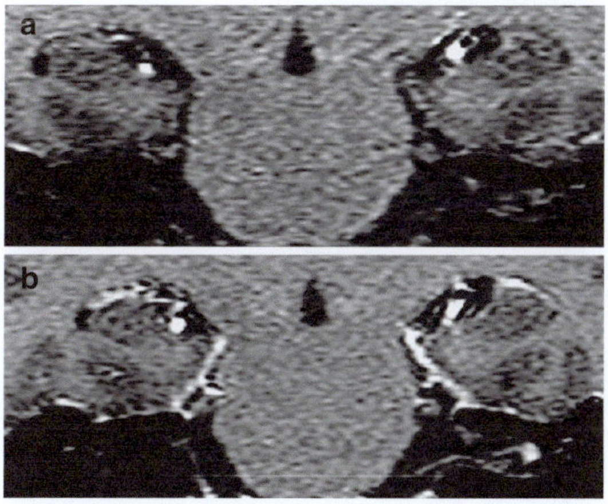

**Fig. 4.7** (**a**, **b**) Small left acoustic neurinoma: high-definition SE T1 sequence (matrix 512, thickness 1.5 mm). Unenhanced (**a**) and contrast-enhanced (**b**) images

the same technique as with 1.5 T imagers but with shorter TR and TE due to the shorter T2 relaxation times (Fig. 4.8). High spatial resolution FSE-weighted images are especially effective at 3.0 T as they provide more anatomical detail and better contrast due to the greater SNR, which allows to employ thinner slices and broader matrices (Figs. 4.9, 4.10, 4.11, 4.12 and 4.13) [7–9, 18]. Even better images are obtained with inverted contrast FSE T2 sequences (Fig. 4.14).

In practice, the greater SNR may be attenuated by the increased deposition of RF energy, which in turn requires long TR or pulse refocalization angles well below 180°. This lower SNR can, however, be compensated for by the higher field strength. In addition, the broader bandwidth, smaller echo space, shorter minimum TR and TE and shorter FSE sequences employed at higher field strengths result in improved image quality, artefact reduction and enhanced diagnostic performance in much shorter examination times, to the benefit of patients.

These sequences allow excellent visualization of the basal or mesencephalic nuclei, by virtue of their iron content, despite the intrinsically lower sensitivity of FSE to magnetic susceptibility in 3.0 T compared with 1.5 T systems [3].

Different signal features are also seen in brain haemorrhage, which at 3.0 T is characterized by greater hypointensity in the acute and early subacute phases [19]. With SNR and signal intensity being roughly similar at both field intensities, correct dating of the haemorrhage is usually feasible. Only in the acute phase can bleeding be erroneously construed as early subacute haemorrhage [19].

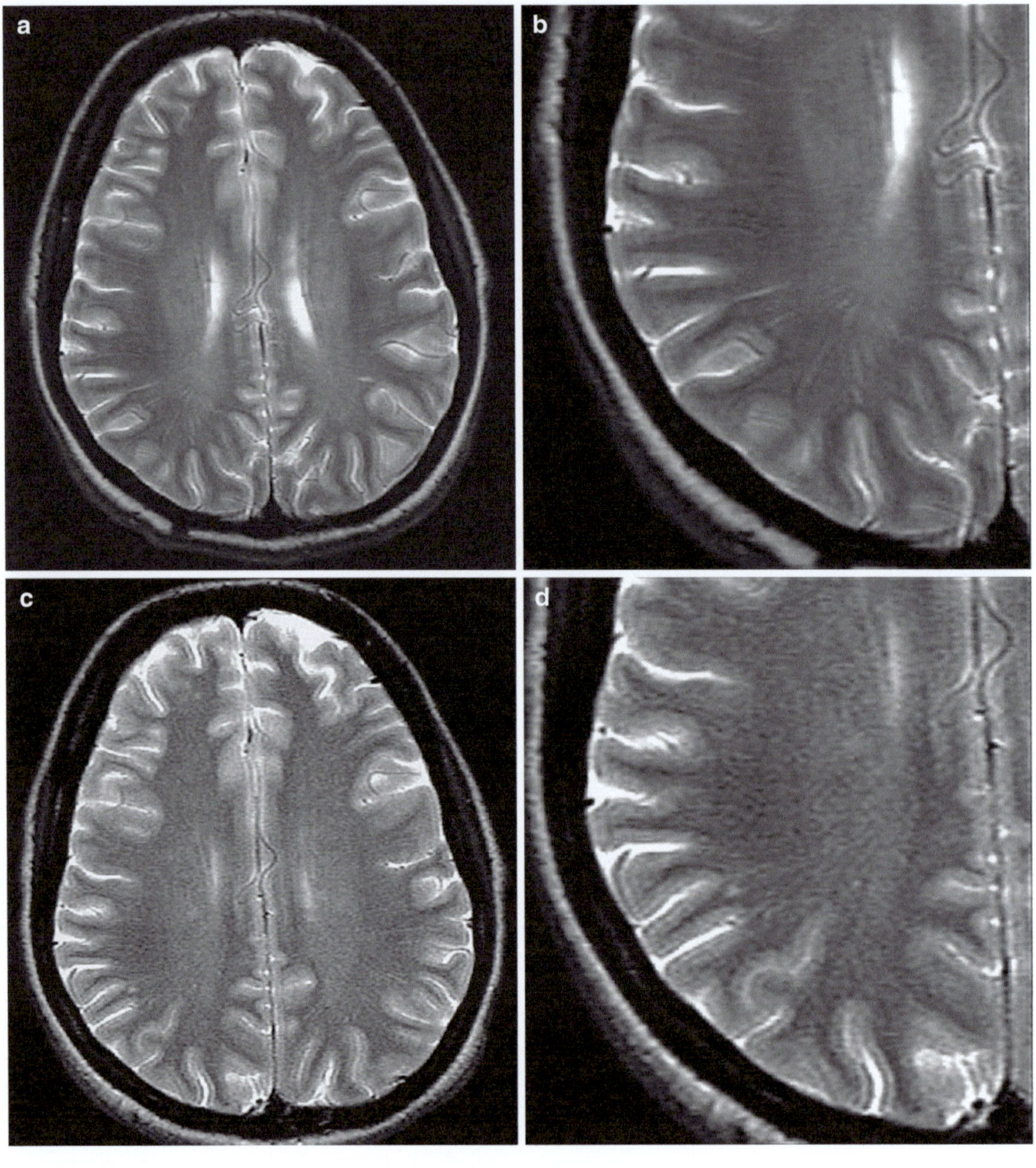


**Fig. 4.8** T2 imaging: comparison between the same FSE T2 sequence at 3.0 T (**a**, **b** zoom) and 1.5 T (**c**, **d** zoom). Anatomical detail and contrast resolution are greater in (**a**) and (**b**)

T2 images can also be acquired with GE (T2*) sequences like CISS (constructive interference in the steady state), which is particularly suited to investigations of the inner ear. 3D CISS offers high-resolution images of the inner ear and labyrinth with greater SNR than other T2-weighted sequences used to study this area (e.g. fast-recovery FSE) (Fig. 4.15) [20].

### 4.1.3 FLAIR Imaging

FLAIR sequences, which are generally included in all imaging protocols, are also sharper and more sensitive at 3.0 T by virtue of their reduced slice thickness and broader matrices, especially in detecting small lesions. Greater sensitivity is also afforded by the longer TE required in relation

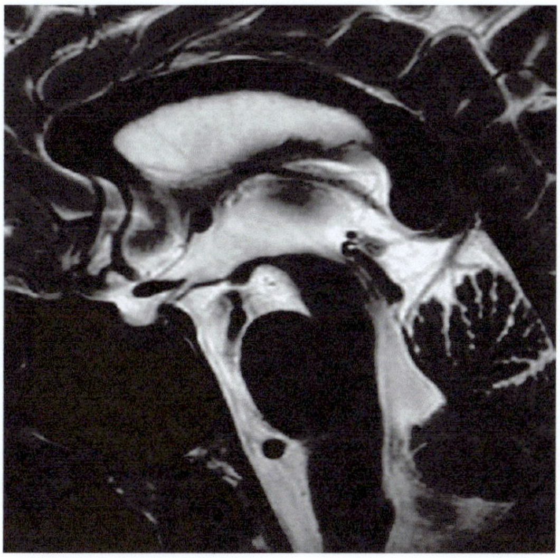

**Fig. 4.9** High-definition FSE T2 image of the median sections of the brain

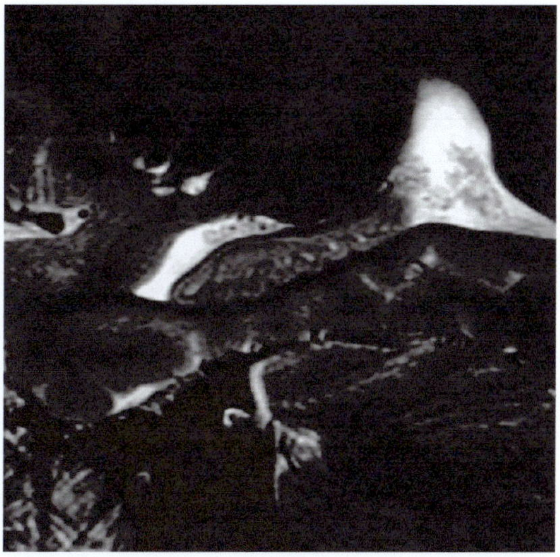

**Fig. 4.10** High-definition FSE T2 image of the hippocampus

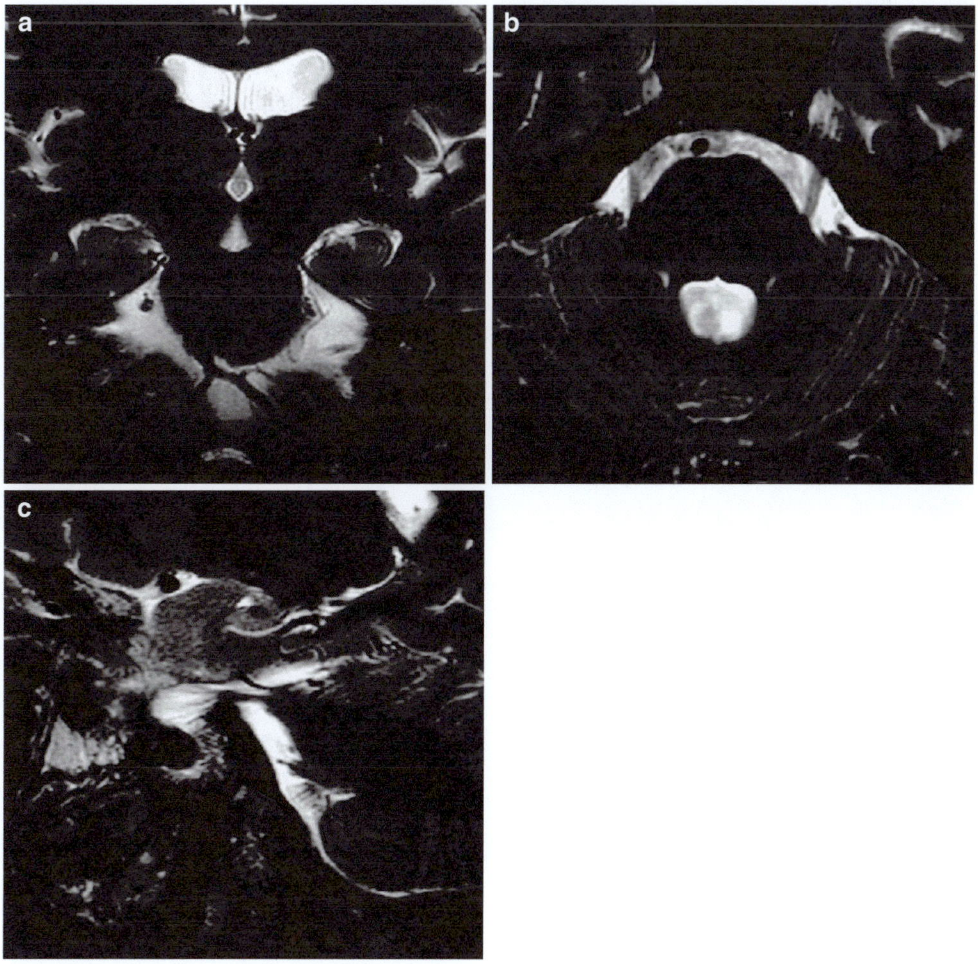


**Fig. 4.11** High-definition FSE T2 image of the fifth cranial nerve in coronal (**a**), axial (**b**) and parasagittal (**c**) section

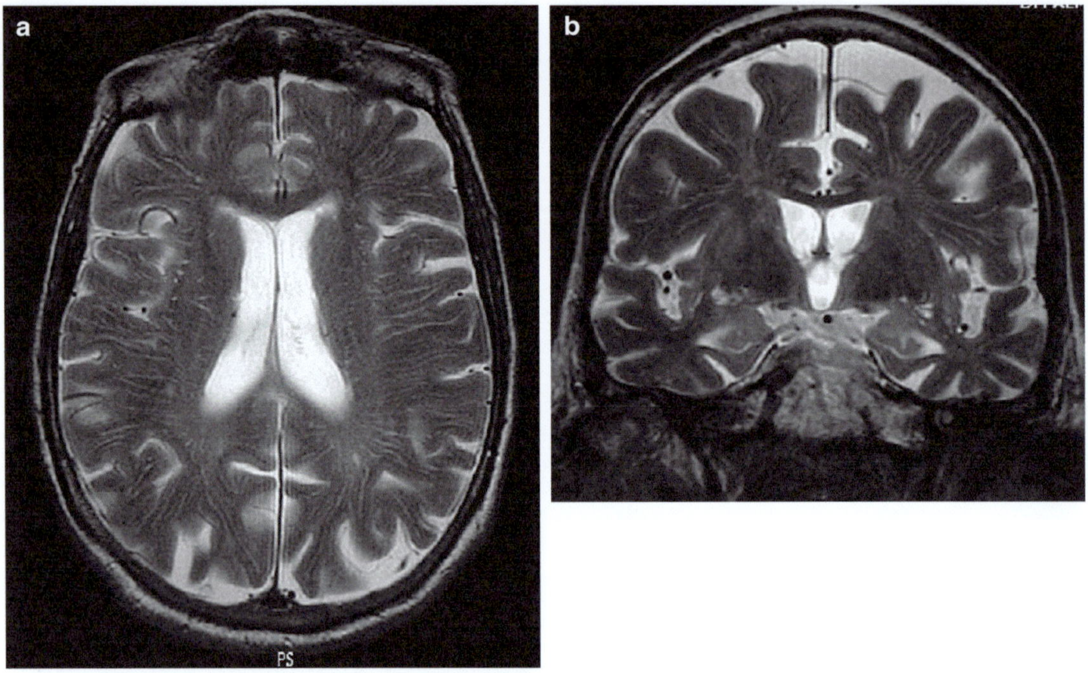


**Fig. 4.12** (**a**, **b**) FSE T2 imaging. The excellent detail of this sequence allows visualization of the perivascular (Virchow-Robin) spaces at the level of the bi-hemispheric cortico-subcortical junction. Axial (**a**) and coronal (**b**) views

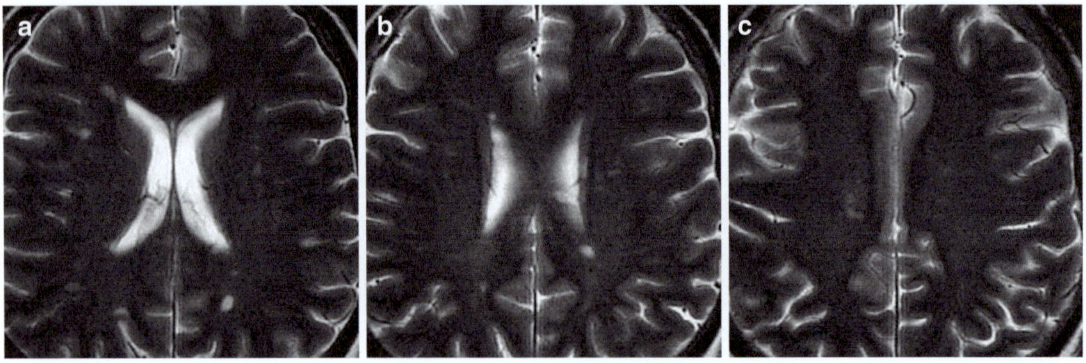


**Fig. 4.13** Multiple sclerosis: (**a**–**c**) FSE T2 sequence

to 3.0 T relaxation times, allowing good contrast and acceptable noise levels (Figs. 4.16, 4.17 and 4.18). Indeed, detection of small lesions requires CNR, rather than SNR, optimization, which is obtained using longer TE (120 ms).

The basic lack of difference in CSF T1 between 1.5 T and 3.0 T entails that a similar inversion time (IT) is required to suppress the fluid signal (around 2250 ms) at both field strengths [3]. This does not apply to other IR sequences, neither those that seek to enhance contrast between different tissues (e.g. between white and grey matter) nor those using fat suppression, where T1 must be increased by 25–40 %.

The white matter, especially periventricular, areas that are physiologically hyperintense at 1.5 T enhance even more strongly on 3.0 T images, requiring great caution in distinguishing them from diseases like amyotrophic lateral sclerosis [7].

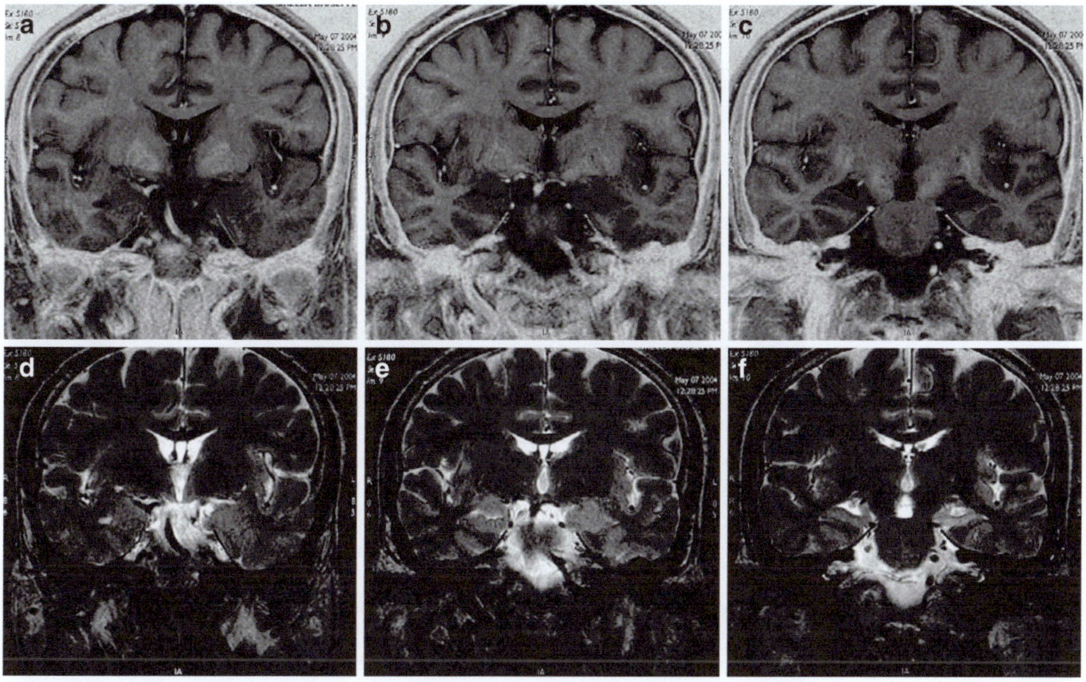


**Fig. 4.14** High-definition FSE T2 sequence (matrix 512×320, thickness 3 mm, ZIP 1024) acquired with (**a–c**) and without (**d–f**) inverted contrast: coronal view. Note the excellent anatomical detail of both hippocampi

The semeiological features described for grey nuclei and recent haemorrhage also apply to FLAIR sequences (Figs. 4.19 and 4.20) [3, 19].

A major drawback of high-field imaging is a larger number of pulsation artefacts, especially in the posterior fossa, probably due to higher blood flow magnetization. The adoption of broader saturation bands does not address the problem because of difficulties with the head coil, but recently developed new coils or new software (parallel imaging) are expected to diminish its impact.

### 4.1.4 Susceptibility-Weighted Imaging

Susceptibility-weighted imaging (SWI) represents a new type of contrast that is complementary to conventional spin-density-, T1- and T2-weighted imaging methods.

SWI is a high-spatial-resolution 3D gradient-echo MR imaging technique (extremely sensitive to susceptibility changes) with phase post-processing that accentuates the paramagnetic properties of blood products and is very sensitive in the detection of intravascular venous deoxygenated blood as well as extravascular blood products. It was originally referred to high-resolution blood oxygen level-dependent venography, because of its broader application than evaluating venous structures. It is also quite sensitive to the presence of other substances such as iron, some forms of calcification and air [21].

SWI exploits the loss of signal intensity created by disturbance of a homogeneous magnetic field. These disturbances can be caused by various paramagnetic, ferromagnetic or diamagnetic substances such as air/tissue or air/bone interfaces. As spins encounter heterogeneity in the local magnetic field, they precess at different rates and cause overall signal-intensity loss in T2*-weighted (i.e. gradient-echo) images. Sensitivity to susceptibility effects increase as one progresses from fast spin-echo to routine spin-echo to gradient-echo techniques, from T1

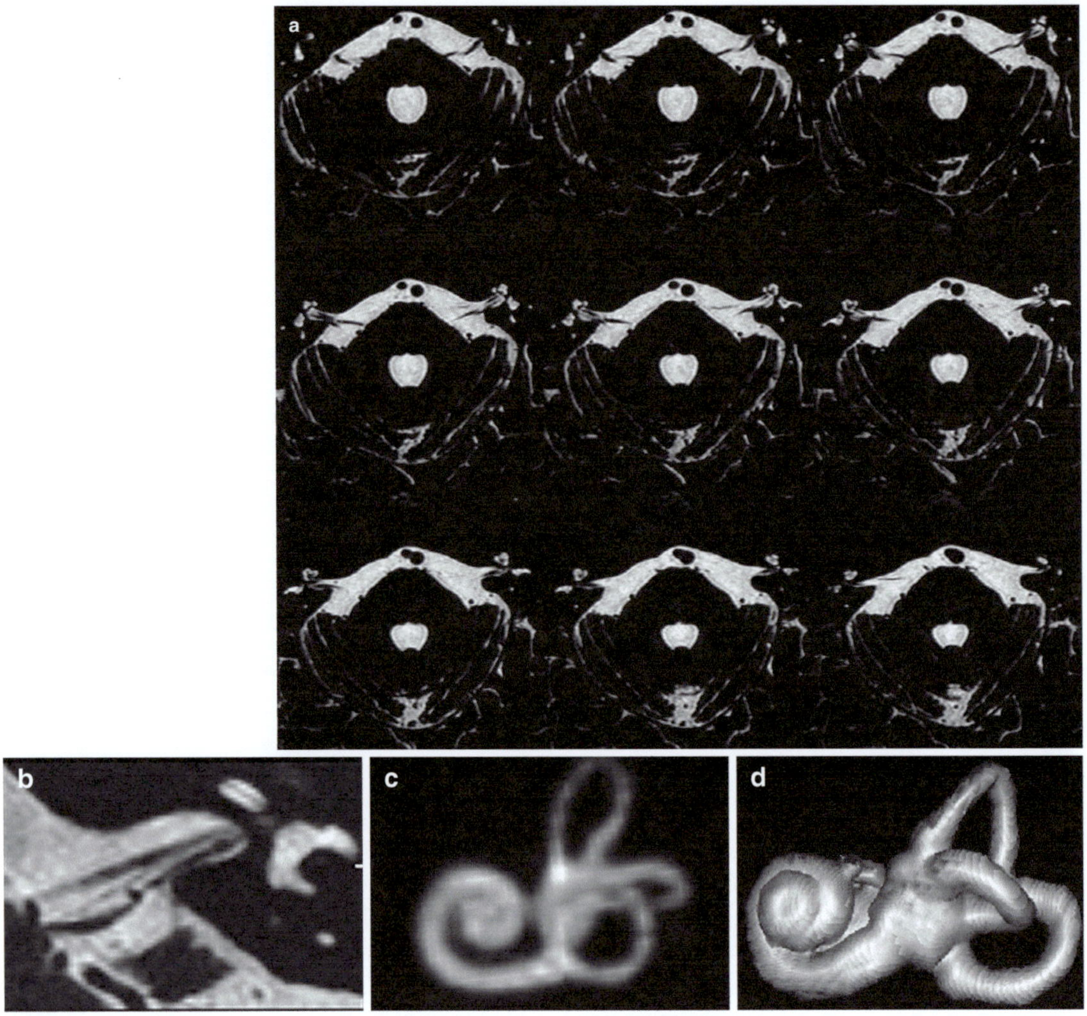


**Fig. 4.15** (**a**) High-definition study of the inner ear using a 3D FIESTA sequence (TR 4.3, TE 1.5, flip angle 50°, BW62 kHz, FOV 170, slice thickness 0.6 mm, matrix 256×256, ZIP 512, 2 NEX, 4:43). Single partitions (**a**), (cont.) detail (**b**), MIP image (**c**), post-processing with volume rendering (**d**)

to T2 to T2*weighting, from short to long echo times and from lower to higher field strengths [22, 23].

Application of a magnetic field to the brain generates an induced field that depends on the applied magnetic field and on the magnetic susceptibility of molecules within the brain. Magnetic susceptibility variations are higher at the interface of two regions, and signal intensity changes are also dependent on other factors, including haematocrit, deoxyhemoglobin concentration, red blood cell integrity, clot structure, molecular diffusion, pH, temperature, field strength, voxel size, previous contrast material use, blood flow and vessel orientation [24].

The term "SWI" implies full use of magnitude and phase information and is not simply a T2* imaging approach.

SWI plays an important role in the diagnostic evaluation and management of acute stroke. In addition, it also plays an important role in the imaging of patients with chronic arterial occlusion and in understanding the effects of chronic infarction, like incomplete infarction and cortical laminar necrosis. The haemodynamic status and oxygen extraction fraction can

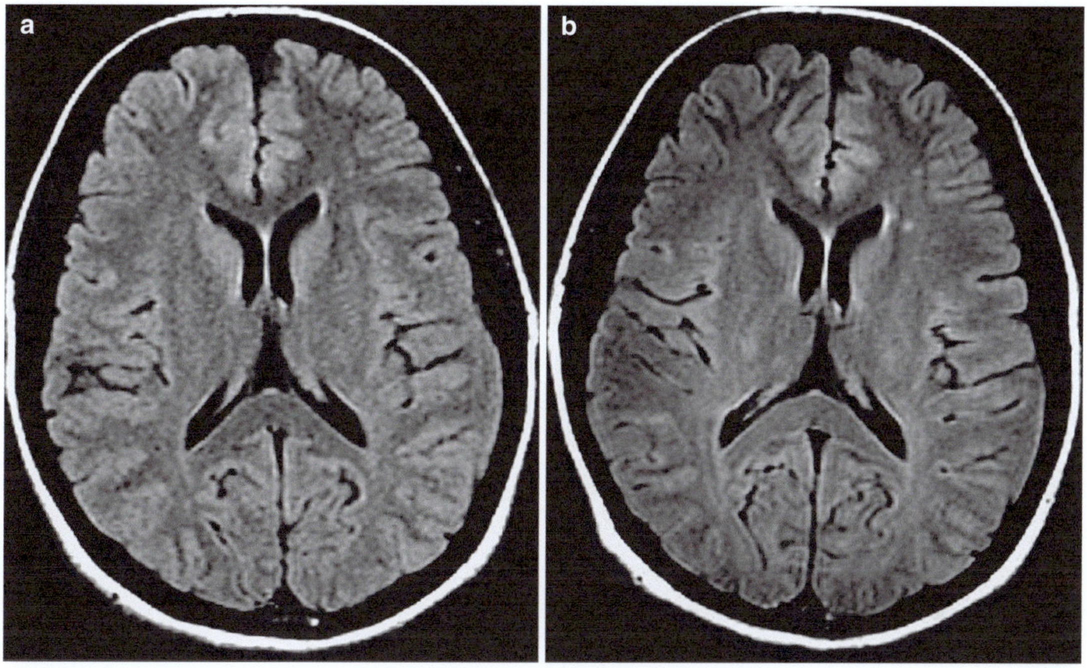


**Fig. 4.16** FLAIR T2 image acquired at 3.0 T (**a**) and1.5 T(**b**). Use of broader matrices and thinner slices at 3.0 T (**a**) disclosed small lesions difficult to identify at 1.5 T (**b**)

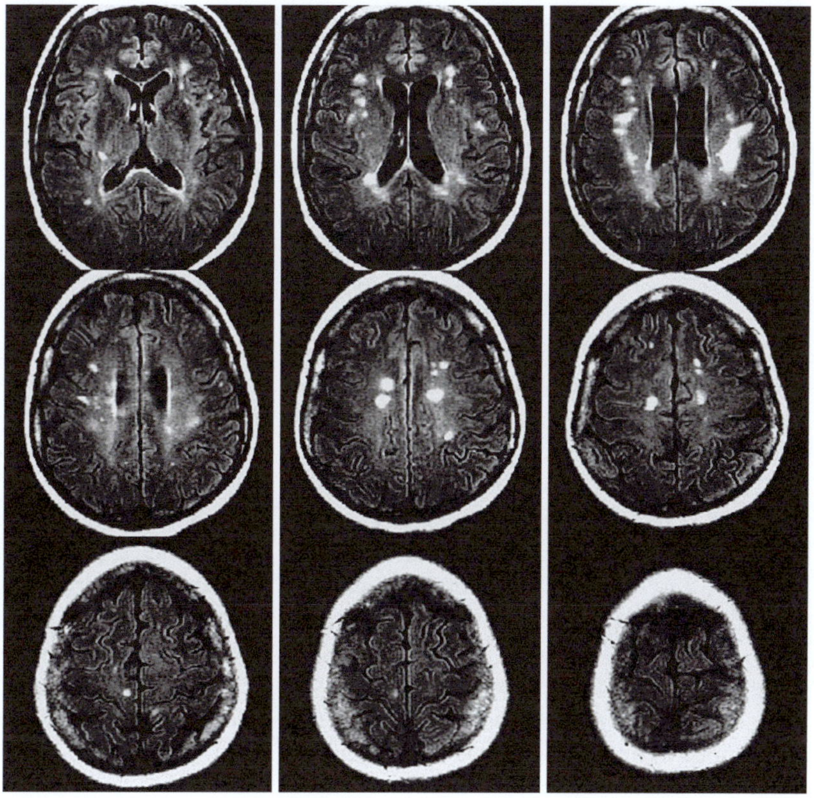

**Fig. 4.17** Multiple sclerosis: image acquired using a FLAIR T2 sequence

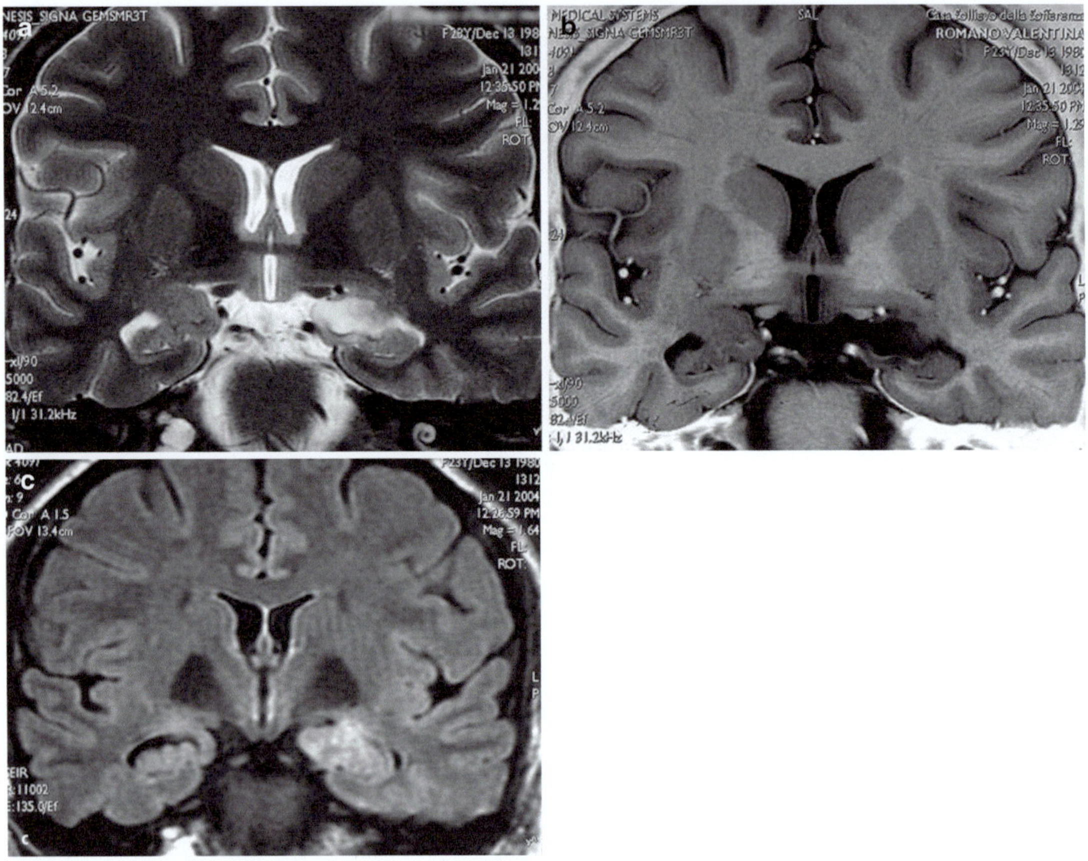


**Fig. 4.18** Left hippocampal lesion on FSE T2 (**a**), "inverted contrast" FSE T2 (**b**) and FLAIR (**c**) sequences. The signal alteration is best appreciated in (**c**). Optimum anatomical cortical-subcortical detail in (**b**)

also be evaluated. SWI is useful in evaluating cerebral venous sinus thrombosis by demonstrating the haemorrhagic venous infarction and thrombus in the sinus and the cortical veins, as well as secondary phenomena like venous stasis in the form of engorged cortical and transmedullary veins and collateral slow flow. Low-flow vascular malformations that are not visualized well on conventional sequences are depicted in exquisite detail along with the venous components on SWI. SWI is used for evaluating cavernomas, developmental venous anomalies, telangiactasias, dural arteriovenous fistulas and the various components of arteriovenous malformations. It has also evolved as a noninvasive technique for evaluating various anomalies of the venous system without administering contrast. Vasculopathies and vasculitis are associated with cerebral microbleeds which are detected on SWI. On the basis of the additional information provided by SWI, it can be included in the routine brain imaging protocol [25].

### 4.1.5 Parallel Imaging

Parallel imaging offers a number of advantages, like faster examination times, when applied to standard MR protocols. Rather than relying on rapid gradient switching to speed acquisition, parallel imaging uses clever algorithms and radio-frequency technology to acquire smaller data sets, specifically by undersampling *k*-space [26–29].

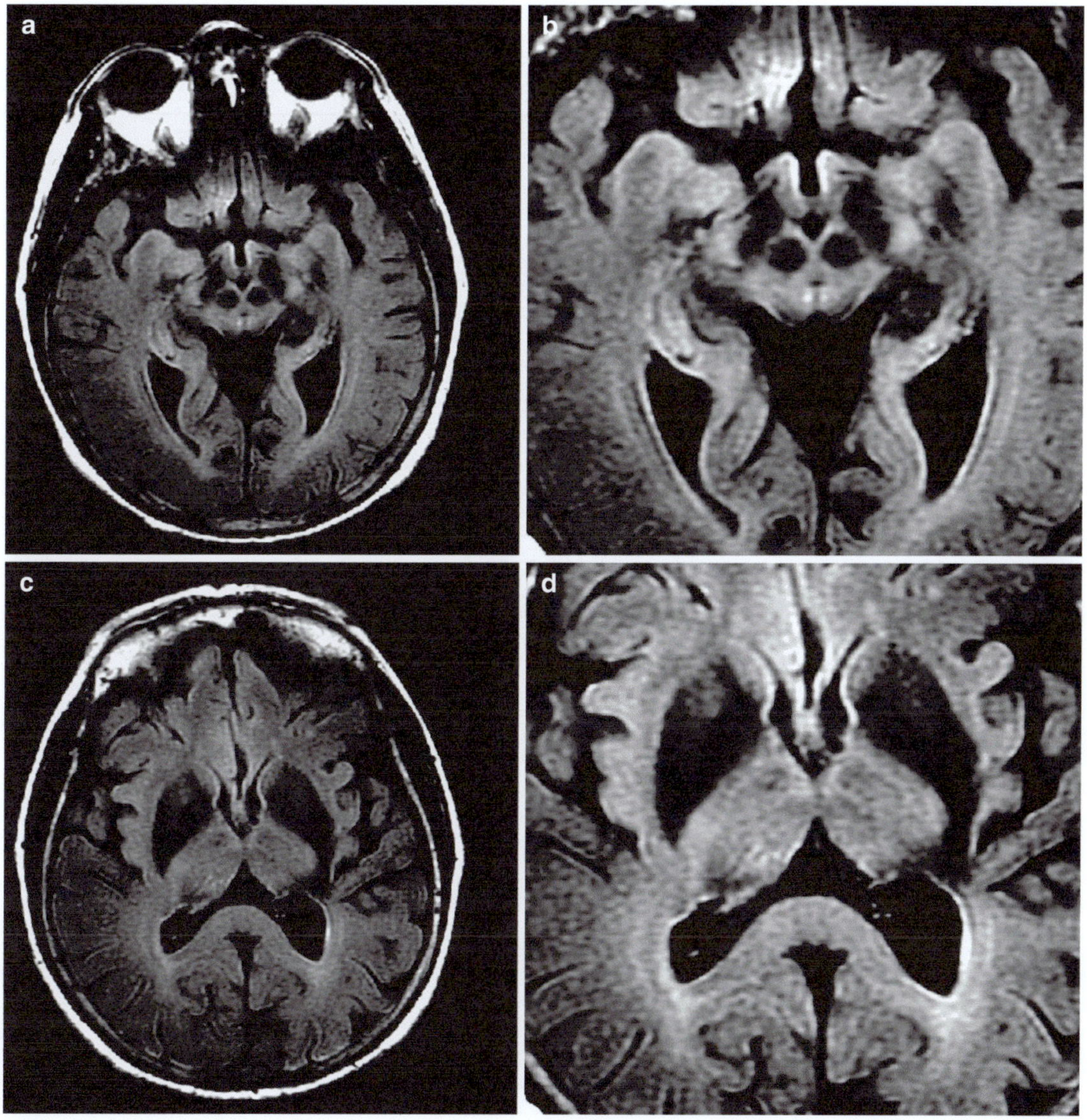


**Fig. 4.19** FLAIR sequence: note the low signal of mesencephalic nuclei (**a**, zoom in **b**) and brain base (**c**, zoom in **d**) due to their iron content

The basis of parallel imaging is the use of the spatial information of the radio-frequency field that is associated with the individual elements of an RF coil array and the use of this information in concert with conventional gradient-based image encoding. Therefore fewer phase-encoding steps have to be performed. It improves data acquisition speeds beyond what can be achieved with conventional non-parallel approaches without imposing additional stress on the gradients (Fig. 4.21). With this method, fully encoded images are reconstructed from undersampled data sets, yielding large savings in scan time. On the other hand, the reductions in scan time incur a cost in both the complexity of the scan and the signal-to-noise ratio (SNR) of the final image [30]. The complexity of the scan arises from the fact that all parallel MRI

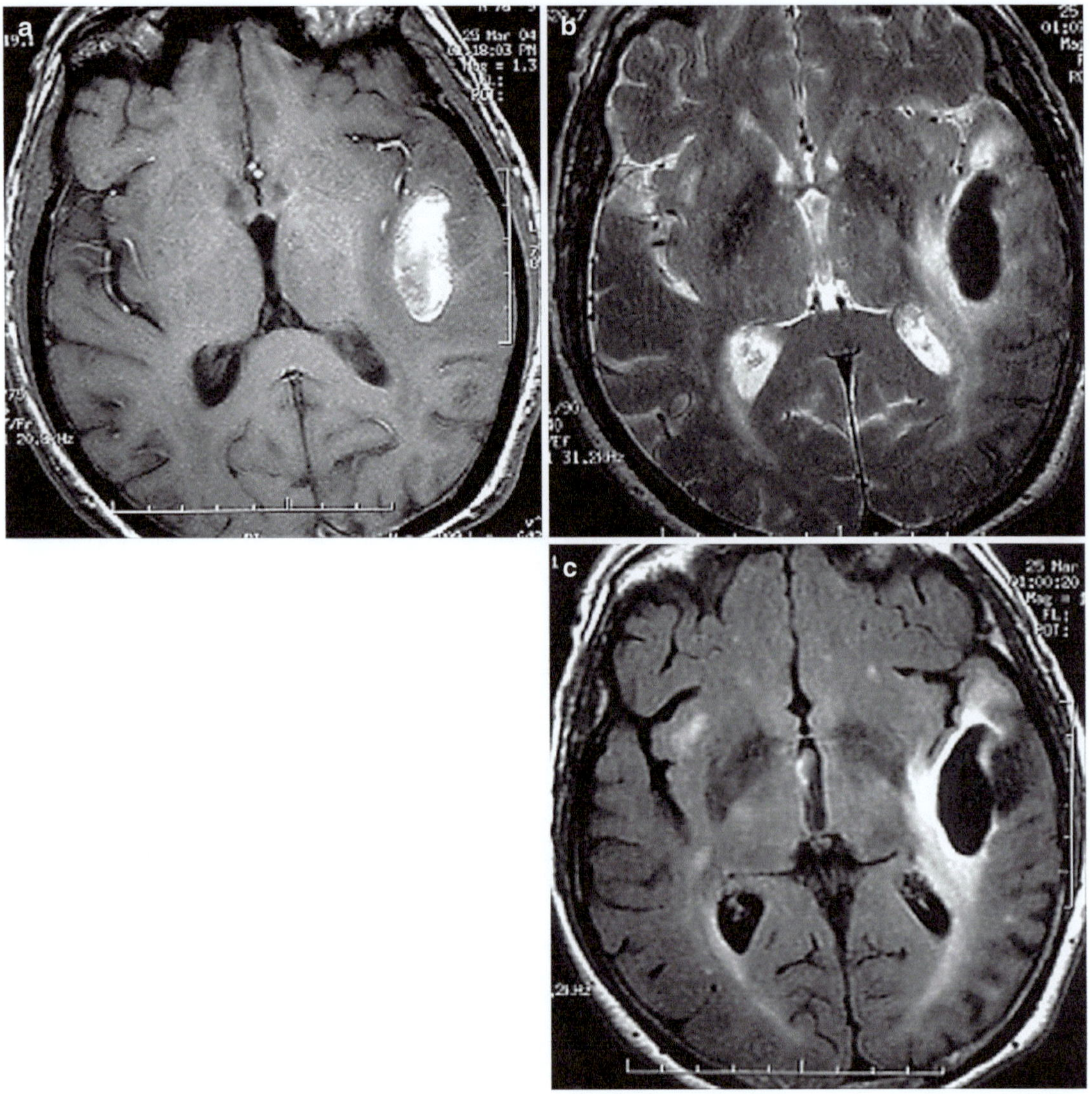

**Fig. 4.20** (**a–c**) Recent intraparenchymal haematoma. FSE T1 (**a**), FSE T2 (**b**) and FLAIR (**c**) acquisitions. Excellent depiction of the lesion and surrounding parenchyma in (**c**)

techniques rely on the knowledge of coil sensitivities, which necessitates some form of calibration. In addition, the SNR loss of every image takes place for two reasons. First, there is a reduction in the temporal averaging of noise associated with the fact that fewer *k*-space points are used in the reconstruction. This leads to an SNR loss proportional to the square root of the reduction in scan time. This has the same effect as in conventional imaging with rectangular FOV. Second, there is amplification of noise because, unlike in conventional Fourier imaging, the transformations used in coil-encoded image reconstruction are not unitary. This leads to an additional spatially dependent source of SNR loss that is quantified by the so-called geometry factor [31]. It is this geometry-associated loss that can be ameliorated through good coil array design and complex algorithms of reconstruction.

Parallel imaging (PI) methods can be categorized into two groups. In the first the missing

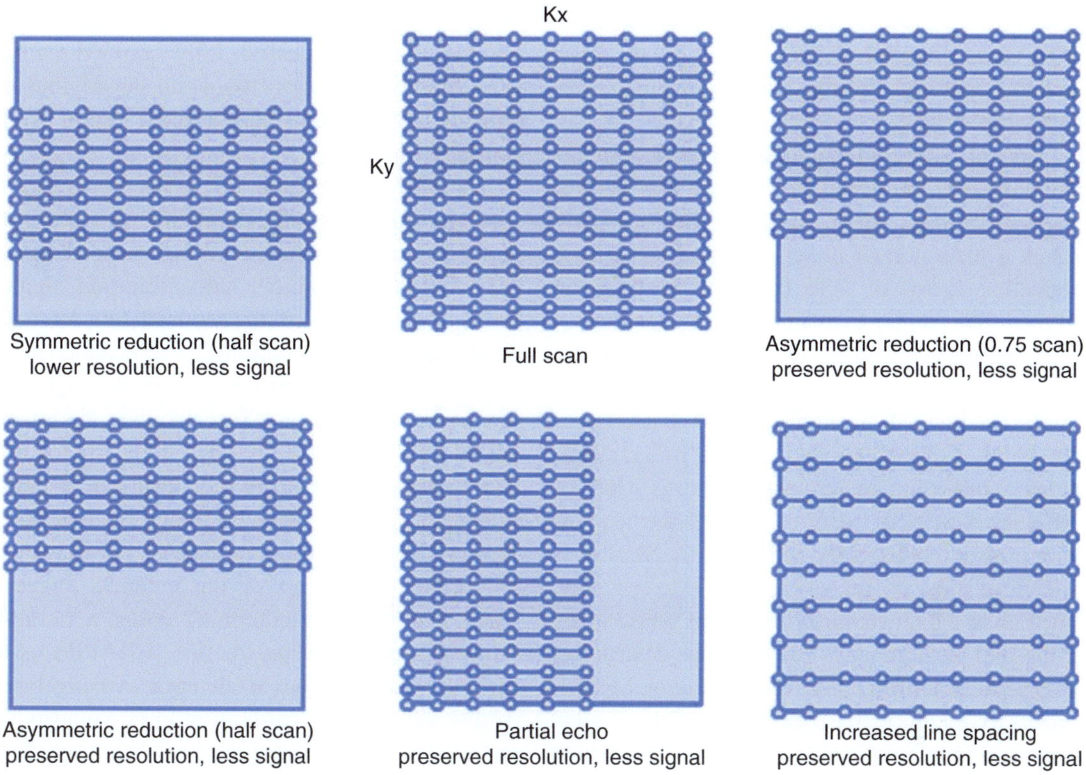


**Fig. 4.21** Basics of *k*-space for faster MRI: MRI can be performed faster by acquiring fewer *k*-lines per MR image. (Courtesy of GE Healthcare Technologies)

*k*-space lines are calculated before Fourier transforming the data, and this kind of algorithm is called simultaneous acquisition of spatial harmonics (SMASH) [32]. It can be truly considered to be the start of a new approach in MRI technology. The third generation of this algorithm is the GeneRalized Auto-calibrating Partially Parallel Acquisition (GRAPPA) that is now available for clinical routine imaging. The second type of PI method first reconstructs images with reduced FOV for all receiver coil elements and then blends these different images, by utilizing the knowledge of the spatial distribution of individual coil sensitivity, into one image with full FOV. The algorithm of this second type is called SENSitive Encoding (SENSE), and the modified algorithm mSENSE is also available as packages on clinical scanners.

Parallel imaging, regardless of in which domain image reconstruction is performed, requires some additional information about the spatial coil sensitivities; in other words providing information about which part of the FOV is covered by each coil element or from which area the coil does receive its MR signal. A homogeneous sample will present itself with a different signal intensity depending on the distance from the coil (principle of reciprocity) [33]. For PI the coil sensitivity information can be acquired as a separate scan or, typical for the GRAPPA and mSENSE algorithm, by additionally acquiring some of the missing data lines in the centre of *k*-space (so-called reference or autocalibration lines) integrated into the acquisition.

In parallel imaging the acceleration of imaging is due to the reduced number of phase-encoding lines that need to be acquired to form an image at a given FOV and resolution. The lines are replaced by exploiting the spatial information that is inherent in the spatially variable sensitivity of an array of surface coils. The number of receiver elements determines the maximum time reduction factor (*R*), which indicates the level of improvement to acquisition speed [34]. With an acceleration factor of 2, only every other line in *k*-space is acquired, and the imaging is virtually cut in half.

Several different techniques for parallel imaging have been proposed by different MR system vendors (ASSET, IPAT, SENSE); they currently allow a reduction of phase-encoding steps by a reduction factor of 2 to 6 (and recently even higher). We can try to examine them separately.

Sensitivity encoding (SENSE) is a parallel imaging technique that trades signal-to-noise for speed. Just as *S*/*N* is reduced by 40 % whenever the number of excitations is halved in a conventional spin-echo image, the same is true of SENSE: A SENSE factor of 2 halves the acquisition time and reduces the *S*/*N* by 40 %. SENSE is therefore most useful when there is excess *S*/*N*, such as at 3 T. It requires the use of phase-array coils, and the number of coil elements determines the theoretical limit on the SENSE factor. SENSE works by intentionally reducing the field of view and the number of phasing-encoding steps, which in turn reduces the acquisition time. This would normally lead to wraparound artefact, or "aliasing", but because the local sensitivity of each coil in the phase array is known, the aliasing can be unwrapped.

SENSE uses the knowledge of coil intensity (sensitivity) profiles to reconstruct undersampled data sets, post-Fourier transform [35]. Sensitivity assessment requires that low-resolution, fully Fourier-encoded reference images are obtained with each array element and with a body coil prior to parallel imaging. Element-wise division of the array references by the body coil references yields raw sensitivity maps. This means that body coil homogeneity forms the basis of homogeneity correction accomplished by SENSE reconstruction [34]. Raw sensitivity maps are refined by a fitting procedure that performs noise elimination and sensitivity extrapolation. Regions that do not contribute signal, according to the references, are automatically excluded from SENSE reconstruction. Another form of SENSE is modified SENSE (mSENSE). The difference is that mSENSE uses autocalibration and does not require a reference scan to calculate sensitivity maps [36]. This is achieved by splitting *k*-space into two regions: a central, fully sampled region from which information about coil sensitivities is derived and an outer undersampled region as in generic SENSE.

The other technique is GRAPPA (generalized autocalibrating partially parallel acquisition); it performs reconstruction in the *k*-space domain [37]. GRAPPA acquires autocalibration signal (ACS) lines along with the reduced data set, and no reference scan is required. The scanner uses the signal lines to estimate a series of weighting functions, which are used to calculate the unacquired lines. When all lines are reconstructed for a particular coil, a Fourier transform can be used to generate the uncombined image for that coil. This process is repeated for each coil of the array to produce a full set of uncombined images, which can then be combined using a normal "sum of squares" reconstruction. GRAPPA uses several blocks of data to fit each missing line. Additional acquired calibration lines can also be included to improve image quality.

*The advantages of using this kind of technique are considerable* The SENSE-mediated reduction of acquisition time can be traded for improved temporal and spatial resolution of any given pulse sequences, without change of image contrast. In addition to the mere increase in image acquisition speed, the reduction of phase-encoding steps brings two further advantages [38]: First, in single-shot EPI applications that are usually used for diffusion imaging, diffusion tensor imaging or functional BOLD-contrast MR studies, SENSE helps to shorten the echo train length in proportion to the reduction factor. The shorter echo train also reduces the phase errors during the EPI readout and the susceptibility effects such as image distortions and blurring. In addition, the shorter echo train translates into a significantly higher SNR.

PI helps to shorten the length of the echo train without loss of spatial resolution in single-shot turbo/fast spin echo (HASTE, SSFSE) too [37]. These sequences often suffer from image artefacts because of their long echo train and can appear blurred because of the T2-related signal decay during the readout of echo train. Second, SENSE helps to reduce RF deposition (regular phase encoding requires an RF pulse for every step). This is extremely helpful for high-field imaging where specific absorption rate (SAR) increases with the square of $B_0$. The higher the field strength, the more energy patients absorb with excessive heating of the patient. In fact SENSE can also decrease the number of echoes in TSE sequences at a given spatial resolution and thus reduce the specific absorption rate. Acceleration factors of up to six are feasible because of the intrinsically high SNR obtained at 3 T [39]. The combination of SENSE with 3 T makes an ideal partnership for optimized high-field MR protocols [40].

The shorter examination time obtained with parallel imaging is therefore useful for claustrophobic patients and patients who find it difficult to remain still.

Using GRAPPA it is possible to take cervical scans with fewer motion artefacts, because GRAPPA provides a greater signal and less ghosting than mSENSE [34].

While the maximum number of parallel receive channels on clinical scanners is currently in the vicinity of eight, Zhu et al. [41] presented a 32-element receive-coil array and a volumetric paradigm that address the SNR challenge at high accelerations. Each system represents the integration of multiple sets of MR electronics, including analog-to-digital converters and digital data pipelines, into a single system. All receivers in the system multiple sets of electronics were synchronized to each other, which in effect expanded the number of parallel receivers to a total of 32. Pulse sequences were adapted to work with the synchronization mechanism, and custom software was developed to facilitate scan control and data communication.

Parallel imaging facilitates trade-offs between acquisition time, spatial coverage and image SNR, which has significant implications for the volumetric paradigm. While acquisition time tends to increase linearly with the expansion of volume coverage using a multislice approach, a more manageable time increase can be expected of the same expansion using a parallel imaging-based volumetric approach [41].

## References


1. Schwindt W, Kugel H, Bachmann R et al (2003) Magnetic resonance imaging protocols for examination of the neurocranium at 3 T. Eur Radiol 13:2170–2179
2. Wansapura JP, Holland SK, Dunn RS et al (1999) NMR relaxation times in the human brain at 3.0 T. J Magn Reson Imaging 9:531–538
3. Frayne R, Goodyear BG, Dickhoff P et al (2003) Magnetic resonance imaging at 3.0 Tesla: challenges and advantages in clinical neurological imaging. Invest Radiol 38(7):385–402
4. Scarabino T, Nemore F, Giannatempo GM et al (2004) Semeiological features of 3.0 T MR imaging: what changes at high magnetic field. Riv Neuroradiol 17:755–764
5. Scarabino T, Nemore F, Giannatempo GM et al (2004) 3.0 T imaging. Riv Neuroradiol 17:765–776
6. Norris DG (2003) High field human imaging. J Magn Reson Imaging 18:519–529
7. Scarabino T, Giannatempo GM, Nemore F et al (2003) RM 3.0 Tesla. II parte: L'imaging morfo-funzionale cerebrale. Radiol Med 105:150–161
8. Scarabino T, Nemore F, Giannatempo GM et al (2003) Risonanza Magnetica 3.0 Tesla. Riv Neuroradiol 16(Suppl):314–315
9. Scarabino T, Nemore F, Giannatempo GM et al (2003) 3.0 T magnetic resonance in neuroradiology. Eur J Radiol 48:154–164
10. Takahashi M, Uematsu H, Hatabu H (2003) MR imaging at high magnetic fields. Eur J Radiol 46:45–52
11. Noebauer-Huhmann I, Ba-Ssalamah A, Mlynarik V et al (2002) Magnetic resonance imaging contrast enhancement of brain tumors at 3 T versus 1.5 T. Invest Radiol 37(3):114–119
12. Trattnig S, Ba-Ssalamah A, Noebauer-Huhmann IM et al (2003) MR contrast agent at high field MRI (3 Tesla). Top Magn Reson Imaging 14(5):365–375
13. Buerk BM, Pulido JS, Chiong I et al (2004) Vascular perfusion of choroidal melanoma by 3.0 Tesla magnetic resonance imaging. Trans Am Ophthalmol Soc 102:209–215
14. Sicotte NL, Voskuhl RR, Bouvier S et al (2003) Comparison of multiple sclerosis lesions at 1.5 T and 3.0 Tesla. Invest Radiol 38(7):423–427
15. Kim DS, Garwood M (2003) High field magnetic resonance techniques for brain research. Curr Opin Neurobiol 13:612–619
16. Krautmacher C, Tschamps H, Traeber F et al (2003) 3.0 T MR imaging of contrast-enhancing brain tumors: intra-individual study comparing standard and half standard dose at 3.0 T with standard dose at 1.5 T. Eur Radiol 1381:222

17. Karlberg M, Annertz M, Magnusson M (2004) Acute vestibular neuritis visualized by 3-T magnetic resonance imaging with high-dose gadolinium. Arch Otolaryngol Head Neck Surg 130(2):229–232
18. Nakada T (2003) Clinical experience on 3.0 T systems in Niigata, 1996 to 2002. Invest Radiol 38(7):377–384
19. Allkemper T, Tombach B, Schwindt W et al (2004) Acute and subacute intracerebral hemorrhages: comparison of MR imaging at 1.5 T and 3.0 T – initial experience. Radiology 232(3):874–881
20. Lane JI, Ward H, Witte RJ et al (2004) 3-T imaging of the cochlear nerve and labyrinth in cochlear-implant candidates: 3 D fast recovery fast spin echo versus 3 D constructive interference in the steady state techniques. Am J Neuroradiol 25(4):618–622
21. Tong KA, Ashwal S, Obenaus A, Nickerson JP, Kido D, Haacke EM (2008) Susceptibility-weighted MR imaging: a review of clinical applications in children. AJNR Am J Neuroradiol 29(1):9–17
22. Haacke EM, Xu Y, Cheng YC, Reichenbach JR (2004) Susceptibility weighted imaging (SWI). Magn Reson Med 52(3):612–618
23. Reichenbach JR, Venkatesan R, Schillinger DJ, Kido DK, Haacke EM (1997) Small vessels in the human brain: MR venography with deoxyhemoglobin as an intrinsic contrast agent. Radiology 204(1):272–277
24. Hermier M, Nighoghossian N (2004) Contribution of susceptibility-weighted imaging to acute stroke assessment. Stroke 35(8):1989–1994
25. Hingwala D, Kesavadas C, Thomas B, Kapilamoorthy TR (2010) Clinical utility of susceptibility-weighted imaging in vascular diseases of the brain. Neurol India 58(4):602–607
26. Hutchinson M, Raff U (1988) Fast MRI data acquisition using multiple detectors. Magn Reson Med 6(1):87–91
27. Ra JG, Rim CY (1993) Fast imaging using subencoding data sets from multiple detectors. Magn Reson Med 30(1):142–145
28. Roemer PB, Edelstein WA et al (1990) The NMR phase array. Magn Reson Med 16(2):192–225
29. Sodickson DK, Manning WJ (1999) Simultaneous acquisition of spatial harmonics (SMASH): fast imaging with radiofrequency coil arrays. Magn Reson Med 42(5):952–962
30. Ohlinger MA, Grant AK et al (2003) Ultimate intrinsic signal-to-noise ratio for parallel MRI: electromagnetic field considerations. Magn Reson Med 50:1018–1030
31. Pipe JG (1999) Motion correction with PROPELLER MRI: application to head motion and free-breathing cardiac imaging. Magn Reson Med 42:963–969
32. Sodickson DK (2000) Tailored SMASH image reconstruction for robust in vivo parallel MR imaging. Magn Reson Med 44:243–251
33. Insko EK, Elliott MA et al (1998) Generalized reciprocity. J Magn Reson 131:111–117
34. Little MW, Mcrobbie DW (2004) Parallel imaging improves scan speed. Diagn Imaging Eur 5:29–35
35. Pruessmann KP, Weiger M et al (1999) SENSE: sensitivity encoding for fast MRI. Magn Reson Med 42(5):952–962
36. Wang J, Kluge T, et al. (2001) Parallel acquisition techniques with modified SENSE reconstruction mSENSE. Presented at the First Würzburg Workshop on Parallel Imaging. Würzburg, Germany, 7–10 November 2001, p 92
37. Griswold MA, Jakob PM et al (2002) Generalized autocalibrating partially parallel acquisition (GRAPPA). Magn Reson Med 47(6):1202–1210
38. Kuhl CK (2004) Parallel imaging in neuroradiology. ASNR Proceedings: 181–182
39. Gieseke J, Manka C et al (2003) Diffusiongewichtete MRT Aufnahmen mit SENSE bei 3 T. Fortschr Roentgenstr 175:202
40. Lewin M, Carlesso N et al (2000) Tat-peptide-derivatized magnetic nanoparticles allow in vivo tracking and recovery of progenitor cells. Nat Biotechnol 18:410–414
41. Zhu Y, Hardy CJ et al (2004) Highly parallel volumetric imaging with a 32-element RF coil array. Magn Reson Med 52:869–877

# 5 3.0 T MR Angiography

Tommaso Scarabino, Saverio Pollice, Giuseppe Maria Giannatempo, Michelangelo Nasuto, Rosario Francesco Balzano, and Teresa Popolizio

Magnetic resonance angiography (MRA) is a well-established non-invasive technique for imaging the intracranial vasculature, particularly large calibre arteries and veins, and detecting changes in vessel calibre and/or course (Figs. 5.1 and 5.2). It is generally performed without administration of paramagnetic contrast media.

Drawbacks with respect to conventional angiography are lower spatial and, above all, temporal resolution. The quality of MR angiographic images has recently been improved even in lower field systems by the advent of surface or phased array coils with a higher signal/noise ratio (SNR) and shorter echo times (TE) made possible by stronger gradients, new pulse sequences with optimized SNR and longer acquisition times (given that a fourfold increase in examination time doubles the SNR).

T. Scarabino (✉) • S. Pollice
Department of Radiology and Neuroradiology, PO "L. Bonomo" Hospital, Andria (BT), Italy
e-mail: tscarabino@hotmail.com

G.M. Giannatempo • M. Nasuto • R.F. Balzano
T. Popolizio
Department of Radiology and Neuroradiology, IRCCS "Casa Sollievo della Sofferenza", San Giovanni Rotondo (FG), Italy

## 5.1 MRA Techniques

Although there are several approaches to visualizing the intracranial vessels with MR, the two most widely used techniques are time-of-flight (TOF) and phase-contrast (PC) MRA.

In TOF MRA, which is usually performed using a flow-compensated gradient-refocused sequence, stationary tissues are saturated and thus have low signal intensity. However, blood upstream of the imaging volume is unsaturated. When this blood flows into the imaging volume, it is bright compared with the stationary background tissue [1].

For vessels coursing within the acquired section, the inflow effect becomes less effective, reducing intravascular signal to the level of the surrounding stationary spins. Potential difficulties in TOF MRA may therefore arise in situations where larger sections of vessels lie within a section and also in situations where turbulent flow is present, as this also suppresses bright intravascular signal.

In TOF MRA, vessels appear bright independent of the flow direction. Hence, arteries and veins cannot be differentiated. Flow in a particular direction can, however, be saturated using spatial flow presaturation bands. Spins being washed into the slice from the presaturation area will not carry any magnetization, and no inflow enhancement occurs [2]. These saturation bands can thus be used to obtain selective TOF angiograms or venograms.



T. Scarabino et al. (eds.), *High Field Brain MRI*, DOI 10.1007/978-3-319-44174-0_5

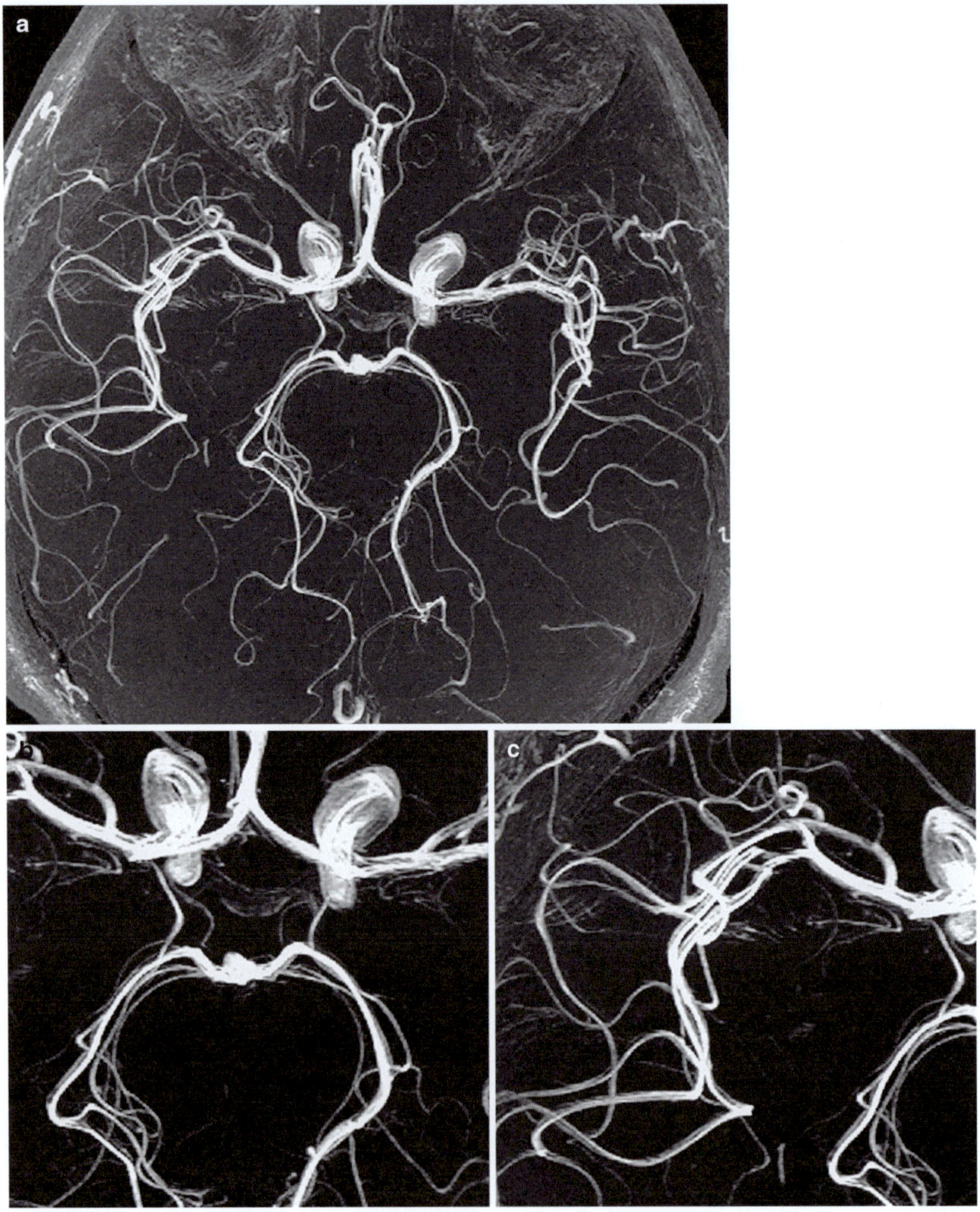


**Fig. 5.1** Normal arterial circulation: high-definition 3D TOF image at 3.0 T (matrix 1024×512, FOV 240 mm, slice thickness 1 mm) (**a**); detail of the circle of Willis, especially of the posterior circle (**b**); also note detail of the right middle cerebral artery branches (**c**)

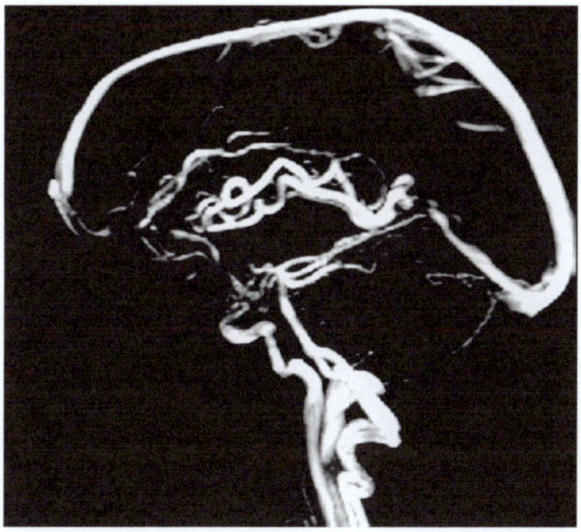

**Fig. 5.2** Normal venous cerebral circulation: 3D PC study at 3.0 T

Unlike TOF MRA, PC MRA utilizes phase shifts as blood flows in the presence of flow-encoding bipolar gradients. On phase-difference images, the signal phase intensity is proportional to velocity, resulting in suppression of the stationary background tissue. The flow-encoding gradients can be applied in any one or multiple directions depending on the desired flow sensitivity [1]. This technique is thus a direct velocity map, where the voxel intensity values are proportional to the actual flow velocity in a particular flow direction.

Because the typical imaging time of these conventional MRA techniques is between 2 and 8 min, neither technique is able to demonstrate the dynamics of cerebral blood flow. Moreover, both techniques are prone to artefacts resulting from slow, turbulent or complex blood flow.

Most of the problems associated with TOF MRA and PC MRA can be overcome with contrast-enhanced MRA (CE-MRA) [1, 3]. Three-dimensional CE-MRA fundamentally differs from other vascular MR imaging strategies in that it is not flow dependent. Blood signal is derived from the T1-shortening effect of the dynamically infused paramagnetic contrast. Hence, arterial contrast is based on the difference in T1 relaxation between blood and surrounding tissue [4]. As a result, problems associated with slow flow and turbulence-induced signal voids are overcome. The technique allows a small number of slices oriented in the plane of the vessels of interest to image an extensive region of vascular anatomy in a short period of time [5]. With this technique, a temporal resolution of about one image in 20 s has become possible, enabling selective demonstration of the early arterial and late venous phase [5–7].

MRA images are best interpreted on an independent workstation with 3D reconstruction capabilities. In addition to perusal of the original sections, diagnoses should be based on a combination of maximum intensity projection (MIP) images and interactive 3D multiplanar reformations (MPR). The MPR technique permits cross-sectional visualization of the vessels in any plane. Venous overlap can effectively be compensated, and the course of tortuous vessels can easily be reconstructed. This represents an advantage even over conventional catheter angiography. Surface-rendering algorithms as well as virtual angioscopic reconstructions are useful mainly for demonstration purpose.

## 5.2 3.0 T MRA

3.0 T MRA offers significant advantages (Figs. 5.3, 5.4, 5.5 and 5.6) [8–11].

First of all, it allows to perform all the angiographic sequences applied routinely in clinical practice with lower field systems, such as 2D and 3D TOF and PC, as well as ultrafast dynamic sequences after administration of a bolus of contrast agent (CE-MRA).

Similarly to standard brain MRI, the technical parameters of MRA sequences also need to be optimized at higher magnetic fields (Table 5.1).

The higher SNR improves scan quality largely through wider acquisition matrices (up to 1024) without giving rise to significantly grainy images [12–15]. In addition, the change in T1 relaxation time, i.e. the increased T1,

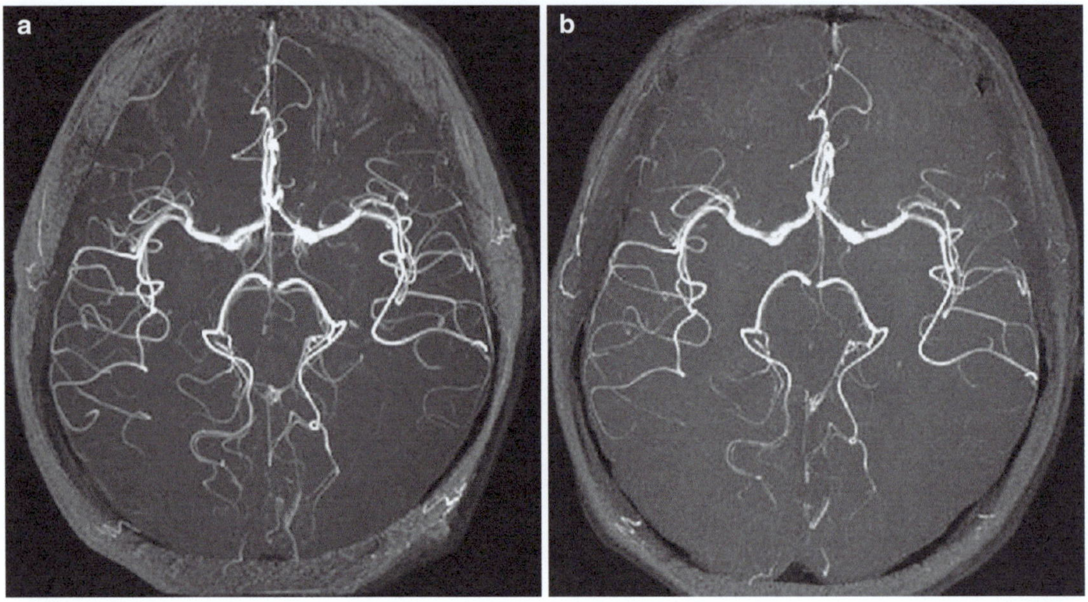


**Fig. 5.3** Normal arterial cerebral circulation imaged using the same 3D TOF sequence at 3.0 T (**a**) and1.5 T (**b**). In (**a**), vessel conspicuity is greater than in (**b**), yielding better and more detailed depiction of superficial, smaller calibre vessels

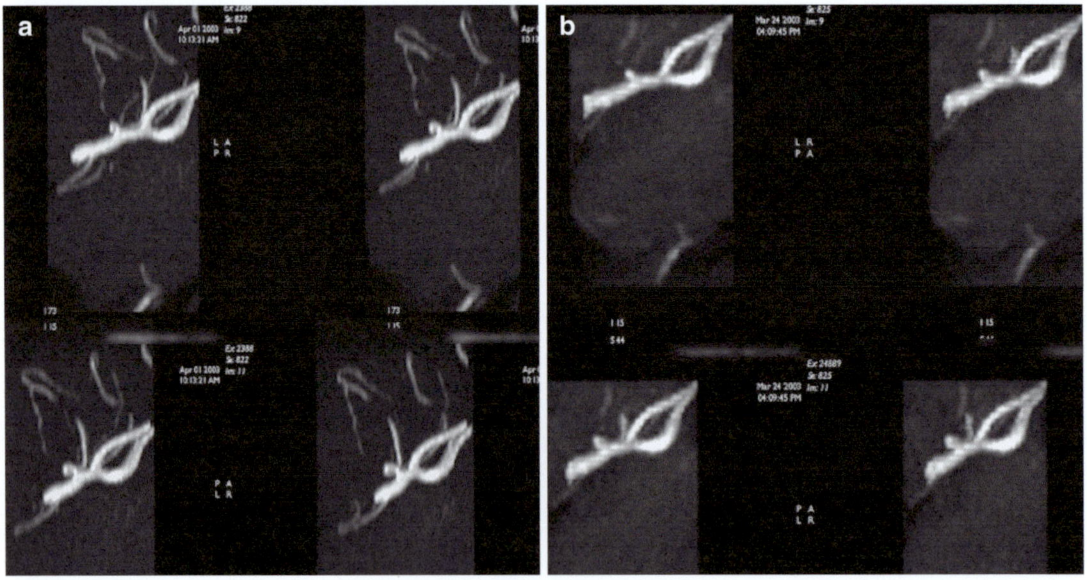


**Fig. 5.4** Coiling of a branch of the right middle cerebral artery studied with a 3D TOF sequence at 3.0 T (**a**) and 1.5 T(**b**). The coil is better depicted in (**a**) than in (**b**), where the image mimics a small aneurysm

yields greater background stationary tissue suppression due to decreased R1 (the rate of longitudinal or spin-lattice relaxation), and greater flow enhancement since blood R1 is roughly constant, thus improving vessel-tissue contrast [12, 16, 17].

This advantage makes the application of magnetization transfer less effective than it is with

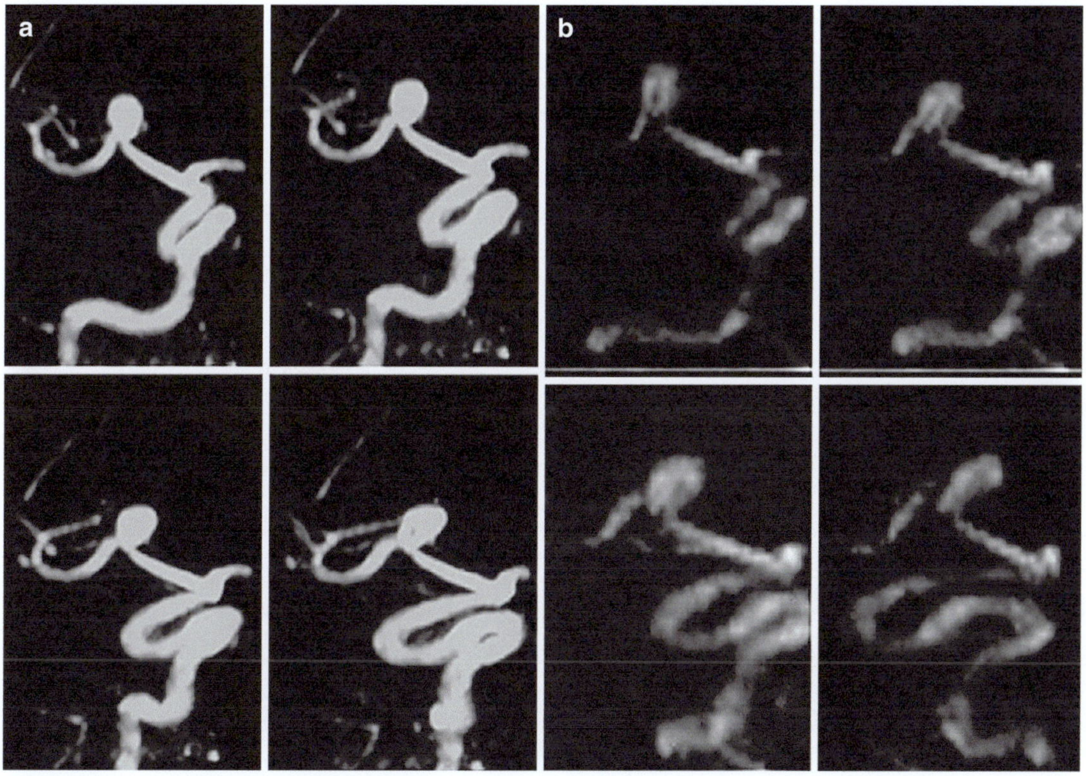


**Fig. 5.5** Sacciform aneurysm of middle cerebral artery imaged using the same 3D TOF sequence performed at 3.0 T (**a**) and 1.5 T (**b**). The sacciform vascular dilatation is depicted in greater detail and exhibits a more intense signal in (**a**) than in (**b**)

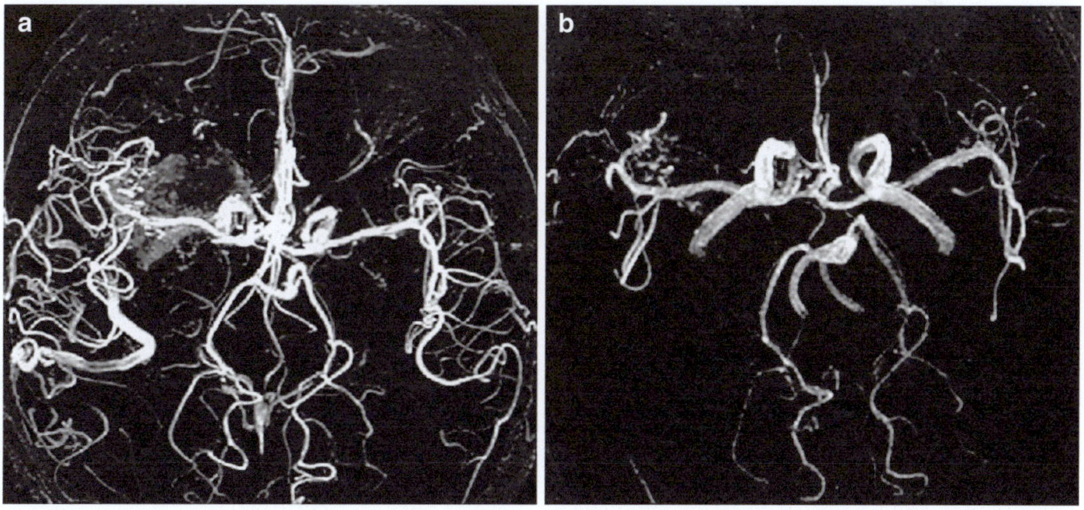


**Fig. 5.6** Large right arteriovenous malformation: unenhanced 3D TOF images acquired at 3.0 T (**a**) and 1.5 T (**b**). Greater background suppression and flow enhancement afford better spatial depiction of the malformation at 3.0 T

**Table 5.1** Optimization of technical parameters of MRA sequences at higher magnetic fields

| Sequence | TR (ms) | TE (ms) | Other parameters (TI, FA, ZIP) | Slice thickness (mm) | No. of slices | FOV | Matrix | NEX | Examination time (min:s) |
|---|---|---|---|---|---|---|---|---|---|
| 3D*TOF* / 1.5T | 30 | 6.9 | FA 30 | 1.2 | 32 | 24 | 352×224 | 1 | 3:08 |
| 3D*TOF* / 3.0T | 26 | Min | FA 20<br>ZIP 512<br>ZIP 2 | 1.4 | 60 | 16 | 288×224 | 1 | 5:53 |
| *HD*3D*TOF* / 3.0T | 30 | Min | FA 20<br>ZIP 1024<br>ZIP 2 | 1.4 | 48 | 19 | 384×320 | 1 | 6:18 |
| 2D*TOF* / 1.5T | Min | Min | 70 | 1.5 | | 23 | 256×224 | 1 | Variable in relation to number of slices |
| 2D*TOF* / 3.0T | Min | Min | 50 | 1.4 | | 22 | 256×192 | 1 | Variable in relation to number of slices |
| 3D*PC* / 1.5T | 33 | | 20 | 50 | | 20 | 256×192 | 8 | 3:23 |
| 3D*PC* / 1.0T | 30 | | 20 | 35 | | 22 | 256×224 | 6 | 2:41 |

1.5 T systems [18, 19] and is mainly evident when using 3D TOF sequences, since the short TR usually saturates stationary tissue but not circulating blood [20], and the tag persists over a longer time. These effects afford greater vessel detail and conspicuity, especially with regard to small calibre structures, including surface vessels not clearly depicted on 1.5 T images (Figs. 5.7, 5.8, 5.9, 5.10, 5.11 and 5.12) [21, 22].

For the same reasons, 3.0 T MRA appears to be a promising technique to enhance vessel conspicuity in neonatal intracranial vessels or to further reduce scanning time [23]. Neonatal brain vessels are small; they exhibit lower blood flow velocity than adult vessels and frequently have a turbulent flow. MRA protocols therefore need to be adapted to the specific needs and features of these patients, e.g. by reducing acquisition time to prevent motion artefacts, by using low flip angles and out-of-phase imaging better to saturate subcutaneous fat (which sometimes masks vessels on 3D MIP sequences) and by implementing ramped RF pulse and multiple thin volume strategies to visualize the intravascular signal at distal cortical branches.

Since the relaxivity of paramagnetic contrast media remains largely unchanged at higher magnetic field strengths, contrast administration further improves 3.0 T imaging given that its high SNR can be transformed into spatial resolution: resolution of 300 μm on the plane of section and of 400 μm on the slice thickness, i.e. 300×300×400 interpolated voxels (ZIP 4 and ZIP 1024) (Fig. 5.13).

Dynamic techniques, which afford shorter acquisition times, further contribute to improving contrast-enhanced MRA.

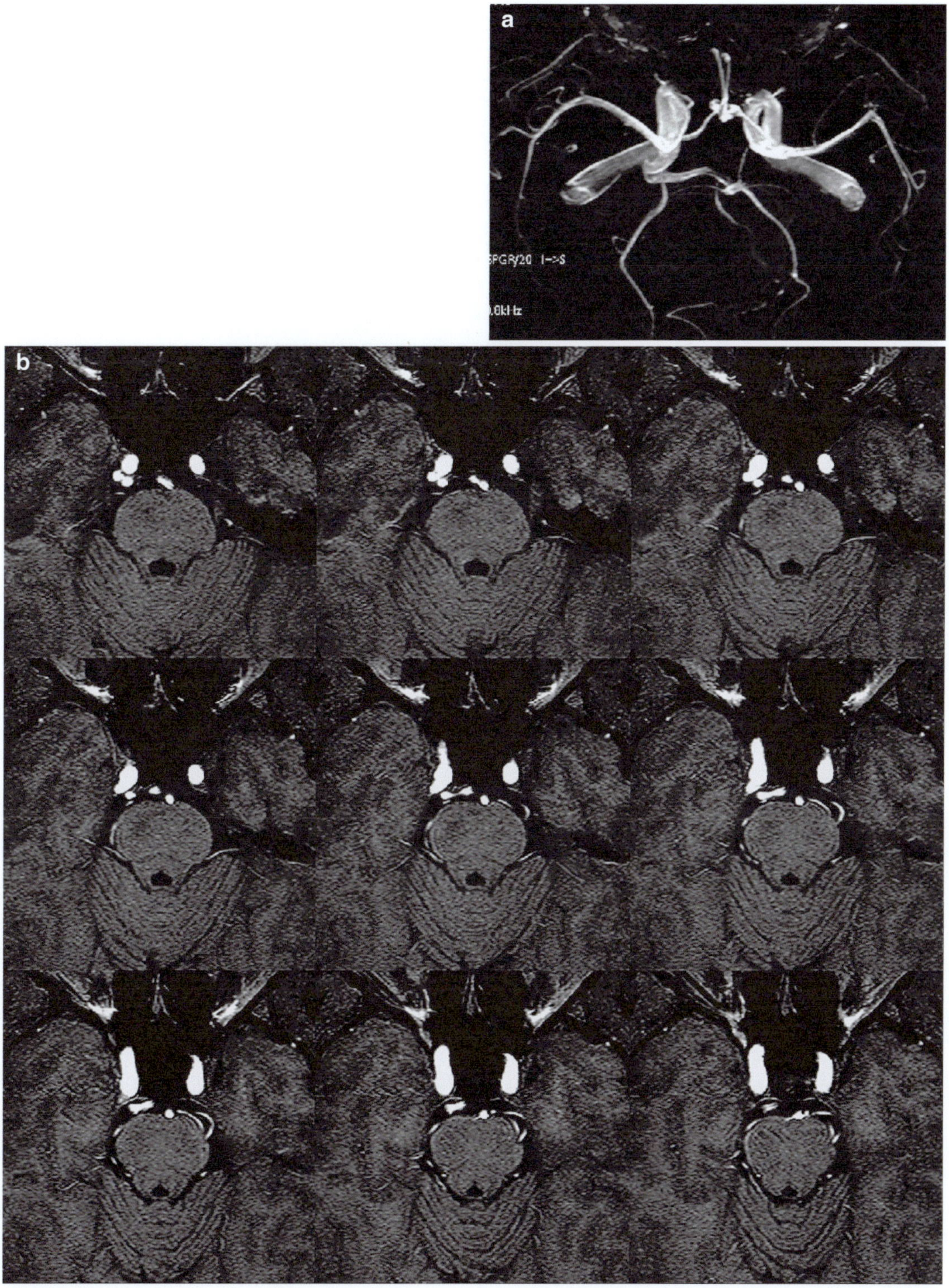

**Fig. 5.7** Vestigial artery: unenhanced 3D TOF study at 3.0 T. MIP image (**a**), single partitions (**b**)

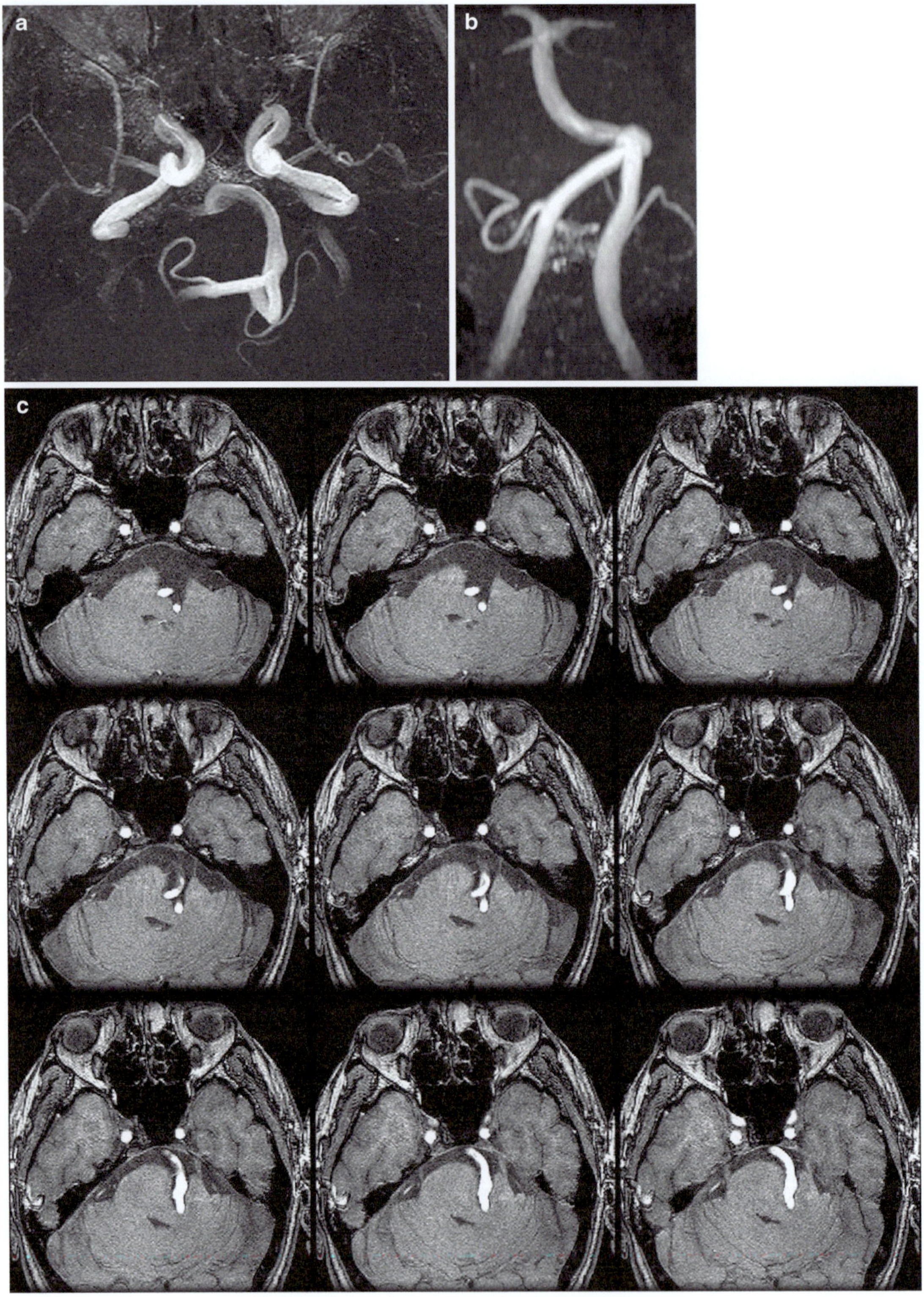


**Fig. 5.8** Neurovascular conflict: 3D TOF unenhanced study at 3.0 T. MIP images (**a**, **b**), single partitions (**c**)

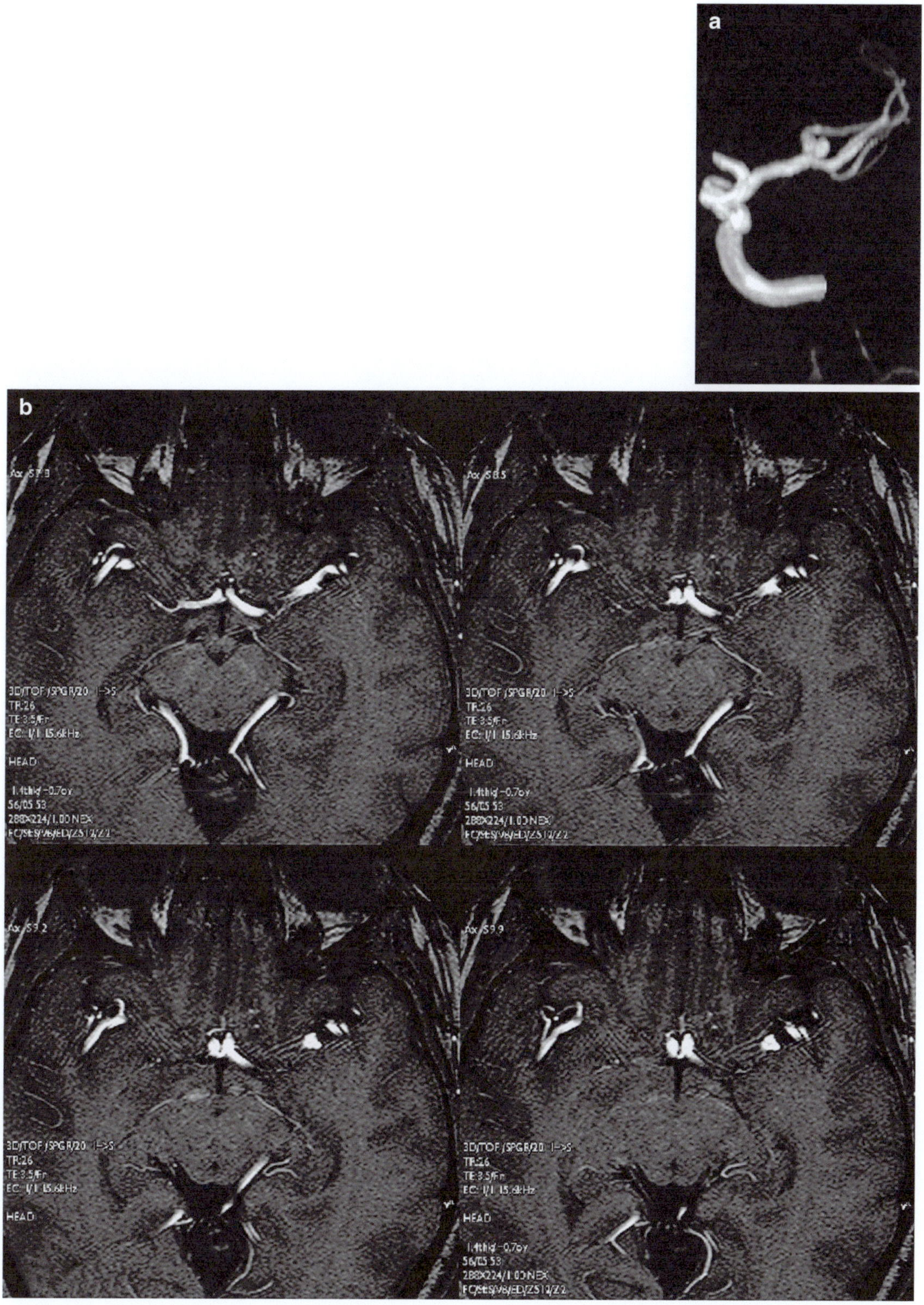


**Fig. 5.9** Small berry aneurysm of left middle cerebral artery: 3D TOF study at 3.0 T. MIP image (**a**), single partitions (**b**)

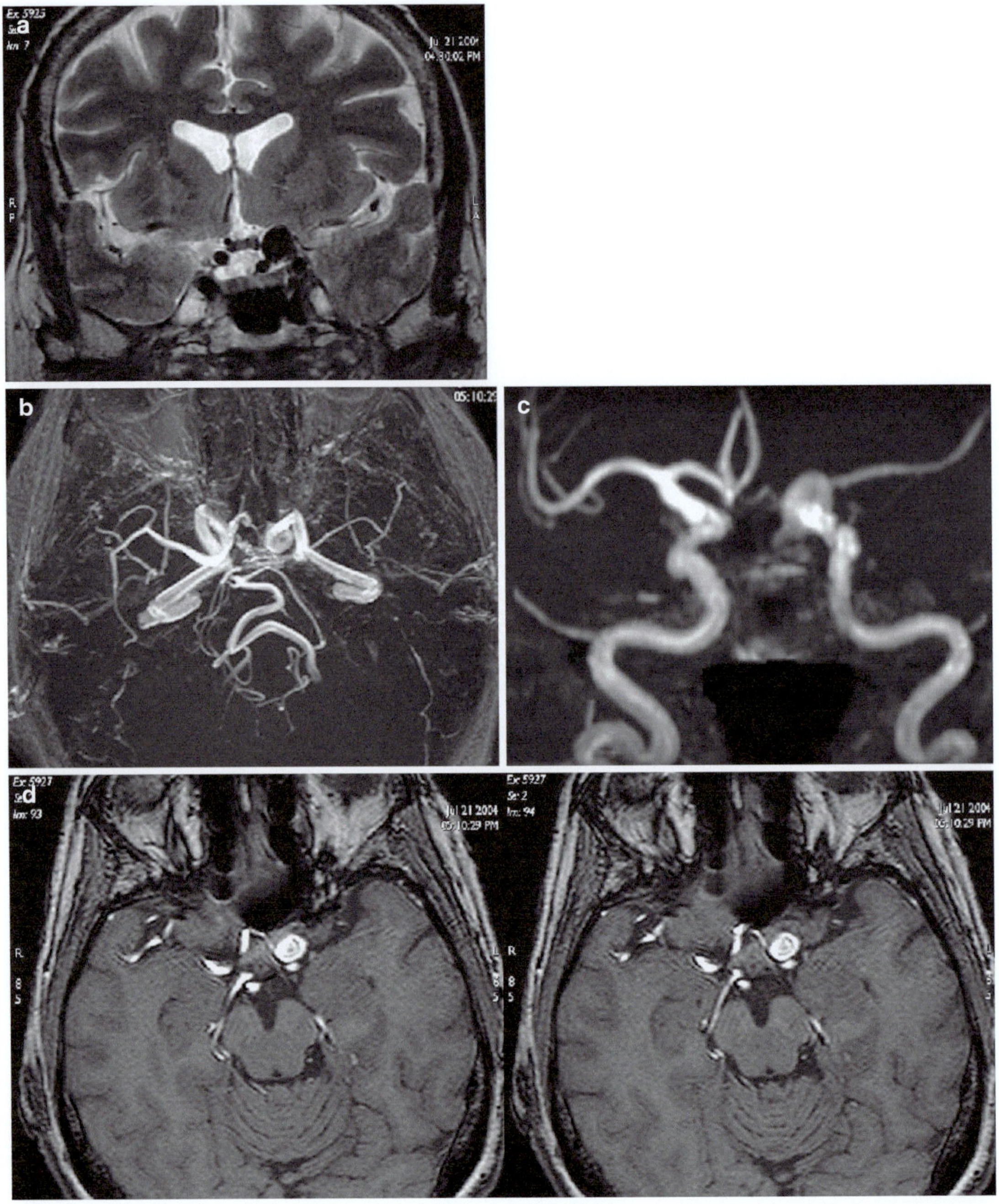

**Fig. 5.10** Small berry aneurysm of the supraclinoid stretch of the left carotid siphon. Standard MRI, FSE T2 sequence (**a**); 3D TOF, axial and coronal MIP images (**b**, **c**); single partitions (**d**)

Additional gains are obtained with parallel imaging, which significantly reduces examination times and increases anatomical coverage providing the same image quality. In this case, a TOF sequence is usually applied with a wide matrix and hence greater spatial resolution [24].

Finally, although the deflection and torsion movements of biomedical devices (such as the aneurysm clips commonly used in interventional and therapeutic neuroradiological procedures) and resulting susceptibility artefacts increase at higher magnetic field strength, the newer devices

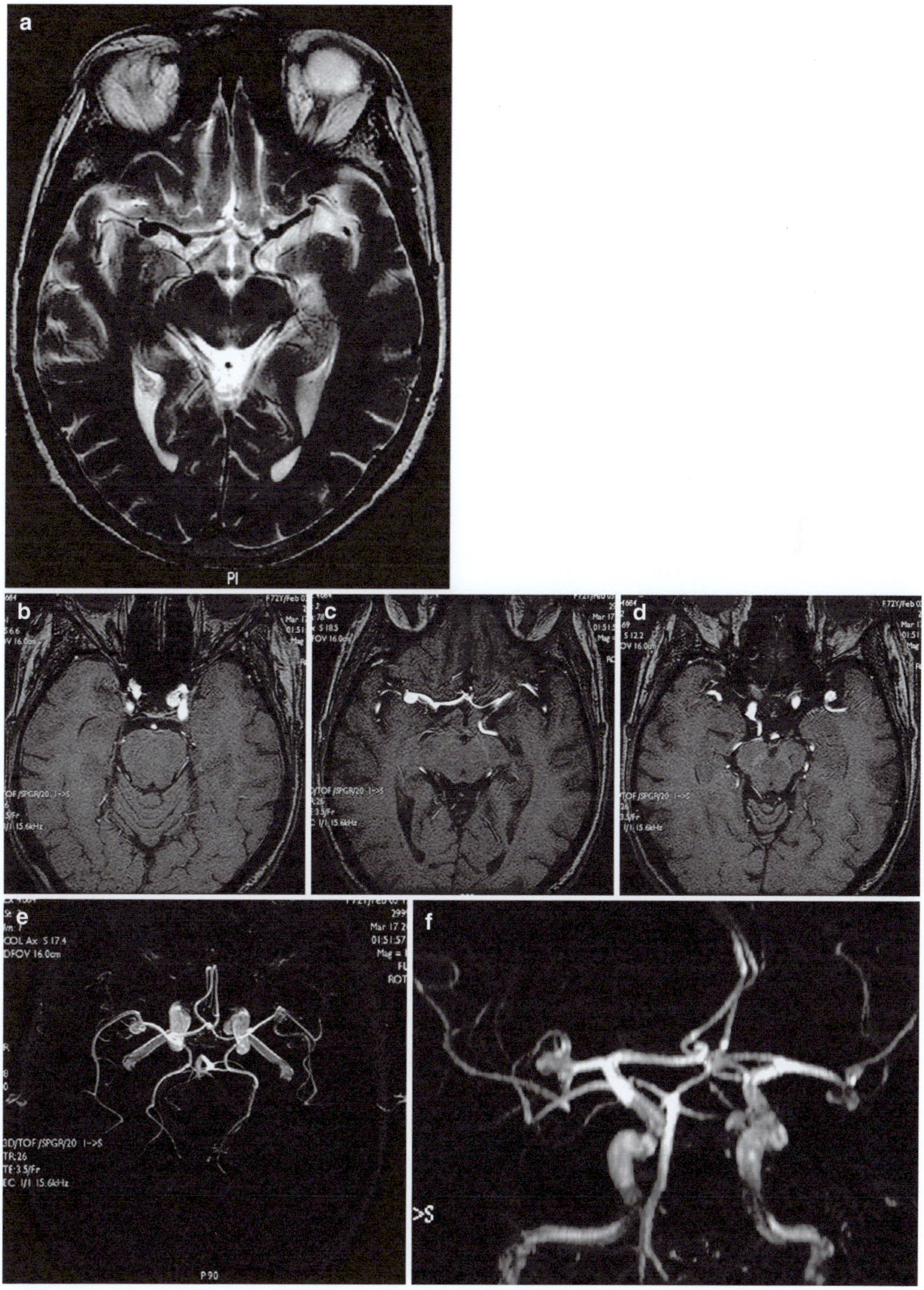


**Fig. 5.11** Small, multiple aneurysms (left carotid siphon, middle cerebral arteries bilaterally). Standard MRI, FSE T2 sequence (**a**); 3D TOF, single partitions (**b–d**), axial and coronal MIP images (**e, f**)

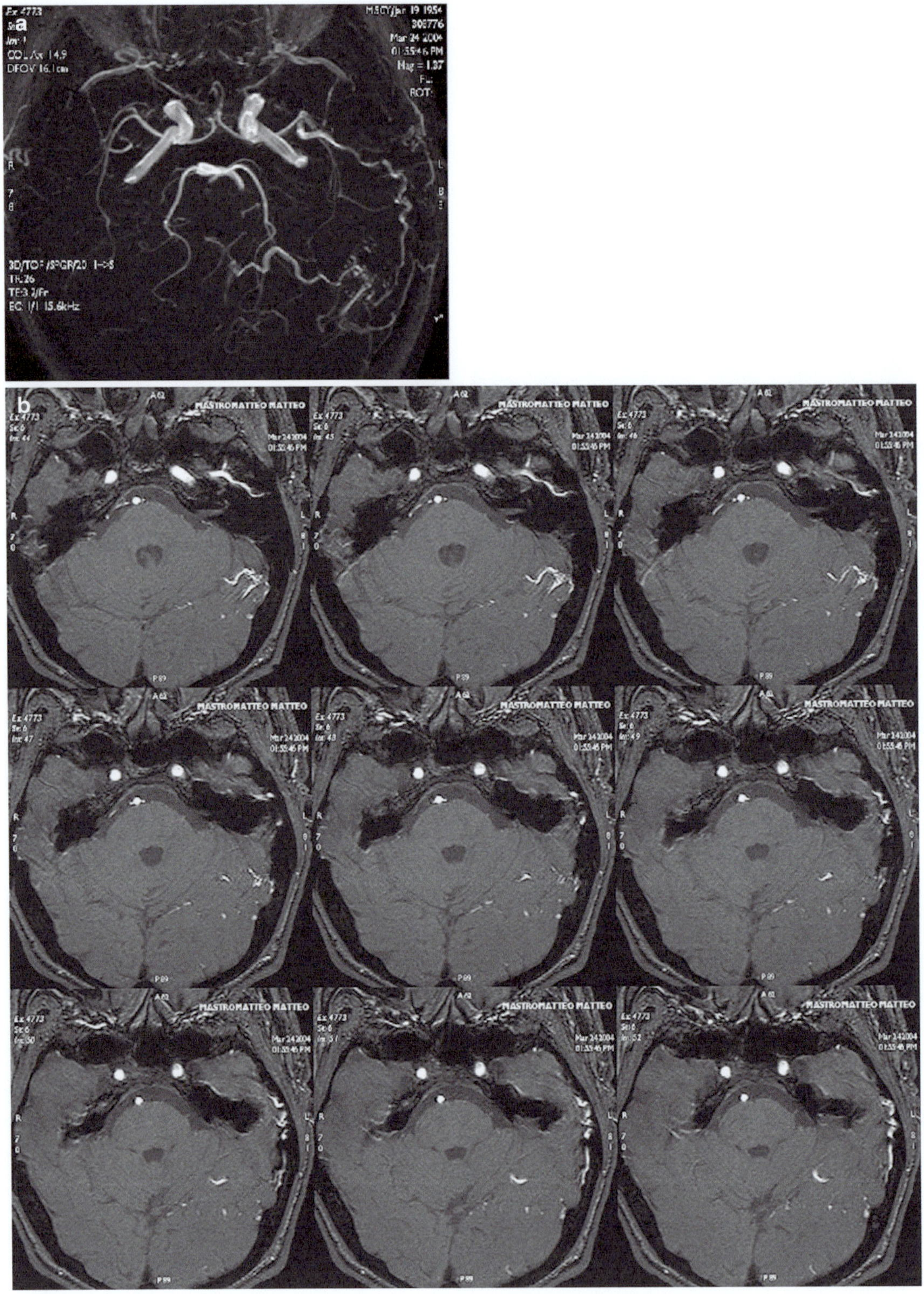

**Fig. 5.12** Left arteriovenous malformation at the convexity: unenhanced 3D TOF study at 3.0 T. MIP image (**a**), single partitions (**b**)

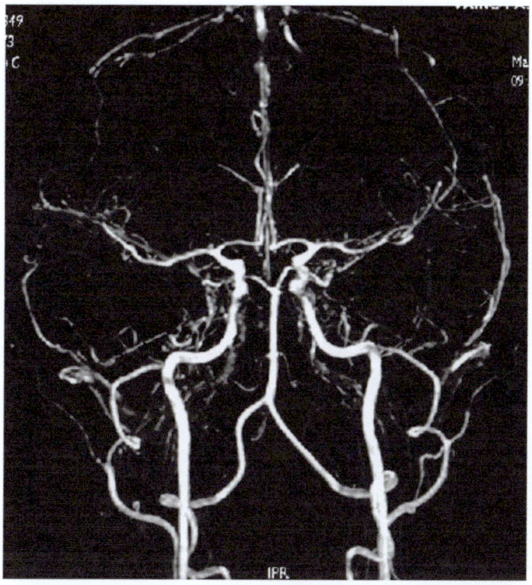

Fig. 5.13 Normal arterial cerebral circulation: contrast-enhanced coronal view at 3.0 T

appear to entail no particular safety or compatibility risk [25, 26]. Patients with tested biomedical implants can therefore safely undergo 3.0 T MRA [27, 28].

### Conclusion

The advantages offered by 3.0 T systems make MRA superior even to digital subtraction angiography, especially for studying atherosclerotic disease and vascular malformations like aneurysms, despite its lower spatial resolution. Digital angiography is increasingly being reserved for interventional and therapeutic rather than diagnostic applications (Figs. 5.14, 5.15, 5.16, 5.17 and 5.18) [29]. Overall 3 tesla MRA has a better diagnostic performance with respect to studies performed with lower field scanner [30].

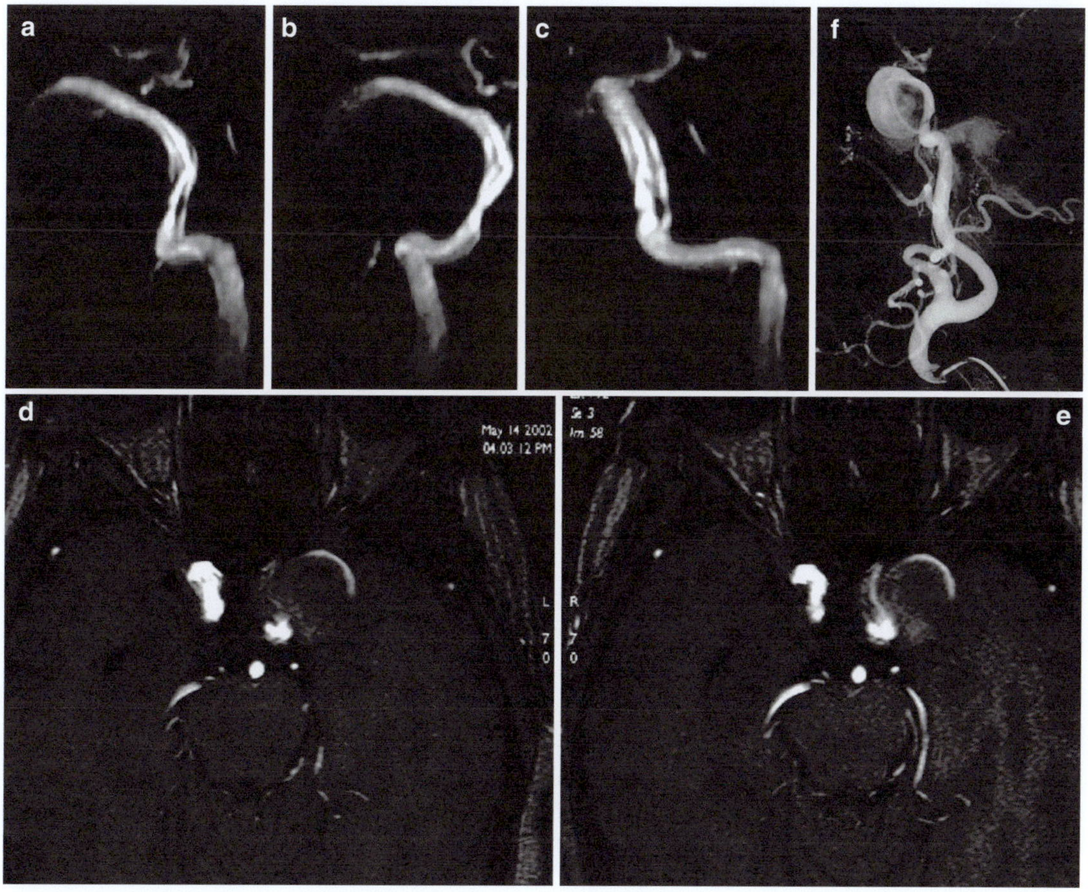


Fig. 5.14 Giant aneurysm with turbulent flow in the intracavernous segment of the left internal carotid artery: 3D TOF study at 3.0 T. MIP images (**a–c**), single partitions (**d**, **e**), digital angiography (**f**)

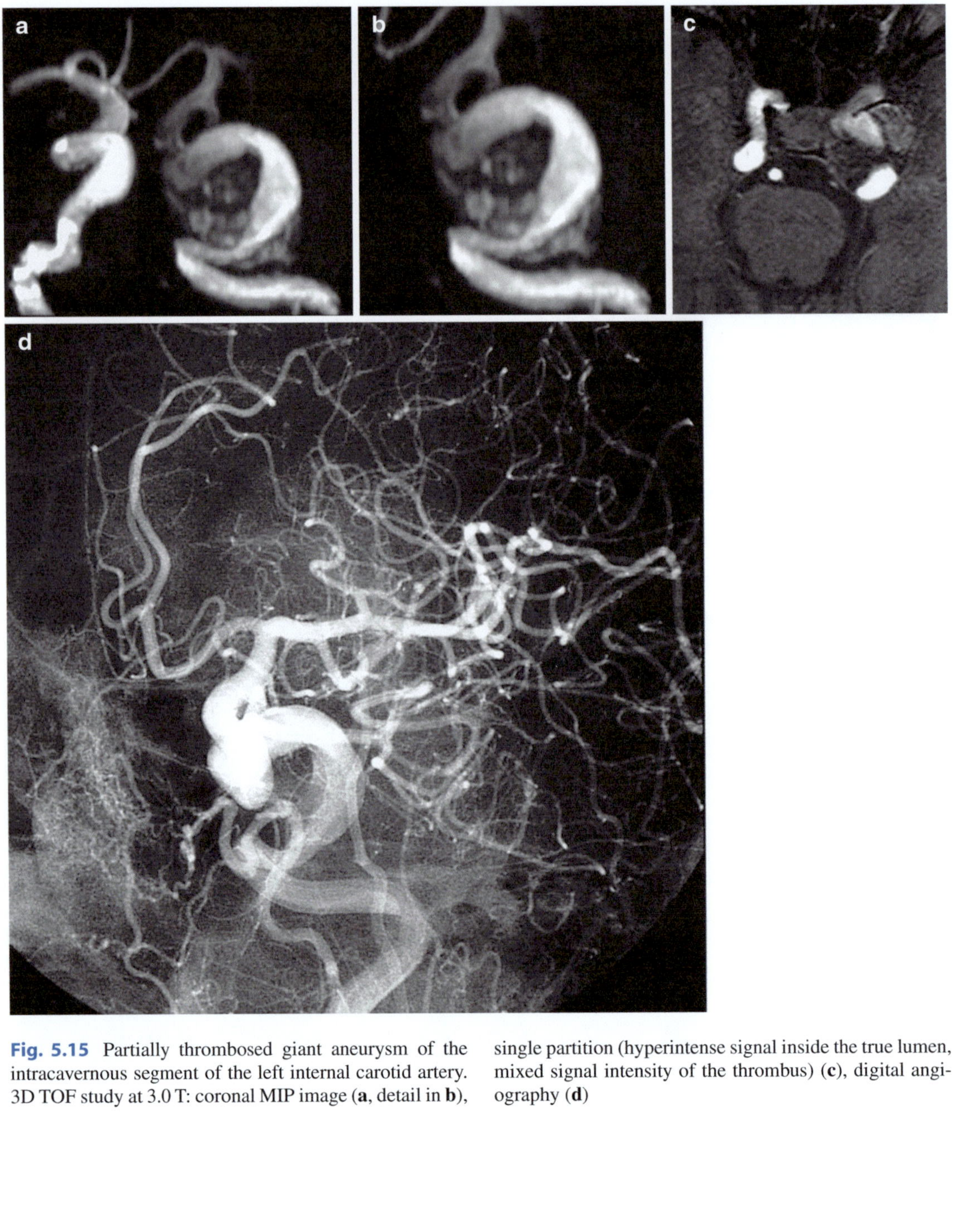


**Fig. 5.15** Partially thrombosed giant aneurysm of the intracavernous segment of the left internal carotid artery. 3D TOF study at 3.0 T: coronal MIP image (**a**, detail in **b**), single partition (hyperintense signal inside the true lumen, mixed signal intensity of the thrombus) (**c**), digital angiography (**d**)

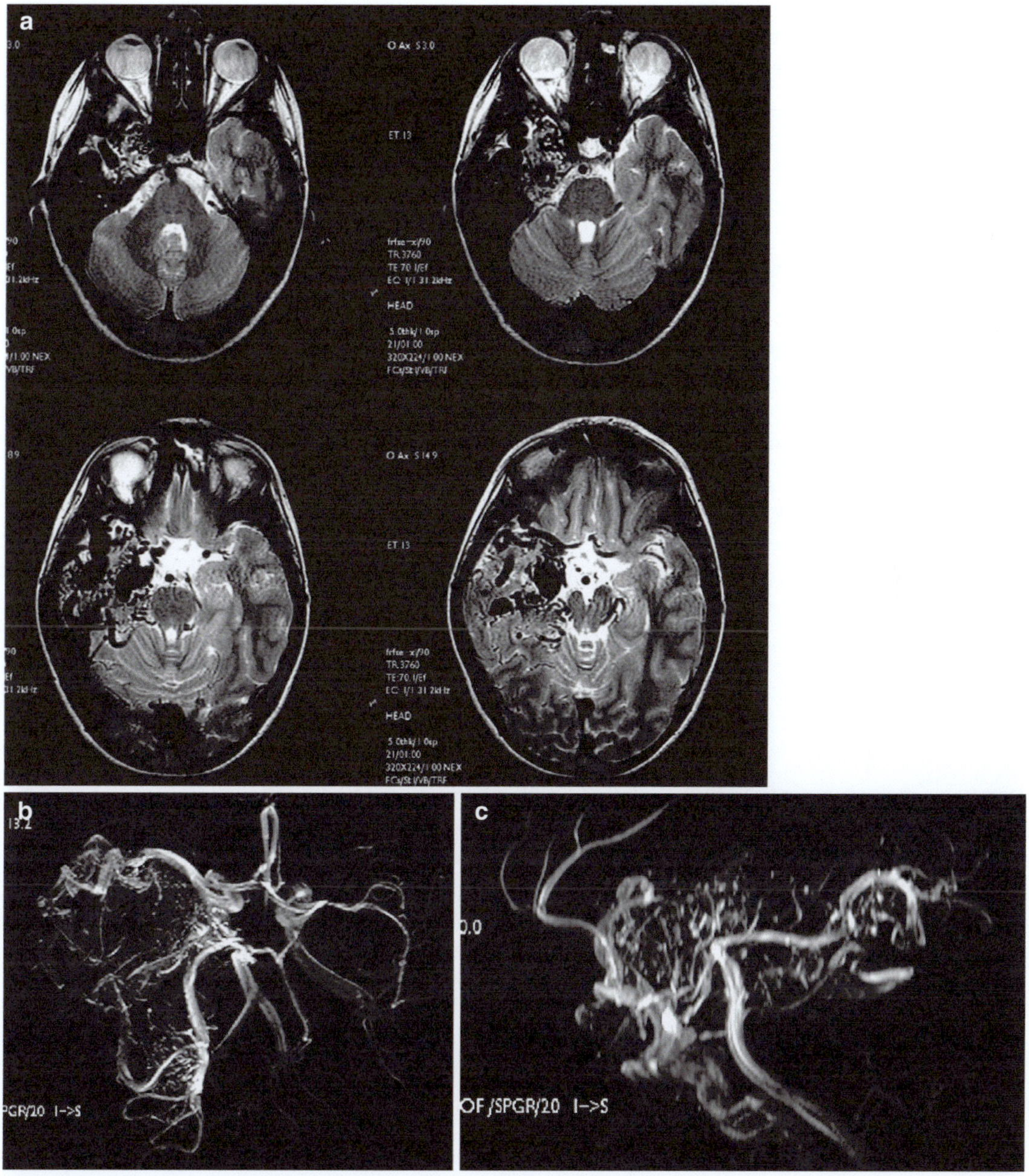


**Fig. 5.16** Bulky right temporal arteriovenous malformation: standard MRI T2 FSE study (**a**), 3D TOF axial and sagittal MIP images (**b**, **c**)

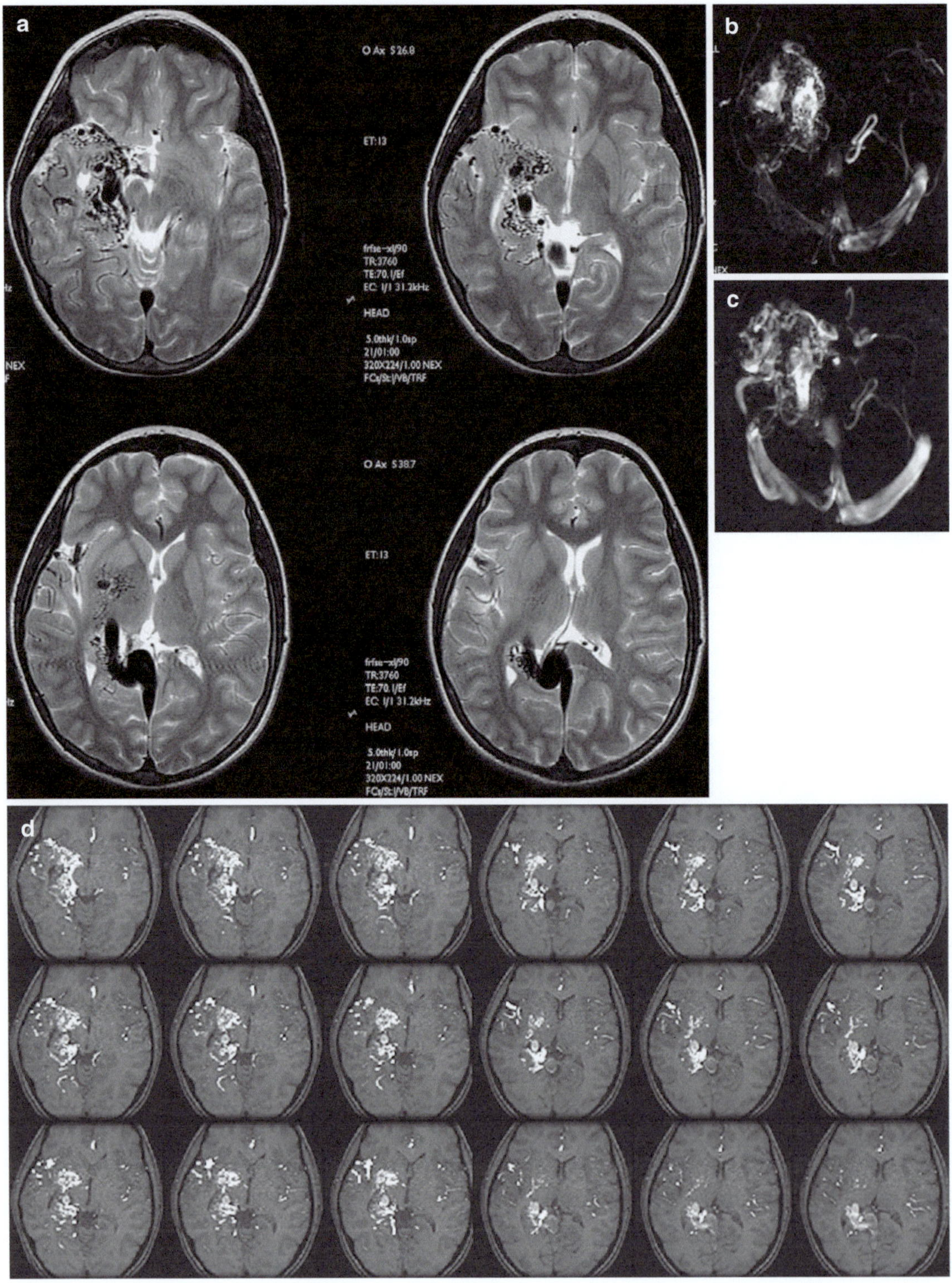


**Fig. 5.17** Right arteriovenous malformation: 3D PC and TOF obtained at 3.0 T. T2 FSE image (**a**), MIP PC image with 20 cm/s (**b**), with 90 cm/s (**c**), single 3D TOF partitions (**d**)

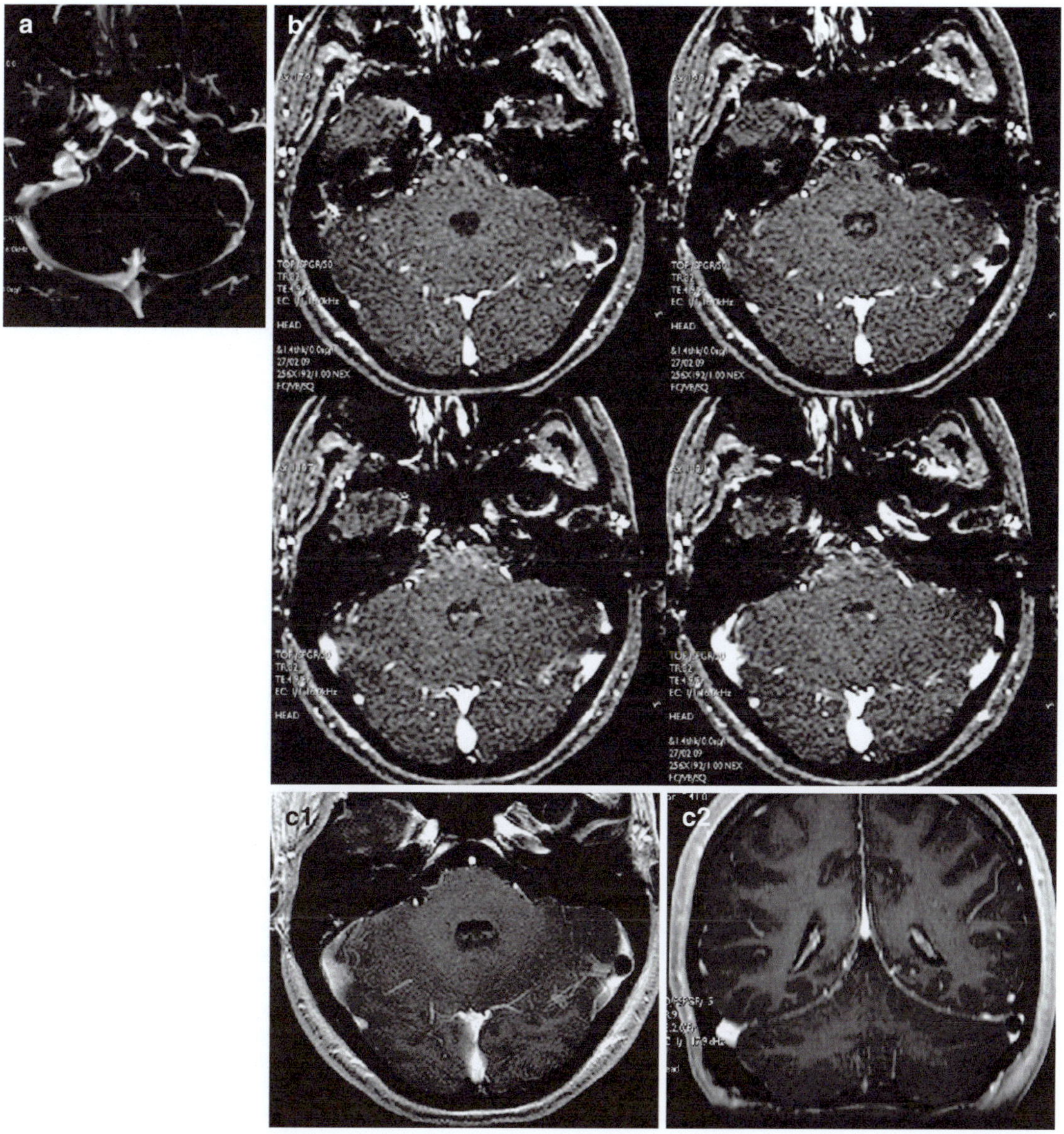

**Fig. 5.18** Circumscribed thrombosis of left transverse sinus. Contrast-enhanced 3D TOF 3.0 T study: MIP image (**a**), single contrast-enhanced partitions (**b**), contrast-enhanced T1 SE images (**c**)

## References


1. Krings T, Hans FJ, Moeller-Hartmann W et al (2002) Time of flight, phase contrast and contrast enhanced magnetic resonance angiography for pre-interventional determination of aneurysm size, configuration, and neck morphology in an aneurysm model in rabbits. Neurosci Lett 326:46–50
2. Lenz GW, Haacke E, Masaryk TJ et al (1988) In plane vascular imaging: pulse sequences design and strategy. Radiology 166:876–882
3. Zou Z, MA L, Cheng L, Cay Y, Meng X (2008) Time resolved contras enhanced MR angiography of intracranial lesions. J Magn Reson Imaging 27:692-699
4. Prince MR, Yucel EK, Kaufmann JA et al (1993) Dynamic gadolinium-enhanced three dimensional abdominal MR arteriography. J Magn Reson Imaging 3:877–881
5. Leung DA, Mckinnon GC, Davis CP et al (1996) Breath-hold contrast-enhanced 3 D MR angiography. Radiology 201:569–571
6. Prince MR, Narasimhan DL, Jacoby WT (1996) Three-dimensional gadolinium-enhanced MR

angiography of the thoracic aorta. Am J Roentgenol 166:1387–1397
7. Prince MR, Narasimham DL, Stanley JC (1995) Breath-hold gadolinium-enhanced MR angiography of the abdominal aorta and its major branches. Radiology 197:785–792
8. Scarabino T, Giannatempo GM, Nemore F et al (2003) RM 3.0 Tesla. II parte: L'imaging morfo-funzionale cerebrale. Radiol Med 105:150–161
9. Scarabino T, Nemore F, Giannatempo GM et al (2003) Risonanza Magnetica 3.0 Tesla. Riv Neuroradiol 16(Suppl):314–315
10. Scarabino T, Nemore F, Giannatempo GM et al (2003) 3.0 T magnetic resonance in neuroradiology. Eur J Radiol 48:154–164
11. Scarabino T, Nemore F, Giannatempo GM et al (2004) 3.0 T MR angiography. Riv Neuroradiol 17:777–783
12. Huang BY, Castillo M (2009) Neurovascular imaging at 1.5 tesla versus 3.0 tesla. Magn Reson Clin N Am 17(1):29–46
13. Frayne R, Goodyear BG, Dickhoff, et al. (2003) Magnetic resonance imaging at 3.0 tesla: challenges and advantages in clinical neurological imaging. Invest Radiol 38(7): 385–402
14. Scarabino T, Nemore F, Giannatempo GM et al (2004) Semeiological features of 3.0 T MR imaging: what changes at high magnetic field. Riv Neuroradiol 17:755–764
15. Takahashi M, Uematsu H, Hatabu H (2003) MR imaging at high magnetic fields. Eur J Radiol 46: 45–52
16. Norris DG (2003) High field human imaging. J Magn Reson Imaging 18:519–529
17. Alvarez-Linera J (2008) 3T MRI : Advances in brain imaging. Eur J Radiol 67:415–426
18. Thomas SD, Al-Kwifi O, Emery DJ et al (2002) Application of magnetization transfer at 3.0 T in three-dimensional time-of-flight magnetic resonance angiography of the intracranial arteries. J Magn Reson Imaging 15:479–483
19. Parker DL, Buswell HR, Goodrick KC et al (1995) The application of magnetization transfer to MR angiography with reduced total power. Magn Reson Med 34:283–286
20. Al-Kwifi O, Emery DJ, Wilman AH (2002) Vessel contrast at 3.0 T in time-of-flight magnetic resonance angiography of the intracranial and carotid arteries. Magn Reson Imaging 20:181–187
21. Bernstein MA, Huston J 3rd, Lin C et al (2001) High-resolution intracranial and cervical MRA at 3.0 T: technical considerations and initial experience. Magn Reson Med 46:955–962
22. Reichenbach JR, Barth M, Haacke EM et al (2000) High resolution MR venography at 3.0 Tesla. J Comput Assist Tomogr 24:949–957
23. Rutherford M, Malamateniou C, Zeka J et al (2004) MR imaging of the neonatal brain at 3 Tesla. Eur J Paediatr Neurol 8:281–289
24. Willinek WA, Gieseke J, von Falkenhausen M et al (2004) Sensitivity encoding (SENSE) for high spatial resolution time-of-flight MR angiography of the intracranial arteries at 3.0 T. Rofo 176:21–26
25. Kaufmann TJ, Huston J 3rd, Cloft HJ et al (2010) A prospective trial of 3 T and 1.5 T time of flight and contrast enhanced MR angiography in the follow up of coiled intracranial aneurysm. AJNR Am J Neuroradiol 31(5):912–918
26. Sommer T, Maintz D, Schmiedel A et al (2004) High field MR imaging: magnetic field interactions of aneurysm clips, coronary artery stents and iliac artery stents with a 3.0 Tesla MR system. Rofo 176(5): 731–738
27. Schaafsma JD, Velthuis BK, Majoie CB et al (2010 Jul) (2010) Intracranial aneurysm treated with coil replacement: test characteristics of follow up MR angiography – Multicenter study. Radiology 256(1): 209–218
28. Shellock FG, Gounis M, Wakhloo A (2005) Detachable coil for cerebral aneurysms: in vitro evaluation of magnetic field interaction, heating, and artifacts at 3 T. AJNR 26:363–366
29. Gibbs GF, Huston J 3rd, Bernstein MA et al (2004) Improved image quality of intracranial aneurysms: 3.0-T versus 1.5-T time-of-fight MR angiography. Am J Neuroradiol 25(1):84–87
30. Anna MH, Sailer MD et al (2014) Diagnosing intracranial aneurysms with MR angiography: systematic review and meta-analysis. Stroke 45(1):119–126

# 3.0 T MR Spectroscopy

6

Michela Tosetti, Timo Schirmer, Valentina D'Alesio, Alfonzo Di Costanzo, Tommaso Scarabino, Teresa Popolizio, Rosario Francesco Balzano, and Marco Perri

Magnetic resonance spectroscopy (MRS) is a non-invasive technique that can be used to measure the concentrations of different low-molecular-weight chemicals. The technique is based on the same physical principles as magnetic resonance imaging (MRI), i.e. the detection of energy exchanges between external magnetic fields and specific nuclei within atoms. The principal differences between MRI and MRS lie in the different use of frequency, phase and signal amplitude as carriers of information:

- In MRI, frequency and phase are used to encode the spatial coordinates, while the signal amplitude of the signal is translated into a grey value of the resulting image (Fig. 6.1a).
- In MRS, phase and frequency are used to identify spectral patterns unique to specific metabolites, while the amplitude is used as a scale for the concentration of these metabolites (Fig. 6.1b).

The information obtained during MRS experiments, usually acquired as a series of FIDs, spin echoes or stimulated echoes in the time domain, is displayed graphically as a spectrum in the frequency domain with individual peaks representing the various chemical compounds. The diagnostic ability of MRS can be increased by improving the spectral quality through changes in hardware and software and/or by improving the analytical approach aiming for objective absolute concentration measurements.

MRS should be performed as an adjunct to MRI gain additional information for a reliable clinical diagnosis: while conventional MRI provides anatomical images of the brain, MRS provides functional information related to its underlying dynamic physiology.

## 6.1 Spectroscopy Basics

MRS has been demonstrated in vivo for different nuclei, including $^{1}H$, $^{31}P$, $^{13}C$, $^{15}N$, $^{19}F$ and $^{23}Na$. While most of these nuclei are very difficult to detect, $^{1}H$ and $^{31}P$ are available in the human brain in significant concentrations and have the appropriate physical configuration to be detected

M. Tosetti
"IRCCS Stella Maris Foundation", Pisa, Italy

T. Schirmer
GE Healtcare Technologies, Monaco, Germany

V. D'Alesio
"Radiosurgery Center Malzoni Hospital", Agropoli (SA), Italy

A. Di Costanzo
Department of Health Sciences, University of Molise, Campobasso, Italy

T. Scarabino
Department of Radiology and Neuroradiology, PO "L. Bonomo" Hospital, Andria (BT), Italy

T. Popolizio (✉) • R.F. Balzano • M. Perri
Department of Radiology and Neuroradiology, San Giovanni Rotondo (FG), Italy
e-mail: t.popolizio1@gmail.com



T. Scarabino et al. (eds.), *High Field Brain MRI*, DOI 10.1007/978-3-319-44174-0_6

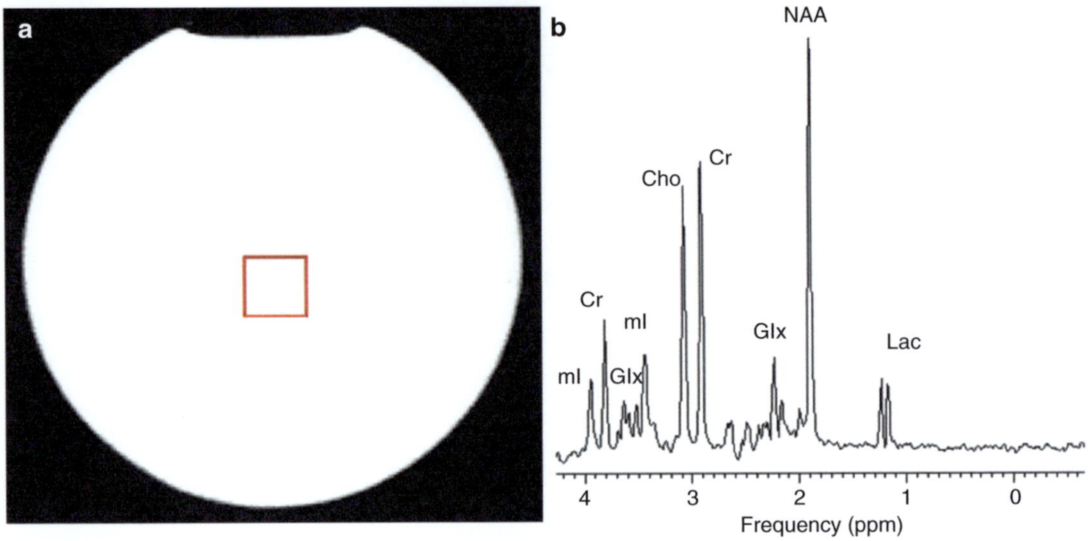


**Fig. 6.1** (**a**) MRI of a phantom containing main brain metabolites dissolved in a water-based, pH-buffered stock solution. (**b**) Spectrum acquired from the VOI prescribed in **a** using volume-selective spectroscopy sequence with PRESS excitation (TR: 2000 ms, TE: 35 ms)

by MRS. Besides the technical prerequisites, $^{1}$H and $^{31}$P are prominent candidates for clinical studies also from a biochemical viewpoint, as they allow in vivo investigation of some of the processes involved in brain metabolism. For instance, $^{31}$P-MRS has been the first to be applied to medicine in vivo and can be used to evaluate brain energy metabolism by directly and non-invasively measuring ATP, PCr or Pi concentrations. While $^{31}$P-MRS was the first spectroscopic technique to be applied in vivo, the main nucleus studied today in neurospectroscopy is $^{1}$H, which provides information on markers of neurons, myelin, energy metabolism and other metabolically active compounds. Besides its important clinical role, $^{1}$H spectroscopy is also less technically demanding as it uses hardware employed for standard MRI and provides a higher signal/noise ratio (SNR) [1, 3].

### 6.1.1 Proton MRS in Neuroradiology

Proton magnetic resonance spectroscopy of the brain reveals specific biochemical information about cerebral metabolites, which may support clinical diagnosis and enhance the understanding of neurological disorders. Analysis of the resonance signals of low-molecular-weight brain metabolites (concentrations in mmol) provides information on metabolite concentrations and makes it possible to correlate their modifications with various pathological conditions. The high diagnostic specificity of MRS enables the biochemical changes that accompany various diseases to be detected, as well as disease characterization, sometimes diagnosis and monitoring. At 1.5 T the main metabolites detected vary according to the acquisition parameters (TR, TE) and type of pulse sequence adopted (STEAM, PRESS). 1.5 T brain MRS currently has a number of clinical applications, including the characterization of cerebral tumours and the monitoring of their treatment (e.g. radiation necrosis versus recurrence tumour), epilepsy, infection, stroke, multiple sclerosis (MS), trauma and neurodegenerative processes, such as Alzheimer's and Parkinson's diseases [2–5], and allows to diagnose several hereditary and acquired brain metabolic disorders such as Canavan's disease [6], brain creatine deficiency syndromes [7, 8], adrenoleukodystrophy [9] and hepatic encephalopathy [10].

However, despite the demonstrated ability of MRS to detect neurochemical changes and to be technically feasible to study the brain in vivo, there are no standardized techniques for acquiring and interpreting MRS spectra, and little high-quality direct evidence of its influence on diagnosis and therapeutic decision-making is available. Its specificity, diagnostic and prognostic value needs to be improved, and especially its sensitivity to disease markers, all of which can be achieved at higher magnetic field.

In the recent past, high magnetic field MR systems, particularly 3 T instruments, have proliferated with FDA "non-significant risk" clearance [11] and have replaced 1.5 T in many clinical and research applications now performed with these magnets [12]. 1.5 T fields have long been seen as the standard, but the development of 3 T and higher-field technology suggests that the concept of "high field" may be a moving target. Indeed, NMR spectrographs operating at magnetic fields of 14–21 T are routinely used for in vitro structural studies of complex molecules. The development of in vivo high-field MRS has however been delayed by safety considerations, hardware limitations (such as the availability of wide-bore magnets), high-performance gradients and methods to correct magnetic field inhomogeneity [12, 19]. MRS like other advanced MR techniques to study the brain (e.g. angiography, diffusion, perfusion and functional imaging) should considerably benefit from the greater SNR and contrast/noise ratio and the increased spatial and temporal resolution provided by high-field systems [11–18].

Several studies comparing brain $^{1}$H-MRS at different field strengths in the same subjects using the same experimental parameters have demonstrated the usefulness of high-field $^{1}$H-MRS [19–25]. Its advantages rest on greater SNR and spectral resolution, which afford greater spatial and temporal resolution and enable the acquisition of high-quality, easily quantifiable spectra in acceptable acquisition times. In addition to improved measurement precision of common metabolites, such as *N*-acetylaspartate (NAA), choline (Cho), creatine/phosphocreatine (Cr/PCr), *myo*-inositol (mI) and when present lactic acid (Lac) and lipids (Lip), high-field systems allow the high-resolution measurement of other metabolites, such as glutamate (Glu), glutamine (Gln), glutathione (GSH), $\gamma$-aminobutyric acid (GABA), *scyllo*-inositol (ScyI), aspartate (Asp), taurine (Tau), *N*-acetylaspartylglutamate (NAAG) and glucose (Glc), thus extending the range of metabolic information. However, these advantages may be hampered by intrinsic field-dependent technical difficulties, such as increased T2 signal decay, chemical shift dispersion errors, J-modulation anomalies, increased magnetic susceptibility, eddy current artefacts, limitations in the design of homogeneous and sensitive radiofrequency coils, magnetic field instabilities and safety issues. Several studies have demonstrated that these limitations can be overcome, suggesting that optimization of high-field $^{1}$H-MRS can lead to its broader application in clinical research and diagnosis.

Table 6.1 summarizes several metabolites involved in brain biochemistry detectable with $^{1}$H-MRS. Besides the most prominent resonances of NAA, choline and creatine, a variety of other resonances might or might not be present in a spectrum depending on its type and quality as well as disease. This list is not complete, in that several metabolites are only observed in the rare cases when their concentrations are several times higher than normal, while metabolites such as alcohol and propylene glycol are not present in normal brain metabolism but may be found in certain patients. For a full list of detectable metabolites, the reader required to interpret spectra with unusual resonances is referred to the literature.

### 6.1.2 MR Spectroscopy: Quality and Resolution

While the $^{1}$H protons bound to the $H_2O$ molecule provide basically the whole signal used for MR imaging, the high water signal is one of the most disrupting elements in MRS, since the molecules of interest are found at much lower concentrations, yielding signal amplitudes more than 1000-fold smaller than the signal of

**Table 6.1** Some of the primary resonances found in [1]Hbrain spectroscopy and corresponding chemical shifts (in ppm)

| Brain metabolites detected on $^1$H MRS | | |
|---|---|---|
| Compound | Abbreviation | Frequency (ppm) |
| Alanine | Ala | 1.48, 3.78 |
| Aspartate | Asp | 3.9, 2.69, 2.82 |
| Choline | Cho | 3.22 (4.05, 3.54) |
| Creatine/phosphocreatine | Cr/PCr | 3.03, 3.95 |
| $\gamma$-Aminobutyric acid | GABA | 2.31, 1.91, 3.01 |
| Glucose | Glc | 3.43, 3.84 (...) |
| Glutamate | Glu | 3.77, 2.06, 2.38 |
| Glutamine | Gln | 3.71, 2.15, 2.46 |
| Glycine | Gly | 3.56 |
| Lactate | Lac | 1.33 |
| *myo*-Inositol | mI | 3.56, 4.06 |
| *N*-Acetylaspartate | NAA | 2.02 |
| *scyllo*-Inositol | ScyI | 3.35 |
| Taurine | Tau | 3.44, 3.38, 3.32, 3.27 |

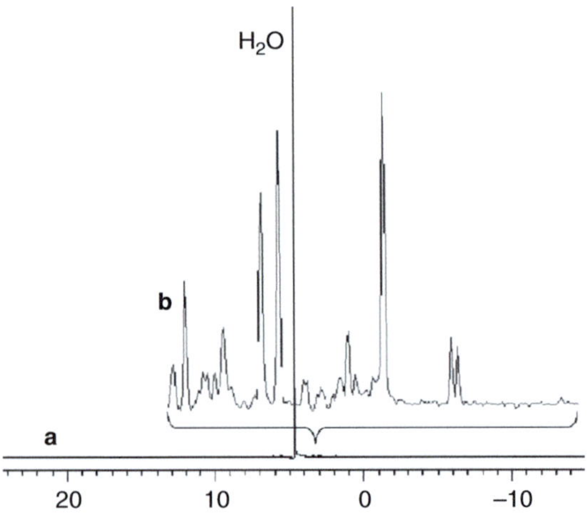


**Fig. 6.2** *a* Full water signal of a phantom spectrum containing the main brain metabolites compared to the metabolite signal *b* several orders of magnitude smaller than the water signal

water (Fig. 6.2). Thus the quality of a spectrum, which is usually measured as SNR, and its resolution, which includes the spectral, spatial and temporal dimensions, play a major role in the applicability and acceptance of MR spectroscopy.

#### 6.1.2.1 Signal/Noise Ratio

The SNR is based on several variables, the most important of which are of course signal intensity (where Cr is often used as the reference) and the underlying noise of a spectroscopy experiment. The dependencies of signal intensity and noise can be divided into two categories:

1. Dependencies which cannot be affected by the user and which are given by fixed natural constants. The corresponding SNR shall be called $SNR_{int}$.
2. Dependencies that can be altered by modifying the acquisition parameters. The corresponding SNR shall be called $SNR_{Exp}$.

The most important factors for $SNR_{int}$ in an $^1$H-MRS experiment are to be aware of the number of protons contributing to the total signal $N$, the field strength of the static magnetic field $B_0$ and the relaxation properties of a specific metabolite. With a direct, linear proportionality of $SNR_{int}$ to $N$ and $B_0$, these parameters define the intrinsic SNR available for the spectroscopy experiment, which means that an increase in $B_0$ from 1.5 to 3.0 T will theoretically boost the SNR by a factor of two. This achievable SNR will always be degraded by the natural phenomena of relaxation, expressed as an exponential signal decay after full excitation with the relaxation constants T2 and exponential return of the spin system into thermal equilibrium with the time constant T1.

For a given sample in a specific MR scanner, the value of $SNR_{int}$ is fixed, and its limitations cannot be overcome. Beside these factors, there are others which can be optimized by the user and which contribute to the final SNR. The main parameters to be considered by the user are the type of sequence, the number of signal averages *N*, the sample volume (VOI) and the echo and repetition times (TE, TR).

The SNR gain obtained from the intensity increase from 1.5 to 3.0 T can for instance be used to decrease the acquisition volume by a factor of two. On the other hand, reduction of the acquisition volume by a factor of two at a constant field strength would require to increase the number of averages by factor of four to maintain the SNR. In addition, T1 relaxation times increase with higher field strength, leading to increased signal saturation for a given repetition time, and T2 relaxation times decrease. Therefore, the theoretical doubling of SNR cannot be achieved, due to the use of repetition times (TR) in the order of the T1 decay times (and not infinitely long) and echo times (TE) in the order of the metabolite T2 decay times [25–28].

Comparison of different experimental settings thus requires careful analysis of all parameters to avoid errors and misinterpretations (Fig. 6.3).

### 6.1.2.2 Spatial and Temporal Resolution

The achievable quality of a spectrum identified by its SNR is directly related to the size of the sample volume (VOI) and the acquisition time, defined by the number of signal averages *N* multiplied by the repetition time (TR), as described in the paragraph above. Thus the SNR is usually the limiting factor for spatial and temporal resolution in a clinical setting, where the time of acquisition is usually restricted by logistical, technical, financial and ethical aspects.

Spectra can be acquired from a single-voxel or a multidimensional grid of spectra, which are generally referred to as chemical shift or spectroscopic images (CSI, SI) (Fig. 6.4). Unlike the ca. 1 $mm^3$ resolution that can be achieved with routine MRI, $^1$H-MRS studies have been performed with a spatial resolution of 8 ml and an acquisition time of 3–5 min per single-voxel acquisition and 2–4 ml for CSI in 5–10 min [29].

The greater ability to detect smaller lesions afforded by advanced MRI technologies can involve an increased need for greater spatial resolution of single-voxel spectroscopy and CSI experiments. Whereas the poor SNR of 1.5 T magnets prevented the acquisition of single-voxel spectra with a spatial resolution significantly

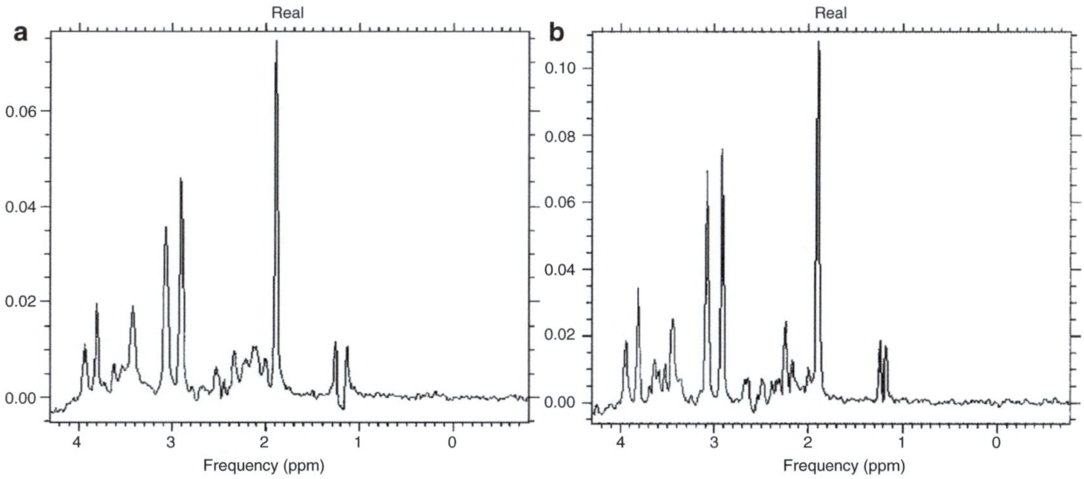


**Fig. 6.3** Spectra acquired on the same phantom containing the main brain metabolites at 1.5 T (**a**) and at 3.0 T (**b**) using the same sequence parameters (PRESS: TR, 2000 ms; TE, 35 ms), showing the increased SNR; the improved spectral resolution, in particular, between 2 and 2.6 ppm; and the different peak ratio between the main metabolites due to the different relaxation times of individual metabolites at different field strengths

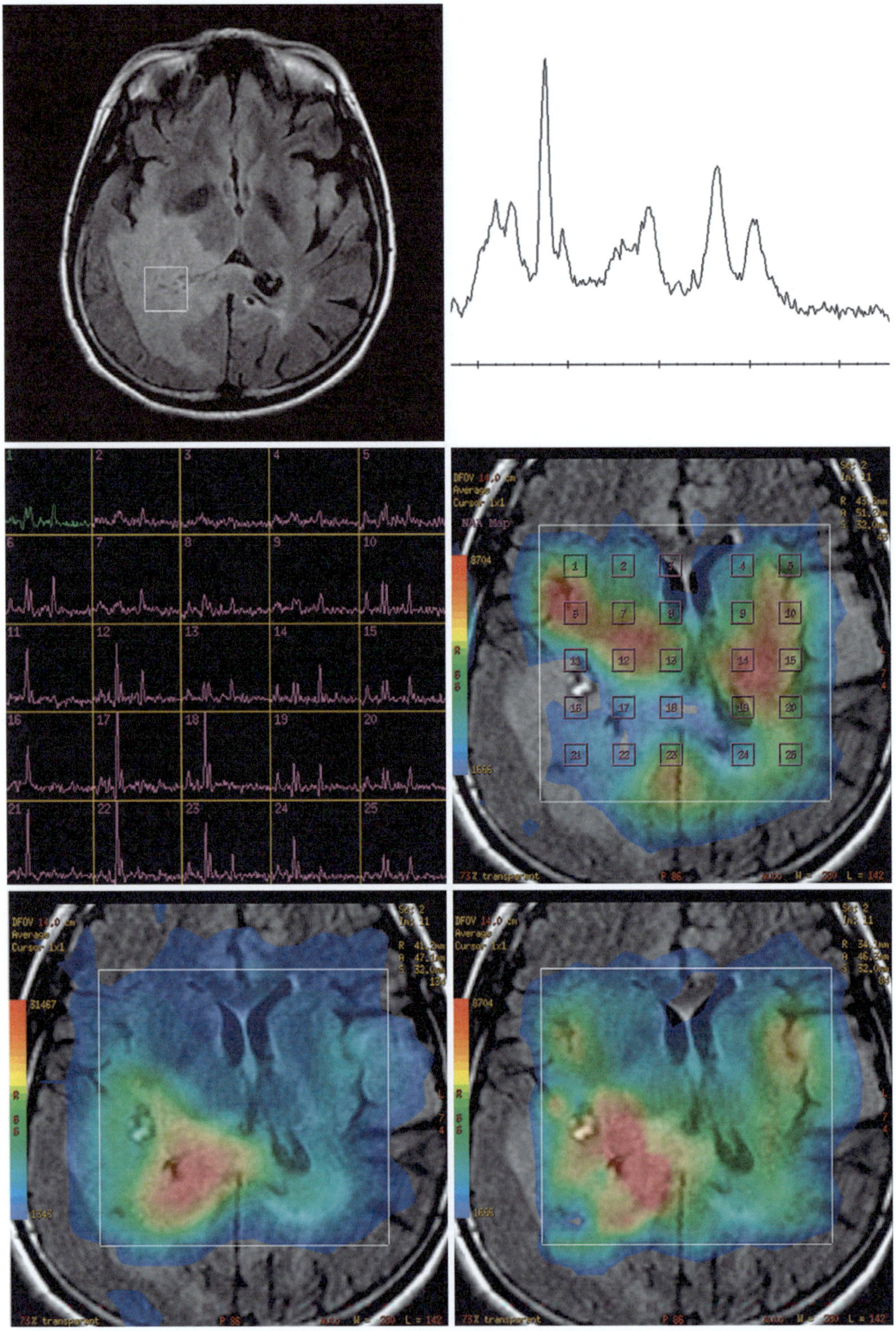

**Fig. 6.4** Whereas a single-voxel spectrum usually provides good-quality, high SNR data but limited to a small region, a CSI acquisition will yield a grid of spectra, which are often prone to artefacts or low SNR, which can be translated into metabolite maps (Images courtesy of Charité, Virchow Clinic, Berlin, Germany)

below 4–8 ml or chemical shift images with a spatial resolution of less than 2 ml, lower spatial resolutions are becoming feasible at 3 T.

The direct matching of metabolic and anatomical information would obviously be of clinical importance since it could improve the sensitivity and specificity of diagnosis. Higher-resolution SI can enable to distinguish between different anatomical structures, between normal and pathological tissue or between different pathological structures (e.g. heterogeneous tumours, SM plaques, etc.). In patients with brain tumour, for example, high-resolution SI could differentiate healthy oedematous from affected tissue as well as normal from normal-appearing hippocampus in patients with temporal lobe epilepsy. At 3 T and higher field intensities, voxel volumes of 1 $cm^3$ and lower can be obtained with still good intrinsic SNR and acceptable acquisition times [29, 30].

Higher field strengths have also considerably ameliorated resolution time reducing examination times which had limited the application of $^1$H-MRS to clinical research. The advantages of shorter examinations for patients, radiologists, technicians and hospital administrators are obvious. At high magnetic fields, larger brain volumes can be studied overtimes similar to current single-voxel protocols using multivoxel 2D or 3D $^1$H-SI sequences. In multivoxel 3D spectroscopy experiments, the time of acquisition has been reduced to 25 %, retaining the lowest SNR of 1.5 T at 3 T [24, 28, 29]. Shorter times allow multinuclear MRS to determine the metabolic changes coupled to neuronal activity.

Besides the clinical advantages, high spatial and temporal resolution also have some striking technical features. Next to the SNR, the linewidths of the individual peaks are responsible for the qualitative appearance of a spectrum. The linewidth is defined by the T2 relaxation time of the metabolite and the local field in homogeneities, where the inhomogeneities can be the dominating factor of a resulting T2*. As local inhomogeneities will decrease with smaller voxel volumes, T2* increases, resulting in a noticeable decrease of linewidths, improving spectral quality, especially for voxels with a volume smaller than 0.75 $cm^3$ [30].

Another factor degrading spectral quality is the stability of the consecutively acquired signal averages. Patient motion, magnet drifts and the instability of other system components can interfere with the acquisition of MRS data, yielding broadened metabolite peaks or other artefacts. Thus keeping the acquisition times as short as possible, spectral quality can significantly be improved.

#### 6.1.2.3 Spectral Resolution

Spectral resolution essentially refers to the ability to distinguish adjacent peaks in a spectrum of individual peaks. The resonance frequency $\omega$ of a specific metabolite is defined by the static magnetic field $B_0$ and a shielding factor $\sigma$, defined by the geometric structure of the molecule shielding the nuclei from the external magnetic field and referred to as chemical shift. The chemical shift is field independent, for every metabolite characteristic unit measured as parts per million (ppm). The resonance frequency $\omega(\sigma, B_0)$ of a specific metabolite is defined by:

$$\omega = \gamma \cdot B_0 \cdot (1 - \sigma)$$

where $\gamma$ is the gyromagnetic ratio of the nucleus studied. The spectral distance $\Delta\omega$ between two peaks with chemical shifts $\sigma_1$ and $\sigma_2$ can be expressed using the above equation as:

$$\Delta\omega = \gamma \cdot B_0 \cdot (\sigma_2 - \sigma_1)$$

This means that the spectral distance $\Delta\omega$ for two identical metabolites will be twice as much at 3.0 T compared to 1.5 T (Fig. 6.5a).

This gain in spectral resolution with higher field strengths will allow for improved differentiation between peaks that might overlap at lower field strengths. It is necessary to adjust some sequence parameters to make full use of this gain in spectral resolution. The achieved resolution of the raw data acquired is defined by the sampling scheme used. A given number of points are sampled with a specific sampling rate to get a good digital representation of the MR signal. Typically at 1.5 T, a spectroscopy signal is sampled with 2048 points and a sampling rate of 2500 Hz, which is equivalent to a sampling interval of 0.4 ms

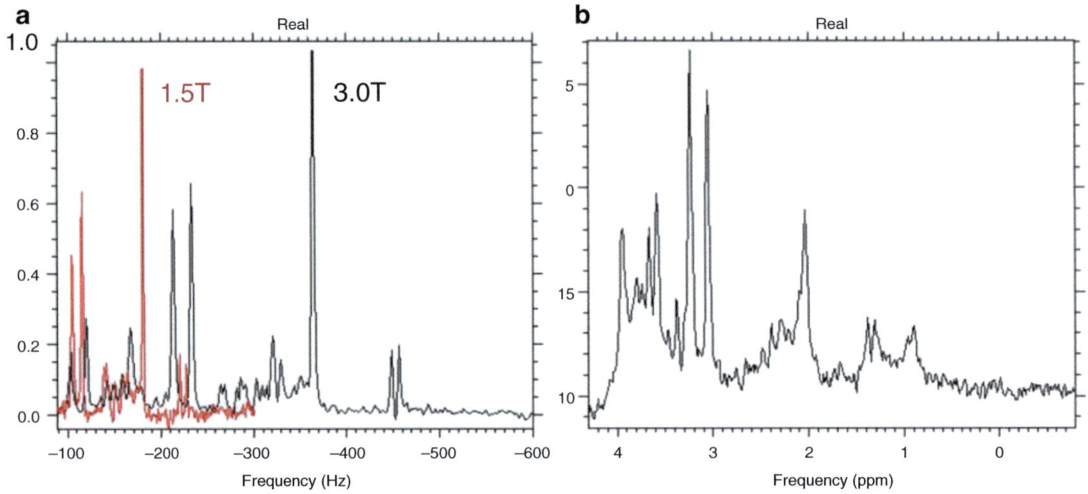


**Fig. 6.5** The frequency resolution between individual peaks increases as a proportion of field strength. This means that the spectral distance $\Delta\omega$ for two identical metabolites will be twice as much at 3.0 T compared to 1.5 T (**a**), and therefore in abnormal tissue, it is possible to resolve different close resonance signals such as glycine at 3.56 ppm from *myo*-inositol at 3.55 ppm and to achieve a better detection of scyllo-inositol (3.35 ppm) (**b**)

between each point, yielding a total sampling time of 819.2 ms in which the acquisition window is opened. This kind of resolution is recommended at 1.5 T to cover most of the spectral information and sample long enough to see the signal decay down to the noise level. To cover exactly the same spectral information at 3.0 T, it is necessary to double the sampling rate to 5000 Hz, which for these settings is equivalent to a sampling interval of 0.2 ms between points. At a constant number of 2084 points sampled, the acquisition window is open for an overall 409.6 ms of sampling time. This sampling window can be so short, especially for phantom experiments, that a significant amount of signal is left at the end of the sampling interval. This can cause artefacts, known as ringing artefacts, in the reconstructed spectrum.

Even though the above considerations are usually of minor importance to the clinical user, they show that a direct one-to-one comparison of MR spectroscopy experiments at different field strengths can be misleading. If exactly the same parameters for sampling rate and number of points are used, the quality of the spectrum acquired at higher field strength is always degraded. If the parameters are adjusted, the comparison is no longer one to one anymore.

Spectral resolution also depends on the attainable linewidths, which are a function of field-dependent T2 relaxation times and field homogeneity. However, higher-field MR scanners can improve the resolution between peaks as shown above, allowing a more accurate identification and quantification of each metabolite [22–25, 27]. Despite shorter T2 relaxation times and increased field inhomogeneity, the chemical shift doubling at 3 T yields better spectral resolution. At 1.5 T, the quantification of NAA, Cho, Cr, Lac and other metabolites such as mI has been feasible [1–4], while Glu and Gln are closely coupled and present extensive spectral overlap at this field intensity, making peak assignments and quantitative measurements difficult and subject to considerable uncertainty. At 3.0 T the increase in chemical shift is reflected, for instance, in improved baseline separation of Cho and Cr, which are only 0.2 ppm apart, and in slightly better resolution of Glu/Gln region, between 2.05 and 2.5 ppm. Furthermore the presence of abnormal metabolites such as Phe at 7.36 ppm (Fig. 6.6) or the differentiation of glycine at 3.56 ppm from *myo*-inositol at 3.55 ppm (Fig. 6.5b) can be confirmed with more confidence.

Significantly improved spectral resolution was also demonstrated in the quantification of J-coupled metabolites, such as glutamate, glutamine and GABA and the detection of glucose at

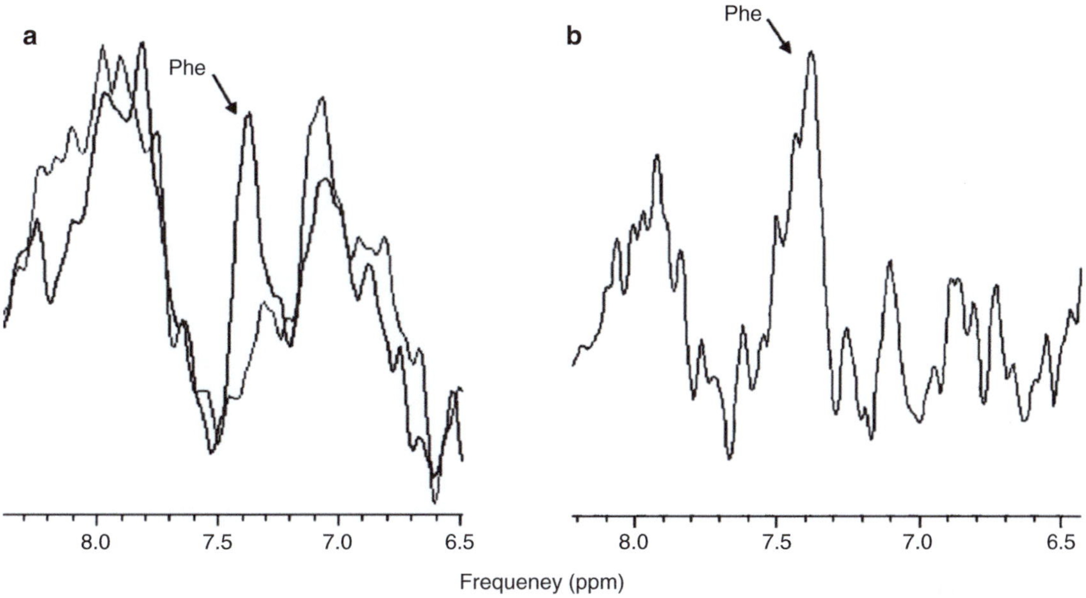


**Fig. 6.6** Detection of phenylalanine (Phe) at 7.36 ppm in a patient affected by phenylketonuria (PKU). With respect to the MRS study conducted with the 1.5 T system (**a**) to detect the Phe signal, it is mandatory to use a VOI of 32 cc and to compare two signals in a follow-up therapeutic study. At 3 T (**b**), the Phe signal is detectable and can be analysed due to the increased SNR and the better spatial resolution. In fact, use of a smaller VOI (8 cc) reduced the line broadening effects, allowing Phe to be better resolved with respect to histidine and homocarnosine at 7.05, 7.8 and 8.02 ppm, to the amide proton of NAA at 7.9 ppm and due to the reduction in the macromolecular contributions (MM) at 7.3 ppm

3.48 ppm and 5.23 ppm, without using glucose infusion [17, 18, 27, 31].

The previous paragraphs have shown that spectral quality is always a compromise between SNR and the spatial, spectral and temporal resolutions. The relations cannot be expressed in a simple formula, and even though systems with higher field strength provide the required basis for a trend to higher resolutions or SNR, experimental settings have to be carefully weighted against each other to provide the optimum raw data required for further analysis.

## 6.2 Spectroscopy Artefacts and Pitfalls

### 6.2.1 Magnetic Susceptibility and $B_0$ and $B_1$ Inhomogeneities

Different materials placed in a homogeneous magnetic field (e.g. in an MR scanner) affect the magnetic field in different ways according to their magnetic susceptibility. For instance, water has weak negative susceptibility; namely, it develops a small magnetization that acts to counteract the external field, while bone and air have near-zero susceptibility with little effect on the magnetic field. When a structure composed of materials of different susceptibility, such as the head, is placed in the bore, the magnetic field becomes distorted and inhomogeneous [32]. At higher magnetic fields, microscopic susceptibility from paramagnetic substances and blood products and macroscopic susceptibility at the level of air-tissue and tissue-bone interfaces, such as near the air-filled sinuses and skull base, are sensibly increased. Consequently, magnetic field inhomogeneity and susceptibility artefacts will make it more difficult to obtain good-quality spectra, especially from lesions near the skull base or close to the calvaria. These problems can be alleviated mainly by the following expedients: using higher spatial resolution, optimizing RF pulse and coil designs [33, 34], improving automatic local shimming methods [35, 36] and undistorting the images using magnetic field maps [32]. Spectral distortion and loss in SNR may also be caused by eddy currents, which are more apparent at higher field strength due to increased speed and power of gradient coils. These eddy currents can create an additional magnetic field of duration much longer than the original gradient pulse that generated them [37], even though these effects can be reduced by dedicated hardware and software designs [38].

Field inhomogeneity, measured in Hz, has been found to be similar at 1.5 T and 3.0 T in phantom studies, but comparison of the linewidth and T2 values in vivo shows that the inhomogeneity contribution to the linewidth is greater at 3.0 T than at 1.5 T. For all three main metabolites (NAA, Cr and Cho), the average of the difference between the experimental linewidth and the estimated natural linewidth was 0.95 Hz at 1.5 T and 2.66 Hz at 3 T [39]. Improved high-order shimming techniques may help to minimize this term at higher field strengths [40].

Another important effect found at 3.0 T is related to $B_1$ inhomogeneities, usually referred to as dielectric resonance. As soon as the sample size approaches the dimension of the RF wavelength, the RF field becomes inhomogeneous. This can be observed as bright spots in the central area of head, body or phantom images acquired at 3.0 T and above. In MRS experiments, this effect makes it difficult or impossible to define the appropriate transmitter gain going along with the required flip angle, which will locally vary significantly, to apply the reciprocity theorem for spectrum quantification.

## 6.2.2 Chemical Shift Misregistration and J-Modulation Artefacts

The spatial location of a signal is usually encoded by a volume-selective excitation. With three consecutive excitation pulses, the signal is first selectively excited in a slice, with a second pulse focused on a row inside the slice and finally selectively excited inside the volume of interest with a last, third pulse. The excitation performed by 90° and 180° excitation pulses used in a PRESS or STEAM sequence suffers from a frequency-dependent spatial misregistration known as the chemical shift error. While ideally all spins of every metabolite inside a VOI would be excited by the same pulse angle, the excitation varies across the metabolites and their localization. As a compromise NAA is often used as the reference for the VOI, so that all NAA protons are fully excited inside the selected VOI, while, for instance, the excited volume of metabolites right of the NAA would be shifted by a few millimetres to the right and upwards (Fig.6.7). The size and location of chemical shift errors are influenced by a number of factors, including the field strength [41]. At higher magnetic fields, the selective pulses used for MRS volume localization go along with increased volume misregistration. This problem can be minimized by several techniques, where the use of outer volume suppression techniques with very selective saturation pulses has shown to be very promising [42].

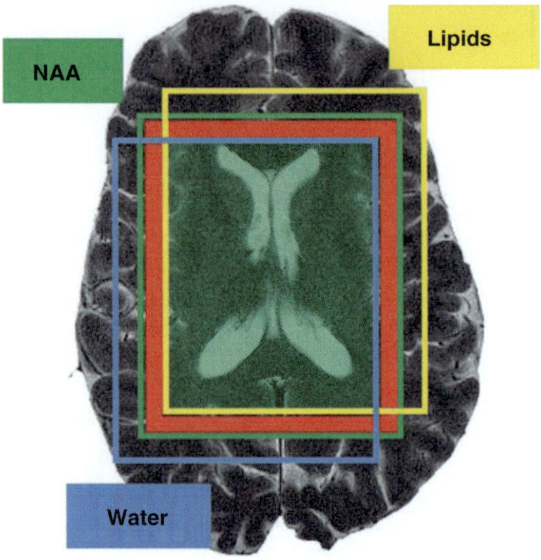


**Fig. 6.7** Voxel misregistration due to chemical shift error caused by spatially varying, frequency-dependent differences of excitation. The different metabolites are only in a subset of the whole excitation volume (*red plus green area*) and equally excited (*green area*), while certain metabolites are or are not excited inside or outside the ROI, which can have a significant impact on the achieved qualitative and quantitative results

J-modulation anomalies for homonuclear-coupled resonances represent another difficulty more frequently encountered at higher magnetic fields. For molecules such as lactate, the extreme separation of the coupled resonances (a doublet at 1.33 ppm due to methyl protons and a quartet at 4.1 due to methine protons) will result in incomplete inversion of the coupled spin over a large portion of the selected volume, resulting in anomalous intensity losses, which are a function of position. This effect can be overcome by some methods, each presenting advantages and disadvantages [43].

### 6.2.3 Magnetic Field Stability and Radiofrequency Coil Efficiency

The temporal variation of the metabolite signal, especially during long examinations, strongly impairs the quality of the resulting spectra. Besides the usual patient motion, the reason for this instability can be found in the drift of the main magnetic field, which particularly affects high-field systems due to the higher technical demands for these magnets. The observable magnet drift over a long spectroscopy experiment can be within the order of the linewidth that can be achieved in $^{1}$H-MRS. Spectral distortions due to temporal signal instabilities can be efficiently compensated for by the use of a correction algorithm on the basis of phase and frequency post-correction of the time-resolved raw data or by using additional signals from interleaved acquisition with a navigator scan [44].

A further hurdle for clinical spectroscopy at high field is the difficulty in building high-sensitivity, high-homogeneity volume coils. Since RF penetration into tissues becomes more demanding [45], the problems become striking for large structures, where achieving satisfactory field homogeneity is difficult. An inadequate RF coil may sacrifice the SNR gained with the greater field strength. To address these problems, some technical strategies have been proposed leading to a second generation of head coils for 3.0 T and 4.0 T systems [45–47]. Further improvements can be expected with the development of new multi-element coil arrays, low temperature coils and new concepts of coil designs for volume resonators.

## 6.3 MR Spectroscopy Quantification and Analysis

Quantification of metabolites is one of the major challenges in current clinical MR spectroscopy. At higher field strength, the increase in SNR and spectral resolution helps to improve the reliability and reproducibility of the quantitative results. The improvement has been striking for some metabolites, such as Glu, Gln and GABA, suggesting that multiplet resolution is as important in spectral quantification as SNR [15, 16, 23]. Still, all the difficulties and pitfalls known from quantitative analysis of spectra acquired at 1.5 T, especially when trying to determine absolute concentrations, apply to spectra acquired at 3.0 T. The challenges of quantitative spectroscopy are twofold, as in a first step a variety of methods can be used to determine the integral under the individual peaks, which is known to be proportional to the concentrations, and then to translate the value of the integral thus determined into true concentration. While the first is more of a statistical and mathematical problem, albeit quite a large one, where all methods applied should yield similar results, the second step can adopt conceptually different approaches that can yield very different results. Apart from the statistical methods, there are two conceptually different techniques to approach a quantitative output MR spectroscopy:

1. The use of a reference as a standard to normalize the results
2. The use of the so-called reciprocity theorem to translate signal intensity directly into an absolute concentration value

There is no agreement on which method should be employed in which cases, but use of a reference has become an established method, at least as a significant set of results. There are several signals that can be used as a reference:

historically, creatine has been used as a reference, as in the majority of the neurological diseases studied with $^{1}$H-MRS the Cr concentration has been shown to be constant up to the reliability of the method. On the other hand, a mounting body of findings where Cr is not constant is leading to the exploration of further reference markers. One of these markers is the internal water signal. Since the mmol concentration of water from healthy brain tissue is known, the metabolite signal can be normalized using the water signal as a reference. This method has disadvantages, as it does not take atrophy into consideration, even though there are methods to correct, for instance, for CSF contamination. If no internal signal is available, an external reference like a small phantom close to the sample volume has been suggested. This requires good $B_0$ and also RF homogeneity, which is not always given. While the use of internal references works as well for 1.5 and 3.0 T, the use of an external signal is more difficult. Due to the properties of wave propagation, it is nearly impossible to achieve homogeneous RF excitation over a large FOV with 3.0 T systems. It would be necessary to acquire the spectrum of the VOI inside the patient followed by an acquisition of an external reference while keeping all acquisition parameters constant.

This also yields to a problem related to the second conceptual approach using the reciprocity theorem to quantify in absolute units. The use of the theorem requires knowing the exact transmitter gain, e.g. defined by the RF energy needed to apply a 90° pulse, and receiver gains used to amplify and digitize the signal. Whereas this works well at 1.5 T, acquisitions at higher field strengths are impaired by dielectric resonance due to $B_1$ inhomogeneities.

Additional to the analytical approach, the decrease in the intrinsic individual metabolic T1 and T2 relaxation times has to be well thought out [39], particularly if metabolite concentrations are to be expressed as absolute concentrations. The "normal" metabolite ratios observed at 1.5 T are, therefore, different at higher magnetic fields, and it is essential to gather new normative data when switching to a different field strength.

Despite all the qualitative arguments speaking for MR systems with higher field strength, the quantification of the resulting spectra can be much more demanding, and some of the methods well established at 1.5 T might not even be applicable at all.

## 6.4 Advanced Spectroscopy Sequences and Applications

### 6.4.1 Spectral Editing

Even though their concentration levels limit the number of detectable metabolites with in vivo spectroscopy, there are still a dozen or more metabolites contributing to the total spectrum. Due to signal overlaps and complicated spectral patterns, most of these metabolites cannot easily be differentiated from each other and have to be treated as metabolite groups like the Glx-components glutamine, glutamate and GABA or just as baseline disturbances like most of the macromolecules.

Any technique simplifying or selectively changing the appearance of a spectrum can be considered a spectral editing technique. Most clinical $^{1}$H spectroscopy sequences have several of these techniques in common like CHESS water or lipid suppression or spatially selective excitation. In this chapter, all the techniques that allow to simplify a spectrum by focusing on a subset of specific metabolites will be discussed under spectral editing. Increasing the echo time TE is the simplest approach, where only metabolites with long T2 relaxation times will contribute to the spectrum.

Most of the advanced spectral editing techniques rely on the phenomenon of either homonuclear or heteronuclear spin coupling. Spin coupling, also known as J-coupling, is responsible for several of the spectral patterns of individual metabolites observable in spectroscopy, like the doublet of lactate or the multiplet of

GABA. Even though J-coupling itself is independent of the field strength $B_0$, several of the editing sequences cannot be applied with clinical 1.5 T scanners. A sufficient spectral resolution and usually high signal when aiming for low concentrated metabolites are prerequisites for successful spectral editing.

In vivo measurements of cerebral GABA, for example, are limited by its low concentration and by the presence of the significantly overlapping resonances at GABA-2 (2.3 ppm) from Glx, at GABA-3 (1.9 ppm) from NAA and at GABA-4 (3.0 ppm) from the methyl group of creatine. Fortunately, the methyl group of creatine is not subject to the effects of J-coupling. This allows it to be suppressed or separated using a variety of spectroscopic techniques, such as J-editing [48–52], 2D J-resolved spectroscopy [39, 53], longitudinal scalar order difference editing [54] and multiple quantum filtering [55, 56]. These methods selectively prepare GABA-3 and GABA-4 into a steady state while suppressing the dominant overlapping creatine signal at 3.0 ppm. The GABA-4 can be made visible by further advanced processing, which can include signal averaging or subtraction. The result is a single signal assigned to GABA as shown in Fig. 6.8, even though a significant amount of co-edited resonances from macromolecules, such as glutathione at 2.87–2.94 ppm, are included.

Another application of the J-coupled editing technique is in the detection of glutamate (Glu), which gives rise to a complex proton spectrum characterized by the coupled spins of the C2–C4 hydrogen nuclei. At the moderate field strength of 1.5 T, the in vivo brain spectrum in the respective spectral ranges exhibits poor resolution and, despite the relatively high brain Glu concentration of 7–12 mmol/l, low sensitivity due to substantial contributions by glutamine (Gln). In conventional spectroscopy sequences, the resonances in this range are therefore mostly assigned to a mixture of Glu and Gln (and sometimes

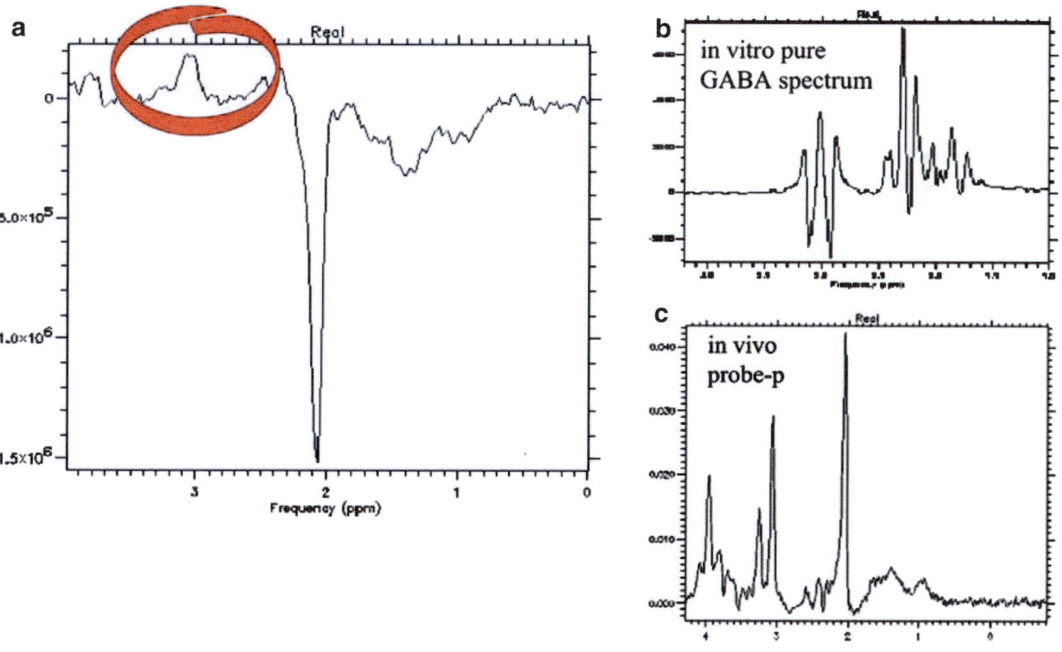


**Fig. 6.8** In vivo GABA spectrum (**a**) acquired with use of a specific editing sequence. Due to the complicated spectral pattern (**b**) and the overlay of GABA with other metabolites (**c**), advanced acquisition techniques are required for successful detection of GABA (Image courtesy of Ruber International Hospital, Madrid, Spain)

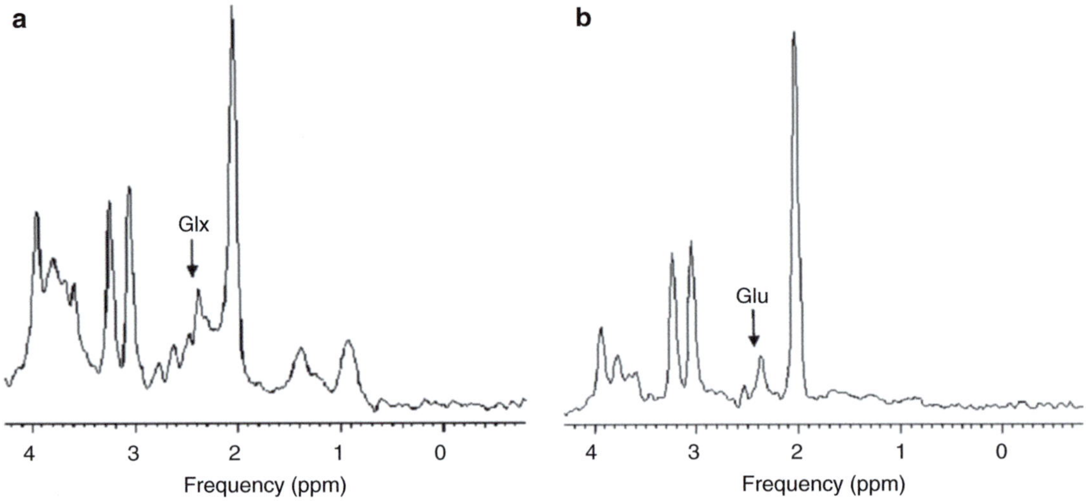


**Fig. 6.9** Spectra obtained from grey matter in a healthy subject using PRESS (**a**) and TE-averaged PRESS (**b**) sequences. In conventional spectroscopy sequences (**a**), the resonances between 2 and 2.6 ppm are assigned to a mixture of glutamate (Glu) and glutamine (Gln), designated Glx. At 3 T, a TE-averaged PRESS data acquisition gives an unobstructed single-line response for glutamate at 2.38 ppm (**b**)

GABA), summarized as Glx-components. A method to accurately measure the tissue level of brain glutamate at 3 T is based on a TE-averaged PRESS data acquisition, which gives an unobstructed single-line response for glutamate at 2.38 ppm (Fig. 6.9). The sequence is based on a modification of the standard asymmetric single-voxel PRESS sequence with equidistant TE increments ranging from 35 to 195 ms [57].This sequence also provides a sensitive method to measure the other metabolites and their effective T2 relaxation rates for uncoupled spins [58, 59].

### 6.4.2 Fast Acquisition Techniques

Fast acquisition techniques are usually restricted to techniques for multidimensional spectroscopic imaging (CSI). While the acquisition time in a CSI experiment is mainly defined by the number of phased-encoding steps used for encoding the spatial information, the time for a single-voxel experiment is proportional to the number of signal averages and the repetition time TR. None of the techniques used to decrease the time needed to cover the *k*-space for spectroscopic imaging can be directly applied to single-voxel spectroscopy.

Different fast CSI acquisition techniques make use of increased gradient performance and specific *k*-space trajectories to acquire the full spatial and spectral information in a reduced amount of time. These techniques utilize approaches initially developed for conventional fast imaging methods and include echoplanar spectroscopic imaging (EPSI, PEPSI) [60, 61], spiral acquisitions [62] or recently developed fly-back techniques [63].

Some of the techniques described above are very hardware demanding, and an alternative approach, with very little or no extra hardware requirements, uses a method commonly known as parallel imaging. These techniques work with dedicated coil arrays, using the known $B_1$ field distribution of every coil element to reduce the number of required phased-encoding steps for full encoding of the required spatial information. Parallel imaging techniques have successfully been applied to spectroscopic imaging, even though post-processing is very demanding, and the complex nature of the spectroscopic data makes the resulting spectra prone to artefacts or quality losses.

Even though all the techniques enable a significant reduction in acquisition time, down to less than 15 min for a full brain metabolite map, the resulting spectra always suffer from reduced SNR compared, for instance, to conventional PRESS chemical shift imaging. To regain this SNR, multiple averaging would be required, preventing the acceptance of these approaches for clinical applications. Greater field strengths with higher intrinsic SNR may in the future open new prospects for the use of these methods.

### 6.4.3 High Spatial Resolution Spectroscopy

The ability of improved MRI technologies to detect smaller lesions may involve a greater need for higher spatial resolution in single-voxel spectroscopy and CSI experiments. Whereas the poor SNR of 1.5 T magnets prevented the acquisition of single-voxel spectra with a spatial resolution significantly below 4–8 ml or chemical shift images with a spatial resolution of less than 2 ml, lower spatial resolutions are becoming feasible at 3.0 T.

A specific application requiring lower resolution is the MR spectroscopic study of small animals. These studies are usually performed on dedicated animal systems, which offer ideal conditions. However, given their increasing diffusion, researchers are interested in using whole-body high-field MR systems for animal studies both for reasons of cost reduction and to perform direct comparisons of animal and human data. This requires new techniques that allow to achieve the highest possible spatial resolution and obtain conclusive data from brain structures that are several orders of magnitude smaller than the human brain while keeping examination times short to minimize animal mortality [64].

Recent studies have shown that proton spectroscopy, for instance, of newborn rat brain in a 3.0 T whole-body scanner using a standard clinical spectroscopy protocol is feasible. Irrespective of field strength, the RF resonator for signal transmission and reception plays a major role in the quality that can be achieved. A coil with a size close to that of the object to be studied is usually appropriate, like the small birdcage resonator shown in Fig. 6.10 designed for brain studies of newborn rats. If the transfer of results from animal experiments to human in vivo studies is going to be explored, similar acquisition protocols would be appropriate to achieve comparable results. While maintaining these prerequisites, single-voxel spectra can be acquired of volumes

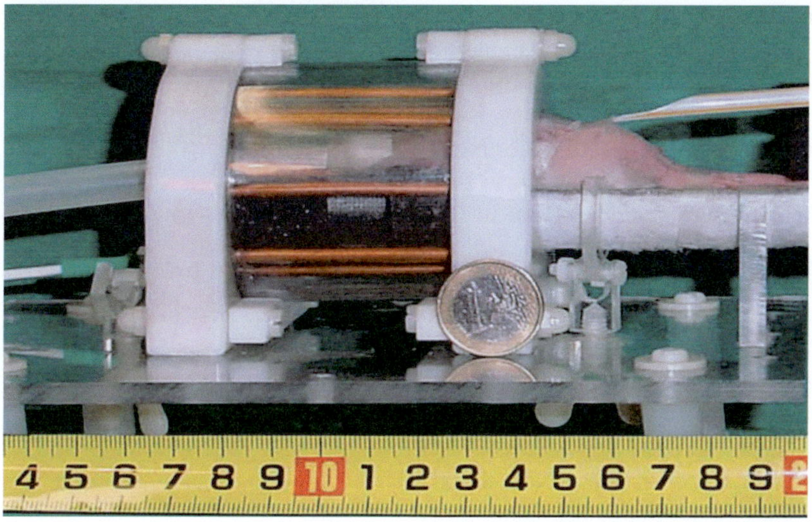


**Fig. 6.10** Dedicated linear volume resonator (Flick Engineering Solutions, the Netherlands) designed for newborn rat brain MR studies in a conventional clinical 3.0 T MR scanner (Image courtesy of University Children's Hospital, Zurich, Switzerland)

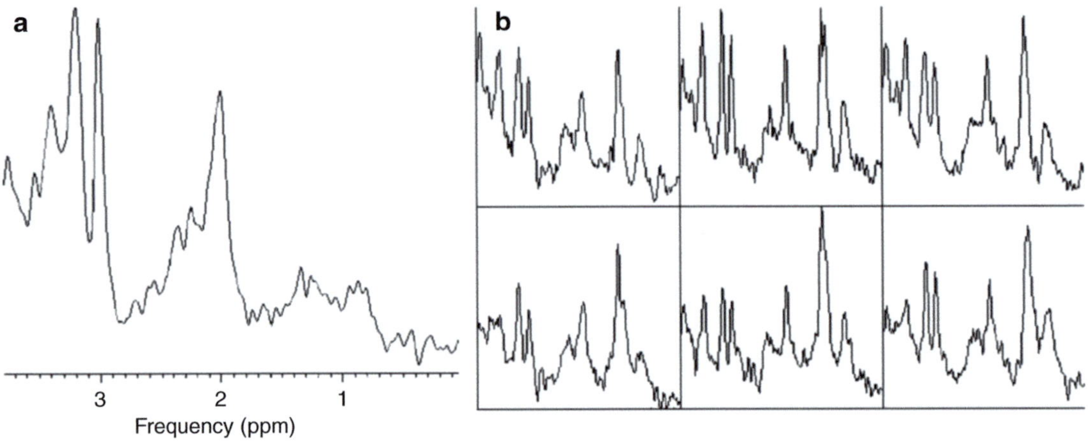


**Fig. 6.11** High-resolution single-voxel spectrum (**a**) with a spatial resolution of 0.2 ml and high-resolution CSI (**b**) with a spatial resolution of 0.04 ml acquired from a newborn rat brain in a conventional clinical whole-body 3.0 T scanner

as small as about 0.2 ml and CSI spectra with a spatial resolution of 0.04 ml, both with an acquisition time of less than 10 min (Fig. 6.11).

### Conclusions

The utilization of high-field MR systems for clinical spectroscopy studies involves a variety of improvements and advantages which enable the use of new and advanced acquisition techniques that raise the diagnostic accuracy of MR spectroscopy above the desired threshold. At the same time, the higher field strength can also carry disadvantages and limitations that may degrade its usefulness. At the time of the introduction of clinical 3.0 T scanners, results were often unsatisfactory and performances for some applications were poorer than those obtained with the well-optimized clinical 1.5 T scanners. However, most problems with 3 T systems have been or are being addressed by the research community and the manufacturers with the development of sophisticated technical strategies, pulse sequences and/or processing algorithms.

Higher field strength will improve MR imaging thanks to the greater SNR, but will also experience some image degradation due to the increased frequency distance between fat and water. By contrast, MR spectroscopy will gain from both the increased SNR and the increased spectral resolution. Thus spectroscopy is and will be one of the key applications of MR systems with field strength of 3.0 T and above, despite the current problems. The various strategies illustrated above should allow these problems to be overcome and make higher magnetic field scanners the workhorse for all brain MR applications in the near future.

## References

1. Smith ICP, Stewart LC (2002) Magnetic resonance spectroscopy in medicine: clinical impact. Prog Nucl Magn Reson Spectrosc 40(1):1–34
2. Bonavita S, Di Salle F, Tedeschi G (1999) Proton MRS in neurological disorders. Eur J Radiol 30(2):125–131
3. Ross B, Bluml S (2001) Magnetic resonance spectroscopy of the human brain. Anat Rec 265(2):54–84
4. Di Costanzo A, Trojsi F, Tosetti M et al (2007) Proton MR spectroscopy of the brain at 3 T: an update. Eur Radiol 7:1651–1662
5. Burtscher IM, Holtås S (2001) Proton MR spectroscopy in clinical routine. J Magn Reson Imaging 13(5):732–737
6. Grodd W, Krageloh-Mann I et al (1990) In vivo assessment of *N*-acetylaspartate in brain spongy degeneration (Canavan's disease) by proton spectroscopy. Lancet 336:437–438
7. Stöckler S, Hanefeld F, Frahm J (1996) Creatine replacement therapy in guanidinoacetate methyltransferase deficiency, a novel inborn error of metabolism. Lancet 348:789–790

8. Bianchi MC, Tosetti M, Fornai F et al (2000) Reversible brain creatine deficiency in two sisters with normal blood creatine level. Ann Neurol 47:511–513
9. Kruse B, Barker PB, Van Zijl PC et al (1994) Multislice proton magnetic resonance spectroscopic imaging in X-linked adrenoleukodystrophy. Ann Neurol 36:595–608
10. Ross BD, Jacobson S, Villamil F et al (1994) Subclinical hepatic encephalopathy: proton MR spectroscopic abnormalities. Radiology 193:457–463
11. Guidance for significant risk investigations. US CDRH, FDA, DHHS. 29 Sept 1997
12. Takahashi M, Uematsu H, Hatabu H (2003) MR imaging at high magnetic fields. Eur J Radiol 46(1):45–52
13. Kangarlu A, Burgess RE, Zhu H et al (1999) Cognitive, cardiac, and physiological safety studies in ultra high field magnetic resonance imaging. Magn Reson Imaging 17(10):1407–1416
14. Ding XQ, Lanfermann H (2015) Whole brain 1H-Spectroscopy: a developing technique for advanced analysis of cerebral metabolism. Clin Neuroradiol 25:245–250
15. Lally N, An L, Banerjee D et al (2016) Reliability of 7 T (1) H-MRS measured human prefrontal cortex glutamate, glutamine, and glutathione signals using an adapted echo time optimized PRESS sequence: A between- and within-sessions investigation. J Magn Reson Imaging 43(1):88–98
16. Ganji SK, An Z, Banerjee A et al (2014) Measurement of regional variation of GABA in the human brain by optimized point-resolved spectroscopy at 7T in vivo. NMR Biomed 27(10):1167–1175
17. Donadieu M, Le Fur Y, Lecocq A et al (2016) Metabolic voxel-based analysis of the complete human brain using fast 3D-MRSI: proof of concept in multiple sclerosis. J Magn Reson Imaging 44(2):411–419
18. Jiru F, Skoch A, Wagnerova D et al (2016) The age dependence of T2 relaxation times of N-acetyl aspartate, creatine and choline in the human brain at 3 and 4 T. NMR Biomed 29(3):284–292
19. Vaughan JT, Garwood M, Collins CM et al (2001) 7T vs 4 T: RF power, homogeneity and signal-to-noise comparison in head images. Magn Reson Med 46(1):24–30
20. Uematsu H, Dougherty L, Takahashi M et al (2003) A direct comparison of signal behavior between 4.0 and 1.5 T: a phantom study. Eur J Radiol 45(2):154–159
21. Posse S, Cuenod CA, Risinger R et al (1995) Anomalous transverse relaxation in $^1$H spectroscopy in human brain at 4 Tesla. Magn Reson Med 33(2):246–252
22. Gruetter R, Weisdorf SA, Rajanayagan V et al (1998) Resolution improvements in in vivo $^1$HNMR spectra with increased magnetic field strength. J Magn Reson 135(1):260–264
23. Bartha R, Drost DJ, Menon RS, Williamson PC (2000) Comparison of the quantification precision of human short echo time $^1$H spectroscopy at 1.5 and 4.0 Tesla. Magn Reson Med 44(2):185–192
24. Gonen O, Gruber S, Li BSY et al (2001) Multivoxel 3D proton spectroscopy in the brain at 1.5 versus 3.0 T: signal-to-noise ratio and resolution comparison. Am J Neuroradiol 22(9):1727–1731
25. Barker PB, Hearshen DO, Boska MD (2001) Single-voxel proton MRS of the human brain at 1.5 T and 3.0 T. Magn Reson Med 45(5):765–769
26. Ocali O, Atalar E (1998) Ultimate intrinsic signal-to-noise ratioinMRI. Magn Reson Med 39(3):462–473
27. Tká I, Andersen P, Adriany G et al (2001) Invivo $^1$HNMR spectroscopy of the human brain at 7 T. Magn Reson Med 46(3):451–456
28. Hetherington HP, Pan JW, Chu WJ et al (1997) Biological and clinical MRS at ultra-high field. NMR Biomed 10(8):360–371
29. Gruber S, Mlynárik V, Moser E (2003) High-resolution 3D proton spectroscopic imaging of the human brain at 3 T: SNR issues and application for anatomy-matched voxel sizes. Magn Reson Med 49(2):299–306
30. Li BSY, Regal J, Gonen O (2001) SNR versus resolution in 3D $^1$H MRS of the human brain at high magnetic fields. Magn Reson Med 46(6):1049–1053
31. Kim DS, Garwood M (2003) High-field magnetic resonance techniques for brain research. Curr Opin Neurobiol 13(5):612–619
32. Cusack R, Brett M, Osswald K (2003) An evaluation of the use of magnetic field maps to undistort echo-planar images. Neuroimage 18(1):127–142
33. Stenger VA, Boada FE, Noll DC (2000) Three-dimensional tailored RF pulses for the reduction of susceptibility artifacts in $T^*_2$-weighted functional MRI. Magn Reson Med 44(4):525–531
34. Alecci M, Collins CM, Smith MB, Jezzard P (2001) Radio frequency magnetic field mapping of a 3 Tesla birdcage coil: experimental and theoretical dependence on sample properties. Magn Reson Med 46(2):379–385
35. Pfeuffer J, Tká I, Provencher SW, Gruetter R (1999) Toward an in vivo neurochemical profile: quantification of 18 metabolites in short-echo-time $^1$H NMR spectra of the rat brain. J Magn Reson 141(1):104–120
36. Gu H, Feng H, Zhan W et al (2002) Single-shot interleaved z-shim EPI with optimized compensation for signal losses due to susceptibility-induced field inhomogeneity at 3 T. Neuroimage 17(3):1358–1364
37. Klose U (1990) In vivo proton spectroscopy in presence of eddy currents. Magn Reson Med 14(1):26–30
38. Gach HM, Lowe IJ, Madio DP et al (1998) A programmable pre-emphasis system. Magn Reson Med 40(3):427–431
39. Mlynárik V, Gruber S, Moser E (2001) Proton $T_1$ and $T_2$ relaxation times of human brain metabolites at 3 Tesla. NMR Biomed 14(5):325–331
40. Michaeli S, Garwood M, Zhu XH et al (2002) Proton T2 relaxation study of water, *N*-acetylaspartate, and creatine in human brain using Hahn and Carr-Purcell

spin echoes at 4 T and 7 T. Magn Reson Med 47(4):629–633
41. Parizel PM, van Hasselt BA, van den Hauwe L et al (1994) Understanding chemical shift induced boundary artefacts as a function of field strength: influence of imaging parameters (bandwidth, field-of-view, and matrix size). Eur J Radiol 18(3):158–164
42. Hood MN, Ho VB, Smirniotopoulos JG, Szumowski J (1999) Chemical shift: the artifact and clinical tool revisited. Radiographics 19(2):357–371
43. Kelley DAC, Wald LL, Star-Lack JM (1999) Lactate detection at 3 T:compensating J coupling effects with BASING. J Magn Reson Imaging 9(5):732–737
44. Thiel T, Czisch M, Elbel GK, Hennig J (2002) Phase coherent averaging in magnetic resonance spectroscopy using interleaved navigator scans: compensation of motion artifacts and magnetic field instabilities. Magn Reson Med 47(6):1077–1082
45. Zhang X, Uurbil K, Chen W (2001) Microstrip RF surface coil design for extremely high-field MRI and spectroscopy. Magn Reson Med 46(3):443–450
46. Alecci M, Collins CM, Wilson J et al (2003) Theoretical and experimental evaluation of detached endcaps for 3 T birdcage coils. Magn Reson Med 49(2):363–370
47. Wright AC, Song HK, Wehrli FW (2001) In vivo MR micro imaging with conventional radiofrequency coils cooled to 77 degrees K. Magn Reson Med 43(2):163–169
48. Rothman DL, Petroff OAC, Behar KL, Mattson RH (1993) Localized 1H NMR measurement of $\gamma$-aminobutyric acid in human brain in vivo. Proc Natl Acad Sci U S A 90:5662–5666
49. Keltner JR, Wald LL, Christensen JD et al (1996) A technique for detecting GABA in the human brain with PRESS localization and optimized refocusing spectral editing radiofrequency pulses. Magn Reson Med 36:458–461
50. Hetherington HP, Newcomer BR, Pan JW (1998) Measurement of human cerebral GABA at 4.1 T using numerically optimized editing pulses. Magn Reson Med 39:6–10
51. Mescher M, Merkle H, Kirsch J et al (1998) Simultaneous in vivo spectra editing and water suppression. NMR Biomed 11:266–272
52. Henry PG, Dautry C, Hantraye P, Bloch G (2001) Brain GABA editing without macromolecule contamination. Magn Reson Med 45(3):517–520
53. Ke Y, Cohen BM, Bang JY et al (2000) Assessment of GABA concentration in human brain using two-dimensional proton magnetic resonance spectroscopy. Psychiatry Res 100:169–178
54. de Graaf RA, Rothman DL (2001) Detection of gammaaminobutyric acid (GABA) by longitudinal scalar order difference editing. J Magn Reson 152(1):124–131
55. Keltner JR, Wald LL, Frederick B, Renshaw P (1997) In vivo detection of GABA in human brain using a localized double-quantum filter technique. Magn Reson Med 37:366–371
56. Shen J, Shungu DC, Rothman DL (1999) In vivo chemical shift imaging of $\gamma$-aminobutyric acid in the human brain. Magn Reson Med 41:35–42
57. Hurd R, Sailasuta N, Srinivasan R et al (2004) Measurement of brain glutamate using TE-averaged PRESS at 3 T. Magn Reson Med 51(3):435–440
58. Hancu I, Zimmerman EA, Sailasuta N, Hurd RE (2005) 1H MR spectroscopy using TE averaged PRESS: a more sensitive technique to detect neurodegeneration associated with Alzheimer's disease. Magn Reson Med 53(4):777–782
59. Srinivasan R, Sailasuta N, Hurd R et al (1994) Evidence of elevated glutamate in multiple sclerosis using magnetic resonance spectroscopy at 3 T. Brain 128(5):1016–1025
60. Posse S, DeCarli C, Le Bihan D (1994) Three-dimensional echo-planar MR spectroscopic imaging at short echo times in the human brain. Radiology 192(3):733–738
61. Guimaraes AR, Baker JR, Jenkins BG et al (1999) Echoplanar chemical shift imaging. Magn Reson Med 41(5):877–882
62. Adalsteinsson E, Spielman DM (1999) Spatially resolved two-dimensional spectroscopy. Magn Reson Med 41(1):8–12
63. Dydak U, Pruessmann KP, Weiger M et al (2003) Parallel spectroscopic imaging with spin-echo trains. Magn Reson Med 50(1):196–200
64. Dydak U, Weiger M, Pruessmann KP et al (2001) Sensitivity-encoded spectroscopic imaging. Magn Reson Med 46:713–722

# 3.0 T Diffusion Studies

# 7

Armando Tartaro, Antonio Ferretti, Simone Salice, and Piero Chiacchiaretta

## 7.1 Introduction

Diffusion refers to the random translational motion of molecules, also called Brownian motion, resulting from the thermal energy carried by these molecules [1]. In the human body, we mostly consider diffusion of water molecules. In pure water, the average displacement of water molecules caused by diffusion is about 20 μm in a time interval comparable to typical MRI sequences timing parameters (50 ms). These microscopic random displacements of water molecules produce a tiny, but detectable, change in the MRI signal obtained with dedicated sequences. The basic principle to render the MRI signal sensitive to the diffusion process is to add a strong linear field gradient to the imaging sequence. As a spin move randomly in this non-uniform magnetic field, there are corresponding random changes in its precession frequency leading to additional dephasing and greater signal loss with respect to the same signal acquired without the applied gradient.

A. Tartaro (✉) • A. Ferretti • S. Salice
P. Chiacchiaretta
Department of Neuroscience Imaging and Clinical Sciences – Institute of Advanced Biomedical Technologies, "G. D'Annunzio" University, Chieti (PE), Italy
e-mail: armando.tartaro@gmail.com

In biological systems, the presence of membranes, macromolecules and other components hinders the movement of water molecules. Thus, quantification and characterization of water diffusion in the different tissues of the human body can provide useful informations about tissue structure and integrity.

It is a remarkable fact that diffusion MRI has the ability to probe tissue structure at a spatial scale that is much smaller than the voxel size of the acquired images.

In this regard, water offers several advantages with respect to other soluble molecules that also exhibit Brownian diffusion. Indeed, besides the high concentration of its MRI visible nucleus ($^1H$) in biological tissue, the small dimensions of water molecules permit an easy access to most biological compartments (cell walls, membranes, intracellular organs, macromolecules), making the diffusion process very sensitive to the structural organization of tissues at the microscopic level.

Diffusion in a particular tissue may be restricted in any direction in a similar way (isotropic diffusion, e.g. in CSF) or more in one particular direction (anisotropic diffusion, e.g. in white matter).

Diffusion measurements are generally expressed as the effective displacement in space of the water molecules in a certain time interval [2].

To understand the quantification of diffusion, we can refer to a group of molecules initially



T. Scarabino et al. (eds.), *High Field Brain MRI*, DOI 10.1007/978-3-319-44174-0_7

concentrated at one point. After a time t, the molecules will have expanded in the three dimensions according to Einstein's equation of diffusion:

$$r^2 = 6 \cdot D \cdot t \tag{7.1}$$

where $r$ is the average displacement and $D$ is the diffusion coefficient. A typical value for the brain is $D = 0.001\ mm^2/s$.

One of the primary clinical applications of diffusion MRI is in stroke disease, where changes in diffusion-weighted MRI (DWI) are visible at earlier stages of injury development when compared to conventional $T_2$-weighted MRI [3, 4]. Moreover, advanced applications of DWI such as diffusion tensor imaging (DTI) provide a powerful tool to map white matter fibre bundles, allowing the investigation of structural connectivity of the brain that complements fMRI studies of functional connectivity [5–7].

## 7.2 Diffusion MRI Measurements

The basic principle to make the MRI signal sensitive to the diffusion process is based on the addition of a pair of strong bipolar gradient pulses to the acquisition sequence [8]. The second gradient is oriented in the same spatial direction but has inverse polarity with respect to the first gradient (Fig. 7.1). The net effect of this gradient pair is to restore the phase coherence of stationary spins, while the randomly diffusing spins experience a phase coherence loss proportional to their displacement in the gradient direction. In practice, the most commonly implemented acquisition modality is the Stejskal-Tanner spin-echo scheme. With a spin-echo acquisition, the principle is the same, but the two gradients have the same polarity and are applied symmetrically on both sides of the 180° refocusing pulse. In the case of free diffusion, with a Gaussian distribution of spin phases, the signal is attenuated by a factor $A$ that depends on the value of $D$ and sequence parameters [9]:

$$A = e^{-bD} \tag{7.2}$$

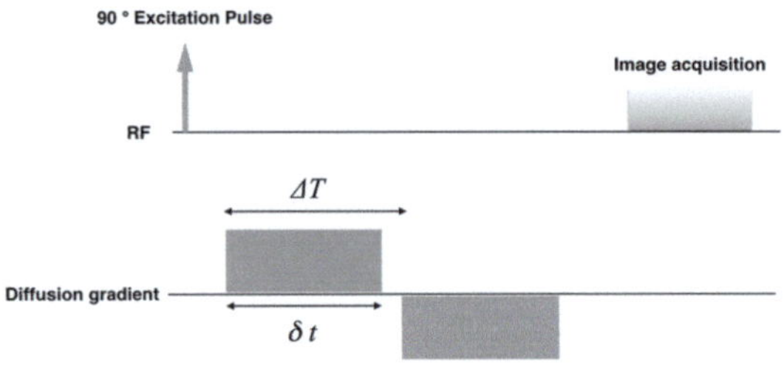


**Fig. 7.1** Schematic of the bipolar gradient pulse making the MRI signal sensitive to diffusion. The timing parameters have the same meaning of those appearing in formula 7.3

In particular, the factor $b$ is an experimental parameter that depends on the strength and duration of the applied gradient pulses:

$$b = (\gamma G \delta t)^2 (\Delta T - \delta t / 3) \tag{7.3}$$

where $\gamma$ is the gyromagnetic ratio, G is the strength of the diffusion gradients, $\delta t$ is the duration of the diffusion gradients and $\Delta T$ is the interval between the start of the diffusion gradients [8, 10, 11].

The net signal in a diffusion-sensitized MR image is

$$S = S_0 e^{-bD} \tag{7.4}$$

where $S_0$ is the signal obtained without the application of the diffusion gradients, i.e. with $b = 0$. The diffusion coefficient $D$ can then be calculated by acquiring an image with no diffusion gradients applied ($b = 0$) and the same image with a large value of $b$. The ratio of the two signals is the attenuation factor $A$ from which $D$ can be derived using the relation (7.2). This calculation is performed voxel by voxel producing an image of $D$ that is usually called a map of the apparent diffusion coefficient (ADC). Note that the signal (4) in the DWI image itself contains also other weighting (e.g. a certain $T_2$ weighting in the $S_0$ term). However, if the same echo time is used for both the low and high $b$ value, the $T_2$ effects cancel out, and the obtained ADC map is a quantitative measure of the diffusion characteristics of local tissues. In practice the low $b$ value is often selected slightly greater than 0 to eliminate the effects of large vessels and flow [12], while for the high $b$ value image, a typical value is $b = 1000$ s/mm$^2$, producing a measurable attenuation of the signal and then a good signal-to-noise ratio for the derived ADC map.

Equation (7.2) is strictly valid for free diffusion in a simple medium (e.g. pure water), leading to a Gaussian distribution of the molecular random displacements. In most biological tissue, the picture is more complex, and the diffusion of water molecules takes place in a multicompartment environment, each characterized by its own diffusion coefficient.

For example, intracellular water has a significantly smaller diffusion coefficient than extracellular water. If the exchange of water molecules between the two compartments is fast compared to the timing of the MRI experiment (fast exchange regime), the tissue behaves like a uniform medium with a diffusion coefficient equal to the weighted mean of the two diffusion coefficients:

$$D_{mean} = v_e D_e + v_i D_i \tag{7.5}$$

where the weights ve and vi are the volume fractions of the two compartments (about 20 % for the extracellular space and 80 % for the intracellular space).

Instead, if a diffusing water molecule remains in the same compartment during the MRI measurement (slow exchange regime), the dependence of the attenuation factor on the b value deviates from eq. (7.2) and is better represented by a biexponential form [13]:

$$A = v_e e^{-bD_e} + v_i e^{-bD_i} \tag{7.6}$$

where ve and vi are again the volume fractions of the two compartments. In this case, measurements with many *b* values are required to fully characterize multicompartment diffusion in a tissue. The presence of tissue structures, such as cell membranes, has also other effects on diffusion. These structures act like barriers, restricting the diffusion phenomenon. Considering for simplicity a single compartment (e.g. the intracellular space enclosed by a membrane), the diffusion of water molecules will be restricted by the membrane in the sense that after a certain diffusion time, a fraction of the molecules reaching the barrier will bounce back rather than diffusing past. The result is that the apparent D is smaller than expected when measured with longer diffusion times. Furthermore, the shape of the distribution of random displacements of diffusing water molecules is no longer Gaussian as in free diffusion, compromising the validity of eq. (7.2). Advanced approaches have been developed exploiting the effects of restriction on diffusion to probe the structural composition of tissues. One approach, called *diffusion spectrum imaging* (DSI), showed promise to infer structural information from complex tissue architecture as micrometric interdigitating muscle fibres and crossing axonal fibres [14]. However, with DSI, many *b* values and consequently long acquisition times are needed to collect sufficient data for a full evaluation of the local diffusion characteristics. Another approach, called *diffusion kurtosis imaging* (DKI), provides a quantitative estimate of how the distribution of random displacements in restricted diffusion differs from a Gaussian [15]. This technique is less time-consuming since it requires a limited number of *b* values and may provide a powerful tool to investigate neural tissue in both health and disease [16, 17].

## 7.3 Non-EPI Diffusion-Weighted Imaging

Echo-planar diffusion-weighted imaging (EP-DWI) sequences are more sensitive to image artefacts than conventional imaging sequences because of two main reasons. Firstly, in EP-DWI, every second echo is acquired under a negative gradient. Consequently, any imperfection in the acquired signal (e.g. eddy current, heterogeneity of the radiofrequency receive path, etc.) leads to an alternate line variation in the raw data, resulting in a ghost image shifted by half of the field of view after Fourier transformation (*N/2* ghosting). Secondly, in EP-DWI, acquisition time is longer. Hence, the longer readout period can cause several artefacts: large fat-water shift, geometric distortions due to Bo inhomogeneity, signal loss due to dephasing and resolution loss due to filter effect by T2* [18].

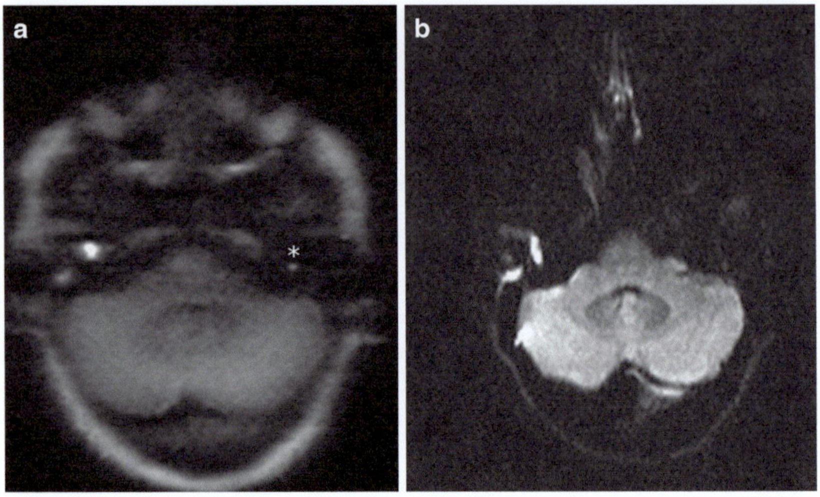


**Fig. 7.2** Bilateral cholesteatoma in a 38-year-old patient. (**a**) Axial non EPI T2 HASTE DWI shows diffuse hyperintensity of the right middle ear. A less than 3mm wide hyperintensity is also appreciable in the left middle ear (asterisk). (**b**) Axial EPI DWI is contaminated by artefact due to bone-air-soft tissues interfaces. The small hyperintensity in the left middle ear is not demonstrable

EPI artefacts are common in areas of great field inhomogeneity and multiple bone-air-soft tissues interfaces, causing frequent diagnostic issues in case of pathology affecting the skull base.

Very high specificity of DWI technique for keratin-containing lesions affecting the skull base (cholesteatoma and epidermoid cyst) has prompted MR imaging vendors to develop fast spin-echo-based non-EPI DWI techniques in order to reduce false negatives due to susceptibility artefacts.

These techniques include Half-Fourier acquisition single-shot turbo spin-echo (HASTE) DWI (Siemens Medical Solutions, Erlangen, Germany), periodically rotated overlapping parallel lines with enhanced reconstruction (PROPELLER) DWI (GE Healthcare. Milwaukee, WI, USA), single-shot turbo spin-echo DWI, BLADE (Siemens Medical Solutions) and multishot DWI turbo spin echo.

Thanks to lesser susceptibility artefacts than EPI DWI techniques, thinner sections and higher imaging matrices, non-EPI DWI techniques have been proposed for detection of residual cholesteatoma as small as 2 mm after middle ear surgery (Fig. 7.2) [19], for detection of congenital cholesteatoma and in cases of acquired cholesteatomas in which clinical signs, otoscopic findings and CT are not sufficient for final diagnosis [20].

## 7.4 Diffusion Tensor Imaging (DTI)

An important consideration in all DWI techniques is the effect of the tissue anisotropy and the orientation of the bipolar gradient pulses on the signal attenuation. If the tissue is isotropic, water diffuses in any direction in a similar way, and the orientation of the gradient pulses does not affect the measured ADC. In anisotropic tissues, such as in white matter fibre bundles, diffusion is less restricted along the fibre direction than perpendicularly to the fibres. In this case gradient pulses along different directions will give a different attenuation of the MRI signal, potentially producing false identifications of affected areas. In order to fully characterize diffusion properties in most biological tissues and make the results independent of the gradient directions, $D$ must be represented by a tensor rather than a single number:

$$\mathbf{D} = \begin{pmatrix} D_{xx} & D_{xy} & D_{xz} \\ D_{yx} & D_{yy} & D_{yz} \\ D_{zx} & D_{zy} & D_{zz} \end{pmatrix} \quad (7.7)$$

With this mathematical formalism, the diffusion coefficient along a direction $u = (u_x, u_y, u_z)$ is given by

$$D = \mathbf{u}^T \mathbf{D} \mathbf{u} \quad (7.8)$$

where the superscript T indicates the transpose. The diffusion tensor is symmetric, so there are only six independent quantities. The minimum amount of data required to measure $D$ consists of an image acquired with $b = 0$ and six images acquired with a high $b$ value (typically $b = 1000$ s/mm$^2$) but with the gradient pulses applied along six different directions [22]. The specific values of these six quantities depend on the coordinate system used, i.e. the system defined by the orientation of the scanner gradients. However, the measured tensor $D$ can be transformed in a diagonal tensor $D_d$ that describes diffusivity in a particular coordinate system called the principal axes:

$$\mathbf{D_d} = \begin{pmatrix} D_1 & 0 & 0 \\ 0 & D_2 & 0 \\ 0 & 0 & D_3 \end{pmatrix} \quad (7.9)$$

The diagonal elements of $D_d$ represent the diffusivity along the principal axes. Two diffusion metrics are commonly derived using these tensor components: the mean diffusivity (MD), given by

$$MD = (D_1 + D_2 + D_3)/3 \quad (7.10)$$

and the fractional anisotropy (FA) given by

$$FA = \sqrt{\frac{3}{2}} \frac{\sqrt{\left[(D_1 - MD)^2 + (D_2 - MD)^2 + (D_3 - MD)^2\right]}}{\sqrt{D_1^2 + D_2^2 + D_3^2}} \quad (7.11)$$

FA varies from zero (no anisotropy) to one (the diffusivity along one principal axis is much larger with respect to the other two).

The fractional anisotropy is the most commonly used metric to capture the degree of anisotropy and is calculated voxelwise to obtain FA maps [23].

DTI has now evolved in a powerful tool to map white matter fibre tracts in basic studies of brain function and structure [24, 25]. Diffusion is strongly anisotropic in white matter regions, with a $D$ value along fibres ten times larger than the $D$ value in a direction perpendicular to the fibres. Local fibre orientation is determined considering the principal axis corresponding to the largest diffusivity value in the diagonal tensor. Then fibre tract mapping is obtained graphically, connecting these vectors across voxels. The resulting paths can be visualized on standard brain images to show white matter connections. To increase the precision of orientation estimate, DTI acquisition for fibre-tracking studies is usually performed with more than the minimum set of six gradient directions required to measure the diffusion tensor. A number of 30 directions for the high $b$ value and five images (to increase SNR) for $b = 0$ is quite common, while 60 or more directions are used in advanced setups.

The reconstruction of these pathways is carried out using mainly two algorithms: deterministic or probabilistic. The deterministic approach assumes a single orientation at each voxel, starting with a seed point and then determining the path to the next voxel on the basis of the local fibre orientation. The probabilistic approach assumes a distribution of orientations and try to make decisions about pathway directions and branching. A major challenge for fibre-tracking algorithms and DTI in general is represented by voxels containing crossing fibre bundles. In this case the simple diffusion tensor model can fail in detecting this more complex situation. Advanced methods such as high angular resolution diffusion imaging (HARDI) and Q-ball imaging have been developed to deal with this complexity [26, 27]. Furthermore, advanced diffusion models such as the composite hindered and restricted water diffusion (CHARMED) model and the neurite orientation dispersion and density imaging (NODDI) technique have shown promise to study the microstructural complexity of dendrites and axons in vivo, providing more specific markers of neurites microstructure than fractional anisotropy and other indices derived from standard DTI [27, 28].

## References


1. Einstein A (1905) On the movement of small particles suspended in stationary liquids required by the molecular-kinetic theory of heat. Ann Phys 17:549–560
2. Le Bihan D (1988) Intravoxel incoherent motion imaging using steady-state free precession. Magn Reson Med 7:346–351
3. Baird AE, Warach S (1998) Magnetic resonance imaging of acute stroke. J Cereb Blood Flow Metab 18:583–609
4. Moseley ME, Cohen Y, Mintorovitch J et al (1990) Early detection of regional cerebral ischemia in cats: comparison of diffusion – and T2- weighted MRI and spectroscopy. Magn Reson Med 14:330–346
5. Mukherjee P, Berman JI, Chung SW et al (2008) Diffusion tensor MR imaging and fiber tractography: theoretic underpinnings. AJNR Am J Neuroradiol 29:632–641
6. Choudhri AF, Chin EM, Blitz AM et al (2014) Diffusion tensor imaging of cerebral white matter: technique, anatomy, and pathologic patterns. Radiol Clin North Am 52:413–425
7. Basser PJ, Mattiello J, LeBihan D (1994) MR diffusion tensor spectroscopy and imaging. Biophys J 66:259–267
8. Stejskal EO, Tanner JE (1965) Spin-diffusion measurements: spin echoes in the presence of a time-dependent field gradient. J Chem Phys 42:288–292
9. Le Bihan D (1991) Molecular diffusion nuclear magnetic resonance imaging. Magn Reson Q 7:1–30
10. Yang E, Nucifora PG, Melhem ER (2011) Diffusion MR imaging: basic principles. Neuroimaging Clin N Am 21:1–25
11. Mori S, Tournier JD (2014) Introduction to diffusion tensor imaging and higher order models. Elsevier/Academic Press, Amsterdam Boston
12. Melhem ER, Mori S, Mukundan G et al (2002) Diffusion tensor MR imaging of the brain and white matter tractography. AJR Am J Roentgenol 178:3–16
13. Buxton RB (2009) Introduction to functional magnetic resonance imaging principles and techniques. Second edition Cambridge University Press
14. Wedeen VJ, Hagmann P, Tseng WY et al (2005) Mapping complex tissue architecture with diffusion spectrum magnetic resonance imaging. Magn Reson Med 54:1377–1386
15. Jensen JH, Helpern JA, Ramani A et al (2005) Diffusional kurtosis imaging: the quantification of non-Gaussian water diffusion by means of magnetic resonance imaging. Magn Reson Med 53:1432–1440
16. Hui ES, Cheung MM, Qi L et al (2008) Towards better MR characterization of neural tissues using directional diffusion kurtosis analysis. Neuroimage 42:122–134
17. Marrale, M., Collura, G., Brai, M. et al. Clin Neuroradiol (2015). doi:10.1007/s00062-015-0469-9
18. Fisher H, Ladebeck R (1998) Echo-planar imaging image artifacts. In: Schmitt F, Stehling MK, Turner R (eds) Echo-planar imaging: theory, technique and application. Springer, New York, pp. 179–200
19. De Foer B, Vercruysse JP, Bernaerts A et al (2008) Detection of postoperative residual cholesteatoma with non-echo-planar diffusion-weighted magnetic resonance imaging. Otol Neurotol 29(4): 513–517
20. Más-Estellés F, Mateos-Fernández M, Carrascosa-Bisquert B, Facal de Castro F, Puchades-Román I, Morera-Pérez C (2012) Contemporary non-echo-planar diffusion-weighted imaging of middle ear cholesteatomas. Radiographics 32(4):1197–1213
21. Basser PJ, Pierpaoli C (1998) A simplified method to measure the diffusion tensor from seven MR images. Magn Reson Med 39:928–34
22. Pierpaoli C, Basser PJ (1996) Toward a quantitative assessment of diffusion anisotropy. Magn Reson Med 36:893–906
23. Mori S, Zhang J (2006) Principles of diffusion tensor imaging and its applications to basic neuroscience research. Neuron 51:527–539
24. Vorona GA, Berman JI (2015) Review of diffusion tensor imaging and its application in children. Pediatr Radiol 45:S375–S381
25. Tuch DS (2004) Q-ball imaging. Magn Reson Med 52:1358–1372
26. Tuch DS, Weisskoff RM, Belliveau JW et al (1999) High angular resolution diffusion imaging of the human brain. In Seventh Meeting of the International Society for Magnetic Resonance in Medicine, Philadelphia, p. 321
27. Assaf Y, Basser PJ (2005) Composite hindered and restricted model of diffusion (CHARMED) MR imaging of the human brain. Neuroimage 27:48–58
28. Zhang H, Schneider T, Wheeler-Kingshott CA, Alexander DC (2012) NODDI: practical in vivo neurite orientation dispersion and density imaging of the human brain. Neuroimage 61(4):1000–1016

# Nerve Pathways with MR Tractography

**8**

Maria Eugenia Caligiuri, Andrea Cherubini, Carlo Cosentino, Francesco Amato, Tommaso Scarabino, and Umberto Sabatini

The neuroradiological interpretation of magnetic resonance (MR) images relies on a complex semeiotics that is based on the morphological and signal characteristics of normal and pathological brain tissue and on the detailed knowledge of the ultrastructural and functional organization of the central nervous system (CNS). In the brain, the study of cortical organization is facilitated by the presence on its surface of fissures, which divide it into lobes, and sulci, which circumscribe in each lobe a number of convolutions or gyri. Identification of subcortical nuclei, grey matter formations lying deep in the hemispheres, is also facilitated by their characteristic morphology, their symmetric position with respect to the midline and the presence of well-defined white matter structures such as the internal, external and extreme capsule that mark their borders.

Detailed evaluation of white matter structure is more challenging than the study of cortical organization, because it does not exhibit anatomical landmarks except the contiguous cortical gyri, the ventricular systems and the base nuclei; however, white matter contains fibres with distinct anatomical courses and functional significance that include projection, association and commissural systems. Identification of nerve fibre bundles is essential in neurophysiology and in studying CNS diseases. Furthermore, knowledge of the spatial relationship between fibres and lesions requiring surgical treatment is crucial in order to preserve white matter functional pathways and the activities they promote.

Conventional and morphometric MR techniques provide an accurate representation of the brain's macroscopic anatomy, but they do not carry detailed information on white matter structure. By contrast, the study of the anisotropic diffusion of water molecules (diffusion tensor imaging; DTI) [1] and tractography (fibre tracking) provide data on white matter microscopic organization and allow the reconstruction of axonal tracts using diffusion-weighted MR images [2–6]. Since tractography is currently the sole

M.E. Caligiuri • A. Cherubini
Institute of Molecular Bioimaging and Physiology of the National Research Council (IBFM-CNR), Catanzaro, Italy

C. Cosentino • F. Amato
Faculty of Biomedical Engineering, Magna Graecia University, Catanzaro, Italy

T. Scarabino
Department of Radiology and Neuroradiology, PO "L. Bonomo" Hospital, Andria (BT), Italy

U. Sabatini (✉)
Institute of Neuroradiology, Magna Graecia University, Catanzaro, Italy
e-mail: u.sabatini@hsantalucia.it



T. Scarabino et al. (eds.), *High Field Brain MRI*, DOI 10.1007/978-3-319-44174-0_8

method affording non-invasive study of the 3D architecture of axons in vivo, it has potential applications to several fields of neurology and neurophysiology to visualize and quantify physiological mechanisms and pathological processes.

Herein we illustrate the main methods for modelling diffusion-weighted MR images and for performing tractography and discuss their enormous potential and current limitations.

## 8.1 Basic Principles

A brief overview of the structural characteristics of nerve tissue is helpful for understanding the rationale behind diffusion studies. While grey matter is made up of cells, principally neuronal soma, white matter is mainly composed of myelinated axons with a specific orientation. Axons have a mean diameter of ~20 μm and may form parallel bundles of varying thickness.

The rationale behind DTI and tractography is that the random movement of water molecules in tissues (diffusion) is restricted by the presence of cell structures (Fig. 8.1). As a consequence, diffusion perpendicular to axon bundles is hindered by axonal cell membranes and myelin sheaths [7, 8] whereas it is unrestricted along them. Within axons water is surrounded by cell membranes and myelin sheaths; again, its diffusion will be greater parallel to the fibres. Longitudinally oriented axoplasmic neurofilaments do not seem to restrict diffusion [9]. Tissues like cerebral white matter, which possess a microscopic architecture characterized by a specific spatial orientation, will thus exhibit different diffusion values in the different spatial directions. When diffusion exhibits a preferential direction, it is termed anisotropic.

The diffusion of water molecules in biological tissues can be measured using MR gradients and diffusion-weighted sequences. The acquisition technique consists of "tagging" the water molecules with a very short gradient. Tagged molecules acquire a magnetization and a phase that depend on their spatial position. The natural phenomenon of diffusion causes the displacement of these molecules to areas containing molecules with different magnetization and phase. The presence in a region of signals with different magnetization and phase results in an overall lower signal intensity, as the signal of the diffusing molecules reduces the one of local molecules. Therefore, increasing diffusion of the water molecules induces a reduction in tissue signal. The study of diffusion anisotropy uses the same image

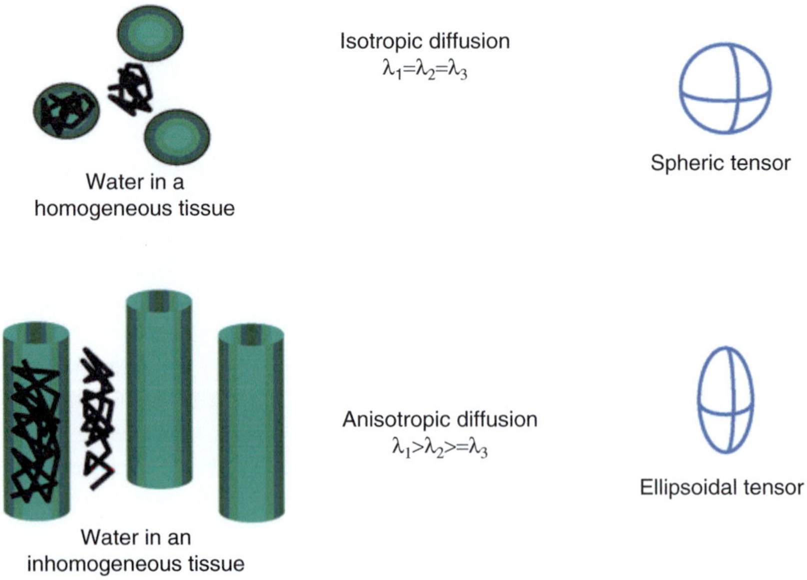


**Fig. 8.1** Representation of the physical bases of the reconstruction of the diffusion tensor. In homogeneous tissues, the three eigenvalues have similar values, and the tensor is spherical. In tissues where barriers restrict water diffusion in a particular direction, the tensor is an ellipsoid, and the direction corresponding to the principal eigenvalue represents the direction of the fibres

acquisition strategies as clinical diffusion studies. Indeed, water molecule diffusion data are actually generated as anisotropic data, because all acquisitions read diffusion along a given spatial direction, coinciding with the direction of the magnetic field gradient used. In clinical diffusion studies, the direction information is lost through the averaging of diffusion values along the three spatial axes; this simplifies the detection of pathological changes in the diffusion coefficient, which are independent of fibre direction.

In DTI studies, this information is retained, and the prevalence of diffusion along a direction, e.g. along a fibre bundle, can be expressed in terms of anisotropy. The degree of anisotropy can be quantified using the diffusion tensor [9–11]. A tensor is a complex mathematical entity [12]; when measured with MR, it may be represented in matrix form using data from diffusion-weighted images to obtain parameters like fractional anisotropy (FA) and the apparent diffusion coefficient (ADC), better known nowadays as mean diffusivity (MD) [13]. The diffusion tensor also contains much additional information. In particular, an algebraic procedure called diagonalization makes it possible to obtain for each image voxel three eigenvalues ($\lambda_1$, $\lambda_2$, $\lambda_3$) representing the values of diffusion along three spatial directions (eigenvectors). If in a given voxel the three values are similar ($\lambda_1 \sim \lambda_2 \sim \lambda_3$), as in all grey matter, the water diffuses in a similar manner in all directions and its diffusion in the voxel is called isotropic. If, by contrast, one of the three eigenvalues is much greater than the other two, as in white matter, water diffuses more easily along the direction corresponding to that eigenvalue, and its diffusion in the voxel is anisotropic.

It is worth noting that, unlike MR parameters such as relaxation times, those obtained from the diffusion tensor do not depend directly on the magnetic field and can thus be measured and directly compared between high- and low-field acquisitions. In practice, whereas T1 and T2, and thus the relevant images, change as a function of the magnetic field, water diffusion in a given space is the same at 1.5, 3.0 and even 7.0 T. Diffusion studies thus fully benefit from the greater signal/noise ratio (SNR) of high-field magnets.

## 8.2 Image Acquisition

Calculation of the diffusion tensor requires acquisition of a set of MR images using suitable diffusion-weighted sequences. Echo-planar sequences with different gradient directions and intensities are the more appropriate for these applications and are those most commonly used [1, 14, 15].

Diffusion weighting involves a general reduction in signal intensity, which increases the greater the diffusion of water. This magnifies the SNR problems shared by all MR acquisitions and makes it difficult to obtain images with very high spatial resolution. Currently, the best spatial resolution that can be achieved is rarely less than 1 mm, particularly along the slice-encoding direction, but the use of high magnetic fields (3.0 T or greater) and parallel imaging can further enhance resolution [16]. Diffusion weighting depends on gradient intensity, which is usually denominated *b* factor and is measured in s/mm$^2$. In theory, increasing *b* values should be used to calculate MD; in practice, limitations in the gradients used in clinical practice, specific absorption rate and times of acquisition have led to the prevalent use of only two *b* values, one virtually null (no diffusion weighting) and the second high (1000 s/mm$^2$ or greater). A *b* value slightly greater than 0 (~20) is used to remove the effects of large vessels. The minimum set of images to be acquired for a DTI study includes six different diffusion-weighted directions (with $b$ = 1000 or greater) and a non-diffusion-weighted scan ($b$ = 0). The minimum set may be acquired several times to improve the SNR, whereas acquisitions with different *b* values for each direction are unnecessary as well as inefficient in terms of SNR [11]. More accurate evaluation of the diffusion coefficient *D* from two acquisitions has been demonstrated using two values of *b* differing by $\sim 1/D$, which in the brain entails that $b2 - b1 <$ 1000–1500 s/mm$^2$ [11, 17]. If more than two acquisitions are performed to optimize the SNR, the theory of error propagation states that it is more convenient to obtain multiple acquisitions at the two $b$ values selected than to use a broader range of $b$ values [11].

Acquisitions of $b$ values in a range, rather than a pair ($b = 0$ and $b = 1000$), can however provide interesting information [18, 19]. Although a single MD value is usually assigned at each tissue voxel, most tissues are indeed made up of separate compartments, each bearing its distinct value of MD. Brain tissue comprises at least two compartments, a fast-diffusion intracellular compartment and a slower-diffusion extracellular compartment. The MD depends on the range of $b$ values used, because low values (1000) are more sensitive to fast-diffusion components and thus to the structural features of the interstitium, than to those of axon fibres. Ideally, the different tissue compartments should be studied separately using several different $b$ values and then fitted with a multi-exponential function. However, since slow-diffusion compartments can be studied only with high $b$ values and favourable SNRs, this is difficult to achieve.

Simulation studies [20] confirmed the notion that higher $b$ values allow the attainment of shaper angular diffusion profiles, which are more sensitive to the orientation of fibres. In particular, by increasing the $b$ value from 1000 to 3000 s/mm$^2$, the minimal resolvable angle between fibre bundles was reduced from about 45 to 30°, independently from the number of diffusion-encoding gradient orientations. Instead, increasing the $b$ value to 5000 s/mm$^2$ did not improve the diffusion model further.

The number of directions offering the best compromise between a reliably reconstructed tensor (multiple directions) and long acquisition times is still debated. In a given voxel, if the fibres are all oriented along the same axis, sampling of the angular diffusion space along a limited set of directions (at least six) is not a problem. However, large portions of white matter are characterized by complex fibre configurations [21], and for this reason the diffusion-weighted signal needs to be acquired along a larger number of unique orientations in order to obtain an accurate reconstruction of fibre orientation distribution functions. Even in the case of a single direction of the fibres within a voxel, a high number of sampling directions would be needed, since the orientation of this direction might change from voxel to voxel.

Besides increasing the precision (reproducibility) in reconstructing fibre orientation distribution functions, a higher number of unique sampling orientations will also reduce the extent to which the variance in an estimate of a given parameter depends on the orientation of the structure. For example, while from a mathematical standpoint at least six different directions plus a low $b$ value acquisition are required in order to fit the diffusion tensor model, it has been shown that for a statistically rotationally invariant reconstruction (such that the variance in tensor-derived parameters is independent of the orientation of the tensor) at least 30 directions uniformly distributed over the sphere are needed [22]. Currently, most researchers use 6 to 90 different directions, with considerable differences in acquisition times and uncertain benefit. A sequence with 68 directions, $b = 100$ and 1000 s/mm$^2$, and a cubic voxel of 2.3 mm lasts about 13 min, but actually takes much longer because image averaging to obtain an acceptable SNR requires multiple acquisitions. Here, a large role is played by acquisition conditions, particularly magnetic field intensity and the availability of parallel imaging to improve the SNR.

High-angular resolution techniques (HARDI; [23]), which require a much greater number of directions (even 252 or more), benefit from favourable conditions of field intensity and high coil sensitivity. A drawback of HARDI techniques is their requirement for a greater number of diffusion-encoded acquisitions compared to DTI, leading to an increase in acquisition time. In addition, these techniques often use a substantial amount of the acquisition sequence duration for the diffusion-encoding gradients, resulting in long repetition and scan times. For example, a typical 60-direction, 60-slice whole-brain Q-ball acquisition can take up to 10 min to complete the diffusion and slice encoding, while a 257-direction whole-brain diffusion spectrum imaging scan lasts as long as 45 min. The length of these acquisitions limits their utility in clinical and research studies. In order to overcome this limitation, several approaches have been developed, such as conventional accelerated 2D parallel imaging approaches and simultaneous multi-slice approaches for single-shot echo-planar imaging. With 2D parallel imaging [24], the number of phase-encoding steps can be decreased by a factor up to 4, thus significantly reducing image distortion and blurring. Despite allowing for an improved image quality, this reduction in echo train length does not translate to a significant reduction in acquisition time because of the large fixed diffusion-encoding time blocks [25]. On the other hand, multi-slice approaches can reduce scan time by a factor equal to the number of excited slices, which are diffusion-encoded with the same diffusion gradients, and readout simultaneously. Methods developed according to this approach include wideband imaging [26, 27], simultaneous image refocusing (SIR) [28, 29] and parallel image reconstruction-based multi-slice imaging [30–34]. Unfortunately, these techniques suffer from significant artefact and/or SNR loss: the wideband approach suffers from a large voxel tilting artefact, while the SIR technique necessarily lengthens the readout period of the echo-planar imaging, thus increasing echo time and susceptibility-induced image distortions. On the other hand, multi-slice imaging techniques based on parallel image reconstruction can lead to a large SNR penalty related to the g-factor, since the aliased slices are generally close to each other due to a comparatively small field of view (FOV) in the slice direction. Several attempts have been developed to solve these issues, such as the controlled aliasing in parallel imaging results in higher acceleration (CAIPIRINHA) technique [30] and the blipped-CAIPI method [34].

As mentioned above, the diffusion tensor basically provides two types of information: a quantitative estimate of diffusion anisotropy and the spatial orientation of fibres (Fig. 8.2). These data are interesting but "local", i.e. they regard a single voxel. Tractography uses these microscopic data to obtain "global" information and reconstruct macroscopic fibre tracts.

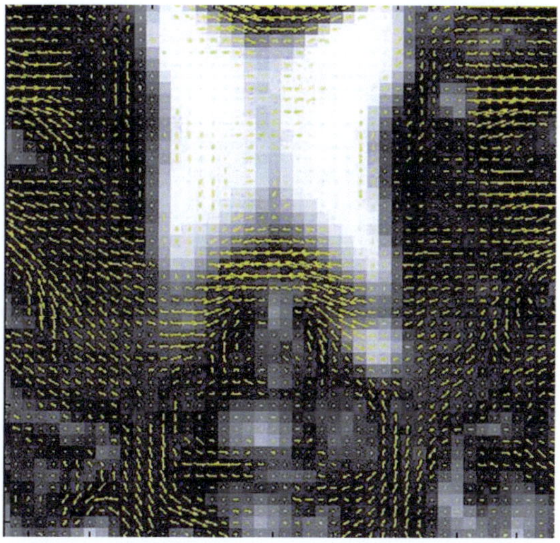

**Fig. 8.2** Diffusion tensor. Projection in the image plane of the principal eigenvector. Vectors are represented by *double-headed arrows* because diffusion data provide the direction, not the orientation of diffusion

## 8.3 Fibre-Tracking Techniques

### 8.3.1 Line Propagation Algorithm: Deterministic Tractography

The voxel grid of an MR image may be compared to a chessboard: selecting a number of adjacent voxels that form a trajectory is like drawing a line on the chessboard (Fig. 8.3). The algorithm used to draw this trajectory in most fibre-tracking techniques involves selecting an initial point (seed point) that is highlighted on the image and then moving to the next nearest voxel, which in turn is highlighted, along the prevalent anisotropic direction, until a condition that halts this process arises (stopping criterion). The differences among these, line propagation, algorithms lie in the way in which the information contained in the voxels nearest to the one being examined with the algorithm (nearest neighbours approach) is used by the algorithm itself to draw the likeliest trajectories and minimize noise.

Since digital images are represented on discrete fields, the vector will often point to an area straddling at least two adjacent voxels, requiring a choice from one or more possible trajectories. In such cases, the selected tract will be a mere

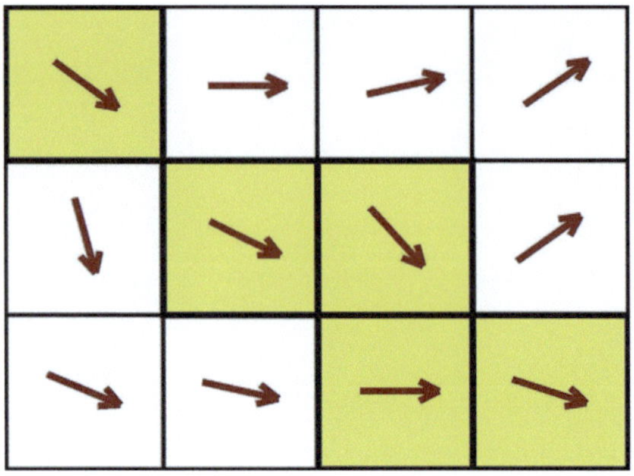

**Fig. 8.3** Propagation of a fibre in a vector field. The *yellow pixels* represent the course of the reconstructed fibre

approximation of the information contained in the diffusion data, irrespective of the trajectory that has been selected.

The first researchers to reconstruct a white matter fibre tract successfully [35, 36] solved this problem using propagation in a continuous numerical field – where the coordinates can be expressed as decimal values – each time approximating the coordinates of the line to those of the nearest voxel. This simple but fairly rough method can be improved by applying a tract curvature threshold. Assuming that the course of a fibre tract exhibits only reasonably soft curves, whenever two possible trajectories present, the less curved one is selected, while sharp curves (e.g. >60°) are excluded. Line propagation algorithms may require vector interpolation (direction and eigenvalue) at the point of arrival of the previous step, which usually straddles two or more voxels and therefore does not directly correspond to a measured value. Interpolation is a mathematical operation that makes it possible to obtain the value of a point from those of surrounding points. In the simpler algorithms, the vectors corresponding to the neighbouring voxels are interpolated, while the more sophisticated ones directly interpolate the diffusion tensor and calculate a new vector [6]. Interpolation enables more uniform paths to be obtained with respect to the algorithms that do not employ them and is less sensitive to noise, although the additional calculations considerably increase computation time.

### 8.3.2 Global Algorithms

The algorithms of this class use a radically different approach. In fact, whereas the line propagation algorithms use only local information (i.e. the data contained in a voxel and in those nearest to it), these techniques employ the information in a global way by applying a mathematical function that reproduces the structural characteristics of the fibre tracts. For instance, the physical analogy used for the fast marching technique [37–39] is that of an ink drop falling on adsorbent tissue. The stain extends faster along the direction of the tissue fibres than perpendicular to them. Assuming a vector field indicating the directions in which the ink spreads, a speed function for front propagation can be defined on the basis of the fibres' anisotropy value. This function reflects the fact that propagation is fastest along fibres and slowest perpendicular to them and makes it possible to calculate the "shape" of the stain from any point at any given time. Its contours may be compared to the isobars of meteorological charts and, in the case of a vector field of DTI data, they represent a sort of map of the likelihood of connection starting from a given point. Using this technique, the course of the fibres coincides with the faster route, hence its name.

Another physical analogy, well known in the field of numerical simulations as the "travelling salesman problem", can help explain another class of methods. A travelling salesman needs to find the optimum route passing through all the towns where he will be calling. One solution is to define a function, e.g. petrol consumption or time, and find the route that minimizes it. Using DTI data, the function ensuring global energy minimization is related to paths along the direction of the field vectors, while those associated with greater energy expenditure are perpendicular to them [40]. Calculation of the value of the function for all possible trajectories makes it possible to identify the course that minimizes the energy function. However, methods like simulated annealing allow the solution to be found rapidly without calculating the energy for all the possible courses while minimizing the effect of noise.

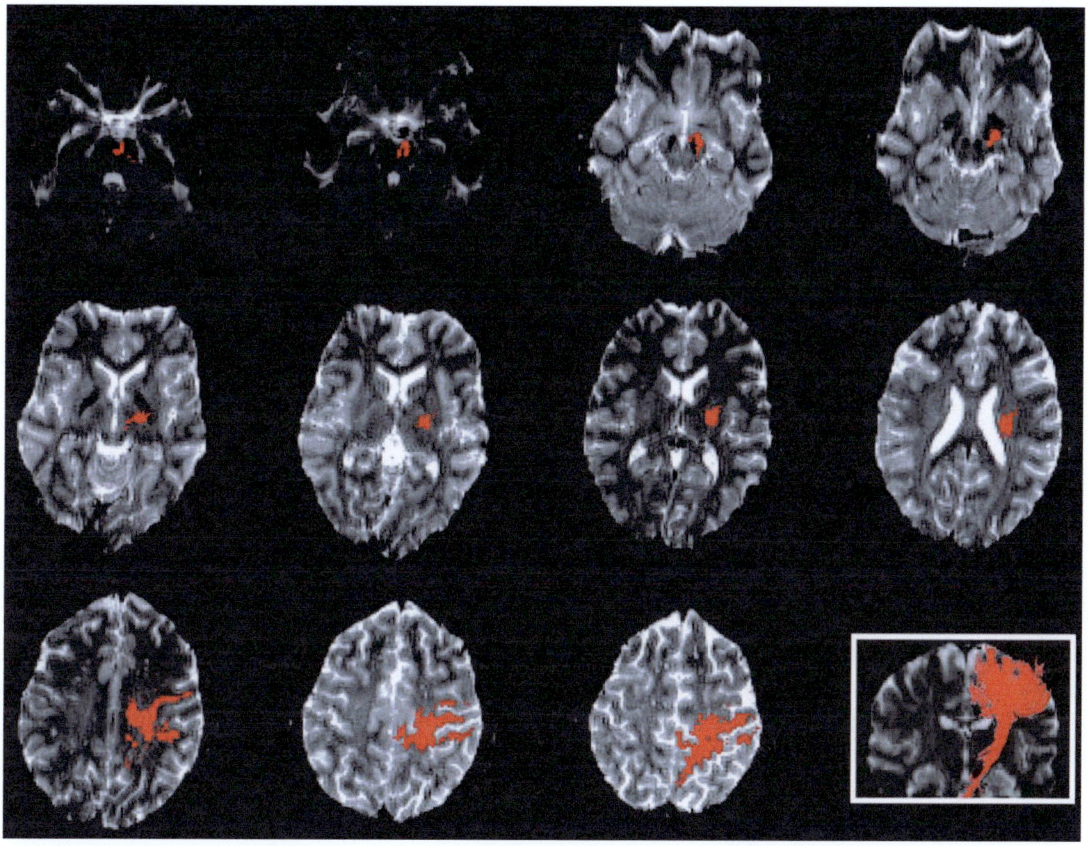

**Fig. 8.4** Fibre reconstruction with a line propagation algorithm (left pyramidal tract in *red*), superimposed on axial T2-weighted images. *Lower right corner:* 3D reconstruction of the same tract overlaid on a coronal image

Global methods have two main advantages. First, they can provide a semi-quantitative estimate of the level of connectivity between two points or regions. In fact, fibres like those shown in Fig. 8.4 provide a visual representation of the bundles, but not a "value" of the connection [41], for instance, between two activation areas shown on functional MR. Secondly, they are less affected by the typical limitations of line propagation algorithms (addressed below). However, the level of calculation required to implement them is often close to the computational capacity of current processors, and they are still in an early phase of development compared with the more common line propagation algorithms (Fig. 8.5).

Halfway between deterministic (line propagation) and global algorithms are the Monte Carlo probabilistic methods [42–44]. With these techniques, thus named for their similarity to gambling, each time the tract is propagated from one voxel to the next, the various directions are given a probability value depending on the diffusion values measured. It is assumed that by repeating the line propagation a large number of times, the course that has been selected most often will correspond to the actual trajectory of the fibre.

To date, several deterministic (line propagation) and probabilistic tractography algorithms have been developed, some of which can be applied not only to DTI data but also on orientation distribution functions reconstructed on HARDI data. The most commonly used deterministic algorithm is the "fibre assignment by continuous tracking" (FACT; [36]), which is computationally leaner and requires minutes to perform whole-brain tractography for a single

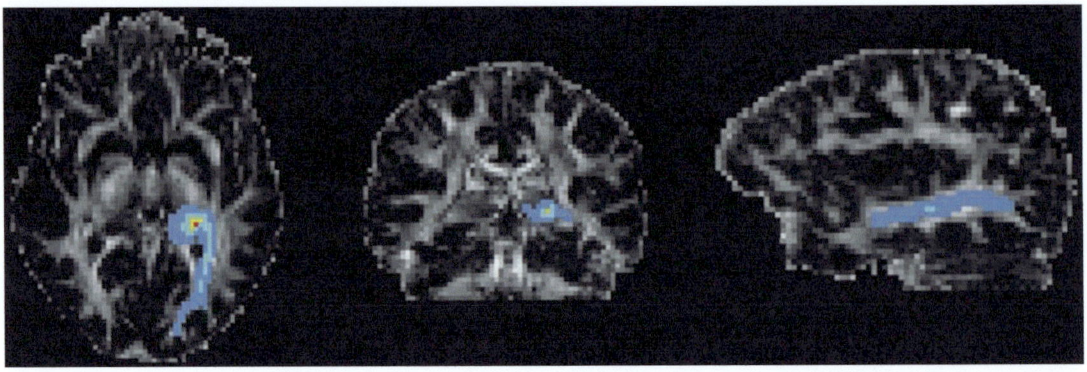

**Fig. 8.5** Connectivity map generated using a Monte Carlo algorithm. Overlay on a fractional anisotropy map. Fractional anisotropy is derived from the diffusion tensor and represents white matter distribution. Colours represent the likelihood of connection with the seed point in the left lateral geniculate nucleus, according to an intensity scale

subject. For what concerns probabilistic tractography, the most commonly used approach relies on the combination of two steps [44, 45]: first, a Bayesian method for assessing the most appropriate number of fibre orientations at each voxel is performed; subsequently, probabilistic tractography through the complex orientation fields is carried out. The main advantage of this approach is that the Bayesian step allows the modelling of crossing fibres, which makes this approach more sensitive to secondary or subordinate pathways. Each voxel is modelled as an isotropic compartment (ball: "round" tensor with all eigenvalues equal) and one or several anisotropic compartments (sticks: "thin" tensors with only one non-zero eigenvalue).

However, the obtainable accuracy in identifying complex fibre configurations based on DTI data is limited [21], and HARDI approaches might be more suitable to this scope, even if their application in clinical routine is heavily limited by the long acquisition times.

### 8.3.3 Seed Point

A factor requiring careful consideration is the initial point of tract propagation, as this choice influences the relative effect of noise on the propagation itself. In the earliest approaches, a frequently adopted solution was to use a number of equidistant seed points arranged on a grid space. This reduced the variance connected with the arbitrary choice of the seed point. An acceptance criterion was applied to avoid selecting voxels not containing fibres. To date, the most frequently used condition is a minimum FA value ensuring the presence of a distinct fibre at the seed point. It is worth stressing that, since the directions identified in each voxel by the diffusion tensor do not have an orientation (see Fig. 8.2), a forward and a backward pathway, lying on the same straight line but running in opposite directions, are consistently generated at seed points.

More recently, because of the development of reliable brain atlases of cortical, subcortical and white matter structures, the definition of seed points has changed. In fact, by using these templates, cortical and subcortical region of interest can be automatically identified on the individual MR scan and used as seeds for tract reconstruction.

### 8.3.4 Stopping Criteria

All fibre-tracking algorithms that use a seed point require a stopping criterion to terminate the propagation process. The most intuitive criterion is the FA value itself; in grey matter FA is low (0.1–0.2 on a 0–1 scale), so the orientation of the principal eigenvector of the diffusion tensor is random and unrelated to that of the fibre tract. A useful stopping criterion may thus be an FA threshold (usually 0.2) below which the propagation is halted, preventing reconstruction of fibres that are not organized into bundles, like grey matter fibres. However, this criterion may also halt the elongation of a line in those white matter voxels, which, albeit containing fibre tracts, have a low FA because of the lack of a main direction (see below).

Another possible stopping criterion is the curvature of the reconstructed fibre tract. The method used to calculate the diffusion tensor assumes the absence in the voxels of sharp curves, in line with the fundamental hypothesis of the Gaussian nature of the diffusion process in all directions. A criterion halting tract propagation in the presence of sharp angles is thus useful, but is difficult to apply to the shorter and more tortuous tracts, where the low spatial resolution of the image does not enable reconstruction of the real course of the fibres.

### 8.3.5 Waypoints and Termination Points

When one is interested in using tractography to reconstruct a specific white matter tract, the definition of the seed region alone might not be sufficient. In fact, no tractography algorithm, to date, directly incorporates knowledge on the actual bundles known to connect different regions of the brain, and for this reason erroneous connections might be identified. To account for this limitation, there are two main approaches, both relying on the use of atlases. A frequently used procedure is that of defining not only the starting point (seed), but also a termination region, where the tract of interest is known to have one of its ends, and, eventually, one or more regions where the tract is known to pass (waypoints). These regions may be easily identified on existing MRI atlases (see Fig. 8.6, second row). If a deterministic or probabilistic streamline crosses the waypoints (eventually in a fixed order), it will be retained for the final reconstruction of the tract, otherwise it will be excluded. Of course, also one or more avoidance masks can be defined, implying that if a streamline reaches any of their voxels, it is rejected. Waypoints, avoidance and termination regions have been successfully used in order to create an atlas of the principal fibre bundles of the human brain [47].

The second approach is mainly used in whole-brain tractography (see Fig. 8.6, third row), either deterministic or probabilistic, and consists in automatically assigning each tractography streamline to a specific white matter bundle. This labelling process relies on the correspondence of the anatomical position of the streamline with that of the white matter tracts in an atlas (which in turn could have been constructed using waypoints and termination masks).

### 8.3.6 Tractography-Based Metrics

The ultimate aim of tractography is, of course, to extract quantitative information regarding the brain's structural connections. To this end, there are several metrics that can be extracted from tractography data.

If deterministic tractography is performed, the exact number of streamlines that connect two regions can be calculated and, for example, compared across groups. On the other hand, if probabilistic tractography is used, an analogue measure is calculated, at each voxel, as the fraction of retained streamlines passing through the voxels over all the streamlines generated from the seed region.

Any tractographic reconstruction, appropriately thresholded in order to exclude outliers and normalized by the total number of streamlines, can also be binarized and overlaid on other MRI sequences or maps in order to extract an average value of volume (e.g. from 3D T1-weighted scans) or diffusion metrics (e.g. FA and MD). However, after the development of white matter atlases, similar results can be achieved without performing tractography on the single subjects, but rather extracting the probabilistic map for the

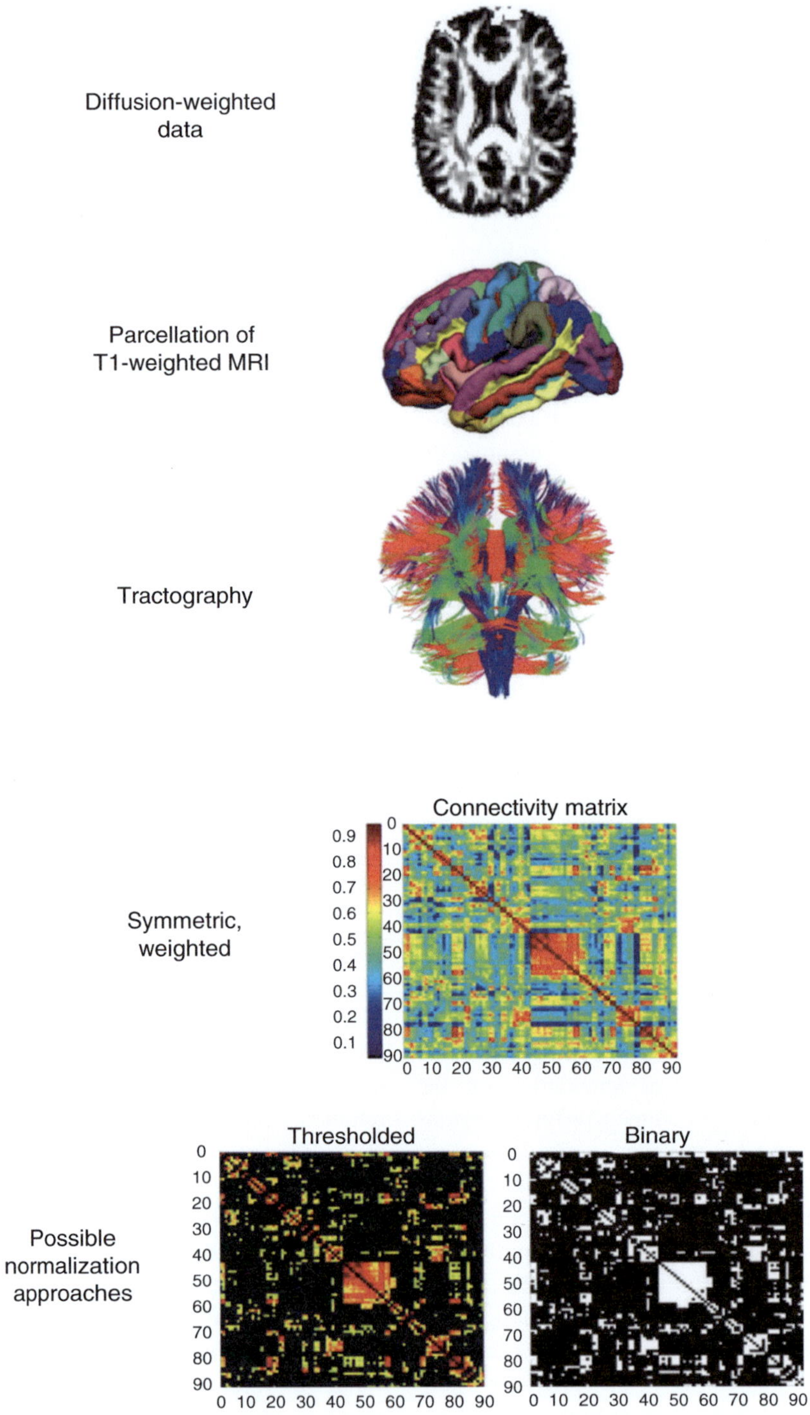


**Fig. 8.6** Typical processing workflow for the reconstruction of whole-brain connectivity and network analysis (Adapted from Filippi et al. [46]). Diffusion-weighted data is used to perform tractography (*first row*). Atlas-based identification of cortical and subcortical brain regions on the individual brain (parcellation, *second row*) can be used to define seeds, targets, waypoints and exclusion masks for fibre tracking (*third row*). By using all the regions defined in the atlas to generate pairwise comparisons, a connectivity matrix is obtained in which the connection strength between all pairs of nodes is contained (*fourth row*). To obtain comparability across different subjects, a normalization step is required (*bottom row*): the matrix can be thresholded, to exclude weak connections, and or binarized, to exclude connection weights from the analysis

region of interest from the atlas itself and registering it on the subject's image.

The most recently introduced method for exploiting tractography data is represented by the application of graph theory to reconstructed fibre bundles, which is known as structural connectomics [48, 49]: this theory considers pairwise brain connections (reconstructed using any fibre-tracking method) with the scope of modelling the brain as a complex network consisting of *nodes* (i.e. regions of the cortex and subcortical nuclei) connected by *edges* (i.e. the white matter bundles). There is a large number of theoretical metrics that can be extracted from graphs in order to quantify network organizational properties both at the global and the local. Here we briefly describe the metrics most frequently used in neuroimaging studies that exploit brain graph analysis [50]. The node *degree* is the number of edges connected to a given node. For each node, the *clustering coefficient* is defined as the ratio of the number of actual connections among the first-degree neighbours to the number of all possible connections. The clustering coefficient indicates the extent to which neighbouring nodes are interconnected to one another, thus reflecting the local efficiency of information transfer of a network. In order to assess the graph distance between nodes, the *shortest path length* is computed by counting the minimum number of edges needed to link any node pair. To measure the centrality of a node (i.e. its importance with respect to the entire network), *node betweenness centrality* is computed as the fraction of all shortest paths that contain the specific node. Similarly, *edge betweenness centrality* measures how influential any given edge is with respect to the entire network and is defined as the fraction of all shortest paths in the network that contain the considered edge. At the graph global level, instead, the *characteristic path length* is calculated as the average of all the shortest path lengths (i.e. across all node pairs), while the *global efficiency*, another frequently used graph metric, is the average of all the inverse shortest path lengths. Both characteristic path length and global efficiency quantify the global integration of the network, with the latter preferred if measuring topological distances in relatively disconnected graphs. Finally, any complex network in graph theory can be decomposed into *modules*. Each module is composed by a set of nodes whose connections with each other are much stronger than their connections to nodes in different modules. To quantify the community structure, the *modularity* metric can be used to assess how strongly nodes in a community interconnect compared to a random graph with the same number of nodes and edges (i.e. a graph where the edges occur at random). Thus, modularity is a statistical quantity related to the extent to which a network is decomposable into such clearly delineated modules.

Whenever applying graph analysis to tractography data, an important aspect to consider is that intrinsic network organizations are better assessed at a specific connection density, as this way it is less influenced by intersubject variability in the total number of reconstructed streamlines. If the appropriate density were not used, each subject's raw connectivity matrix (containing, for each subject, the number of connections between any node pair, see Fig. 8.6, bottom rows) would show substantial differences in connections between regions of interest, based on slight variations in individual anatomy. To normalize the network density, connectivity matrices must be thresholded. The threshold is chosen so that a specified percentage of edges is preserved in the network. Furthermore, by imposing another threshold on edge weights (e.g. fibre density), only the strongest edges are preserved, reducing the likelihood of including spurious connections not supported by evidence [51]. Normalized networks allow for topological properties such as path length and clustering to be quantitatively compared across subjects. Binarization of edges aids this process by ensuring that in addition to the number of edges being identical across subjects, the sum of edge weights is also identical. In recent years, several studies used graph theory to explore the organization of brain circuits in healthy controls and different populations of patients with neurological and psychiatric disorders [46, 52–55].

## 8.4 Limitations of Tractography Techniques and Their Solutions

Also due to their recent introduction, tractography techniques suffer from a number of drawbacks.

### 8.4.1 Noise

Owing to the frequent need for compromising between acquisition time and image quality, the three-dimensional vector field that is obtained using DTI data may contain a high level of noise. Several researchers have tried to quantify the effects of noise on tensor and tract reconstruction [56–61]. Unlike what takes place in standard MR, the noise present in the reconstructed tensor is not directly perceived on images like those of Figs. 8.2 and 8.4, because it affects only the direction of the tracts. Consequently, though exhibiting a consistent distribution of directions, the vectors may indicate slightly different trajectories with respect to the actual anatomy. This type of noise considerably affects fibre tracking, and one of the main problems of line propagation algorithms is that such errors accumulate with increasing distance from the seed point [44]. Therefore, the greater this distance, the higher the risk of deviation of the reconstructed fibre towards an adjacent, unconnected fibre tract. This possibility should always be taken into account when analysing DTI reconstructions, especially of long fibre tracts. SNR optimization is essential to obviate this and other, conceptually related problems. Here, too, the intensity of the magnetic field used and the availability of parallel imaging play a large role.

### 8.4.2 Partial Volume

Different types of tissue may be found in a single voxel (partial volume effects), resulting in a reduction in the value of anisotropy [62]. Partial volume effects constitute a problem for fibre-tracking techniques. The problem may be accentuated in short fibre tracts and in those close to grey matter, where white matter tends to thin out and anisotropy to diminish. Addressing partial volume effects requires spatial resolution to be increased, thus reducing the SNR. As in the previous case, the solution lies in defining the noise level tolerated by the algorithm used and in adjusting the resolution and acquisition time of the MR image.

### 8.4.3 Ultrastructure and Complex Fibre Configurations

DTI provides information on fibre bundles, not on individual axon branches. In addition, the diffusion tensor is unable to model adequately voxels containing more than two axon populations with different directions [63]. For instance, if the relationship among the three eigenvalues of the diffusion tensor is of the type $\lambda_1 = \lambda_2 > \lambda_3$, the FA may still be sufficiently high as to fail to halt a line propagation algorithm, even in the absence of a major direction with an eigenvalue greater than the other two. In this case, the plane defined by the *two* major eigenvectors contains several more or less equivalent directions, leading to error. This problem stems from the nature of the diffusion tensor itself, which being a mere second-order approximation of the diffusion process, cannot adequately represent complex situations like the one described. The tensor line technique partially obviates this problem by selecting, among the directions of the plane defined by the two main eigenvectors, the one minimizing the curvature of the trajectory according to the original direction [59].

These methods do not address the possibility that a dominant direction is not identified in a voxel due to crossing bundles giving rise to different directions. The inability to resolve a single direction within each voxel is a significant general limitation of DTI. In fact, in the millimetre scale of the MR voxel, voxels typically exhibit a number of fibre orientations. Common situations of intra-voxel heterogeneity of orientations may be due to the intersection of different white matter bundles or to the complex architecture of subcortical or junctional fibres. In the presence of fascicles with multiple directions within the same voxel, for example, due to crossing or divergence, DTI will estimate the prevalent direction, which does not necessarily correspond to any actual direction. For instance, if in a voxel a vertical bundle branches off a horizontal bundle, DTI will show the presence of a single direction corresponding to their diagonal, thus failing to represent either.

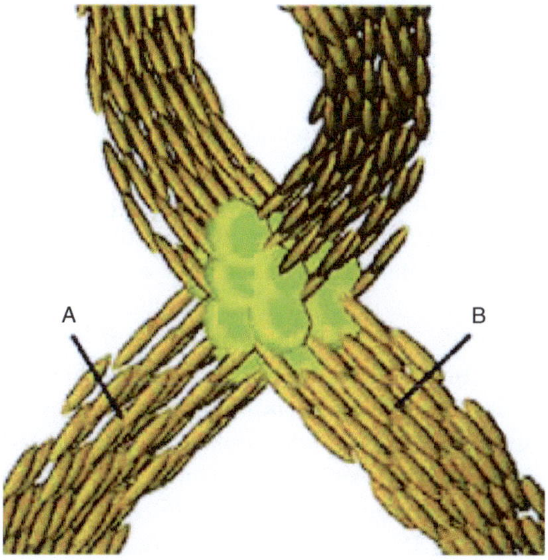


**Fig. 8.7** The crossing of two fibre bundles may result in a spherical diffusion tensor, erroneously indicating an absence of fibres

The standard diffusion tensor reconstruction technique using DTI data cannot resolve this problem. Indeed, even using several different diffusion-weighting directions to reconstruct the tensor, its mathematical nature prevents it from identifying the different directions when, for instance, two or three different bundles cross. The inability of the DTI technique to resolve fibres with multiple directions derives from the assumption of the Gaussian nature of the tensor model, because a Gaussian function has a single directional peak, preventing the recognition of multidirectional diffusion by the tensor model.

Methods capable of using all the diffusion information are HARDI techniques [23], which measure diffusion in several directions with an equal distribution in the three-dimensional space but do not calculate the diffusion tensor. These approaches to the resolution of multiple fibre directions in voxels are based on much more complex models of diffusion in nerve tissue (see Figs. 8.7 and 8.8).

HARDI methods can be categorized on the basis of the approach used to mathematically model the orientation dependence of the

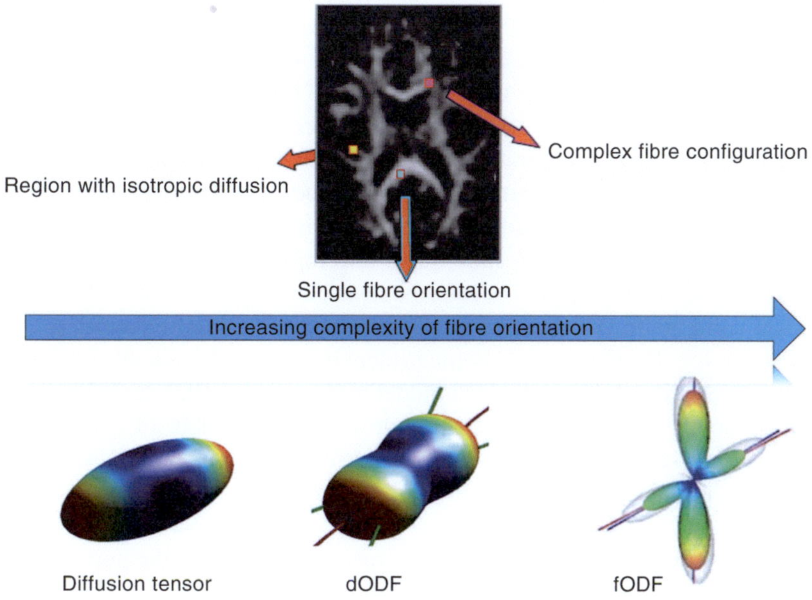


**Fig. 8.8** Possible scenarios of fibre configurations in a voxel. As fibre number per voxel and orientation complexity increase, the diffusion tensor becomes less appropriate for characterizing tissue microstructure, while diffusion or fibre orientation distribution functions (dODF and fODF) provide better performances

diffusion-weighted MR signal. Estimates of fibre orientation are obtained either through the diffusion orientation density function (dODF) or the fibre orientation density function (fODF). The diffusion ODF is a spherical function that, for any point on the sphere, represents the relative number of particles that have diffused along the axis joining that point to the origin. In the case of co-axial fibres, the dODF can be used to infer the orientation of the fibres. However, the dODF will be non-zero in all other directions, since water can also diffuse perpendicular to the fibre direction (albeit hardly). In general, dODF approaches require reconstruction of the diffusion propagator, i.e. the density of the probability that a particle has moved a certain distance within the diffusion time. In principle, and taking into account the limits of acquisition time, these models do not require uncertain model assumptions to be made, which instead needed in fODF methods. However, an implicit modelling does exist in order to make any inferences, and it regards the relationship between the diffusion propagator and the microstructural properties of the tissue of interest (e.g. fibre bundle directions or partial volume). Despite dODF advantages, the exact reconstruction of the entire diffusion propagator is not achievable in practice, due to the limits of most acquisition schemes, which foresee a single *b* value. In such cases, substantial modelling simplifications must be invoked, the most common of which is DTI itself. Reconstructing the diffusion ODF is the aim of approaches such as diffusion spectrum imaging [64] and Q-ball imaging [65]. The original version of the latter had some issues related to spherical coordinates, which have been taken into account in subsequent developments of the method [66, 67], referred to as constant solid angle Q-ball imaging. Other models that employ dODF are multi-compartment models, which extend the single DTI model by summing up the contributions of multiple tensors [68]. Multi-compartment models are currently used in probabilistic tractography on DTI data [44, 45].

The composite hindered and restricted model of diffusion (CHARMED) method [69] combines elements of DTI and Q-ball imaging, thus simultaneously accounting for hindered diffusion in the extracellular space and within cell bodies and for restricted diffusion in the intra-axonal space, respectively. Hindered diffusion is modelled by a diffusion tensor, while restricted diffusion requires special solutions for a cylindrical restricted diffusion space. The parameters of the model need to be estimated from measurements at both low and high *b* values.

In contrast to diffusion propagator and dODF approaches, which essentially describe the diffusion within a voxel, fibre ODF techniques aim at estimating relative fibre density over orientation space. In the case of all fibres being parallel to the x-axis, for example, the true fODF will be a delta function pointing along the x-axis and zero in all other orientations. In this case, only the angular distribution of fibre orientations is inferred from the angular structure of either the signal [70] or of the dODF [20] by spherical deconvolution with a kernel. This kernel is essentially the simplest model of the diffusion properties of a single fibre that the data support (e.g. white matter with the highest anisotropy must contain a single-fibre orientation).

Despite many aspects of the white matter (e.g. axon diameter and packing density) may vary across brain regions, the single-fibre response will only be an approximation that is generalized across the brain. However, fODFs are superior to dODFs with respect to angular resolution and precision.

Reconstructing the fODF is the aim of approaches such as spherical deconvolution [70–74].

Many tract-reconstruction algorithms exploit peaks in the dODF or fODF to propagate white matter trajectories.

It should be emphasized that, even using HARDI techniques, none of these methods is capable of reconstructing nerve fibres or even fibre bundles. As what happens in the case of DTI data, tractography only computes trajectories or pathways through the data, to which a large portion of the nerve fibres should reasonably run in parallel.

The degree of anisotropy can also be estimated directly using HARDI methods without calculating the tensor. In this case, an anisotropy index, the spherical diffusion variance, is used instead of conventional FA. Given that, unlike the tensor, this method is not based on an a priori physical model of diffusion, it has the advantage of not losing any information contained in the data. HARDI and its future developments appear to be very promising, and the evolution of tractography is likely to be based on it even though it requires specialized acquisition sequences, generally longer acquisition times than tensor methods, more complex processing algorithms and, save for *q*-ball imaging, very powerful gradients [40].

### 8.4.4 Error Correction Methods

Tractography may yield anatomical reconstruction errors with any technique. These errors can be minimized using one of two methods of result analysis, one based on functional brain anatomy and one, a probabilistic method, using a standard space of brain coordinates. The first consists of using the anatomical data a priori by requiring a fibre tract to pass through at least two manually selected regions of interest (ROIs) [60, 75]. Using a single ROI, the reconstructed tract is more likely to contain different fibres, some representing trajectories belonging to the tract being studied and others generated by partial volume effects or noise. The latter can be eliminated by selecting multiple ROIs along the fibre tract being reconstructed so as to avoid an erroneous deviation of the reconstruction algorithm from the actual trajectory (Fig. 8.9). This method makes it possible to track simply and non-invasively the position of several tracts with a high level of confidence [60, 75]. Its main drawback is that it cannot reconstruct bundles that are not well documented anatomically [75] and may also exhibit limitations in the presence of fibre deviations induced by brain disease.

The second probabilistic method is based on the assumption that errors induced by partial volume effects or low SNR have a random distribution and are not reproduced consistently if multiple studies of the same object are performed, and their results are superimposed. The same principle underpins a method that uses data from a large sample of subjects in a standard space of brain coordinates (e.g. the Talairach atlas). The first studies applying this method of normalization have yielded a high level of reproducibility for the large fibre bundles, but greater intersubject variability for the smaller bundles [39, 76–78].

### 8.4.5 The Problem of Validation

One of the critical problems in the development of fibre-tracking techniques is that there are no other available methods to assess the course of nerve fibres in vivo or reference standards to which data can be compared. Indeed, knowledge of white matter fibre anatomy derives from post-mortem studies, where even in the best conditions only the main fibre bundles can be followed and the resolution is insufficient to constitute a reference for validation [75].

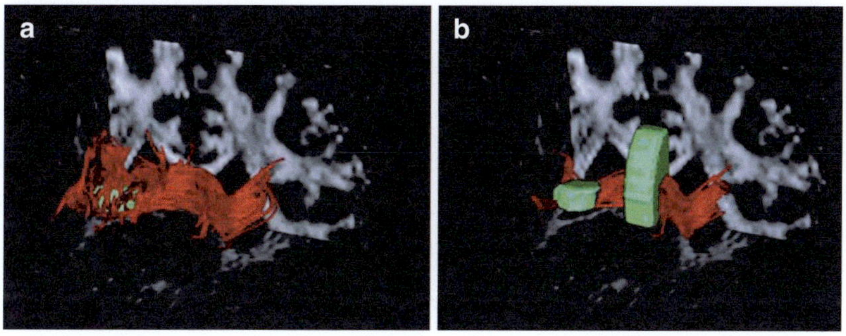


**Fig. 8.9** (**a**, **b**) The use of the multi-ROI approach improves tractographic reconstruction of white matter tracts. Above, the addition of a second ROI (**b**) specifically selects the fibre tract of interest

Ablation studies of animal models make it possible to document the course of axons using specific tracers. Though representing the reference standard for connectivity studies, these data cannot, however, be extended to humans because tracer methods follow single axons at the cell level, and axons may cross different fibre bundles along their course. Owing to the practical impossibility of obtaining adequate statistics for $10^{11}$ neurons, these methods cannot be used to validate effectively data obtained using tractographic techniques.

Despite the limitations outlined above, a good agreement between fibre tracking and anatomy has, however, been demonstrated [39, 76].

Another limitation for DTI-derived results validation is related not only to inter-scanner differences, but also to intra-scanner variability, meaning that diffusion tensor estimation, and subsequent fibre tracking, might be heavily influenced by slight differences even for the same subject undergoing the same MRI protocol at two different times [79]. Estimation of variability sources is currently being addressed also thanks to large, publicly available databases, such as the Alzheimer's Disease Neuroimaging Initiative [80] and the Parkinson's Progression Markers Initiative [81], which provide high-quality MRI data acquired on different scanners, from both patients and healthy subjects and at multiple timepoints. These databases represent a precious resource in order to identify and address those variability sources that largely influence tractography results.

## 8.5 Clinical Applications

The potential clinical applications of tractographic techniques are numerous [82, 83], first and foremost in physiological studies of human CNS, where they enable in vivo identification of the topographic distribution of circuits shown by anatomical primate research and surmised in man.

In neurophysiology, tractography has fostered the development of a new strategy to study brain activity patterns: anatomical connectivity. This technique is based on the possibility of visualizing directly the connections among the brain areas activated during a given task and conceptually complements two other strategies that explore connectivity, i.e. functional connectivity (the study of how two cerebral areas tend to work in a correlated manner) and effective connectivity (the study of the information flow within an active pattern by identifying its direction and orientation). Anatomical connectivity is essential, because it provides evidence for the existence of anatomical connections, which are indispensable elements to confirm and validate the results of functional and effective connectivity studies. An example is the study of the connectivity of the dopaminergic system, which originates in substantia nigra neurons in the pars compacta of the mesencephalon. Tractography has recently made it possible to identify the course of human dopaminergic fibres as far as the corpus striatum (nigrostriatal circuit) and their subsequent cortical distribution (cortico-striatal circuit) [84] (Fig. 8.10).

The use of this method in neurological investigations is obvious, especially in degenerative CNS disease. In Parkinson's disease, MR has a limited role except in the differential diagnosis from other diseases, since its diagnosis is essentially clinical but can only be confirmed by post-mortem histopathological examination. By identifying the dopaminergic fibres at their origin, tractography can quantify the axonal depletion and thus provide an index of disease severity. Another common degenerative disease, Alzheimer's, is characterized already in its early phase by a depletion of temporo-mesial neurons, which can be identified with tractography [85–93]. In Huntington's disease, a neurodegenerative autosomal dominate disorder, MR tractography has shown white matter abnormalities prior to the disease onset [94–96].

In neurophysiology, electrophysiological data – indirect indicators of fibre integrity – could be better interpreted using tractography, which is capable of displaying fibre tracts directly. For instance, corticospinal fibres can be identified and reconstructed with tractography from their

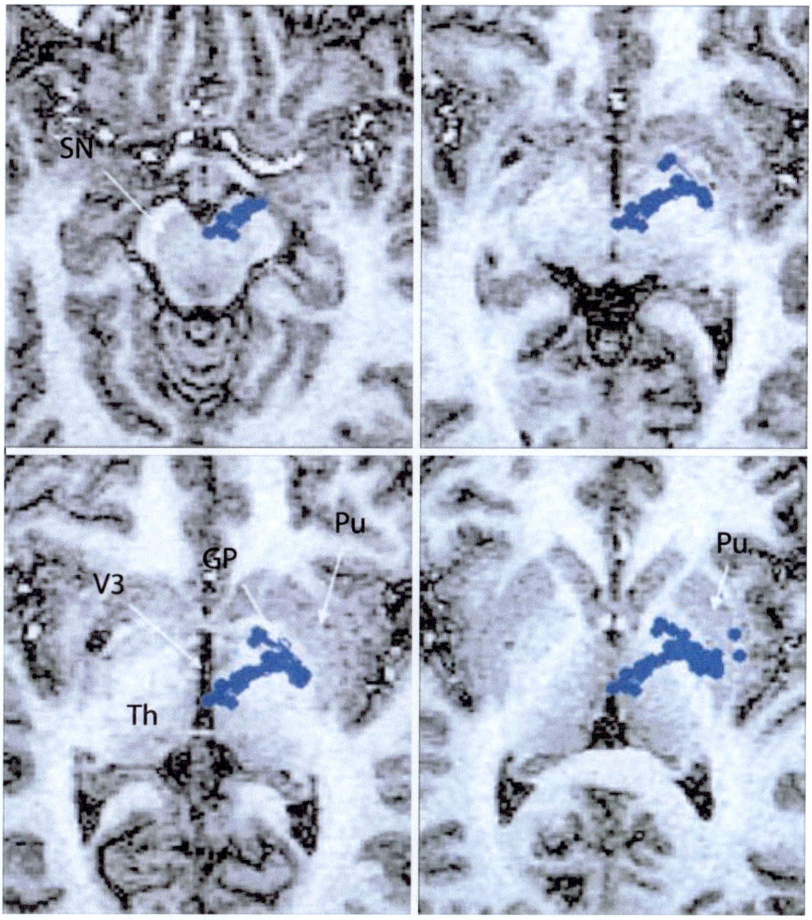


**Fig. 8.10** T1-weighted axial images at the level of the mesencephalon (*upper left*), subthalamic area (*upper right*) and thalamus (*lower left and right*). *Blue points* represent the fibre tract reconstructed from the putamen through globus pallidus, subthalamic area and medial substantia nigra. *GP* globus pallidus, *Pu* putamen, *SN* substantia nigra, *Th* thalamus, *V3* third ventricle (Image from Lehéricy et al. [84])

origin through the centrum semiovale, corona radiata, internal capsule and cerebral peduncle. Identification of this bundle is important in neurological diseases like multiple sclerosis, where demyelination and the consequent axon damage even at a distance from the lesion site can be documented and quantified using these techniques [97–112].

In neurosurgery, knowledge of the course of nerve fibre bundles (Fig. 8.11) and their relationships to the expanding lesion can preserve them from resection [113–123].

Another application of tractography in this field is represented by connectivity-based classification of a seed region. As the name suggests, this method classifies each voxel of the starting region for tractography on the basis of the region of the brain to which it connects with the highest probability. For example, it has been applied to identify areas of the basal ganglia connected to different cortical regions, both in healthy subjects and Parkinson's disease patients [124, 125]. Connectivity-based classification could also be used before and after surgery, in order to assess changes in the connectivity of the region near the surgical breach towards the rest of the brain.

Finally, tractography should be applied to identify and describe the brain plasticity phenomena secondary to CNS lesions. Identification of the axonal loss and consequent impairment of further adjacent or distant circuits, normally not involved in a given function, can offer insights into the complex phenomena underpinning clinical recovery and enable better targeted pharmacological and rehabilitation therapy [126–138].

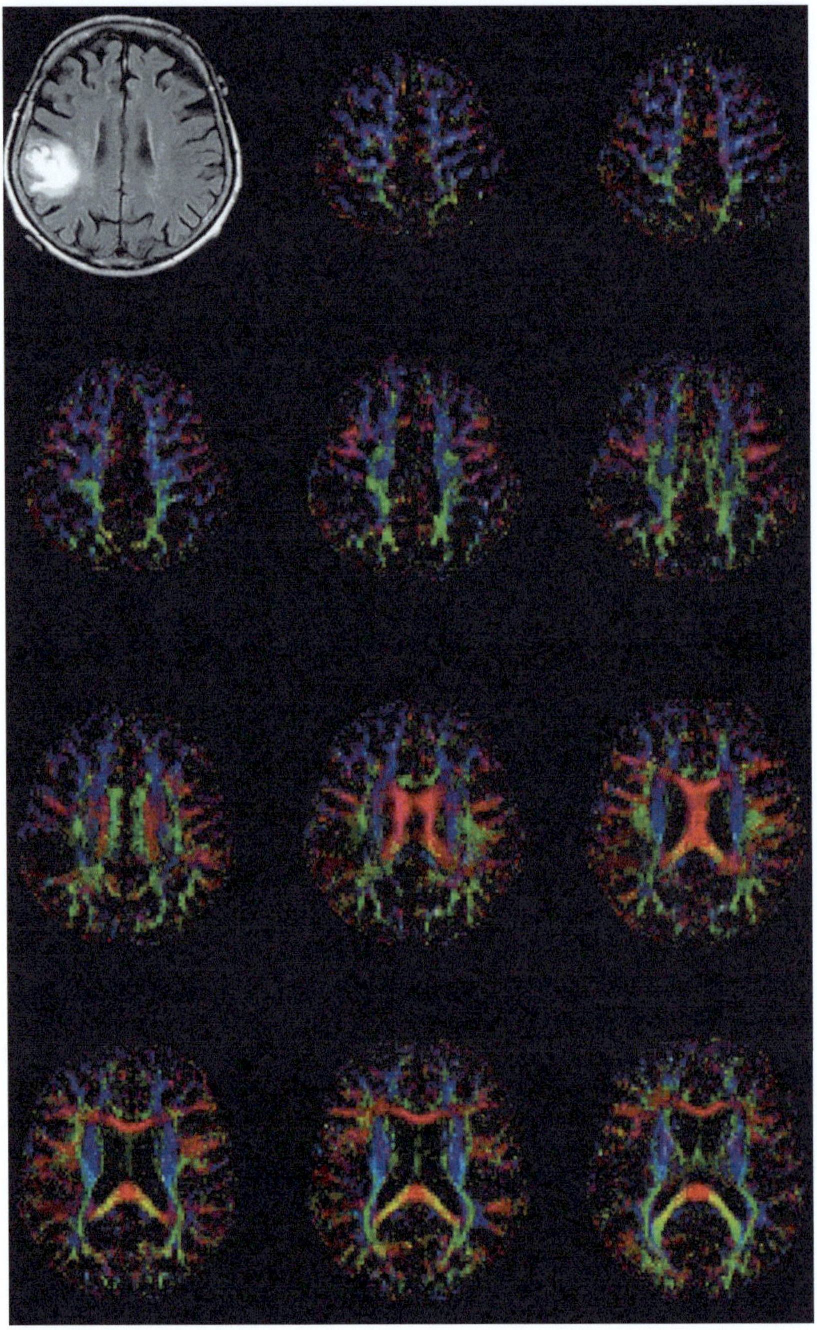

**Fig. 8.11** Axial FLAIR image (*upper left*) compared with fractional anisotropy maps. DTI-based colour orientation map: *red* = *x* direction; *green* = *y* direction; *blue* = *z* direction. A tumour shown in the FLAIR image alters the course of surrounding fibres in several slices, as shown by the DTI data

## Conclusion

We have described the main MR tractographic techniques, which enable in vivo and non-invasive reconstruction of the anatomy of axon fibres, documenting the connections among grey matter areas. Tractography is the natural complement of functional MR, which can depict the activation of these areas. Combined use of these techniques is expected to be performed with increasing frequency in the future [118, 121, 139, 140], and to yield useful results in the study of physiological and pathological CNS mechanisms, enabling better planning and quantification of therapeutic interventions.

## References


1. Basser PJ, Jones DK (2002) Diffusion-tensor MRI: theory, experimental design and data analysis – a technical review. NMR Biomed 15:456–467
2. Basser PJ, Pajevic S, Pierpaoli C et al (2000) In vivo fiber tractography using DT-MRI data. Magn Reson Med 44:625–632
3. Bammer R, Acar B, Moseley ME (2003) In vivo MR tractography using diffusion imaging. Eur J Radiol 45:223–234
4. Mori S, van Zijl PC (2002) Fiber tracking: principles and strategies – a technical review. NMR Biomed 15:468–480
5. Habas C (2004) Basic principles of diffusion tensor MR tractography. J Radiol 85:281–286
6. Conturo TE, Lori NF, Cull TS et al (1999) Tracking neuronal fiber pathways in the living human brain. Proc Natl Acad Sci U S A 96:10422–10427
7. Beaulieu C (2002) The basis of anisotropic water diffusion in the nervous system – a technical review. NMR Biomed 15:435–455
8. Moseley ME, Cohen Y, Kucharczyk J et al (1990) Diffusion-weighted MR imaging of anisotropic water diffusion in cat central nervous system. Radiology 176:439–445
9. Le Bihan D, Mangin JF, Poupon C et al (2001) Diffusion tensor imaging: concepts and applications. J Magn Reson Imaging 13:534–546
10. Basser PJ, Mattiello J, LeBihan D (1994) MR diffusion tensor spectroscopy and imaging. Biophys J 66:259–267
11. Basser PJ, Mattiello J, LeBihan D (1994) Estimation of the effective self-diffusion tensor from the NMR spin echo. J Magn Reson B 103:247–254
12. Batchelor PG, Moakher M, Atkinson D et al (2005) A rigorous framework for diffusion tensor calculus. Magn Reson Med 53:221–225
13. Parker GJ (2004) Analysis of MR diffusion weighted images. Br J Radiol 77 Spec No 2:S176–S185
14. Lori NF, Akbudak E, Shimony JS et al (2002) Diffusion tensor fiber tracking of human brain connectivity: acquisition methods, reliability analysis and biological results. NMR Biomed 15:494–515
15. Assaf Y, Freidlin RZ, Rohde GK et al (2004) New modeling and experimental framework to characterize hindered and restricted water diffusion in brain white matter. Magn Reson Med 52:965–978
16. Nagae-Poetscher LM, Jiang H, Wakana S et al (2004) High-resolution diffusion tensor imaging of the brain stem at 3 T. AJNR 25:1325–1330
17. Burdette JH, Elster AD, Ricci PE (1998) Calculation of apparent diffusion coefficients (ADCs) in brain using two-point and six-point methods. J Comput Assist Tomogr 22:792–794
18. Xing D, Papadakis NG, Huang CL et al (1997) Optimised diffusion weighting for measurement of apparent diffusion coefficient (ADC) in human brain. Magn Reson Imaging 15:771–784
19. Melhem ER, Mori S, Mukundan G et al (2002) Diffusion tensor MR imaging of the brain and white matter tractography. AJR 178:3–16
20. Descoteaux M, Deriche R, Knösche TR, Anwander A (2009) Deterministic and probabilistic tractography based on complex fibre orientation distributions. IEEE Trans Med Imaging 28:269–286
21. Jeurissen B, Leemans A, Tournier J-D et al (2012) Investigating the prevalence of complex fiber configurations in white matter tissue with diffusion magnetic resonance imaging. Hum Brain Mapp 34(11):2747–2766
22. Jones DK (2004) The effect of gradient sampling schemes on measures derived from diffusion tensor MRI: a Monte Carlo study. Magn Reson Med 51: 807–815
23. Daducci A, Canales-Rodriguez EJ, Descoteaux M et al (2013) Quantitative comparison of reconstruction methods for intra-voxel fiber recovery from diffusion MRI. IEEE Trans Med Imaging 33(2): 384–399
24. Griswold MA, Jakob PM, Heidemann RM et al (2002) Generalized autocalibrating partially parallel acquisitions (GRAPPA). Magn Reson Med 47: 1202–1210
25. Setsompop K, Cohen-Adad J, Gagoski BA et al (2012) Improving diffusion MRI using simultaneous multi-slice echo planar imaging. Neuroimage 63(1): 569–580
26. Paley MN, Lee KJ, Wild JM et al (2006) Simultaneous parallel inclined readout image technique. Magn Reson Imaging 24:557–562
27. Weaver JB (1988) Simultaneous multislice acquisition of MR images. Magn Reson Med 8:275–284
28. Feinberg DA, Reese TG, Wedeen VJ (2002) Simultaneous echo refocusing in EPI. Magn Reson Med 48:1–5
29. Reese TG, Benner T, Wang R et al (2009) Halving imaging time of whole brain diffusion spectrum imaging and diffusion tractography using simultaneous image refocusing in EPI. J Magn Reson Imaging 29:517–522
30. Breuer FA, Blaimer M, Heidemann RM et al (2005) Controlled aliasing in parallel imaging results in higher acceleration (CAIPIRINHA) for multi-slice imaging. Magn Reson Med 53:684–691
31. Larkman DJ, Hajnal JV, Herlihy AH et al (2001) Use of multicoil arrays for separation of signal from multiple slices simultaneously excited. J Magn Reson Imaging 13:313–317
32. Moeller S, Yacoub E, Olman CA et al (2010) Multiband multislice GE-EPI at 7 tesla, with 16-fold

acceleration using partial parallel imaging with application to high spatial and temporal whole-brain fMRI. Magn Reson Med 63:1144–1153
33. Nunes RG, Hajnal JV, Golay X, et al. (2006) Simultaneous slice excitation and reconstruction for single shot EPI. Proceedings of the 14th Annual Meeting of ISMRM, Seattle, p. 293
34. Setsompop K, Gagoski BA, Polimeni J et al (2012) Blipped-controlled aliasing in parallel imaging (blipped-CAIPI) for simultaneous multi-slice EPI with reduced g-factor penalty. Magn Reson Med 67:1210–1224
35. Xue R, van Zijl PC, Crain BJ et al (1999) In vivo three-dimensional reconstruction of rat brain axonal projections by diffusion tensor imaging. Magn Reson Med 42:1123–1127
36. Mori S, Crain BJ, Chacko VP et al (1999) Three-dimensional tracking of axonal projections in the brain by magnetic resonance imaging. Ann Neurol 45:265–269
37. Parker GJ, Stephan KE, Barker GJ et al (2002) Initial demonstration of in vivo tracing of axonal projections in the macaque brain and comparison with the human brain using diffusion tensor imaging and fast marching tractography. Neuroimage 15:797–809
38. Parker GJ, Wheeler-Kingshott CA, Barker GJ (2002) Estimating distributed anatomical connectivity using fast marching methods and diffusion tensor imaging. IEEE Trans Med Imaging 21:505–512
39. Ciccarelli O, Toosy AT, Parker GJ et al (2003) Diffusion tractography based group mapping of major white-matter pathways in the human brain. Neuroimage 19:1545–1555
40. Duncan JS, Papademetris X, Yang J et al (2004) Geometric strategies for neuroanatomic analysis from MRI. Neuroimage 23(1):S34–S45
41. Wu YC, Field AS, Chung MK et al (2004) Quantitative analysis of diffusion tensor orientation: theoretical framework. Magn Reson Med 52: 1146–1155
42. Parker GJ, Alexander DC (2003) Probabilistic Monte Carlo based mapping of cerebral connections utilising whole-brain crossing fibre information. Inf Process Med Imaging 18:684–695
43. Parker GJ, Haroon HA, Wheeler-Kingshott CA (2003) A framework for a streamline-based probabilistic index of connectivity (PICo) using a structural interpretation of MRI diffusion measurements. J Magn Reson Imaging 18:242–254
44. Behrens TE, Woolrich MW, Jenkinson M et al (2003) Characterization and propagation of uncertainty in diffusion-weighted MR imaging. Magn Reson Med 50:1077–1088
45. Behrens TE, Berg HJ, Jbabdi S et al (2007) Probabilistic diffusion tractography with multiple fibre orientations: what can we gain? Neuroimage 34(1):144–155
46. Filippi M, van den Heuvel MP, Fornito A et al (2013) Assessment of system dysfunction in the brain through MRI-based connectomics. Lancet Neurol 12:1189–1199
47. de Schotten MT, Ffytche DH, Bizzi A et al (2011) Atlasing location, asymmetry and inter-subject variability of white matter tracts in the human brain with MR diffusion tractography. Neuroimage 54(1): 49–59
48. Hagmann P (2005) From diffusion MRI to brain connectomics. Signal Processing Institute. Ecole Polytechnique Fédérale de Lausanne (EPFL). Lausanne, p 127. doi:10.5075/epfl-thesis-3230
49. Sporns O, Tononi G, Kotter R (2005) The human connectome: a structural description of the human brain. PLoS Comput Biol 1:e42
50. Bullmore E, Sporns O (2009) Complex brain networks: graph theoretical analysis of structural and functional systems. Nat Rev Neurosci 10(3):186–198
51. Wen W, Zhu WL, He Y et al (2011) Discrete neuroanatomical networks are associated with specific cognitive abilities in old age. J Neurosci 31(4):1204–1212
52. Bernhardt BC, Bonilha L, Gross DW (2015) Network analysis for a network disorder: the emerging role of graph theory in the study of epilepsy. Epilepsy Behav 50:162–170
53. Griffa A, Baumann PS, Thiran J-P et al (2013) Structural connectomics in brain diseases. Neuroimage 80:515–526
54. Korgaonkar MS, Fornito A, Williams LM et al (2014) Abnormal structural networks characterize major depressive disorder: a connectome analysis. Biol Psychiatry 76:567–574
55. Phillips DJ, McGlaughlin A, Ruth D et al (2015) Graph theoretic analysis of structural connectivity across the spectrum of Alzheimer's disease: the importance of graph creation methods. NeuroImage Clin 7:377–390
56. Jones DK, Basser PJ (2004) "Squashing peanuts and smashing pumpkins": how noise distorts diffusion-weighted MR data. Magn Reson Med 52:979–993
57. Jones DK (2003) Determining and visualizing uncertainty in estimates of fiber orientation from diffusion tensor MRI. Magn Reson Med 49:7–12
58. Anderson AW (2001) Theoretical analysis of the effects of noise on diffusion tensor imaging. Magn Reson Med 46:1174–1188
59. Lazar M, Weinstein DM, Tsuruda JS et al (2003) White matter tractography using diffusion tensor deflection. Hum Brain Mapp 18:306–321
60. Huang H, Zhang J, van Zijl PC et al (2004) Analysis of noise effects on DTI-based tractography using the brute-force and multi-ROI approach. Magn Reson Med 52:559–565
61. Heim S, Hahn K, Samann PG et al (2004) Assessing DTI data quality using bootstrap analysis. Magn Reson Med 52:582–589
62. Alexander AL, Hasan KM, Lazar M et al (2001) Analysis of partial volume effects in diffusion-tensor MRI. Magn Reson Med 45:770–780
63. Barrick TR, Clark CA (2004) Singularities in diffusion tensor fields and their relevance in white matter fiber tractography. Neuroimage 22:481–491
64. Wedeen VJ, Hagmann P, Tseng WYI et al (2005) Mapping complex tissue architecture with diffusion

spectrum magnetic resonance imaging. Magn Reson Med 54:1377–1386
65. Tuch DS (2004) Q-ball imaging. Magn Reson Med 52:1358–1372
66. Tristán-Vega A, Westin C-F, Aja-Fernández S (2009) Estimation of fiber orientation density probability density functions in high angular resolution diffusion imaging. Neuroimage 47:638–650
67. Aganj I, Lenglet C, Sapiro E et al (2010) Reconstruction of the orientation distribution function in single and multiple shell q-ball imaging with constant solid angle. Magn Reson Med 64:554–566
68. Liu C, Bammer R, Acar B et al (2004) Characterizing non-Gaussian diffusion by using generalized diffusion tensors. Magn Reson Med 51:924–937
69. Assaf Y, Basser P (2005) Composite hindered and restricted model of diffusion (charmed) MR imaging of the human brain. Neuroimage 27:48–58
70. Tournier JD, Calamante F, Gadian DG et al (2004) Direct estimation of the fiber orientation density function from diffusion-weighted MRI data using spherical deconvolution. Neuroimage 23:1176–1185
71. Alexander DC, (2005) Maximum entropy spherical deconvolution for diffusion MRI. In: Christensen GE, Soka M (eds) Information processing in medical imaging, proceedings, pp 76–87
72. Dell'Acqua F, Scifo P, Rizzo G et al (2010) A modified damped Richardson–Lucy algorithm to reduce isotropic background effects in spherical deconvolution. Neuroimage 49:1446–1458
73. Kaden E, Knösche TR, Anwander A (2007) Parametric spherical deconvolution: inferring anatomical connectivity using diffusion MR imaging. Neuroimage 37:474–488
74. Patel V, Shi Y, Thompson PM et al (2010) Mesh-based spherical deconvolution: a flexible approach to reconstruction of non-negative fiber orientation distributions. Neuroimage 51:1071–1081
75. Mori H, Masutani Y, Aoki S et al (2003) Simple visualization of the corticospinal pathway using tractography: one-ROI and two-ROI methods. Nippon Igaku Hoshasen Gakkai Zasshi 63:51–53
76. Ciccarelli O, Parker GJ, Toosy AT et al (2003) From diffusion tractography to quantitative white matter tract measures: a reproducibility study. Neuroimage 18:348–359
77. Catani M, Jones DK, Donato R et al (2003) Occipito-temporal connections in the human brain. Brain 126:2093–2107
78. Holodny AI, Gor DM, Watts R et al (2005) Diffusion-tensor MR tractography of somatotopic organization of corticospinal tracts in the internal capsule: initial anatomic results in contradistinction to prior reports. Radiology 234:649–653
79. Lemkaddem A, Daducci A, Vulliemoz S et al (2012) A multi-center study: intra-scan and inter-scan variability of diffusion spectrum imaging. Neuroimage 62(1):87–94
80. Jack CR, Bernstein MA, Fox NC et al (2008) The Alzheimer's Disease Neuroimaging Initiative (ADNI): MRI methods. J Magn Reson Imaging JMRI 27(4):685–691
81. Marek K, Jennings D, Lasch S et al (2011) The Parkinson Progression Marker Initiative (PPMI). Prog Neurobiol 95(4):629–635
82. Oppenheim C, Rodrigo S, Poupon C et al (2004) Diffusion tensor MR imaging of the brain. Clinical applications. J Radiol 85:287–296
83. Sundgren PC, Dong Q, Gomez-Hassan D et al (2004) Diffusion tensor imaging of the brain: review of clinical applications. Neuroradiology 46:3 39–350
84. Lehericy S, Ducros M, Van de Moortele PF et al (2004) Diffusion tensor fiber tracking shows distinct corticostriatal circuits in humans. Ann Neurol 55:522–529
85. Rose SE, Chen F, Chalk JB et al (2000) Loss of connectivity in Alzheimer's disease: an evaluation of white matter tract integrity with colour coded MR diffusion tensor imaging. J Neurol Neurosurg Psychiatry 69:528–530
86. Bozzali M, Franceschi M, Falini A et al (2001) Quantification of tissue damage in AD using diffusion tensor and magnetization transfer MRI. Neurology 57:1135–1137
87. Bozzali M, Falini A, Franceschi M et al (2002) White matter damage in Alzheimer's disease assessed in vivo using diffusion tensor magnetic resonance imaging. J Neurol Neurosurg Psychiatry 72:742–746
88. Horsfield MA, Jones DK (2002) Applications of diffusion weighted and diffusion tensor MRI to white matter diseases – a review. NMR Biomed 15:570–577
89. Larsson EM, Englund E, Sjobeck M et al (2004) MRI with diffusion tensor imaging post-mortem at 3.0 T in a patient with frontotemporal dementia. Dement Geriatr Cogn Disord 17:316–319
90. Sugihara S, Kinoshita T, Matsusue E et al (2004) Usefulness of diffusion tensor imaging of white matter in Alzheimer disease and vascular dementia. Acta Radiol 45:658–663
91. Sun Y, Du XK, Zhang ZX et al (2004) Relationship between the data from MR-diffusion tensor imaging and the clinical cognitive evaluation in Alzheimer's disease. Zhongguo Yi Xue Ke Xue Yuan Xue Bao 26:134–138
92. Yoshida T, Shiga K, Yoshikawa K et al (2004) White matter loss in the splenium of the corpus callosum in a case of posterior cortical atrophy: a diffusion tensor imaging study. Eur Neurol 52:77–81
93. Sullivan EV, Pfefferbaum A (2003) Diffusion tensor imaging in normal aging and neuropsychiatric disorders. Eur J Radiol 45:244–255
94. Phillips O, Sanchez-Castaneda C, Elifani F et al (2013) Tractography of the corpus callosum in Huntington's disease. PLoS One 8:1–9
95. Phillips O, Squitieri F, Sanchez-Castaneda C et al (2014) Deep white matter in Huntington's disease. PLoS One 23(9):10

96. Phillips O, Squitieri F, Sanchez-Castaneda C et al (2015) The cortispinal tract in Huntington's disease. Cereb Cortex 25(9):2670–2682
97. Rovaris M, Gallo A, Valsasina P et al (2005) Short-term accrual of gray matter pathology in patients with progressive multiple sclerosis: an in vivo study using diffusion tensor MRI. Neuroimage 24:1139–1146
98. Hong YH, Lee KW, Sung JJ et al (2004) Diffusion tensor MRI as a diagnostic tool of upper motor neuron involvement in amyotrophic lateral sclerosis. J Neurol Sci 227:73–78
99. Yin H, Lim CC, Ma L et al (2004) Combined MR spectroscopic imaging and diffusion tensor MRI visualizes corticospinal tract degeneration in amyotrophic lateral sclerosis. J Neurol 251:1249–1254
100. Abe O, Yamada H, Masutani Y et al (2004) Amyotrophic lateral sclerosis: diffusion tensor tractography and voxel-based analysis. NMR Biomed 17:411–416
101. Cassol E, Ranjeva JP, Ibarrola D et al (2004) Diffusion tensor imaging in multiple sclerosis: a tool for monitoring changes in normal-appearing white matter. Mult Scler 10:188–196
102. Ulug AM, Grunewald T, Lin MT et al (2004) Diffusion tensor imaging in the diagnosis of primary lateral sclerosis. J Magn Reson Imaging 19:34–39
103. Rashid W, Hadjiprocopis A, Griffin CM et al (2004) Diffusion tensor imaging of early relapsing-remitting multiple sclerosis with histogram analysis using automated segmentation and brain volume correction. Mult Scler 10:9–15
104. Sach M, Winkler G, Glauche V et al (2004) Diffusion tensor MRI of early upper motor neuron involvement in amyotrophic lateral sclerosis. Brain 127:340–350
105. Ciccarelli O, Werring DJ, Barker GJ et al (2003) A study of the mechanisms of normal-appearing white matter damage in multiple sclerosis using diffusion tensor imaging – evidence of Wallerian degeneration. J Neurol 250:287–292
106. Cercignani M, Bozzali M, Iannucci G et al (2002) Intravoxel and inter-voxel coherence in patients with multiple sclerosis assessed using diffusion tensor MRI. J Neurol 249:875–883
107. Tench CR, Morgan PS, Wilson M et al (2002) White matter mapping using diffusion tensor MRI. Magn Reson Med 47:967–972
108. Guo AC, MacFall JR, Provenzale JM (2002) Multiple sclerosis: diffusion tensor MR imaging for evaluation of normal appearing white matter. Radiology 222:729–736
109. Filippi M, Rocca MA, Falini A et al (2002) Correlations between structural CNS damage and functional MRI changes in primary progressive MS. Neuroimage 15:537–546
110. Assaf Y, Ben-Bashat D, Chapman J et al (2002) High b-value q-space analyzed diffusion-weighted MRI: application to multiple sclerosis. Magn Reson Med 47:115–126
111. Horsfield MA, Larsson HB, Jones DK et al (1998) Diffusion magnetic resonance imaging in multiple sclerosis. J Neurol Neurosurg Psychiatry 64(1):S80–S84
112. Castriota-Scanderbeg A, Tomaiuolo F, Sabatini U et al (2000) Demyelinating plaques in relapsing-remitting and secondary-progressive multiple sclerosis: assessment with diffusion MR imaging. AJNR 21:862–868
113. Nimsky C, Ganslandt O, Hastreiter P et al (2005) Intraoperative diffusion-tensor MR imaging: shifting of white matter tracts during neurosurgical procedures – initial experience. Radiology 234:218–225
114. Wu JS, Zhou LF, Hong XN et al (2003) Role of diffusion tensor imaging in neuronavigation surgery of brain tumors involving pyramidal tracts. Zhonghua Wai Ke Za Zhi 41:662–666
115. Clark CA, Barrick TR, Murphy MM et al (2003) White matter fiber tracking in patients with space-occupying lesions of the brain: a new technique for neurosurgical planning? Neuroimage 20:1601–1608
116. Akai H, Mori H, Aoki S et al (2005) Diffusion tensor tractography of gliomatosis cerebri: fiber tracking through the tumor. J Comput Assist Tomogr 29:127–129
117. Nimsky C, Ganslandt O, Hastreiter P et al (2005) Preoperative and intraoperative diffusion tensor imaging-based fiber tracking in glioma surgery. Neurosurgery 56:130–138
118. Parmar H, Sitoh YY, Yeo TT (2004) Combined magnetic resonance tractography and functional magnetic resonance imaging in evaluation of brain tumors involving the motor system. J Comput Assist Tomogr 28:551–556
119. Kier EL, Staib LH, Davis LM et al (2004) MR imaging of the temporal stem: anatomic dissection tractography of the uncinate fasciculus, inferior occipitofrontal fasciculus, and Meyer's loop of the optic radiation. AJNR 25:677–691
120. Barboriak DP (2003) Imaging of brain tumors with diffusion-weighted and diffusion tensor MR imaging. Magn Reson Imaging Clin N Am 11:379–401
121. Guye M, Parker GJ, Symms M et al (2003) Combined functional MRI and tractography to demonstrate the connectivity of the human primary motor cortex in vivo. Neuroimage 19:1349–1360
122. Holodny AI, Ollenschlager M (2002) Diffusion imaging in brain tumors. Neuroimaging Clin N Am 12:107–124
123. Holodny AI, Schwartz TH, Ollenschleger M et al (2001) Tumor involvement of the corticospinal tract: diffusion magnetic resonance tractography with intraoperative correlation. J Neurosurg 95:1082
124. Leh SE, Ptito A, Chakravarty MM et al (2007) Fronto-striatal connections in the human brain: a probabilistic diffusion tractography study. Neurosci Lett 419:113–118
125. Sharman M, Valabregue R, Perlbarg V et al (2013) Parkinson's disease patients show reduced cortical-

subcortical sensorimotor connectivity. Mov Disord 28(4):447–454
126. Le TH, Mukherjee P, Henry RG et al (2005) Diffusion tensor imaging with three-dimensional fiber tractography of traumatic axonal shearing injury: an imaging correlate for the posterior callosal "disconnection" syndrome: case report. Neurosurgery 56:189
127. Naganawa S, Sato C, Ishihra S et al (2004) Serial evaluation of diffusion tensor brain fiber tracking in a patient with severe diffuse axonal injury. AJNR 25:1553–1556
128. Huisman TA, Schwamm LH, Schaefer PW et al (2004) Diffusion tensor imaging as potential biomarker of white matter injury in diffuse axonal injury. AJNR 25:370–376
129. Huisman TA, Sorensen AG, Hergan K et al (2003) Diffusion-weighted imaging for the evaluation of diffuse axonal injury in closed head injury. J Comput Assist Tomogr 27:5–11
130. Arfanakis K, Haughton VM, Carew JD et al (2002) Diffusion tensor MR imaging in diffuse axonal injury. AJNR 23:794–802
131. Konishi J, Yamada K, Kizu O et al (2005) MR tractography for the evaluation of functional recovery from lenticulostriate infarcts. Neurology 64:108–113
132. Yamada K, Ito H, Nakamura H et al (2004) Stroke patients' evolving symptoms assessed by tractography. J Magn Reson Imaging 20:923–929
133. Munoz Maniega S, Bastin ME, Armitage PA et al (2004) Temporal evolution of water diffusion parameters is different in grey and white matter in human ischaemic stroke. J Neurol Neurosurg Psychiatry 75:1714–1718
134. Thomalla G, Glauche V, Koch MA et al (2004) Diffusion tensor imaging detects early Wallerian degeneration of the pyramidal tract after ischemic stroke. Neuroimage 22:1767–1774
135. Huisman TA (2003) Diffusion-weighted imaging: basic concepts and application in cerebral stroke and head trauma. Eur Radiol 13:2283–2297
136. Kunimatsu A, Aoki S, Masutani Y et al (2003) Three-dimensional white matter tractography by diffusion tensor imaging in ischaemic stroke involving the corticospinal tract. Neuroradiology 45:532–535
137. Sotak CH (2002) The role of diffusion tensor imaging in the evaluation of ischemic brain injury – a review. NMR Biomed 15:561–569
138. Huisman TA, Hawighorst H, Benoit CH et al (2001) Diffusion weighted MRI: ischemic and traumatic injuries of the central nervous system. Radiologe 41:1038–1047
139. Johansen-Berg H, Behrens TE, Sillery E et al (2005) Functional-anatomical validation and individual variation of diffusion tractography-based segmentation of the human thalamus. Cereb Cortex 15:31–39
140. Toosy AT, Ciccarelli O, Parker GJ et al (2004) Characterizing function-structure relationships in the human visual system with functional MRI and diffusion tensor imaging. Neuroimage 21:1452–1463

# 3.0 T Perfusion MRI Dynamic Susceptibility Contrast and Dynamic Contrast-Enhanced Techniques

9

Giuseppe Maria Giannatempo,
Tommaso Scarabino, Teresa Popolizio,
Tullio Parracino, Ettore Serricchio,
and Annalisa Simeone

Cerebral perfusion is the process by which oxygen and glucose are supplied to the brain capillaries through the circulation. Disruption of brain perfusion is found in nearly all types of brain disease, most notably stroke and tumors, but also in neurodegenerative disorders [1–8].

Imaging the regional distribution of cerebral blood flow quantitatively is a diagnostic and technical challenge [3, 7, 9]. $H_2{}^{15}O$ positron emission tomography (PET), which uses a freely diffusible tracer and can quantitate blood flow with relative insensitivity to vascular transit time variations, has been in the past the gold standard of perfusion studies [7, 10].

However, it is an expensive examination entailing radioactive dosing and invasive monitoring, besides having low intrinsic spatial resolution. Moreover, $H_2{}^{15}O$ PET imaging centers are relatively few due to difficulties in staffing and maintaining an on-site cyclotron. Hence the interest is in adapting more widespread imaging modalities, such as magnetic resonance imaging (MRI), to the quantitative measurement of blood flow.

MR perfusion imaging is increasingly being used for the assessment of brain perfusion in several different pathological conditions including ischemic stroke [8, 11–15], neurovascular disease [16–19], brain tumors [20–28], and neurodegenerative disorders [29–35]. In brain tumors, perfusion MRI has been applied to grade gliomas; to distinguish between different tumor types, like primary tumor from solitary metastases or lymphoma; to differentiate radiation necrosis from recurrent tumor [2]; and to discriminate high-grade neoplasms from nonneoplastic lesions like abscess [20–28].

Perfusion MRI has been used in the diagnosis of dementia, including Alzheimer's disease, mild cognitive impairment and non-Alzheimer's dementia [29–34], epilepsy [35], and multiple sclerosis [36].

Unlike angiography, which depicts flow within large vessels, MR perfusion techniques are sensitive to perfusion at such microscopic levels as the capillary bed.

Measurement of tissue perfusion depends on the ability to measure serially the concentration of a tracer in a target organ. Tracers can be divided into exogenous and endogenous. The former include paramagnetic contrast agents, while magnetically labeled blood is currently the sole available endogenous tracer [1, 3]. Obtaining

G.M. Giannatempo (✉) • T. Popolizio • T. Parracino
E. Serricchio • A. Simeone
Department of Radiology and Neuroradiology,
"IRCCS Casa Sollievo della Sofferenza",
San Giovanni Rotondo (FG), Italy
e-mail: giannatempogiuseppe@libero.it

T. Scarabino
Department of Radiology and Neuroradiology,
PO "L. Bonomo" Hospital, Andria (BT), Italy



T. Scarabino et al. (eds.), *High Field Brain MRI*, DOI 10.1007/978-3-319-44174-0_9

**Table 9.1** Three types of perfusion techniques

| | DSC | DCE | ASL |
|---|---|---|---|
| Full term | Dynamic susceptibility contrast | Dynamic contrast enhanced | Arterial spin labeling |
| Bolus handling | Bolus tracking | Bolus passage | Bolus tagging |
| Acquisition point | First pass of contrast agent | Accumulation of contrast agent | Accumulation of tagged blood |
| Exogenous/endogenous | Exogenous | Exogenous | Endogenous |
| Contrast agent | Gadolinium chelate | Gadolinium chelate | Without contrast agent |
| Tracer model | Nondiffusible blood pool tracer | Flow or permeability-limited diffusible tracer | Diffusible tracer |
| Relaxation mechanism | T2/T2* relaxation | T1 relaxation | Magnetic labeled blood T1 relaxation |
| Effect | Increased susceptibility effect | T1-shortening effect | Blood magnetization inversion |
| Signal behavior | Decreased signal | Increased signal | Subtracted signal |

From Jahng et al. [5], modified

hemodynamic parameters from serial measurements of tissue tracer concentrations requires the use of a general model of the way in which the tracer passes through or diffuses in the target organ that takes into account tracer diffusibility from intravascular to extravascular space, volume of distribution, equilibrium, and half-life.

Two main perfusion MRI approaches have been developed: those with and those without the use of an exogenous contrast agent (Table 9.1).

The first group of techniques (exogenous tracer methods) includes dynamic susceptibility contrast (DSC)-MRI and dynamic contrast-enhanced (DCE)-MRI, while the second group (that uses endogenous tracer) includes arterial spin labeling (ASL) [5].

Exogenous tracer methods for perfusion MRI (DSC and DCE) use a model assuming that the tracer is confined to the intravascular compartment and does not diffuse to the extravascular space [1, 3–5]. Both techniques involve the rapid intravenous injection of a magnetic resonance contrast agent (gadolinium chelate) and the serial measurement of induced signal modification. Both DSC and DCE are patterned after tracer kinetic models of tissue perfusion, which utilize a tracer (gadolinium chelate), track the tracer through the tissue, and then analyze its ingress/egress [5].

DSC utilizes the T2* effect of a bolus of gadolinium chelate and measures the transient decrease in signal intensity during the passage of the bolus through the vasculature.

On the other hand, DCE relies on the observation that gadolinium-chelate contrast agents, after the transient T2* effects, cause relative T1 shortening within the blood pool (and within any extravascular space in which the contrast agent accumulates because of leakage across the blood-brain barrier or the blood-tumor barrier), causing the increase in signal intensity [5]. In DCE T1-weighted images are acquired dynamically before, during, and after bolus injection of contrast medium.

Contrast-based perfusion imaging methods require a high-temporal resolution to capture the pass of the bolus, particularly when most of the contrast agent remains intravascular.

Endogenous tracer methods in perfusion MRI (ASL) use a model that assumes that the tracer diffuses freely from the intravascular compartment into the tissue compartment. This model is similar to the one used in PET measuring the regional accumulation of the tracer, which is influenced by regional blood flow and its half-life [1].

In ASL water protons within inflowing arterial blood are magnetically labeled (or "tagged") by application of a special radiofrequency pulse designed to invert spins in a thick slab proximal to the slice of interest [1], taking advantage of using the magnetically labeled blood itself as an endogenous tracer.

By comparing tagged and untagged baseline images, qualitative or quantitative images can be obtained.

The modeling of ASL is similar to that used in the analysis of PET perfusion imaging, since in ASL methods arterial blood water is labeled as an endogenous diffusible tracer that can detect functional deficiencies in a way similar to PET [1] and permitting a quantitative measurement of the real cerebral blood flow, giving absolute values of perfusion of tissue by blood.

This chapter illustrates the gadolinium-based techniques, focusing primarily on the DSC, which currently has greater widespread clinical application than DCE.

## 9.1 Dynamic Susceptibility Contrast (DSC)-MRI

Dynamic susceptibility contrast perfusion (DSC)-MRI, also called dynamic susceptibility-weighted perfusion imaging or first-pass bolus tracking perfusion MRI, is the most widespread, clinically applicable MR technique for estimating cerebral hemodynamic parameters, especially in stroke, but also for tumor imaging and other research applications.

This technique is based on the passage of a bolus of contrast medium through the arterial and capillary circulation and on the transient changes it produces in vessels and surrounding tissues (Fig. 9.1).

Under normal perfusion conditions, in the presence of an intact blood-brain barrier (BBB), the contrast medium remains confined within the vascular network and does not diffuse in the extravascular space. While passing through the cerebral vasculature, a short bolus of contrast material produces local magnetic field inhomogeneities that lead to a reduction in the transverse relaxation time of the tissue. This susceptibility effect can be recorded by a series of ultrafast T2*- or T2-weighted sequences using gradient-echo and spin-echo sequences, respectively. The signal intensity-time curves can be converted to concentration-time curves, which allow the calculation of hemodynamic parameters such as blood volume, blood flow, and transit time (Fig. 9.2).

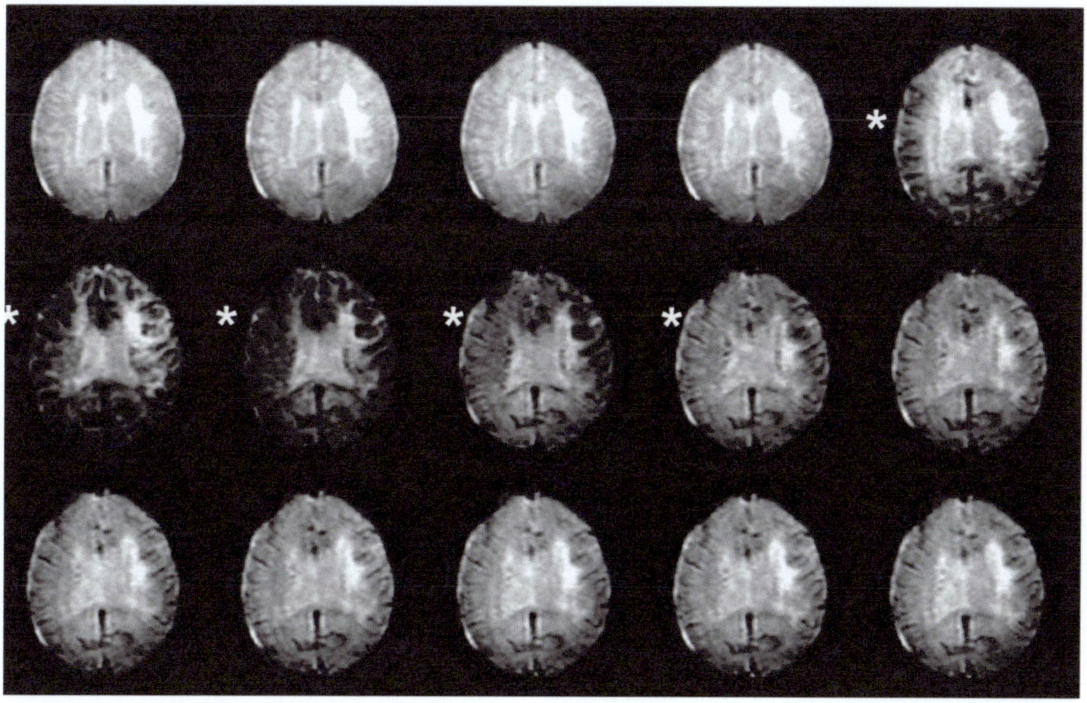


**Fig. 9.1** Series of T2*-weighted images from a single axial slice during the passage of a bolus of contrast agent. When the bolus arrives, it produces signal attenuation (*)

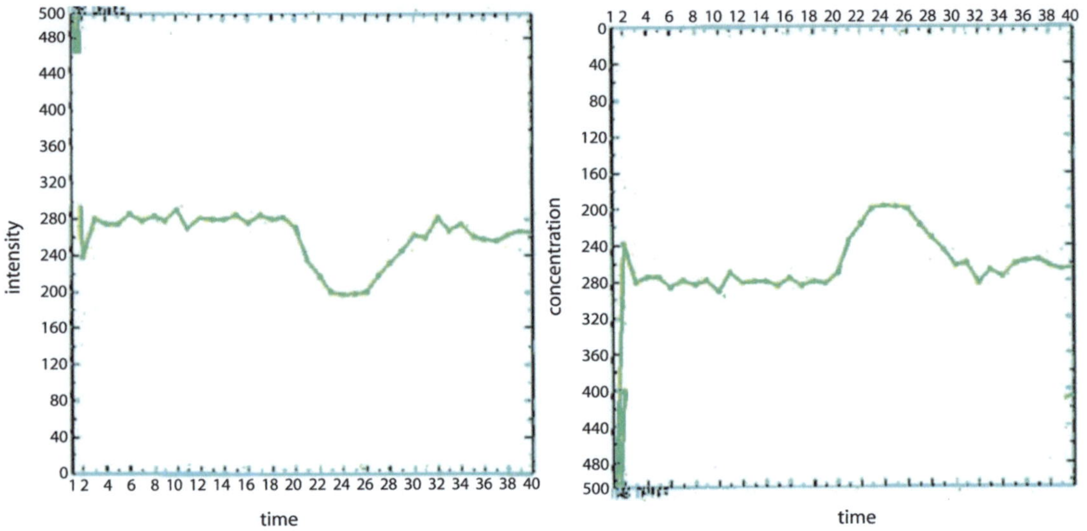


**Fig. 9.2** The inversion proportion between signal drop and concentration of contrast agent permits the calculation of the relative concentration from the signal intensity curve

In pathological perfusion conditions, e.g., hyperacute ischemic lesion, the signal reduction is attenuated or delayed, whereas in brain tumor, the signal varies in relation to grade.

Perfusion imaging requires (1) rapid administration of the contrast agent, (2) acquisition of ultrafast sequences, and (3) post-processing of the native images to calculate the intensity-time curve and obtain perfusion maps.

- Infusion of the gadolinium-chelated agent must be as rapid as possible to ensure correct mixing of the agent with blood and a sharp signal drop profile. This requires using a large intravenous line (18 or, preferably, 16 gauge), an automatic injector, a dose of up to 0.2 mmol/kg of body weight (or less at 3.0 T, see below), and a bolus injection rate of 3–5 ml/s, followed by a 25 ml (range 10–30 ml) saline flush at the same rate, to push the bolus toward the heart.

Bolus injection of the gadolinium chelate should commence after about 20-second delay from the start of the DSC sequence.

- Imaging sequences must be sufficiently fast to allow accurate measurement of the rapidly changing signal from the first pass of the bolus and have adequate temporal resolution ( < 2 s for the entire brain) [1]. The most widely applied imaging sequences for these studies are T2*-weighted gradient-echo single-shot echo-planar imaging (EPI) and T2-weighted spin-echo EPI (Table 9.2).

**Table 9.2** Exogenous agent perfusion techniques: imaging sequences

| | DSC | DCE |
|---|---|---|
| Acquisition | 2D or 3D dynamic acquisition | 2D or 3D dynamic acquisition |
| Sequences | Common: 2D single-shot GE EPI | Common: 3D GE (FSPGR, FLASH, THRIVE) |
| TR | Intermediate TR < 2 s | Shortest TR < 0.5 |
| TE | Intermediate TE = 30–40 ms for GE | Shortest TE < 10 ms |
| Flip angle | Intermediate FA = 60–90° | Small FA = 20° |
| Total scan duration | Relatively short ( < 2 min) | Long ( = 5–6 min) |

From Jahng et al. [5], modified

Spin-echo EPI sequences display excellent sensitivity for the susceptibility effect produced by 5 μm capillaries. Gradient-echo EPI sequences are generally more sensitive up to a vessel diameter of 7 μm. Spin-echo sequences are thus inherently weighted toward the microvasculature and are therefore less sensitive to larger vessels.

Gradient-echo EPI sequences are currently those used most frequently [37–40]. They are characterized by superior sensitivity in detecting the signal change produced by the passage of the contrast material and therefore require smaller doses of the agent. Their drawback is their high sensitivity not only to the microvasculature but also to the macrovasculature, including large arteries and veins on the brain surface. Susceptibility effects are elicited not only by the passage of contrast material but also by hemoglobin degradation products, the interfaces between different tissues, and age-related iron accumulation in the extrapyramidal nuclei. These effects are much more pronounced at high field intensities [40].

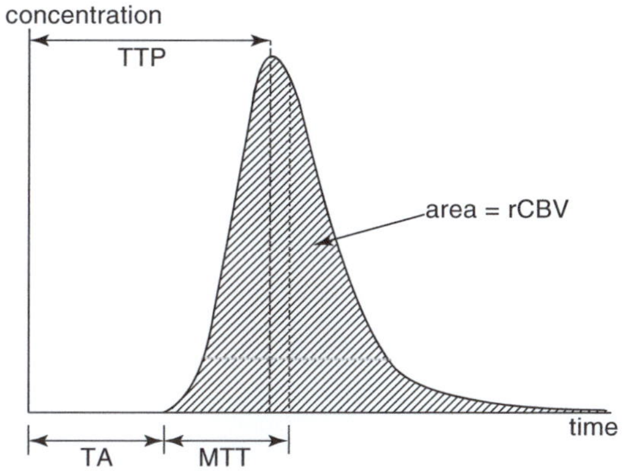


**Fig. 9.3** Concentration-time curve (*rCBV* cerebral blood volume, *MTT* mean transit time, *TA* arrival time, *TTP* time to peak)

- The decrease in signal intensity produced by the passage of a bolus of gadolinium chelate allows a signal intensity-time curve to be obtained by calculating the change in signal intensity in a single voxel (or in a single region of interest) as a function of time. This curve is then converted to an agent concentration-time curve.

The sum of all the concentration-time curves of all the voxels in a given slice generates perfusion maps from which various hemodynamic parameters can be calculated, including cerebral blood volume (CBV), cerebral blood flow (CBF), mean transit time (MTT), and time to peak (TTP) (Figs. 9.3 and 9.4) (Table 9.3).

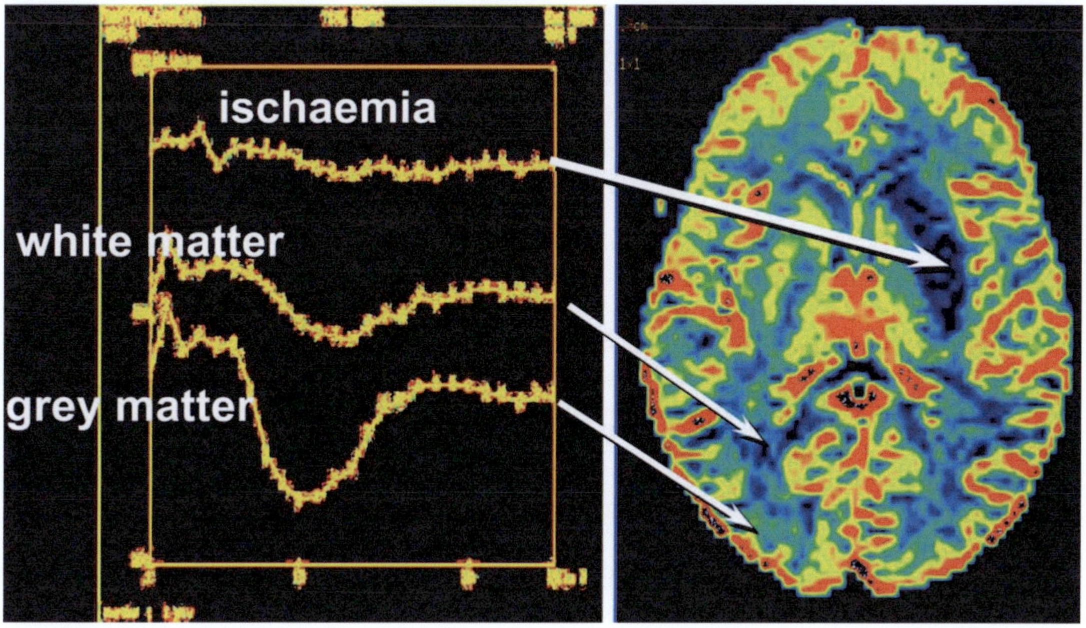


**Fig. 9.4** Intensity-time curves are correlated to cerebral perfusion, better visualized in the CBV map: perfusion is greater in gray than in white matter and is reduced or absent in the ischemic area

**Table 9.3** Exogenous agent perfusion techniques. Mechanism and quantitative parameters

| | DSC | DCE |
|---|---|---|
| Mechanism | Gd distorts magnetic field and reduces T2/T2* around vessel | Gd causes dipole-dipole interactions and produces signal enhancement |
| Quantitative parameters | rCBF<br>CBV<br>MTT | $K^{trans}$<br>$K^{ep}$<br>$V^{e}$<br>$V^{p}$ |

These parameters are dependent on the specific features of the bolus injection (injection rate, amount, and concentration of contrast material) and on specific variables of the patient being imaged (total body vascular volume and cardiac output) [1, 3]. As a result, hemodynamic parameters cannot be directly compared between different subjects and may even differ between examinations of the same individual performed at different times [1, 3].

Thus, relative values can be obtained using an internal standard of reference such as normal-appearing gray or white matter (Figs. 9.5 and 9.6) [1, 3].

For diffuse processes, in which the internal reference may also be affected, absolute quantitation is required. Absolute quantitation of CBV and CBF has been attempted using methods that measure arterial input to the brain, but their accuracy is debated [1, 3].

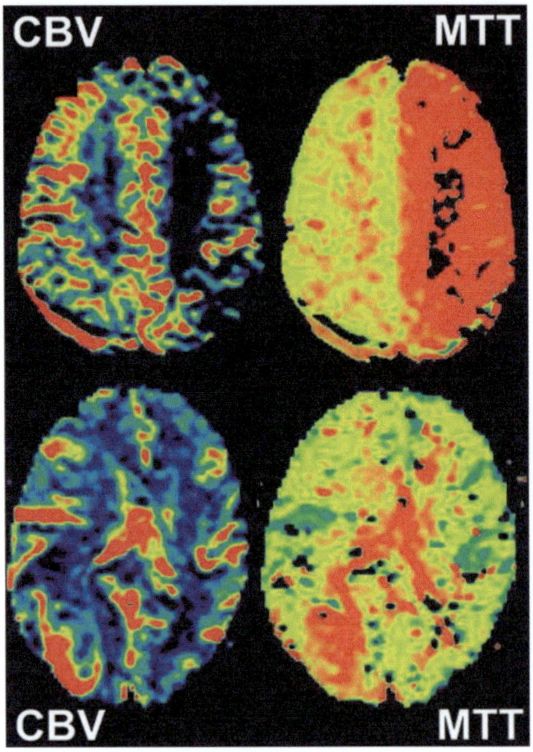


**Fig. 9.5** CBV and MTT maps

### 9.1.1 Cerebral Blood Volume

Cerebral blood volume (CBV) is the fraction of each imaged voxel comprising the intravascular space and therefore the volume of the blood vessels within a volume of brain tissue. It is measured as milliliters of blood per 100 g of tissue; since brain tissue approximates water in density (1 g/mL), this can also be expressed as a percent value.

Typical values for the brain are between 3 % and 5 %. Only a small fraction of CBV is arterial, most of it being divided between capillaries and veins, and its changes are related to autoregulatory vasodilatation of the capillaries and/or veins [6, 7, 38]. CBV is a potentially sensitive indicator of vascular endothelial response to changes in local CBF and tissue metabolism.

Relative CBV can be measured as the area under the curve of the voxel concentration versus time. Absolute CBV can be determined by dividing the area under the curve by a "reference" voxel known to contain 100 % blood, such as the superior sagittal sinus [7, 39].

Unfortunately several technical factors can impair the accuracy of this relatively simple measurement [1, 3, 41]. The first is that dynamic susceptibility contrast arises from spin diffusion in the space surrounding the blood vessels, making it difficult to determine a reference 100 % blood-filled voxel [41]. Secondly, the effects of contrast recirculation must be eliminated or minimized. Thirdly, CBV measurement

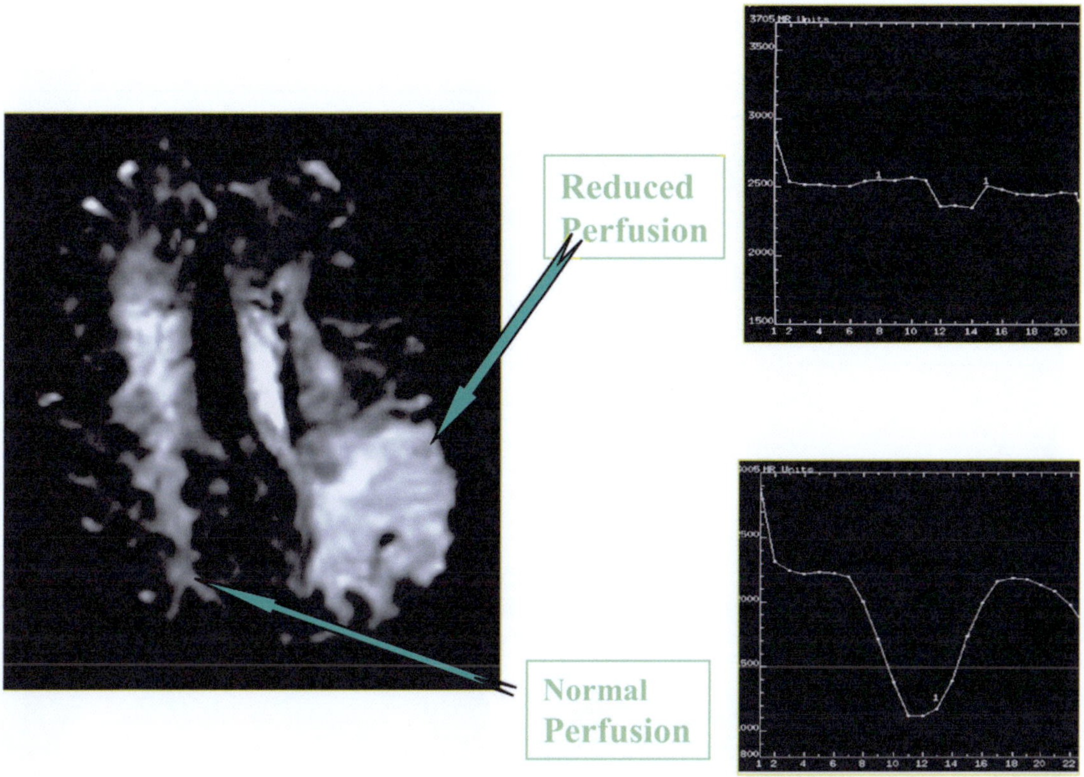


**Fig. 9.6** Intensity-time curves and CBV maps in normal tissue and in focal ischemic area

can be erroneous if the gadolinium chelate leaks through a disrupted BBB. This is of particular concern when imaging tumors, since several tumors cause BBB disruption, yielding a bright signal on post-contrast T1 images [7, 42] (Fig. 9.7).

DSC perfusion MRI model assumes that the contrast agent remains confined in the intravascular space throughout image acquisition. If the BBB is leaky, the DSC data can be compromised as the relative shortening of the T1 of water, due to parenchymal contrast extravasation, counteracts or mutes the T2* effect and the relative signal intensity decreases [8].

Comparative studies have shown that a "preload" of gadolinium chelate, given before the actual bolus dose for DSC data acquisition, can reduce the deleterious impact of a BBB breakdown on the perfusion data [8]. The preload reduces the T1 leakage effects by saturating the leaky tissues with contrast agent, thereby dampening the T1-shortening effects of the main bolus during DCS data acquisition [8].

New molecules, such as superparamagnetic iron-oxide particles, dendritic compounds saturated with gadolinium atoms, or reversible protein-binding gadolinium-based agents, have a longer half-life in blood [7, 43–45]. These so-called "blood pool" agents offer higher SNR for measuring CBV using steady-state susceptibility contrast that circumvents many of the problems outlined earlier.

### 9.1.2 Cerebral Blood Flow

Cerebral blood flow (CBF) is the amount of arterial blood delivered to brain tissue per unit of time. It is most commonly measured as milliliters of blood per 100 g of tissue per minute. Characteristic values for gray matter are

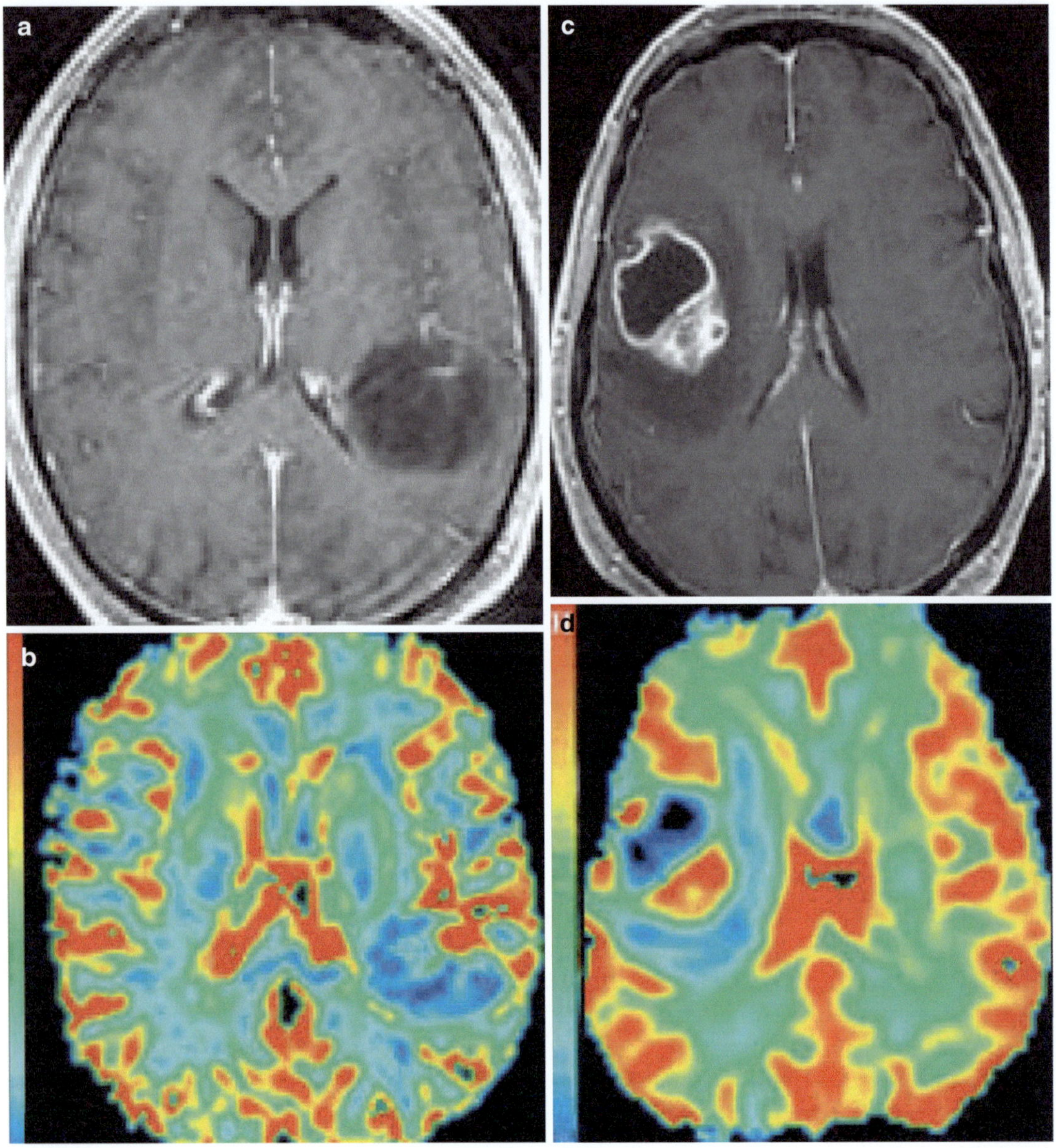


**Fig. 9.7** (**A**, **B**) Low-grade astrocytoma: SE T1 after contrast agent administration (**a**) and CBV map (**b**); (**C**, **D**) glioblastoma: SE T1 after contrast administration (**c**) and CBV map (**d**). The CBV is reduced in the low-grade astrocytoma (**b**) and in the cystic component of the glioblastoma (**d**), whereas it is increased in the solid part of the glioblastoma (**d**)

60 ml/min/100 g and 15 ml/min/100 g for white matter. CBF control is via control of the diameter of the feeding arterioles.

CBF is the primary rate constant controlling the supply of nutrients and removal of waste products from the brain. Below a threshold level, duration multiplied by the absolute CBF level can predict tissue infarction [7].

While CBV measurement with intravascular tracers is relatively straightforward, the measurement of CBF is more challenging [7, 46], as it requires delicate deconvolution methods.

In particular, one method tries to deconvolve the effects of a bolus of finite width (as estimated from the arterial signal near a large feeding vessel, such as the anterior communicating artery). This arterial input function is taken to represent the profile of the bolus at its point of entry into each individual voxel based on the assumption that every voxel has the same arterial input function. This is clearly an oversimplification, and uncertainties about regional changes in the profile and timing of the bolus can cause significant errors in CBF evaluation [7, 47].

Good absolute CBF correlation with $H_2{}^{15}O$ PET has been shown in anesthetized healthy pigs [48], and an excellent relative CBF correlation has been reported in an experimental model of ischemia [49]. However, in diseased brain, where collateral pathways are more common, intravascular tracer CBF measurements that do not account for variations in bolus delay (caused by arterial stenosis and occlusions) and dispersion are inaccurate [7, 46, 50].

### 9.1.3 Mean Transit Time

Mean transit time (MTT) is the average amount of time the blood spends in the capillary bed. A capillary bed is made up of numerous capillaries of different lengths, so the time spent in the tissue has a distribution. The unit of measurement is seconds. Typical values for the normal brain are in the range of 3–5 s, whereas in acute cerebral infarction, MTT is increased.

According to the central volume principle, it is important to note close relationship between the CBF, CBV, and MTT. This relationship is:

$CBF = CBV/MTT.$

This relationship can easily be explained with the simple case of flow through a single capillary. Flow is defined as the motion of a volume of fluid over time and velocity as distance over time. If the distance is measured along the capillary vessel, and the velocity is the speed of the fluid in this vessel, this relationship can be multiplied by the cross-sectional area of the capillary. This converts the distance to a volume and the velocity to a flow.

### 9.1.4 Time to Peak

Time to peak (TTP) is the time the blood takes to reach the maximum intensity, from the start of the bolus injection to the peak concentration of contrast agent; it is defined as the time point of maximum intensity loss after the passage of the contrast agent. It is calculated in seconds and reveals any delays in transit time, enabling quick quantification of perfusion deficits. Ischemic areas are characterized by a delay of tracer arrival and a TTP increase [6, 51, 52]. A study of patients with acute cerebral ischemia postulated that TTP values of 0–3.5 s are related to normal perfusion; values ranging from 3.5 to 7 s may indicate a perfusion disorder, whereas values above 7 s indicate a high risk of ischemic tissue injury and watershed infarcts in border zones [51].

Despite these difficulties in determining the absolute values of volume and flow, relative values of CBV and CBF are extremely useful in clinical practice, especially in stroke evaluation.

It is generally accepted that tissue with abnormalities on both perfusion and diffusion-weighted imaging has already undergone irreversible ischemia.

However, tissue with perfusion abnormalities but normal diffusion is thought to be consistent with reversible ischemia. This area of diffusion-perfusion mismatch, also called ischemic penumbra, is a region of decreased perfusion that is potentially reversible because it is above the critical level for the maintenance of the $Na^+$ $K^+$-ATPase pump [1]. Exact evaluation of the tissue that can be rescued is critical in assessing the risk-benefit ratio of possible therapies, since patients with no mismatch are considered unlikely to benefit from thrombolytic therapy.

Time-dependent perfusion thresholds were first established using $H_2{}^{15}O$ PET to distinguish underperfused tissue evolving toward infarction ( < 12 ml/min per 100 g) from penumbral flow with functionally compromised but viable tissue (12–20 ml/min per 100 g) [1–3].

The exact role of each hemodynamic parameter (CBV, CBF, MTT, and TTP) in the correct evaluation of brain perfusion changes, and which of them is more representative of salvageable tissue and predictive of final infarct size is still debated.

It appears that MTT maps generally show the largest area of abnormality and often overestimate final infarct size, while CBV maps tend to underestimate this size.

In one study comparing CBV maps, CBF maps, and MTT maps with change in size from initial infarct size to final infarct size, a mismatch between initial CBF maps and a diffusion abnormality predicted more often the growth of infarct than did a mismatch between initial CBV maps and diffusion abnormality [41]. In that study, however, CBV maps best correlated with change in infarct size from initial to follow-up imaging [41].

A recent study comparing TTP maps and thresholds in patients with acute ischemia using CBF data acquired with PET, assumed as the gold standard, indicated that TTP is a useful estimate of ischemic injury but entails considerable methodological limitations that have to be considered in routine use of MRI for stroke [52].

Relative TTP maps are only indirect surrogates of CBF and do not represent the best application of MRI perfusion imaging. They are used in clinical routine because they are simple; they clearly delineate hemodynamic alterations, yield satisfactory results compared with quantitative methods, and do not rely on deconvolution algorithms, calibration with PET data, or selection of adequate input functions [52].

However, TTP maps may be inappropriate, since simple visual analysis is more prone to errors related to individual subjectivity [52].

A quantitative observer-independent measure such as TTP thresholds has proved to be more indicative of underperfusion stated by PET for a CBF value of < 20 ml/min per 100 g [52].

The best estimate of penumbral flow was found for a TTP delay of > 4 s (sensitivity 84 %, specificity 77 %); it best identifies the volume of penumbra and should be used to define the mismatch volume. The volume of a TTP delay of > 4 s was correlated with clinical deficit, whereas the volume of a TTP delay between > 5 and > 8 s was strongly associated with infarct growth [52].

The lack of a complete match between PET and TTP thresholds is partly explained by method-specific properties. TTP only yields a relative estimation of CBF as it indicates the time point of maximum signal intensity loss during the passage of the tracer within several seconds. $H_2^{15}O$ PET assesses the "true" CBF as the concentration of a partly diffusible tracer integrated over a scanning time of several minutes. TTP data are therefore more prone to movement artifacts, collateral flow, or individual hemodynamic properties [1, 52].

However, even the TTP threshold with the best sensitivity and specificity seems to include a large portion of tissue with only modest hemodynamic damage; particularly in small ischemia, TTP tends to overestimate the true extent of the "tissue at risk" [52].

## 9.2 High-Field DSC

Currently, most MR perfusion studies are acquired on 1.5 T machines, but MR systems operating at higher-field strengths are increasingly becoming available in clinical practice [4, 5, 8]. In general, imaging at higher magnetic field strengths offers at least a linear SNR increase, but its utilization is impaired by problems related to magnetic susceptibility artifacts.

Since magnetic susceptibility increases with field strength, at 3.0 T image distortion may be critical, particularly if EPI pulse sequences are used, as in most protocols for DSC perfusion studies. In fact, with EPI sequences the tradeoff is increased $B_0$ inhomogeneity and magnetic susceptibility differences at air-tissue interfaces, leading to signal dropout and geometric distortions, most notably in the phase-encode direction [53].

Image quality may thus be severely impaired by distortion and blurring around tissue interfaces, especially in patients who have undergone neurosurgery, and assessment of signal intensity at the passage of a bolus of contrast agent may be inaccurate.

Other drawbacks inherent with T2* susceptibility are systematic overestimation of perfusion because of the different relaxivity of the paramagnetic contrast agent in the larger vessels (from which the input function is obtained) and in capillaries, problems in defining a good input function because of low spatial resolution on T2*-weighted EPI, and finally problems in assessing a damaged BBB. The latter is a critical element in the evaluation of brain tumor perfusion, because relaxivity is different when the contrast agent is confined to a small compartment as opposed to distributed in the interstitial space [54].

In order to minimize these negative effects, the use of rapid 3D fast-field echo T1-weighted or 3D FLASH T1-weighted sequences has recently been proposed [54, 55]. Although acquisition is slower and yields less spatial and temporal resolution than EPI, FLASH seems to suffer less from spatial distortion than EPI, thus yielding a better arterial input function [55].

On the other hand, T2*-weighted contrast-enhanced perfusion imaging using 3.0 T systems offers some potential advantages. In particular, shorter T2 and T2* relaxation times and increased SNR [56, 57] may allow a greater T2* signal drop to be obtained for a given amount of contrast bolus during capillary passage [58].

A study of the feasibility of MR perfusion at 3.0 T demonstrated that image quality of the perfusion source images was not impaired, leading to rating distortion and blurring as minor in most images [8].

This was also true of critical anatomical areas, such as the posterior fossa and the regions close to the base of the skull (e.g., the hippocampus and brainstem) [8]. This is probably due to the use of a multi-shot echo-shifted three-dimensional gradient-echo echo-planar imaging sequence, in which the short echo train length may compensate for the field-dependent increase in susceptibility effects [8, 59–62].

The choice of correct echo time may also affect the performance of DSC perfusion imaging. A work comparing different echo times (ranging from 21 to 45 ms) in DSC perfusion in 17 patients demonstrated that the shortest echo time used yielded the best images [63].

Important benefits have been reported from using EPI sequences in DSC perfusion at 3.0 T with parallel imaging [37], also with the implementation of a multichannel coil array [53], or with the use of spin-echo EPI, as an alternative to gradient-echo EPI [64].

Parallel imaging (PI) techniques such as simultaneous acquisition of spatial harmonics (SMASH), sensitivity encoding (SENSE), or generalized autocalibrating partially parallel acquisition (GRAPPA) allow the shortening of scanning time by reducing the number of phase-encoding steps needed. Correct image reconstruction is achieved by inclusion of additional spatial information obtained from the spatial variation of coil sensitivity of multiple receiver coils. The reduction in encoding time can be used to achieve greater temporal resolution or to increase spatial resolution of the otherwise typically low-resolution dynamic scans [37].

The use of EPI sequences at 3.0 T is ideally suited for combination with PI techniques because the reduced echo train length results in several improvements.

The first benefit is reduction of image distortion and blurring from $B_0$ inhomogeneities produced by the interfaces between tissues and tissue boundaries or by hemorrhage products and surgical material after craniotomy. These image distortions are proportional to the off-resonance frequency produced by the inhomogeneities and inversely proportional to the time necessary to traverse the *k*-space. With PI the sensitivity of EPI to any of these off-resonance artifacts, particularly significant at 3.0 T, can be reduced [37].

Another advantage is the reduction of the influence of T2* relaxation on spatial resolution, also referred to as *k*-space filtering. *k*-space filtering limits the resolution that can be achieved due to signal loss during spatial encoding. At 1.5 T a typical contrast agent reduces the T2* time of brain tissue to 20–40 ms. Therefore encoding steps performed after the actual T2* time contribute little to the *k*-space information, and the image appears as if acquired at much lower resolution. Because of the shorter T2* relaxation at higher field intensities, this effect is even more pronounced at 3.0 T. This effect is also very important for the measurement of the arterial input function. With conventional EPI, the signal inside vessels vanishes completely, and the arterial input function can be detected only around vessels.

Moreover, reduced shot duration in PI allows the acquisition of more slices in the same scanning time, enabling increased coverage of the region being investigated.

Finally, using interleaved EPI sequences, application of PI is also recommended for selecting an appropriate echo time.

The dose of contrast agent also needs to be adjusted to the high-field strength setting. Although structural contrast-enhanced brain imaging at 1.5 T is usually performed with 0.1 mmol/kg of body weight, 0.2 mmol of gadolinium chelate is the most widely used dose and is considered optimal for DSC perfusion studies [65–71], also in case of higher concentrations of gadolinium-based contrast agents (e.g., gadobutrol, Gadovist, Schering, Berlin, Germany) [8, 72]. When this dose (0.2 mmol) was used for DSC perfusion at 3.0 T, the stronger susceptibility effects caused a complete signal void during the first pass of gadolinium, especially in gray matter, affecting the accuracy of signal drop calculation and impairing sensitivity to perfusion deficits [8]; for this reason, a dose of 0.2 mmol is not recommended for high-field perfusion imaging.

A 3.0 T study comparing different doses (0.05, 0.1, and 0.2 mmol) has recommended a dose of 0.1 mmol on the basis both of subjective analysis of the quality of the perfusion maps and of a quantitative assessment of perfusion variables [8] (Fig. 9.8).

### 9.2.1 Dynamic Contrast-Enhanced (DCE)-MRI

Dynamic contrast-enhanced (DCE)-MRI is the other exogenous contrast-based method.

DSC remains the clinical standard among perfusion techniques using a gadolinium chelate, but errors are introduced into the data processing for a variety of reasons, including the difference in relaxivity between tissue and blood pool and the problem inherent in BBB breakdown [8].

Alternative method to DSC-MRI is DCE-MRI. DCE uses metrics to describe the permeability of the BBB and the relationship to the extracellular extravascular space. The same leakage that confounds the DSC perfusion is measured with DCE by using a dynamic T1-weighted sequence.

After the bolus of the contrast agent is injected, hemodynamic signals of DCE depend on the T1 relaxation time and increase because of the T1-shortening effect associated with the paramagnetic contrast agent [5]. DCE uses rapid and repeated T1-weighted images to measure the signal changes as a function of time. T1 weighting is not affected by extravasation. Extracellular contrast agent diffuses from the blood into the extravascular spaces at a rate determinated by tissue perfusion and permeability of the capillaries and their surface area [5].

The resulting signal intensity-time curve reflects a composite of tissue perfusion, vessel permeability, and extravascular-extracellular space [6, 7]. In contrast with conventional (static) T1-weighted contrast-enhanced MRI, which displays contrast enhancement at a single moment, DCE depicts the wash-in, plateau, and the wash-out contrast kinetics of the tissue, thereby providing insight into the nature of the bulk issue properties at the microvascular level [6, 7].

The time course of enhancement is related to the changes depending on physiological parameters of the microvasculature in the lesion and on the volume fractions of the various tissue compartments [5]. Three major factors determine the behavior of contrast medium in tissues after injection: blood perfusion, transport of contrast medium across the vessel walls, and diffusion of contrast agent in the interstitial space [5].

*Protocols.* DCE is usually scanned with a fast T1-weighted imaging sequence with 2D or 3D dynamic acquisition. Gradient-echo sequences are sensitive to all vessel sizes, while spin-echo sequences are more sensitive to small vessels.

3D sequences such as spoiled gradient-recalled echo SPGR (GE Healthcare), T1-weighted fast-field echo T1 FFE (Philips Healthcare), and volumetric interpolated breath-hold examination (VIBE) (Siemens Healthcare) are commonly

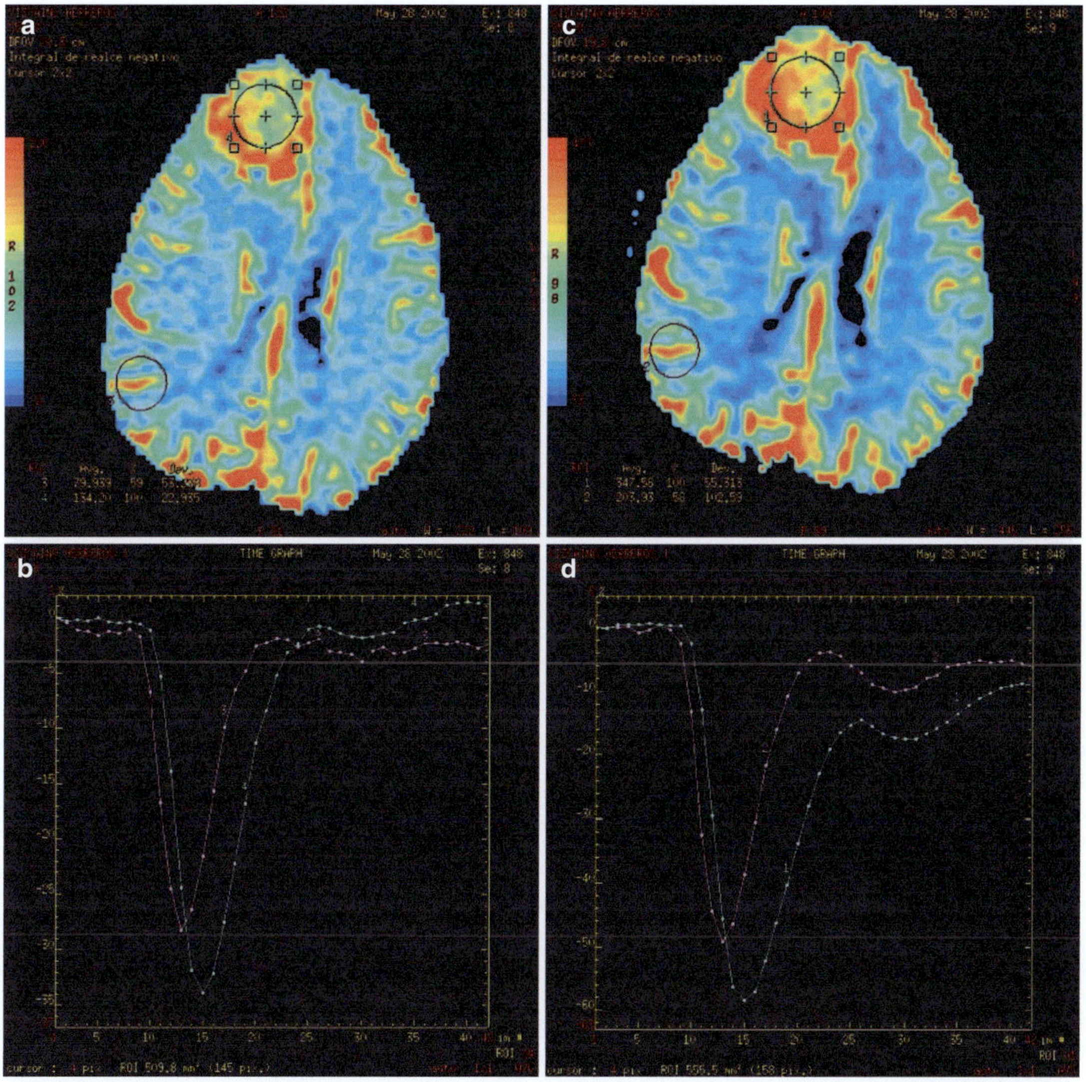


**Fig. 9.8** DSC at 3.0 T. Comparison between two different concentrations of the same dose of contrast agent: 0.5 mmol (**a**, **c**) versus 1.0 mmol (**b**, **d**). At 3.0 T the enhanced magnetic susceptibility requires lower doses and/or lower concentrations than 1.5 T systems. (Courtesy of General Electric)

used. The temporal resolution of the single T1-weighted acquisition should be between 3.5 and 6 seconds depending on the scanner specifics and the field strength used. The injection should start 20 seconds after the start of the DCE sequence with an injection speed of approximately 2–4 mL/s when using the Tofts model and an infusion over 30 seconds when using the Brix model for post-processing the data [6, 7].

The acquisition time depends on the parameters that should be extracted and sum to 3 minutes acquisition to 6–7 min, while acquisition time for DSC is about 60 s.

There are several methods for image interpretation. The simplest method is to examine the signal intensity curves over time for a region of interest. The rate of slope of the wash-in and wash-out curve for multiple regions can be visually assessed, permitting, for instance, to distinguish tumors (rapid curve rise) from radiation necrosis (slow curve rise) [8]. More advanced post-processing involves use of T1 maps and complex pharmacokinetic models.

The latter method is based on a two-compartmental (plasma space and extravascular-extracellular space) pharmacokinetic model. The general steps are perform baseline T1 mapping, acquire DCE images, convert signal intensity data to contrast agent concentration, determine the vascular input function, and perform pharmacokinetic modeling. With pharmacokinetic modeling several metrics are derived: the transfer constant ($K^{trans}$); the fractional volume of the extravascular space ($v_e$); the rate constant $K_{ep}$, where $K_{ep} = K^{trans} / v_e$ ; and the fractional volume of the plasma space ($v_p$). [6, 7].

The most frequently used metric in DCE is $K^{trans}$, which can have different interpretations depending on blood flow and permeability. When there is very high permeability, the flux of the contrast medium is limited only by flow, and thus $K^{trans}$ mainly reflects blood flow [6, 7]. On the contrary, when permeability is low, the gadolinium cannot leak into the extravascular-extracellular space, and thus $K^{trans}$ mainly reflects permeability [6, 7]. Despite this complexity $K^{trans}$ appears to reproducibly measure permeability in glioma patients.

Nowadays DCE is routinely applied in patients with breast, prostate, pelvic, and muscle disease and is also often applied in brain diseases, especially tumors (Table 9.4) [5]. This technique can be used to evaluate tumor grades, the treatment effect of radiotherapy, or in monitoring the response to chemotherapy [5]).

**Table 9.4** Exogenous agent perfusion techniques. Common clinical applications

| | DSC | DCE |
|---|---|---|
| Organs: brain | Brain (most used)<br>Stroke<br>Tumors<br>Neurodegenerative diseases | Brain (less used)<br>Tumors |
| Organs other than the brain | No | Breast (tumors) |
| | No | Prostate (tumors) |
| | No | Pelvic (tumors) |
| | No | Muscle (tumors) |

From Jahng et al. [5], modified

## 9.2.2 Advantages and Disadvantages

DSC imaging is a fast and robust imaging technique that is the most widely used method to measure brain perfusion with MRI [2–8]. The software to post-process the data is widely available and relatively straightforward to use, in evaluating both acute ischemia and brain tumors. DSC provides information that complements traditional structural MRI and is most widely used in clinical practice in diagnosing and managing acute ischemia and brain tumors, offering a valid support in grading gliomas (especially when BBB is intact), differentiating radiation necrosis from recurrent tumor, and selecting biopsy sites for enhancing and non-enhancing tumors. Moreover, the capability to assess tumor angiogenesis may play an important role in the future to assess novel cancer therapies that target blood vessels.

Some limitations of this technique include difficulties to establish absolute quantification of blood flow (relative rather than absolute quantification of CBV), sensitivity to susceptibility artifacts (caused by blood products, calcifications, or metal devices), user dependence in post-processing, and inaccurate estimation of CBV in cases of severe disruption of the BBB [2, 6, 7].

DCE techniques permit to examine the brain microvasculature from a different perspective from DSC, allowing assessment of BBB and microvascular permeability [6, 7].

Important limitations of DCE include complexity in imaging acquisition and pharmacokinetic model post-processing, user dependence, and lack of widely available and easy-to-use post-processing software.

Both methods have some advantages over ASL, including higher SNR that permits imaging at

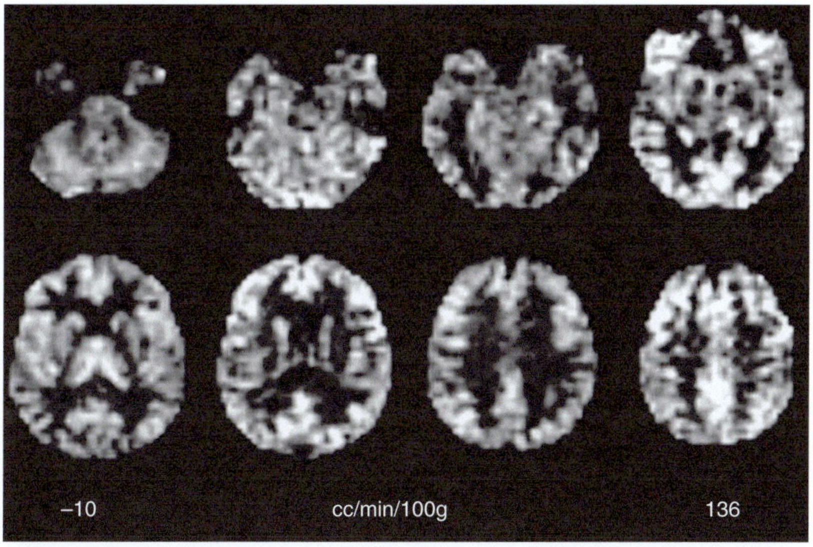


**Fig. 9.9** ASL in normal subject

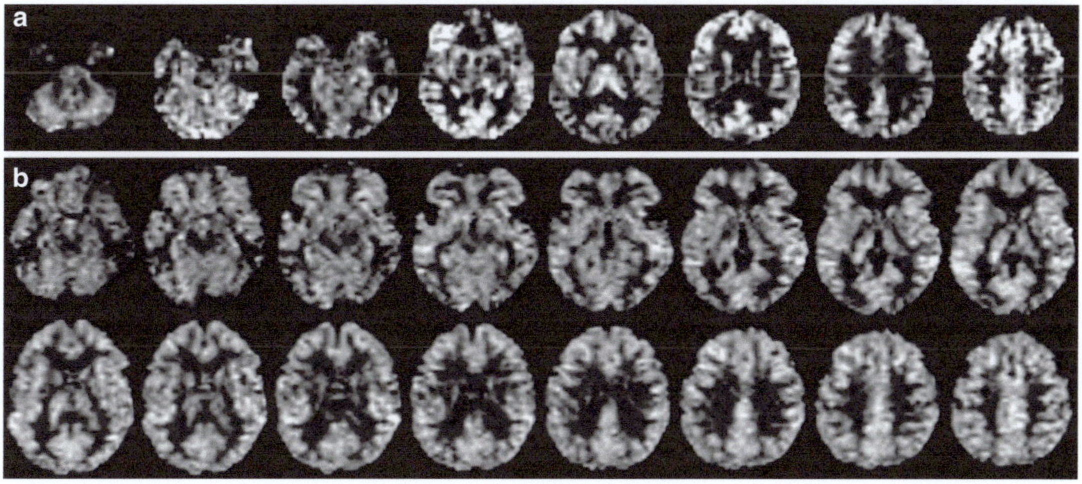


**Fig. 9.10** Comparison between ASL acquired at 1.5T (**a**) and 3.0T (**b**)

higher spatial and temporal resolution (Figs. 9.9 and 9.10). DSC has a scanning time of about 60 s, much shorter in comparing with ASL scanning time of about 4–5 minutes at 3.0 T or 8–10 minutes at 1.5 T [6, 7].

Longer scanning time of ASL causes sensitivity to motion artifacts, which can be a significant problem in uncooperative patients, such as patients with acute stroke or neurodegenerative diseases [6, 7].

On the other hand, ASL offers the advantage to be completely noninvasive, as it does not use contrast agents, which is particularly helpful when repeated measurements are needed or in pediatric patients in which IV access can be difficult.

### 9.2.3 Future Perspectives

In academic centers the application of perfusion techniques has been well established, while its use in routine clinical practice has never been achieved. This is probably due to lack of awareness of perfusion MRI by referring physicians, apparent complexity of perfusion techniques for nonexpert radiologists, lack of reimbursement for perfusion MRI studies, lack of standardized and of optimized perfusion MRI protocols, and lack of simple and of standardized post-processing software [6, 7].

In particular, lack of standardized protocols and of standardized and easy-to-use post-processing software has limited the widespread clinical acceptance of perfusion MRI.

Improvements of image acquisition techniques and standardization of post-processing software may contribute significantly to a greater acceptance of perfusion MRI techniques in the everyday clinical routine.

Technical improvements in the acquisition techniques may come from the broader use of high-field systems [7, 61–63], compressed sensing [7, 64], view sharing, and parallel imaging. Using a higher field provides a substantially higher SNR that one can invest in an improved speed or higher resolution [7, 65].

Compressed sensing has become an important tool for the acceleration of imaging times in MRI and is achieved by enabling the reconstruction of subsampled data. Similarly the applied algorithms can be used to improve both the temporal and the spatial resolution of the DCE-MRI perfusion [7].

View sharing allows a faster acquisition for MR angiography but can also be applied for DCE [7, 66].

The use of parallel imaging enables a significant artifact reduction, the possibility of faster acquisition, and a more robust assessment of the structural and functional parameters [7, 67].

For ASL, the use of higher-field strengths, the use of phased-array coil, and the introduction of fast 3D sequences as an alternative to traditional echo-planar imaging are some technical modifications that may improve SNR and image quality [7, 68–72].

Standardization of an optimized protocol across centers is an important objective, with benefits for the uniform performance and interpretation of perfusion MRI studies.

Efforts such as the Acute Stroke Imaging Standardization Group [7, 73], Stroke Imaging Repository Consortium [7, 74], Radiological Society of North America Quantitative Imaging Biomarkers Alliance [7, 75], the National Cancer Institute Quantitative Imaging Network [7, 76], and Standardization of Acquisition and Post-Processing Study [7, 77] have been created to facilitate the standardization, development, and validation of quantitative imaging biomarkers.

## Conclusions

Perfusion MRI is a valuable and flexible clinical tool enabling the assessment of regional cerebral hemodynamics using a variety of techniques and playing a relevant role in treatment strategies (e.g., in deciding which patient should undergo thrombolysis).

DSC is the most frequently applied technique in clinical practice and uses rapid T2- or T2*-weighted EPI sequences to monitor the first pass of a bolus of gadolinium chelate to calculate semiquantitative maps of relative blood flow, blood volume, and transit time.

The arterial spin labeling technique uses magnetically tagged blood as an endogenous tracer, allowing absolute CBF measurement using the same model as PET. Both techniques benefit from high-field imaging.

Despite disadvantages related to increased susceptibility to field inhomogeneities, the use of high-field imaging, especially in combination with parallel imaging, affords higher SNR and greater sensitivity to the signal drop produced by exogenous tracers, thus permitting use of a smaller dose of contrast agent.

## References

1. Petrella JR, Provenzale JM (2000) MR perfusion imaging of the brain: techniques and applications. AJR Am J Roentgenol 175:207–220
2. Cha S (2009) Dynamic susceptibility-weighted contrast-enhanced perfusion MR imaging in pediatric patients. Neuroimaging Clin N Am. 16(1): 137–147
3. Provenzale JM, Jahan R, Naidich TP, Fox AJ (2003) Assessment of the patient with hyperacute stroke: imaging and therapy. Radiology 229(2):347–359
4. Shiroishi MS, Castellazzi G, Boxerman JL et al (2015) Principles of T2 *-weighted dynamic susceptibility contrast MRI technique in brain tumor imaging. J Magn Reson Imaging. 41(2):296–313

5. Jahng GH, Li KL, Ostergaard L et al (2014) Perfusion magnetic resonance imaging: a comprehensive update on principles and techniques. Korean J Radiol. 15(5):554–577
6. Essig M, Nguyen TB, Shiroishi MS et al (2013) Perfusion MRI: the five most frequently asked clinical questions. AJR Am J Roentgenol. 201(3): W495–W510
7. Essig M, Shiroishi MS, Nguyen TB et al (2013) Perfusion MRI: the five most frequently asked technical questions. AJR Am J Roentgenol. 200(1):24–34
8. McGehee BE, Pollock JM, Maldjian JA (2012) Brain perfusion imaging: How does it work and what should I use? J Magn Reson Imaging. 36(6):1257–1272
9. Viallon M, Cuvinciuc V, Delattre B et al (2015) State-of-the-art MRI techniques in neuroradiology: principles, pitfalls, and clinical applications. Neuroradiology. 57(5):441–467
10. Scarabino T, Nemore F, Giannatempo GM et al (2003) 3.0 T magnetic resonance in neuroradiology. Eur J Radiol 48:154–164
11. Scarabino T, Giannatempo GM, Pollice S et al (2004) 3.0 T perfusion MR imaging. Riv Neuroradiol 17:807–812
12. Provenzale JM, Wintermark M (2008) Optimization of perfusion imaging for acute cerebral ischemia: review of recent clinical trials and recommendations for future studies. AJR Am J Roentgenol. 191(4): 1263–1270
13. Dejobert M, Cazals X, Annan M, et al. (2016) Susceptibility-diffusion mismatch in hyperacute stroke: correlation with perfusion-diffusion mismatch and clinical outcome. J Stroke Cerebrovasc Dis 25(7): 1760–1766.
14. Nael K, Kubal W (2016) Magnetic resonance imaging of acute stroke. Magn Reson Imaging Clin N Am. 24(2):293–304
15. Qian C, Li PC, Jiao Y et al (2016) Precise characterization of the penumbra revealed by MRI: a modified photothrombotic stroke model study. PLos One 11(4):e0153756
16. Schaafs LA, Porter D, Audebert HJ, et al.(2016) Optimising MR perfusion imaging: comparison of different software-based approaches in acute ischaemic stroke. Eur Radiol. [Epub ahead of print] PubMed PMID: 26852218.
17. Mundiyanapurath S, Ringleb PA, Diatschuk S et al (2016) Time-dependent parameter of perfusion imaging as independent predictor of clinical outcome in symptomatic carotid artery stenosis. BMC Neurol 16:50
18. Małowidzka-Serwińska M, Żabicka M, Witkowski A et al (2015) Brain perfusion evaluated by perfusion-weighted magnetic resonance imaging before and after stenting internal carotid artery stenosis in asymptomatic and symptomatic patients. Neurol Neurochir Pol. 49(6):412–420
19. Wang Q, Zhou M, Zhou Y et al (2015) Effects of carotid endarterectomy on cerebral reperfusion and cognitive function in patients with high grade Carotid stenosis: a perfusion weighted magnetic resonance imaging study. Eur J Vasc Endovasc Surg. 50(1): 5–12
20. Kimura M, LC d C Jr (2016) Multiparametric MR imaging in the assessment of brain tumors. Magn Reson Imaging Clin N Am. 24(1):87–122
21. Kickingereder P, Radbruch A, Burth S et al (2016) MR Perfusion-derived hemodynamic parametric response mapping of bevacizumab efficacy in recurrent glioblastoma. Radiology. 279(2):542–552
22. Ho CY, Cardinal JS, Kamer AP et al (2016) Contrast leakage patterns from dynamic susceptibility contrast perfusion MRI in the grading of primary pediatric brain tumors. AJNR Am J Neuroradiol. 37(3):544–551
23. Petr J, Platzek I, Seidlitz A et al (2016) Early and late effects of radiochemotherapy on cerebral blood flow in glioblastoma patients measured with non-invasive perfusion MRI. Radiother Oncol. 118(1):24–28
24. Fouke SJ, Benzinger T, Gibson D et al (2015) The role of imaging in the management of adults with diffuse low grade glioma: a systematic review and evidence-based clinical practice guideline. J Neurooncol. 125(3):457–479
25. Lee KM, Kim EJ, Jahng GH et al (2014) Value of perfusion weighted magnetic resonance imaging in the diagnosis of supratentorial anaplastic astrocytoma. J Korean Neurosurg Soc. 56(3):261–264
26. Mabray MC, Barajas RF Jr, Cha S (2015) Modern brain tumor imaging. Brain Tumor Res Treat 3(1):8–23
27. Barajas RF Jr, Cha S (2014) Benefits of dynamic susceptibility-weighted contrast-enhanced perfusion MRI for glioma diagnosis and therapy. CNS Oncol. 3(6):407–419
28. Essock-Burns E, Phillips JJ, Molinaro AM et al (2013) Comparison of DSC-MRI post-processing techniques in predicting microvascular histopathology in patients newly diagnosed with GBM. J Magn Reson Imaging. 38(2):388–400
29. Binnewijzend MA, Benedictus MR, Kuijer JP et al (2016) Cerebral perfusion in the predementia stages of Alzheimer's disease. Eur Radiol. 26(2):506–514
30. Le Heron CJ, Wright SL, Melzer TR et al (2014) Comparing cerebral perfusion in Alzheimer's disease and Parkinson's disease dementia: an ASL-MRI study. J Cereb Blood Flow Metab. 34(6):964–970
31. Wierenga CE, Hays CC, Zlatar ZZ (2014) Cerebral blood flow measured by arterial spin labeling MRI as a preclinical marker of Alzheimer's disease. J Alzheimers Dis. 42(4):S411–S419
32. Binnewijzend MA, Kuijer JP, van der Flier WM et al (2014) Distinct perfusion patterns in Alzheimer's disease, frontotemporal dementia and dementia with Lewy bodies. Eur Radiol. 24(9):2326–2333
33. Hauser T, Schönknecht P, Thomann PA et al (2013) Regional cerebral perfusion alterations in patients with mild cognitive impairment and Alzheimer disease using dynamic susceptibility contrast MRI. Acad Radiol. 20(6):705–711
34. Park KW, Yoon HJ, Kang DY et al (2012) Regional cerebral blood flow differences in patients with mild

cognitive impairment between those who did and did not develop Alzheimer's disease. Psychiatry Res. 203(2–3):201–206
35. Pizzini FB, Farace P, Manganotti P et al (2013) Cerebral perfusion alterations in epileptic patients during peri-ictal and post-ictal phase: PASL vs DSC-MRI. Magn Reson Imaging. 31(6):1001–1005
36. Koudriavtseva T, Plantone D, Renna R et al (2015) Brain perfusion by arterial spin labeling MRI in multiple sclerosis. J Neurol. 262(7):1769–1771
37. Stollberger R, Fazekas F (2004) Improved perfusion and tracer kinetic imaging using parallel imaging. Top Magn Reson Imaging 15(4):245–254
38. Leenders KL, Perani D, Lammertsma AA et al (1990) Cerebral blood flow, blood volume and oxygen utilization. Normal values and effect of age. Brain 113:27–47
39. Lassen NA, Perl W (1979) Tracer kinetic methods in medical physiology. Raven Press, New York
40. Yamada K, Gonzalez RG, Ostergaard L et al (2002) Iron-induced susceptibility effect at the globus pallidus causes underestimation of flow and volume on dynamic susceptibility contrast-enhanced MR perfusion images. Am J Neuroradiol 23(6):1022–1029
41. Sorensen AG, Copen WA, Ostergaard L et al (1999) Hyperacute stroke: simultaneous measurement of relative cerebral blood volume, relative cerebral blood flow, and mean tissue transit time. Radiology 210:519–527
42. Weisskoff RM, Boxerman JL, Sorensen AG et al (1994) Simultaneous blood volume and permeability mapping using a single Gd-based contrast injection. In: Proceedings of the Society of Magnetic Resonance, 2nd Annual Meeting. CA, San Francisco, p. 279
43. Shen T, Weissleder R, Papisov M et al (1993) Monocrystalline iron oxide nanocompounds (MION): physicochemical properties. Magn Reson Med 29(5):599–604
44. Wiener EC, Brechbiel MW, Brothers H et al (1994) Dendrimer-based metal chelates: a new class of magnetic resonance imaging contrast agents. Magn Reson Med 31(1):1–8
45. Cavagna FM, Maggioni F, Castelli PM et al (1997) Gadolinium chelates with weak binding to serum proteins. A new class of high-efficiency, general purpose contrast agents for magnetic resonance imaging. Invest Radiol 32(12):780–796
46. Lassen NA (1984) Cerebral transit of an intravascular tracer may allow measurement of regional blood volume but not regional blood flow. J Cereb Blood Flow Metab 4(4):633–634
47. Calamante F, Gadian DG, Connelly A (2000) Delay and dispersion effects in dynamic susceptibility contrast MRI: simulations using singular value decomposition. Magn Reson Med 44(3):466–473
48. Ostergaard L, Smith DF, Vestergaard-Poulsen P et al (1998) Absolute cerebral blood flow and blood volume measured by magnetic resonance imaging bolus tracking: comparison with positron emission tomography values. J Cereb Blood Flow Metab 18(4):425–432
49. Sakoh M, Rohl L, Gyldensted C et al (2000) Cerebral blood flow and blood volume measured by magnetic resonance imaging bolus tracking after acute stroke in pigs: comparison with [(15)O]H(2)O positron emission tomography. Stroke 31(8):1958–1964
50. Mukherjee P, Kang HC, Videen TO et al (2003) Measurement of cerebral blood flow in chronic carotid occlusive disease: comparison of dynamic susceptibility contrast perfusion MR imaging with positron emission tomography. Am J Neuroradiol 24(5): 862–871
51. Nasel C, Kronsteiner N, Schindler E et al (2004) Standardized time-to-peak in ischemic and regular cerebral tissue measured with perfusion MR imaging. Am J Neuroradiol 25(6):945–950
52. Sobesky J, Weber OZ, Lenhardt FG et al (2004) Which time-to-peak threshold best identifies penumbral flow? A comparison of perfusion-weighted magnetic resonance imaging and positron emission tomography in acute ischemic stroke. Stroke 35(12):2843–2847
53. Lupo JM, Lee MC, Han ET et al (2005) Feasibility of dynamic susceptibility-weighted perfusion MRI at 3 T using a standard head coil and 8-channel phased-array coil with and without SENSE reconstruction. Proc Intl Soc Mag Reson Med 13:741
54. Larsson HB, Berg HK, Vangberg T et al (2005) Measurement of CBF and PS product in brain tumor patients using T1 w dynamic contrast enhanced MRI at 3 tesla. Proc Intl Soc Mag Reson Med 13:2082
55. Morgan PS, George MS, Kozel FA et al (2005) Dynamic contrast enhanced whole brain perfusion using a rapid 3D T1-weighted sequence at 1.5 T and 3 T. Proc Intl Soc Mag Reson Med 13:1257
56. Wang J, Alsop DC, Li L et al (2002) Comparison of quantitative perfusion imaging using arterial spin labeling at 1.5 and 4.0 Tesla. Magn Reson Med 48:242–254
57. Kruger G, Kastrup A, Glover GH (2001) Neuroimaging at 1.5 T and 3.0 T: comparison of oxygenation-sensitive magnetic resonance imaging. Magn Reson Med 45:595–604
58. Heiland S, Kreibich W, Reith W et al (1998) Comparison of echo-planar sequences for perfusion-weighted MRI: which is best? Neuroradiology 40:216–221
59. Liu G, Sobering G, Duyn J et al (1993) A functional MRI technique combining principles of echo-shifting with a train of observations (PRESTO). Magn Reson Med 30:764–768
60. Mattay VS, Frank JA, Duyn JH et al (1996) Three-dimensional "BURST" functional magnetic resonance imaging: initial clinical applications. Acad Radiol 3(Suppl 2):S379–S383
61. Lee SK (2012) Diffusion tensor and perfusion imaging of brain tumors in high-field MR imaging. Neuroimaging Clin N Am. 22(2):123–134
62. Lövblad KO, Haller S, Pereira VM (2012) Stroke: high-field magnetic resonance imaging. Neuroimaging Clin N Am. 22(2):191–205

63. Prabhakaran V, Nair VA, Austin BP et al (2012) Current status and future perspectives of magnetic resonance high-field imaging: a summary. Neuroimaging Clin N Am 22(2):373–397
64. Han S, Paulsen JL, Zhu G et al (2012) Temporal/spatial resolution improvement of in vivo DCE-MRI with compressed sensing-optimized FLASH. Magn Reson Imaging. 30(6):741–752
65. Attenberger UI, Ingrisch M, Dietrich O et al (2009) Time-resolved 3D pulmonary perfusion MRI: comparison of different k-space acquisition strategies at 1.5 and 3 T. Invest Radiol. 44(9):525–531
66. Le Y, Kroeker R, Kipfer HD et al (2012) Development and evaluation of TWIST Dixon for dynamic contrast-enhanced (DCE) MRI with improved acquisition efficiency and fat suppression. J Magn Reson Imaging. 36(2):483–491
67. Newbould RD, Skare ST, Jochimsen TH et al (2007) Perfusion mapping with multiecho multishot parallel imaging EPI. Magn Reson Med. 58(1):70–81
68. Fernández-Seara MA, Wang Z, Wang J et al (2005 Nov) (2005) Continuous arterial spin labeling perfusion measurements using single shot 3D GRASE at 3 T. Magn Reson Med. 54(5):1241–1247
69. Fernández-Seara MA, Wang J, Wang Z et al (2007) Imaging mesial temporal lobe activation during scene encoding: comparison of fMRI using BOLD and arterial spin labeling. Hum Brain Mapp. 28(12):1391–1400
70. Ye FQ, Frank JA, Weinberger DR (2000) Noise reduction in 3D perfusion imaging by attenuating the static signal in arterial spin tagging (ASSIST). Magn Reson Med. 44(1):92–100
71. Yongbi MN, Fera F, Yang Y et al (2002) Pulsed arterial spin labeling: comparison of multisection baseline and functional MR imaging perfusion signal at 1.5 and 3.0 T: initial results in six subjects. Radiology. 222:569–575
72. Hu LS, Baxter LC, Pinnaduwage DS et al (2010) Optimized preload leakage-correction methods to improve the diagnostic accuracy of dynamic susceptibility-weighted contrast-enhanced perfusion MR imaging in posttreatment gliomas. AJNR Am J Neuroradiol 31:40–48
73. Acute Stroke Imaging Standardization Group-Japan (2012) Website asist.umin.jp/index-e.htm. Accessed 20 Sept 2012
74. Stroke Imaging Repository Consortium (2012) Website, stir.ninds.nih.gov. Accessed 20 Sept 2012
75. Radiological Society of North America Website RSNA. Quantitative Imaging Biomarkers Alliance.(2012) www.rsna.org/QIBA_.aspx.Accessed 20 Sept 2012
76. National Cancer Institute Website. Quantitative Imaging Network. imaging.(2012) cancer.gov/informatics/qin.Accessed 20 Sept 2012
77. University of Erlagen Website. Standardization of Acquisition and Post-Processing Study.(2012) www.neuroradiologie.uk-erlagen.de/e1846/e777/e780/index_ger.html.Accessed 20 Sept 2012

# ASL 3.0 T Perfusion Studies

# 10

Piero Chiacchiaretta, Armando Tartaro,
Simone Salice, and Antonio Ferretti

## 10.1 Introduction

Perfusion refers to the delivery of oxygen, glucose, and other nutrients to tissues by means of blood flow, and its disruption is commonly reported in different pathologies. In particular, changes in brain perfusion is found in most brain diseases, ranging from stroke to neurodegenerative and neoplastic disorders [1–8]. $H_2{}^{15}O$ positron emission tomography (PET) is currently regarded as the gold standard to measure regional cerebral blood flow (CBF) [7–10]. However, PET is an expensive and invasive technique requiring an on-site cyclotron facility and the injection of a radioactive tracer. Furthermore, it suffers from low intrinsic spatial and temporal resolution and low signal-to-noise ratio [11].

Thus, perfusion measurements based on magnetic resonance imaging (MRI) are more often used in the clinical practice, due to the widespread availability of MRI scanners. The most used perfusion MRI technique is dynamic susceptibility contrast (DSC) imaging based on gadolinium as exogenous contrast medium [12]. There are however concerns regarding detrimental effects of gadolinium and other substances in patients with poor renal function [13, 14].

Instead, arterial spin labeling (ASL) is a MRI perfusion technique that uses arterial blood as an endogenous contrast agent by magnetically labeling the blood flowing in the main cerebral feeding arteries with radiofrequency pulses [15, 16]. Since ASL does not require the injection of contrast agents and is implemented by all major MRI systems, it has attracted an increasing interest as an alternative noninvasive technique for quantifying brain perfusion [17, 18]. Quantitative ASL mapping of regional CBF showed good agreement with $H_2{}^{15}O$ PET measurements with good multi-vendor reproducibility, and the number of its clinical applications is continuously growing [19–22]. Indeed, quantitative regional CBF mapping has clinical value in a variety of neurological disorders, such as cerebrovascular disease, epilepsy, neurodegeneration, brain tumors, and pharmacological neuroscience [23, 24]. Furthermore, being completely noninvasive, ASL is also a valuable research tool for basic neuroimaging studies on healthy subjects or aging population [25]. In this regard, ASL offers higher spatial and temporal resolution with respect to both PET and DSC imaging, allowing the possibility to study not only baseline perfusion but also cerebrovascular hemodynamics and

P. Chiacchiaretta • A. Tartaro (✉) • S. Salice
A. Ferretti
Department of Neuroscience Imaging and Clinical Sciences – Institute of Advanced Biomedical Technologies, "G. D'Annunzio" University, Chieti (PE), Italy
e-mail: armando.tartaro@gmail.com



T. Scarabino et al. (eds.), *High Field Brain MRI*, DOI 10.1007/978-3-319-44174-0_10

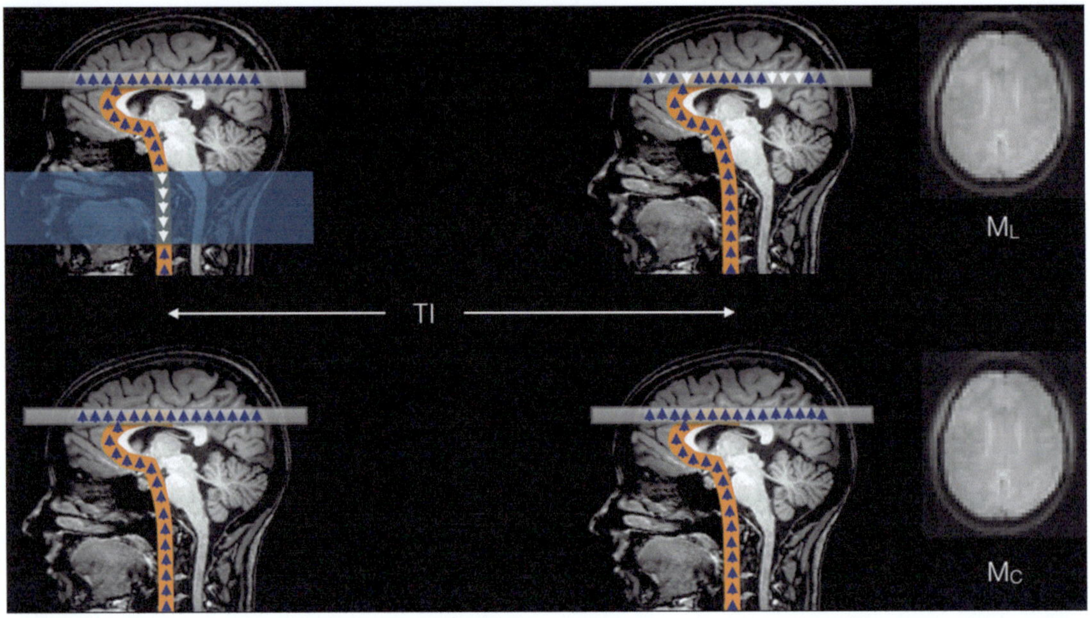


**Fig. 10.1** Arterial spin labeling basic principle. The magnetization of water protons is inverted within a thick slab covering feeding arteries at the base of the head. After a time delay, inserted to allow labeled spins to reach the brain regions of interest, an image is acquired ($M_L$, "label" image). After a few seconds, the image is acquired again without the labeling process ($M_C$, "control" image). Non-labeled spins are represented as upward vectors and the labeled spins as downward vectors. In the label image the number of spins with inverted magnetization will vary according to local blood supply

CBF changes associated to neuronal activity. As a functional magnetic resonance imaging (fMRI) tool, ASL offers some advantages over the more common fMRI technique based on the blood oxygen level dependent (BOLD) effect. In particular, while the BOLD signal [26] is extensively used to map brain function with large sensitivity and good spatial resolution, its limitations as a metric of neuronal activity are well known [27, 28]. Also, because ASL is noninvasive, it can be safely repeated over time, e.g., to track changes in CBF such as those due to disease progression or drug therapy.

## 10.2 ASL Principles

As most methods for CBF quantification, the ASL is based on the principles of compartmental modeling and tracer kinetics. These models describe the dynamics of a tracer as it flows through the arteriocapillary tree (nondiffusible tracers) and eventually exchanges with the tissue (diffusible tracers) prior to venous washout. ASL uses arterial water as an endogenous tracer, which is assumed to freely diffuse from the intravascular compartment into the tissue compartment. This model is similar to the one used in PET measuring the regional accumulation of the radioactive tracer, which is influenced by regional blood flow and its half-life [1]. The fundamental difference is that with ASL the tracer is created just prior image acquisition by magnetically labeling inflowing spins in the brain feeding arteries. This labeling is accomplished by inverting the magnetization of water protons within the arteries at the base of the head [29]. Then, after a time delay that allows labeled spins to reach the brain regions of interest and exchange with the tissue, an image is acquired ($M_L$: "label" image). In this image, the blood water will be in a different magnetization state from that of the static tissue water. The process is shown in Fig. 10.1, representing the non-labeled spins as upward vectors and the labeled spins as downward vectors. After a few

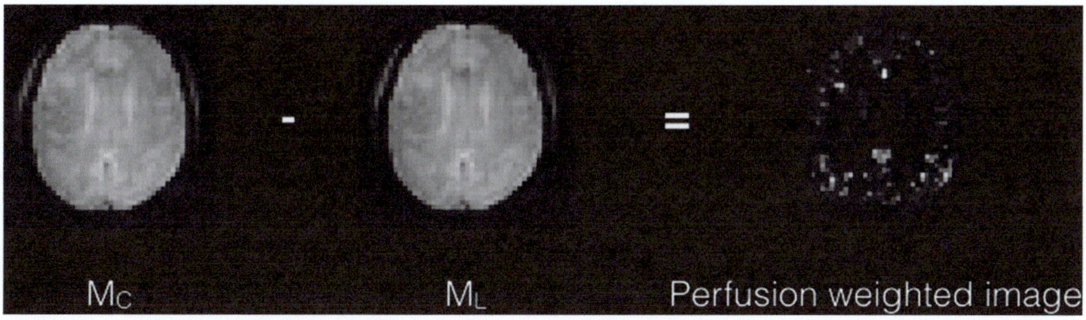


**Fig. 10.2** The magnetization difference between control and label images is proportional to the regional blood flow, since the contribution of static spins cancels out

seconds, the image is acquired again without the labeling process ($M_C$, "control" image). The signal from a given voxel receives contributions from both blood and tissue spins. The tissue static spins in the imaging plane are unaffected by the inversion process; thus, their contribution to the voxel magnetization is the same for control and label images. Spins moving with blood and eventually exchanging with tissue will affect the voxel magnetization differently in the two images: in the label image, the number of spins with inverted magnetization will vary according to local blood supply. The magnetization difference between control and label images will then be proportional to the regional blood flow, since the contribution of static spins cancels out.

Perfusion-weighted images can be generated by the difference between unlabeled and labeled images. In practice, the ASL difference signal ($M_C - M_L$) is a small fraction (about 1 %) of the source image signals, requiring collection of multiple image pairs and averaging to provide adequate signal-to-noise ratio [7]. An example of ASL perfusion-weighted image obtained on a young healthy subject acquiring 35 control-label pairs is shown in Fig. 10.2.

## 10.3 ASL Sequences and Labeling Schemes

Since the original introduction of the basic ASL technique [15, 16], numerous ASL sequences have been developed. The main classification is based on how labeling is achieved, with sequences categorized as either continuous ASL (CASL) or pulsed ASL (PASL), with their own pros and cons. An example of the two labeling methods is shown in Figs. 10.3 and 10.4.

*Continuous ASL (CASL)* In CASL, the magnetization of arterial blood is continuously inverted in the feeding arteries using a combination of a continuous radiofrequency (RF) pulse and a gradient field that define an inversion plane, through a process called adiabatic fast passage [16, 30, 31]. The magnetization of flowing blood is inverted as it crosses this plane, creating an arterial bolus of magnetically labeled blood with a duration equal to the duration of the RF pulse. After the RF pulse is turned off, a post-labeling delay (PLD) is inserted, and the label image is acquired. In the CASL approach, the labeling duration is relatively long (~2 seconds), allowing the creation of a well-defined bolus and a good signal-to-noise ratio. However, a drawback of the long labeling RF pulse used in CASL is represented by its off-resonance influence on the acquired image due to magnetization transfer effects, usually causing signal loss [32]. If these spurious effects are not balanced in the control images, the difference ($M_C - M_L$) would reflect not only the blood flow but also the signal loss due to magnetization transfer effects that are present in $M_L$ but not $M_C$. Different strategies have been developed to balance the magnetization transfer effects on both $M_C$ and $M_L$ images [15, 33]. The basic idea is to apply a RF pulse for the control image as well, designed with the same duration

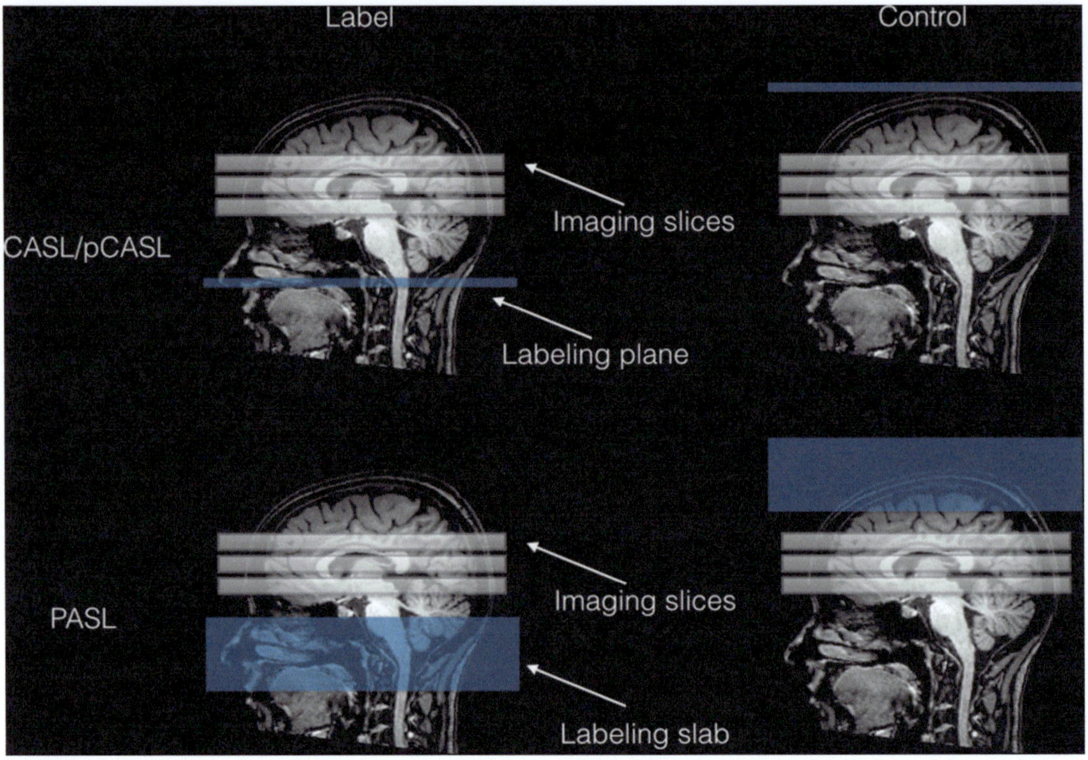


**Fig. 10.3** Schematic representation of the continuous (CASL) and pulsed (PASL) labeling approaches. In CASL, the magnetization of flowing blood is inverted as it crosses the labeling plane, creating an arterial bolus of magnetically labeled blood with a duration equal to the duration of the RF pulse. To compensate off-resonance effects of the long labeling RF pulse, an analogous pulse is applied in the control image on the distal side of the imaging slices, so that no arterial blood is inverted. In PASL, labeling is performed using a single short (~ few ms) RF pulse that invert arterial blood magnetization in a thick slab. As for CASL, off-resonance effects are compensated in the control image applying an inversion slab above the imaging slices

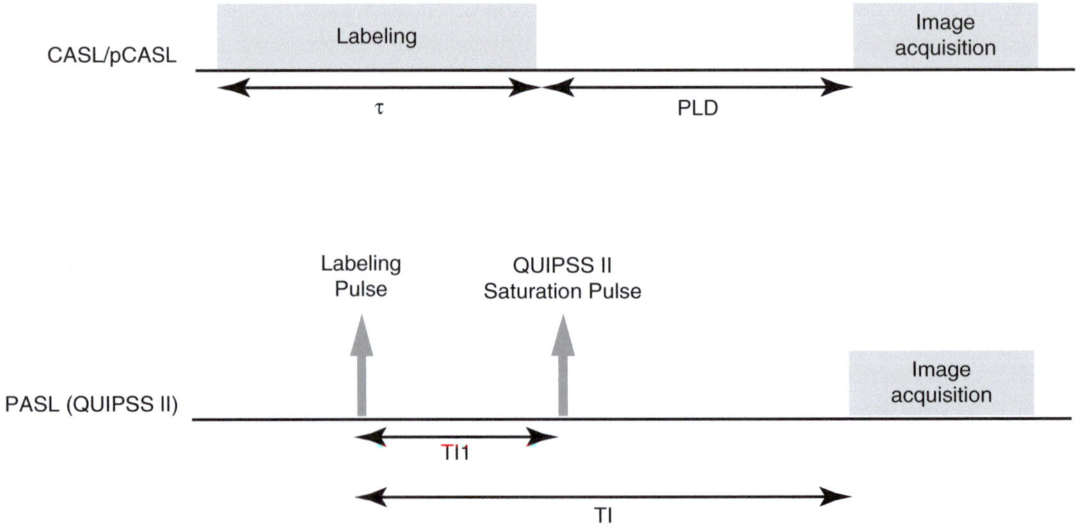


**Fig. 10.4** Schematic diagram of the two ASL sequences, illustrating the labeling parameters described in the main text

as the labeling pulse but applied above the imaged slices so that no inversion is produced on arterial blood (Fig. 10.3). A factor that limited the diffusion of CASL is that the continuous RF pulses are very hardware-demanding and are not supported on most clinical MRI scanners.

*Pulsed ASL (PASL)* In PASL, labeling is performed using a single short (~few ms) RF pulse that inverts arterial blood magnetization in a thick slab. PASL has been implemented with many labeling schemes, differing on how the labeling slab is positioned in control and label images [34]. Here, the early implementation known as EPISTAR (echo-planar imaging and signal targeting with alternating radiofrequency) [35, 36] is described to illustrate the concept. With EPISTAR the labeling band is positioned proximal to the imaging slices, with a small (~1 cm) gap (Fig. 10.3). After a delay to allow the labeled blood to flow into the brain regions, the label images are acquired. As with CASL, the compensation of unwanted effects of the labeling process on the ASL difference image is critical and is accomplished with a proper acquisition of the control image. As shown in Fig. 10.3, the control image is acquired with an inversion pulse applied on a slab placed on the other (distal) side of the imaging slices. Ideally, this control pulse does not label any arterial blood that will flow into the imaging slices but produces off-resonance effects on the static spins similar to those produced by the labeling pulse. Note that with this scheme, venous blood entering from above could actually be labeled by the control pulse and so will appear as focal dark spots, corresponding to veins, in the ASL subtraction image. Unlike CASL, in this basic EPISTAR scheme, there is no control on the duration of the labeled arterial blood bolus. Indeed, in this implementation of pulsed ASL, the bolus duration is determined by the time required for all of the labeled blood to leave the labeling slab, thus depending on the subject physiological state that could influence blood velocity in the feeding arteries of the brain. While this poorly defined arterial bolus has negligible effects on qualitative perfusion-weighted images, it is a critical factor for quantification of CBF in physiological units. In order to control the duration of the arterial bolus of labeled spins, a modified PASL technique known as QUIPSS II is applied [37]. With QUIPSS II, a 90° saturation pulse is applied to the labeling band after the inversion pulse and before the image acquisition. In this approach, the inversion pulse is applied at $t = 0$, the saturation pulse is applied at $TI_1$, and the image is acquired at TI. The saturation pulse is applied to the control image as well to balance off-resonance effects in the ASL signal difference. If $TI_1$ is less than the time required for all of the labeled spins to leave the labeling band, the effect of the saturation pulse is to cut off the end of the arterial bolus, thus producing a well-defined bolus with a duration of $TI_1$.

*Pseudo-Continuous ASL (pCASL)* This approach uses a train of short RF pulses rather than continuous RF to invert the arterial blood spins [38]. Pseudo-continuous ASL has been developed to merge the CASL superior signal-to-noise ratio and the PASL high labeling efficiency without the need of particular demanding hardware [39, 40]. Indeed, the pCASL is emerging as a powerful tool for clinical studies, allowing good reproducibility and reliability with acquisition times of the order of a few minutes and a widespread availability across vendors [21, 41, 42].

## 10.4 Technical Advancements and Readout Strategies

Developments of ASL techniques are growing rapidly, expanding on the original concept to improve signal-to-noise ratio (SNR) and minimize confounding factors. One important addition is represented by the introduction of background suppression pulses that aim at suppressing the static tissue signal in order to improve the SNR of the ASL difference signal [43, 44]. As mentioned before, the signal of interest in ASL is the small difference of two large signals (Mc-ML). Systematic errors on these signals can be as large as the difference signal, thus biasing the CBF estimate. Since both $M_C$ and $M_L$ signals receive the main contribution from static tissue spins, suppression of this background signal can improve the quality of the difference signal. This suppression is achieved with carefully timed spatially selective inversion pulses that are applied to the imaging region prior to the excitation pulse for image acquisition, nulling the static tissue signal over a reasonably wide range of T1 values.

Both three-dimensional (3D) and two-dimensional (2D) readout schemes are applied for ASL image acquisition. For 3D, segmented methods such as RARE or GRASE [45–47] are mostly used, providing optimal SNR and low sensitivity to field inhomogeneity. Since 3D readout approaches require only one excitation pulse per volume, background suppression can be made highly effective, timing the inversion pulses to null the static tissue signal at the excitation time.

For 2D, single-shot EPI and spiral methods are commonly used, with similar performance to one another. Background suppression is less effective for 2D imaging, since the timing of suppression pulses will only be optimal for one or a few slices. However, the residual signal after the partial background suppression can be used for image registration prior to $M_C$-$M_L$ subtraction, reducing the effect of motion artifacts on the ASL difference signal. In general, a short echo time is recommended to reduce T2/T2* weighting, and parallel imaging can be used to achieve both shorter echo times and reduced image distortions in 2D EPI [41]. The application of vascular crushing gradients has also been proposed to reduce vascular artifacts. If the arterial transit time is larger than PLD/TI, bright vascular signals will be evident in the ASL difference image. Vascular crushing gradients work by dephasing the signal from labeled spins that are still present in larger arteries at the time of imaging, thus reducing this type of artifact. This option can be useful in certain applications when large intravascular ASL signals may hide more subtle perfusion-related signals of interest, such as in tumors. However, in other clinical applications, bright intravascular signals due to increased arterial transit time may be a useful indicator, as in the setting of collateral flow and in general for arteriovenous malformation investigations, discouraging the use of vascular crushing gradients in these cases [48–50].

## 10.5 Absolute CBF Quantification

One advantage of the ASL technique is its ability to quantify perfusion in physiological units. In most cases a single PLD/TI ASL sequence is used, with CBF quantification based on a simple model [37, 41, 51]. The basic assumptions of this model require that (i) the entire labeled bolus is delivered to the target tissue, (ii) there is no outflow of labeled blood water, and (iii) labeled spins relax with blood T1 prior image acquisition. With these assumptions, voxel-wise CBF maps in physiological units can be calculated using the following expressions for CASL/pCASL and PASL (QUIPSS II), respectively [37, 51]:

$$\mathrm{CBF} = \frac{6000\lambda\left(M_\mathrm{C} - M_\mathrm{L}\right)e^{\frac{\mathrm{PLD}}{T_\mathrm{1A}}}}{2\alpha T_\mathrm{1A} S_\mathrm{PD}\left(1 - e^{-\frac{\tau}{T_\mathrm{1A}}}\right)}\left[\mathrm{ml/100g/min}\right] \tag{10.1}$$

$$\mathrm{CBF} = \frac{6000\lambda\left(M_\mathrm{C} - M_\mathrm{L}\right)e^{\frac{\mathrm{TI}}{T_\mathrm{1A}}}}{2\alpha\,\mathrm{TI}_1 S_\mathrm{PD}}\left[\mathrm{ml/100g/min}\right] \tag{10.2}$$

where $\lambda$ is the brain/blood partition coefficient; $M_C$ and $M_L$ are the time-averaged signal intensities in the control and label images, respectively; $T_{1A}$ is the longitudinal relaxation time of arterial blood; $\alpha$ is the labeling efficiency; $S_{PD}$ is the signal intensity of a proton density-weighted image; $\tau$ is the label duration; and PLD is the post-labeling delay. TI and $TI_1$ are the previously defined parameters of QUIPSSII PASL. The factor 6000 converts the CBF units from mL/g/s to mL/(100 g)/min.

In principle, to scale the ASL difference signal to absolute CBF units, the signal intensity of the fully relaxed blood is needed. While different methods have been proposed to estimate this value [51–53], a voxel-wise scaling factor obtained from a separately acquired proton density image with a long TR (>5 s) is most commonly used [41]. The signal intensity of blood is then obtained dividing this image by the partition coefficient $\lambda$. Note that, although this coefficient could vary across different tissue types, a brain averaged value is used in practical implementations. Typical values are reported in Table 10.1, together with recommended imaging/labeling parameters [41].

**Table 10.1** Recommended ASL parameters for clinical studies at 3 T

| | |
|---|---|
| pCASL labeling duration ($\tau$) | 1800 ms |
| pCASL post-labeling delay (PLD) | 2000 ms |
| pCASL labeling efficiency ($\alpha$) | 0.85 |
| PASL $TI_1$ | 800 ms |
| PASL TI | 2000 ms |
| PASL labeling efficiency ($\alpha$) | 0.98 |
| Spatial resolution | 3.5 mm × 3.5 mm × 6 mm |
| Scan time | 4 min |
| Blood-brain partition coefficient ($\lambda$) | 0.9 mL/g |
| $T_1$ of arterial blood($T_{1A}$) | 1650 ms |

## 10.6 CBF Quantification in Clinical Studies

While the model at the basis of equations ((10.1) and ((10.2) is simplified, it is considered robust enough to be used as a good compromise in a clinical setting.

A critical sequence parameter for clinical populations is the time delay inserted between labeling and image acquisition that should be long enough to satisfy the first assumption of the CBF quantification model. As explained earlier, this delay is used to allow labeled arterial blood to reach the capillaries. A longer PLD/TI generally reduces the sensitivity of perfusion quantification to uncertainties regarding the precise arrival timing of the labeled blood at different voxels [30, 41]. Note that arterial arrival times may be markedly increased in the diseased brain, suggesting the use of long PLD/TI in clinical populations. However, it should also be considered that longer delays lead to a reduced signal-to-noise ratio, because the magnetic label decays with blood T1 which is comparable with typical PLD values. The choice of PLD is therefore a compromise between acceptable SNR and complete label delivery to ensure that the ASL signal will accurately reflect CBF.

In this regard, ASL perfusion measurements at 3 T are preferred over those at lower fields. Indeed, blood T1 at 3.0 T (1.6–1.8 s) is longer than blood T1 at 1.5 T (1.2–1.4 s), resulting in a better SNR because the label decays more slowly. This also allows the use of longer post-labeling delays to reduce sensitivity to arterial arrival time differences. Furthermore, the increased general SNR at high field can be exploited to decrease scanning time and to acquire higher-resolution images.

As an example of a quantitative CBF map obtained with ASL, Fig. 10.5 shows the results obtained in a recent study investigating the correlation of brain iron accumulation with the severity of vascular damage and cerebral perfusion in Alzheimer disease patients [54].

Methods based on single PLD/TI ASL imaging can provide a rapid and robust measure of CBF that can be made relatively insensitive to ATT with an optimal choice of sequence parameters. However, these methods do not provide measures of ATT or estimates of errors introduced into the CBF measurement by abnormally long ATT values. These aspects are particularly important in some clinical populations, such as patients with steno-occlusive diseases. In these cases, ASL approaches with multiple PLD/TI can be used together with more sophisticated models to fit the data, yielding both CBF and ATT estimates [55–59]. However, these multiple TI/PLD methods are more complex, requiring more measurements and processing, and are therefore not widespread in the standard ASL clinical setting.

In other advanced applications of ASL, labeling is performed on specific arterial vessels for

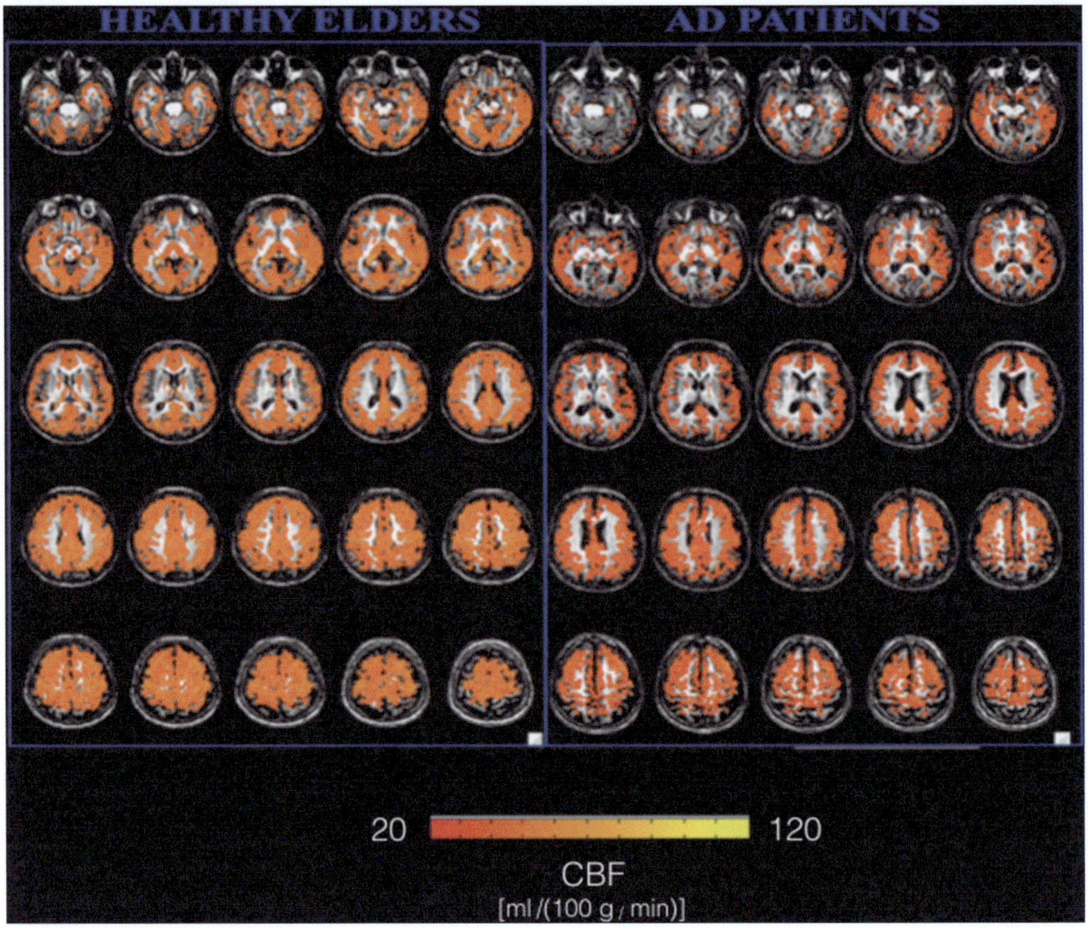


**Fig. 10.5** Quantitative CBF maps showing perfusion levels in a group of AD patients compared to normal elderly

studies requiring regional perfusion territory imaging [60, 61]. Selective labeling may be useful in patients with high-grade or complete vascular occlusion to guide the choice between angioplasty and stenting, to evaluate cerebrovascular bypass grafts, or to estimate the likelihood of an embolic or atherothrombotic source in a patient with multiple bright regions on diffusion-weighted imaging. For example, Hendrikse et al., selecting labeling on the basis of a previous MR angiogram, showed excellent visualization of perfusion territories corresponding to right carotid, left carotid, and posterior circulation [62–64]. It is important to note that the only way to obtain such information previously was invasive catheter angiography. These data may then be helpful to gain a better understanding of vascular dynamics in patients at high risk of stroke or being considered for surgical procedures [65].

## 10.7 Applications of ASL in fMRI

While BOLD fMRI [66–68] has evolved into a powerful tool to study brain function, its limitations as a quantitative technique are well known. Indeed, the BOLD response stems from a complex interplay of changes in CBF, cerebral blood volume (CBV), and oxygen metabolism ($CMRO_2$), and therefore the magnitude of the BOLD signal change is not a direct measure of neural activity [69–72]. This limitation is a major drawback when the research question requires a comparison of fMRI data across groups that may differ in both neural activity and neurovascular coupling [73, 74].

A solution to this problem has been to combine BOLD and ASL imaging within a biophysical model of the BOLD effect in order to disentangle the different physiological variables (e.g., CBF, $CMRO_2$) that link neuronal signaling to changes in MR signal decay via blood deoxyhemoglobin content [75–78]. This approach, termed calibrated BOLD imaging, is very attractive because it offers a noninvasive quantitative measurement of cerebral physiology that can be used, e.g., to characterize long-term changes in brain oxygen metabolism in studies of brain diseases and treatment interventions.

Standard BOLD fMRI based on gradient-echo imaging also suffers from low spatial specificity due to a significant contribution of downside large venous vessels to the functional signal. In addition, the macrovascular contribution introduces a significant nonlinearity in the BOLD response [79]. Although spin-echo imaging was shown to reduce the macrovascular contribution and the corresponding nonlinear effects on the BOLD signal [80–82], the increase in spatial specificity to the capillary bed with this technique was considered significant only at high fields (>7 T) [83, 84]. In this regard, despite a lower sensitivity with respect to standard BOLD, the fMRI technique based on ASL has proved to be a suitable tool for mapping neuronal activity changes induced by motor/cognitive tasks or sensory stimulation [85–87]. In particular, ASL showed higher intrasubject reproducibility and a more accurate spatial localization of neuronal activity than BOLD fMRI even at 3 T due to a lower contribution of macroscopic veins to the functional signal [86].

### Conclusions

Arterial spin labeling is a MRI technique that allows a noninvasive quantification of cerebral blood flow, which is an important physiological parameter in many brain disorders. The technique has been initially validated against other methods that use exogenous contrast agents, such as PET. In the past two decades, ASL has evolved in a powerful tool capable to obtain high-quality whole-brain perfusion images in a few minutes of scanning. With recent technical advances, ASL implementations are now commercially available on all major MRI platforms, offering an attractive methodology to study brain perfusion and function in clinical populations.

## References

1. Petrella JR, Provenzale JM (2000) MR perfusion imaging of the brain: techniques and applications. AJR Am J Roentgenol 175:207–220
2. Cha S (2003) Perfusion MR imaging: basic principles and clinical applications. Magn Reson Imaging Clin N Am 11(3):403–413
3. Provenzale JM, Jahan R, Naidich TP, Fox AJ (2003) Assessment of the patient with hyperacute stroke: imaging and therapy. Radiology 229(2):347–359
4. Scarabino T, Nemore F, Giannatempo GM et al (2003) 3.0 T magnetic resonance in neuroradiology. Eur J Radiol 48:154–164
5. Scarabino T, Giannatempo GM, Pollice S et al (2004) 3.0 T perfusion MR imaging. Riv Neuroradiol 17:807–812
6. Shimony JS (2005) Concepts in perfusion MRI. Syllabus. Int Soc Magn Reson Med 13
7. Zaharchuk G (2005) Frontiers of cerebral perfusion magnetic resonance imaging. Appl Radiol (Suppl to January) (34):100–111
8. Manka C, Traber F, Gieseke J et al (2005) Three-dimensional dynamic susceptibility-weighted perfusion MR imaging at 3.0 T: feasibility and contrast agent dose. Radiology 234(3):869–877
9. Barbier EL, Lamalle L, Decorps M (2001) Methodology of brain perfusion imaging. J Magn Reson Imaging 13(4):496–520
10. Derdeyn CP, TO V, Yundt KD et al (2002) Variability of cerebral blood volume and oxygen extraction: stages of cerebral haemodynamic impairment revisited. Brain 125(3):595–607
11. Chen JJ, Wieckowska M, Meyer E, GB P (2008) Cerebral blood flow measurement using fMRI and PET: across-validation study. Int J Biomed Imaging 2008 :516359. doi:10.1155/2008/516359Article ID
12. Wintermark M, Sesay M, Barbier E et al (2005) Comparative overview of brain perfusion imaging techniques. Stroke 36:e83–e99
13. Penfield JG, Reilly RF Jr (2007) What nephrologists need to know about gadolinium. Nat Clin Pract Nephrol 3:654–668
14. Sadowski EA, Benne LK, Chan MR et al (2007) Nephrogenic systemic fibrosis: risk factors and incidence estimation. Radiology 243:148–157

15. Detre JA, Leigh JS, WIlliams DS, Koretsky AP (1992) Perfusion imaging. Magn Reson Med 23:37–45
16. Williams DS, Detre JA, Leigh JS, Koretsky AP (1992) Magnetic resonance imaging of perfusion using spin-inversion of arterial water. Proc Natl Acad Sci U S A 89:212–216
17. Golay X, Hendrikse J, Lim TC (2004) Perfusion imaging using arterial spin labeling. Top Magn Reson Imaging 15:10–27
18. Hendrikse J, Petersen ET, Golay X (2012) Vascular disorders: insights from arterial spin labeling. Neuroimaging Clin N Am 22:259–269
19. Heijtel DF, Mutsaerts HJ, Bakker E, Schober P, Stevens MF, Petersen ET, van Berckel BN, Majoie CB, Booij J, van Osch MJ, Vanbavel E, Boellaard R, Lammertsma AA, Nederveen AJ (2014) Accuracy and precision of pseudo-continuous arterial spin labeling perfusion during baseline and hypercapnia: a head-to-head comparison with 15O H2O positron emission tomography. Neuroimage 92:182–192
20. Petersen ET, Mouridsen K, Golay X (2010) The QUASAR reproducibility study, part II: results from a multi-center arterial spin labeling test-retest study. Neuroimage 49:104–113
21. Xu G, Rowley HA, Wu G, Alsop DC, Shankaranarayanan A, Dowling M, Christian BT, Oakes TR, Johnson SC (2010) Reliability and precision of pseudo-continuous arterial spin labeling perfusion MRI on 3.0 T and comparison with 15O-water PET in elderly subjects at risk for Alzheimer's disease. NMR Biomed 23:286–293
22. Mutsaerts HJ, van Osch MJ, Zelaya FO, Wang DJ, Nordhøy W, Wang Y, Wastling S, Fernandez-Seara MA, Petersen ET, Pizzini FB, Fallatah S, Hendrikse J, Geier O, Günther M, Golay X, Nederveen AJ, Bjørnerud A, Groote IR (2015) Multi-vendor reliability of arterial spin labeling perfusion MRI using a near-identical sequence: implications for multi-center studies. Neuroimage 113:143–152. doi:10.1016/j.neuroimage.2015.03.043 Epub 2015 Mar 24 PubMed PMID: 25818685
23. Deibler AR, Pollock JM, Kraft RA, Tan H, Burdette JH, Maldjian JA (2008) Arterial spin-labeling in routine clinical practice, part 2: hypoperfusion patterns. AJNR Am J Neuroradiol 29:1235–1241
24. Wang DJ, Chen Y, Fernandez-Seara MA, Detre JA (2011) Potentials and challenges for arterial spin labeling in pharmacological magnetic resonance imaging. J Pharmacol Exp Ther 337:359–366
25. De Vis JB, Hendrikse J, Bhogal A, Adams A, Kappelle LJ, Petersen ET (2015) Age-related changes in brain hemodynamics; a calibrated MRI study. Hum Brain Mapp 36(10):3973–3987
26. Ogawa S, Tank DW, Menon R, Ellermann JM, Kim SG, Merkle H, Ugurbil K (1992) Intrinsic signal changes accompanying sensory stimulation: functional brain mapping with magnetic resonance imaging. Proc Natl Acad Sci U S A 89:5951–5955
27. Buxton RB (2010) Interpreting oxygenation-based neuroimaging signals: the importance and the challenge of understanding brain oxygen metabolism. Front Neuroenerg 2:8. doi:10.3389/fnene.2010.00008
28. VJ S, Vannest J, Lee G, Hernandez-Garcia L, Plante E, Rajagopal A, SK H, CMIND Authorship Consortium (2015) Evidence that neurovascular coupling underlying the BOLD effect increases with age during childhood. Hum Brain Mapp 36(1):1–15
29. Aslan S, Xu F, Wang PL, Uh J, Yezhuvath US, van Osch M, Lu H (2010) Estimation of labeling efficiency in pseudocontinuous arterial spin labeling. Magn Reson Med 63(3):765–771
30. Alsop DC, Detre JA (1996) Reduced transit-time sensitivity in noninvasive magnetic resonance imaging of human cerebral blood flow. J Cereb Blood Flow Metab 16:1236–1249
31. Sardashti M, Schwartzberg DG, Stomp GP, Dixon WT (1990) Spin-labeling angiography of the carotids by presaturation and simplified adiabatic inversion. Magn Reson Med 15:192–200
32. Wolff SD, Balaban RS (1989) Magnetization transfer contrast (MTC) and tissue water proton relaxation in vivo. Magn Reson Med 10:135–144
33. Alsop DC, Detre JA (1998) Multisection cerebral blood flow MRI imaging with continuous arterial spin labeling. Radiology 208:410–416
34. Golay X, Hendrikse J, Lim TCC (2004) Perfusion imaging using arterial spin labeling. Top Magn Reson Imaging 15:10–27
35. Edelman RR, Siewert B, Darby DG et al (1994) Qualitative mapping of cerebral blood flow and functional localization with echo-planar MR imaging and signal targeting with alternating radio frequency. Radiology 192:513–520
36. Edelman RR, Chen Q (1998) EPISTAR MRI: multislice mapping of cerebral blood flow. Magn Reson Med 40:800–805
37. Wong EC, Buxton RB, Frank LR (1998) Quantitative imaging of perfusion using a single subtraction (QUIPSS and QUIPSS II). Magn Reson Med 39:702–708
38. GarciaDM, BazelaireCD, AlsopD (2005) Pseudo-continuous flow driven adiabatic inversion for arterial spin labeling. Scientific Meeting of the International Society for Magnetic Resonance in Medicine, Miami, p. 37
39. Dai W, Garcia D, De Bazelaire C, Alsop DC (2008) Continuous flow-driven inversion for arterial spin labeling using pulsed radio frequency and gradient fields. Magn Reson Med 60:1488–1497
40. Wu WC, Fernandez-Seara M, JA D et al (2007) A theoretical and experimental investigation of the tagging efficiency of pseudocontinuous arterial spin labeling. Magn Reson Med 58:1020–1027
41. Alsop DC, Detre JA, Golay X et al (2015) Recommended implementation of arterial spin-labeled perfusion MRI for clinical applications: a consensus of the ISMRM perfusion study group and the European consortium for ASL in dementia. Magn Reson Med 73:102–116
42. Gevers S, Van Osch MJ, Bokkers RPH et al (2011) Intra- and multicenter reproducibility of pulsed,

continuous and pseudocontinuous arterial spin labeling methods for measuring cerebral perfusion. J Cereb Blood Flow Metab 31:1706–1715
43. Garcia DM, Duhamel G, Alsop DC (2005) Efficiency of inversion pulses for background suppressed arterial spin labeling. Magn Reson Med 54:366–372
44. Lawrence KSS, Frank JA, Bandettini PA et al (2005) Noise reduction in multi-slice arterial spin tagging imaging. Magn Reson Med 53:735–738
45. Vidorreta M, Wang Z, Rodriguez I et al (2012) Comparison of 2D and 3D single-shot ASL perfusion fMRI sequences. Neuroimage 66C:662–671
46. Nielsen JF, Hernandez-Garcia L (2013) Functional perfusion imaging using pseudocontinuous arterial spin labeling with low flip angle segmented 3D spiral readouts. Magn Reson Med 69:382–390
47. Gunther M, Oshio K, Feinberg DA (2005) Single-shot 3D imaging techniques improve arterial spin labeling perfusion measurements. Magn Reson Med 54:491–498
48. Zaharchuk G, Do HM, Marks MP et al (2011) Arterial spin-labeling MRI can identify the presence and intensity of collateral perfusion in patients with moyamoya disease. Stroke 42:2485–2491
49. Le TT, Fischbein NJ, Andre JB et al (2012) Identification of venous signal on arterial spin labeling improves diagnosis of dural arteriovenous fistulas and small arteriovenous malformations. AJNR Am J Neuroradiol 33:61–68
50. Wolf RL, Wang J, Detre JA et al (2008) Arteriovenous shunt visualization in arteriovenous malformations with arterial spin labeling MR imaging. AJNR Am J Neuroradiol 29:681–687
51. Buxton RB, Frank LR, Wong EC et al (1998) A general kinetic model for quantitative perfusion imaging with arterial spin labeling. Magn Reson Med 40:383–396
52. Wong EC, Buxton RB, Frank LR (1997) Implementation of quantitative perfusion imaging techniques for functional brain mapping using pulsed arterial spin labeling. NMR Biomed 10:237–249
53. Wong EC, Buxton RB, Frank LR (1998) A theoretical and experimental comparison of continuous and pulsed arterial spin labeling techniques for quantitative perfusion imaging. Magn Reson Med 40: 348–355
54. MaccaroneM, EspositoR, SaliceS, et al. (2015) Quantitative MR R2* imaging and arterial spin labeling brain perfusion assessment in alzheimer disease. Radiological Society of North America 2015 Scientific Assembly and Annual Meeting, November 29–December 4, 2015, Chicago. archive.rsna.org/2015/15016539.html
55. Gunther M, Bock M, Schad LR (2001) Arterial spin labeling in combination with a Look-Locker sampling strategy: inflow turbo-sampling EPI- FAIR (ITS-FAIR). Magn Reson Med 46:974–984
56. Petersen ET, Lim T, Golay X (2006) Model-free arterial spin labeling quantification approach for perfusion MRI. Magn Reson Med 55:219–232
57. Francis ST, Bowtell R, Gowland PA (2008) Modeling and optimization of Look-Locker spin labeling for measuring perfusion and transit time changes in activation studies taking into account arterial blood volume. Magn Reson Med 59:316–325
58. Dai W, Robson PM, Shankaranarayanan A et al (2012) Reduced resolution transit delay prescan for quantitative continuous arterial spin labeling perfusion imaging. Magn Reson Med 67:1252–1265
59. Wang DJ, Alger JR, Qiao JX et al (2013) Multi-delay multi-parametric arterial spin-labeled perfusion MRI in acute ischemic stroke—comparison with dynamic susceptibility contrast enhanced perfusion imaging. NeuroImage Clin 3:1–7
60. van Laar PJ, van der Grond J, Hendrikse J (2008) Brain perfusion territory imaging: methods and clinical applications of selective arterial spin- labeling MR imaging. Radiology 246:354–364
61. Paiva FF, Tannus A, Silva AC (2007) Measurement of cerebral perfusion territories using arterial spin labelling. NMR Biomed 20:633–642
62. Hendrikse J, van Raamt AF, van der Graaf Y et al (2005) Distribution of cerebral blood flow in the circle of Willis. Radiology 235(1):184–189
63. Hendrikse J, van der Grond J, Lu H et al (2004) Flow territory mapping of the cerebral arteries with regional perfusion MRI. Stroke 35(4):882–887
64. Hendrikse J, van Osch MJ, van der Zwan A et al (2005) Altered flow territories after extracranial to intracranial by- pass surgery: clinical implementation of selective arterial spin labeling MRI. Proc Intl Soc Mag Reson Med 13:1137
65. van Laar PJ, Hendrikse J, Golay X et al (2005) In-vivo flow territory mapping of major brain feeding arteries: a population study with selective arterial spin labeling MRI. Proc Int Soc Mag Reson Med 13:1134
66. Kwong KK, Belliveau JW, Chesler DA et al (1992) Dynamic magnetic resonance imaging of human brain activity during primary sensory stimulation. Proc Natl Acad Sci U S A 89:5675–5679
67. Bandettini PA, Wong EC, Hinks RS et al (1992) Time course EPI of human brain function during task activation. Magn Reson Med 25:390–397
68. Ogawa S, Tank DW, Menon R et al (1992) Intrinsic signal changes accompanying sensory stimulation: functional brain mapping with magnetic resonance imaging. Proc Natl Acad Sci U S A 89:5951–5955
69. Ances BM, Leontiev O, Perthen JE et al (2008) Regional differences in the coupling of cerebral blood flow and oxygen metabolism changes in response to activation: implications for BOLD-fMRI. Neuroimage 39:1510–1521
70. Buxton RB (2010) Interpreting oxygenation-based neuroimaging signals: the importance and the challenge of understanding brain oxygen metabolism. Front Neuroenerg 2:8. http://dx.doi.org/10.3389/fnene.2010.00008
71. Griffeth VEM, Perthen JE, Buxton RB (2011) Prospects for quantitative fMRI: investigating the effects of caffeine on baseline oxygen metabolism and

the response to a visual stimulus in humans. Neuroimage 57:809–816
72. Moradi F, Buracas GT, Buxton RB (2012) Attention strongly increases oxygen metabolic response to stimulus in primary visual cortex. Neuroimage 59:601–607
73. Liu TT (2013) Neurovascular factors in resting-state functional MRI. Neuroimage 80:339–348
74. Mohtasib RS, Lumley G, Goodwin JA et al (2012) Calibrated fMRI during a cognitive Stroop task reveals reduced metabolic response with increasing age. Neuroimage 59:1143–1151
75. Blockley NP, Griffeth VE, Simon AB et al (2013) A review of calibrated blood oxygenation level-dependent (BOLD) methods for the measurement of task-induced changes in brain oxygen metabolism. NMR Biomed 26:987–1003
76. Davis TL, Kwong KK, Weisskoff RM et al (1998) Calibrated functional MRI: mapping the dynamics of oxidative metabolism. Proc Natl Acad Sci U S A 95:1834–1839
77. Wise RG, Harris AD, Stone AJ et al (2013) Measurement of OEF and absolute CMRO2: MRI-based methods using interleaved and combined hypercapnia and hyperoxia. Neuroimage 83:135–147
78. Bulte DP, Kelly M, Germuska M et al (2012) Quantitative measurement of cerebral physiology using respiratory-calibrated MRI. Neuroimage 60:582–591
79. Zhang N, Zhu XH, Chen W (2008) Investigating the source of BOLD nonlinearity in human visual cortex in response to paired visual stimuli. Neuroimage 43:204–212
80. Zhang N, Yacoub E, Zhu XH et al (2009) Linearity of blood-oxygenation-level dependent signal at microvasculature. Neuroimage 48:313–318
81. Chiacchiaretta P, Ferretti A (2015) Resting state BOLD functional connectivity at 3 T: spin echo versus gradient echo EPI. PLoS One 10(3):e0120398. doi:10.1371/journal.pone.0120398
82. Chiacchiaretta P, Romani GL, Ferretti A (2013) Sensitivity of BOLD response to increasing visual contrast: spin echo versus gradient echo EPI. Neuroimage 82:35–43
83. Uludağ K, Müller-Bierl B, Uğurbil K (2009) An integrative model for neuronal activity-induced signal changes for gradient and spin echo functional imaging. Neuroimage 48:150–165
84. Norris DG (2012) Spin-echo fMRI: The poor relation? Neuroimage 62:1109–1115
85. Diekhoff S, Uludag K, Sparing R et al (2011) Functional localization in the human brain: gradient-echo, spin-echo, and arterial spin-labeling fMRI compared with neuronavigated TMS. Hum BrainMapp 32:341–357
86. Raoult H, Petr J, Bannier EC et al (2011) Arterial spin labeling for motor activation mapping at 3 T with a 32-channel coil: reproducibility and spatial accuracy in comparison with BOLD fMRI. Neuroimage 58:157–167
87. Tjandra T, Brooks JC, Figueiredo P et al (2005) Quantitative assessment of the reproducibility of functional activation measured with BOLD and MR perfusion imaging: implications for clinical trial design. Neuroimage 27:393–401

# Functional MRI at 3.0 Tesla

# 11

Daniela Cevolani, Raffaele Agati,
Francesco Di Salle, and Marco Leonardi

## 11.1 Introduction

Since 1936, Pauling and Coryell [1] had discovered that the magnetic susceptibility of hemoglobin changed as a function of whether it was bound to oxygen or not: oxyhemoglobin had magnetic moment zero, whereas deoxyhemoglobin was paramagnetic.

However, it was in 1990 that Seiji Ogawa [2] and colleagues demonstrated, in vivo and by a 7 Tesla magnetic resonance (MR) apparatus, a particular phenomenon called blood oxygenation level dependent (hence the acronym BOLD). By using anesthetized rats and gradient echo T2* images, they showed that, when rats inhaled 100 % oxygen, brain vessels were scarcely detectable at MR; otherwise, when the mixture inhaled was progressively depleted of oxygen, brain vessels were progressively and clearly detected as darker lines. The authors noted that "… the image contrast was caused by the magnetic susceptibility difference between the blood, with paramagnetic deoxyhemoglobin, and the surrounding tissues" and concluded "… gradient echo images of the brain at high fields give a high image contrast which is sensitive to the blood oxygenation level…," but they also deduced "When some region in a brain is much more active than other regions, the active region could show darker lines [the vessels] in the image, because of the increased level of deoxyhemoglobin resulting from higher hemoglobin consumption." This last deduction was later proved not to be completely true, as we will see later on.

Previously (1880s), an Italian physiologist, Angelo Mosso, studied cerebral fluxes and brain pulsations in patients with skull defects: he noted an increase of brain pulsations, when subjects were engaged in tasks as mathematical calculations and deduced that mental activity was accompanied by a local increase of blood flow. To overwhelm the problem of measuring brain blood flow in healthy subjects, with normal skulls, Mosso devised the so-called human circulation balance [3, 4]; this is described as a "delicately balanced table that could tip downwards either at the head or the foot if the weight of either end increased" [5]. When a subject is lying relaxed on the balance, the balance is in equilibrium; when the subject begins to think (to

D. Cevolani (✉)
Department of Specialized Diagnostics and Experimental Health - Department of Neuroradiology, University of Bologna, Bologna, Italy
e-mail: daniela.cevolani@unibo.it

R. Agati • M. Leonardi
Department of Neuroradiology, Bellaria Hospital - University of Bologna, Bologna, Italy
e-mail: raffaele.agati@ausl.bo.it

F. Di Salle
Department of Neuroradiology, University of Salerno, Salerno, Italy



T. Scarabino et al. (eds.), *High Field Brain MRI*, DOI 10.1007/978-3-319-44174-0_11

emotional or mathematical tasks), the balance tilts toward the head, because neural activity causes an increased blood afflux (and weight) to the brain. The work of Mosso was recently replicated by some authors [6], who used modern technologies and gained the same results, demonstrating the validity of Mosso's results.

In those years, two neurophysiologists, Charles Smart Roy and Charles Scott Sherrington [7], suggested a correlation between cerebral circulation and metabolism and focused attention particularly on some acid products (e.g., lactic acid), because of their capability to cause enormous local vasodilation even if they were given in very small amounts. They hypothesized an "... automatic mechanism ..." with "... no rise of pressure in the systemic arteries..." and "... by which the blood-supply of any part of the cerebral tissue is varied in accordance with the activity of the chemical changes which underlie the functional action of that part...." They concluded "... the brain possesses an intrinsic mechanism by which its vascular supply can be varied locally in correspondence with local variations of functional activity," which we now call "local autoregulation of cerebral flow."

Even if all the background was ready to clarify the phenomena at the basis of BOLD signal, nevertheless the time was not ripe to develop and apply these concepts. Moreover, a luminary physiologist of the time, Leonard Hill, stated that no relationship existed between cerebral activity and cerebral circulation [8, 9].

It needs to go up to 1928, to find another work on the subject. In that year, John Farquar Fulton, a neurophysiologist and neurosurgeon, published a study [10] on a patient with an arteriovenous malformation, which eroded the occipital bone. The patient complained a murmur inside his head, which was increasing when he was reading or using his eyes. Objectively, it was characterized by a bruit, which increased every time visual activity increased (e.g., from the dark to the light, from rest to reading). The author concluded that "... localized increase in vascularity of the brain occurs under appropriate sensory stimulation, or, more specifically, it is probable that visual activity in man is associated with an increase in the vascularity of the occipital lobes...."

We will need to wait until 1948, to have a method to quantify the regional cerebral blood flow in humans [11].

## 11.2 Genesis of the BOLD Signal

Today, we know the sequence of events occurring during the genesis of the BOLD signal, which is the following (Fig. 11.1). Some activated neurons fire in a certain area of the cerebral cortex, generating spikes. This activity, and the corresponding $Na^+$ and $K^+$ movements, activates the $Na^+$-$K^+$ pump, which burns metabolic energy and hence adenosine triphosphate (ATP). Metabolic pathways intervening in the synthesis of new ATP cause an increase in both oxygen (from hemoglobin of red blood cells) and glucose (from plasma) consumption. It should be noted that neural metabolism is only aerobic and nervous tissue has no stores of either oxygen or glucose (differently from glycogen in the skeletal muscle). Consequently, any oxygen demand could only be extracted from the oxyhemoglobin, which, in turns, becomes deoxyhemoglobin and acquires paramagnetic properties, in the area where neurons increased their firing rate.

Neuronal firing gives also rise to synaptic activity, and, during synaptic activity, neurotransmitters are released together with other substances as ADP, $H^+$, $K^+$, and nitric oxide (NO). All these substances, but especially NO, are powerful vasodilators [12, 13]. The mechanism at the basis of the neurovascular coupling seems to be the action of NO (possibly mediated by astrocytes) on the precapillary sphincters, where it causes smooth muscle sphincters to relax: the upstream arterial pressure gives rise to important sphincters vasodilation, with consequent huge inflow of oxygenate blood. The spatial extension of vasodilation involves a volume of 1–3 $mm^3$ (spatial resolution), an area corresponding to the local anatomy of the terminal microvascular bed, which is similar, but non equal, to the neuronal firing area (the first is far wider). The latency

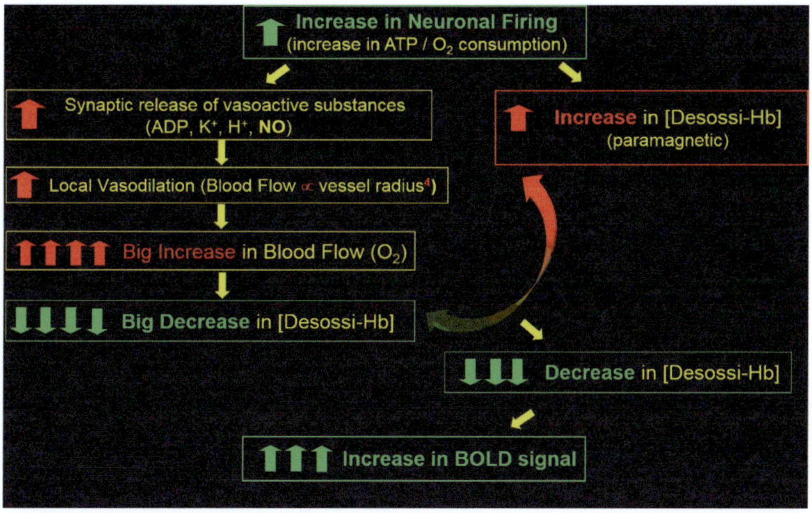


**Fig. 11.1** Schematic view of the events occurring in the genesis of BOLD signal. Explanations in the text

(temporal resolution) of the vasodilation is of some seconds, the time necessary for NO to be released by synaptic activity, to diffuse in the interstitial space, to reach sphincters, and to transduce the signal in smooth muscle relaxation The vasodilation consequent a neuronal firing is also called "neurovascular coupling."

Deoxyhemoglobin production and vasodilation are two phenomena not proportional: vasodilation is largely prevalent compared to the increase in oxygen utilization [14]. Consequently, the increase in blood flow is huge with respect to deoxyhemoglobin production. The local increased supply of arterial oxygenated blood dilutes the deoxyhemoglobin concentration in the capillary and venular side of the area where neural activity was increased. The dilution is so important that deoxyhemoglobin concentration reaches values well below those at rest. When we consider gradient echo images of the brain at MR high fields (T2*), such a reduction in paramagnetic deoxyhemoglobin gives rise to a clear-cut local signal increase.

At this point, we may give an answer to a previous question: why the last Ogawa and coll. deduction was not completely true? Because, in their anesthetized rats, there was no possible local vasodilation induced by any neuronal activity. As a matter of fact, when you analyze a BOLD signal in an unanesthetized subject, you have to take into account not only deoxyhemoglobin increase, consequent to neural activity, but also, and especially, arterial blood flow increase, triggered by synaptic activity.

Summing up, BOLD signal is an indirect phenomenon, not generated by neuronal spikes per se, but derived from the physicochemical and physiological consequences of neuronal firing and synaptic activity. It mirrors neuronal activity, but has far less spatial (mm instead of μm) and temporal (seconds instead of ms) resolution.

## 11.3 Hemodynamic Response

The hemodynamic response (HDR) describes the time course of the BOLD signal, generated by an activated cortical area and acquired by an MR EPI GE T2* sequence (Fig. 11.2). It was described for the first time in 1995 [15] and is usually plotted as a % signal change during time. It consists in a curve starting with a small initial negativity (dip), followed by a steep rise, which reaches a peak in 2–3 s. If the stimulus is short, the signal returns to the baseline, after the peak. If the stimulus is longer, the increase is higher

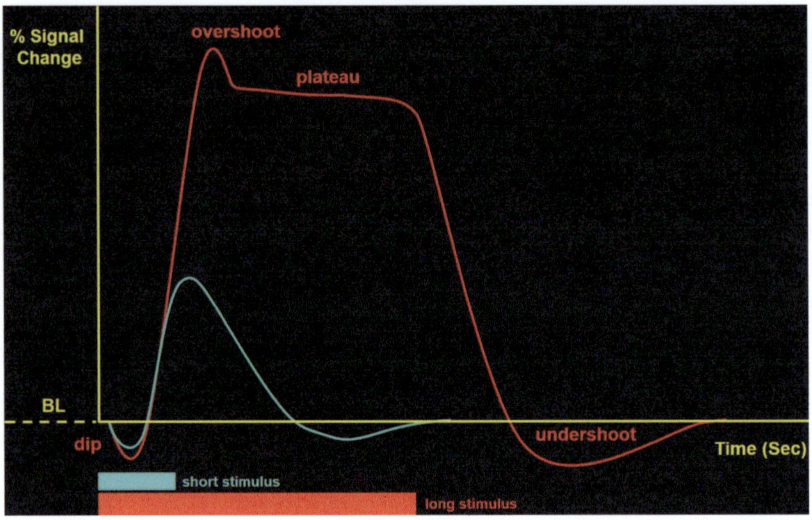


**Fig. 11.2** Time course of hemodynamic response (HDR): responses appear different depending on stimulus duration. When stimulus is short (short blue bar), the curve is smaller in height and duration (*blue curve*); when stimulus is longer (*long red bar*), the curve, besides being taller and longer, shows a dip, a plateau, an overshoot, and an undershoot (*red curve*)

and continues with a plateau, preceded by an extra peak (overshoot). After the end of the stimulus, with a latency of 2–3 s, a drop occurs, which continues beyond the baseline and becomes negative (undershoot poststimulus).

Three variables are at the basis of the described time course: (1) deoxyhemoglobin concentration (and oxygen consumption), (2) local cerebral blood flow (CBF), and (3) cerebral blood volume (CBV).

The initial dip is very small: its intensity is in the order of magnitude of 0.5–1.0 % of the whole BOLD signal (it often is not detectable in 1.5 Tesla systems). It is very spatially localized and corresponds to neuronal firing. It occurs in the gray matter only and is due to the local increase in the deoxyhemoglobin concentration. Since few seconds are needed for the local vasodilation to begin, in the early phase, the increased oxygen consumption, due to the raised neuronal firing, is not matched with the increase in CBF (hence in oxyhemoglobin) and the paramagnetic deoxyhemoglobin prevails, giving rise to a negative signal. As soon as vasodilation begins, the huge oxygenated blood flow predominates over the locally produced deoxyhemoglobin, and the curve inverts its slope, increases very quickly, and goes beyond the zero up to reach the peak just 5–8 s after the beginning of the event (Fig. 11.3). The so-called

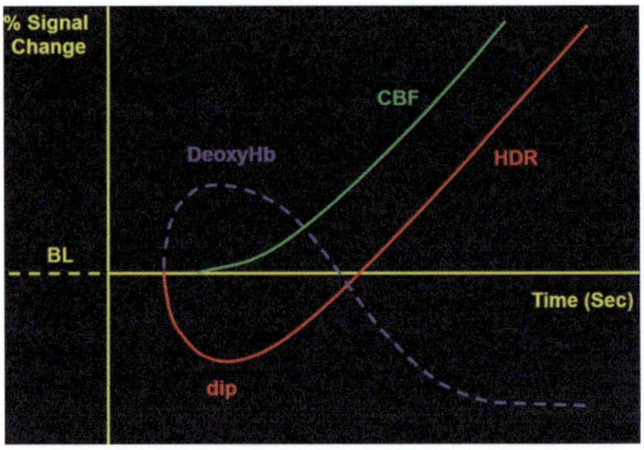


**Fig. 11.3** Events characterizing the dip. The initial decrease in hemodynamic response (HDR, *red*) is due to a mismatch between deoxyhemoglobin concentration (*violet*) and cerebral blood flow (CBF, *green*). At this initial stage, local vasodilation is still not occurred. The increased oxygen consumption, due to increased neuronal firing, gives rise to a local increase in deoxyhemoglobin concentration, with consequent signal decrease. A soon as vasodilation occurs, the big local increase in CBF (and hence in oxyhemoglobin) dilutes deoxyhemoglobin and the signal rapidly increases

BOLD effect is usually referred to this positive response: it is more spatially diffuse, with respect to the area of neuronal firing, because it involves capillaries and venules and has a lower spatial resolution. The local increase in CBF, besides increasing oxyhemoglobin concentration, produces an increase also in CBV, whose dynamic is slower than the other phenomena described. When the stimulation ends, neuronal firing ceases and also local vasodilation ceases, but with a latency of 2–3 s. The curve drops off toward the baseline, goes beyond it, and becomes negative (undershoot). Overshoot and undershoot are both due to the disproportion between CBV and CBF, whose dynamics are faster than that of CBV [16]. When stimulation begins, CBF increases faster than CBV, with a relative increase of oxyhemoglobin (overshoot); when stimulation ends, CBF regains baseline values faster than that of CBV, this time with a relative increase of deoxyhemoglobin (undershoot). The undershoot amplitude is often a function of the stimulus duration; usually it takes 1–2 min to regain the baseline.

Given a stimulus of a definite intensity, if the neuronal firing rate increases, also the height of the plateau will increase; if the stimulus duration increases, also the duration of the plateau will increase, but only to a limited extent. This because neural firing tends to decrease with time, owing to the phenomenon of adaptation. This happens after 15–20 s of continuative stimulation. The knowledge of HDR is of capital importance in setting the duration and the timing of stimulations, to obtain a reliable BOLD signal, as we will see in a little while.

## 11.4 How to Recognize BOLD Signal From Baseline

The BOLD signal resulting from a single stimulation has a very low intensity with respect to the baseline, in the order of 1 %, for a 50 % change in CBF at 1.5 T and of 5–10 % at 3.0 T. Such a signal has an amplitude in the order or magnitude of the experimental error (±10 %) and is not strong enough to be distinct from the background noise with certainty. Consequently, nor can brain activated areas be defined with certainty.

Some strategies can be employed to increase BOLD signal intensity, so that to make its interpretation more reliable: (1) to protract the stimulation, (2) to repeat the stimulation in the single subject, and (3) to repeat the stimulation in many subjects. Their application depends on the aims established by the operator. We have already seen that the stimulation cannot be prolonged more than 20 s, except at expense of neuronal adaptation and decrease of the signal intensity. To repeat stimulations, in single or many subjects (population studies), has otherwise the problem of variability. Anyhow, measures have to be repeated many times, to allow sufficient averaging.

The easiest way to set the duration and timing of a stimulation is the classic block paradigm, in which periods of stimulations are alternated to periods of rest (see also Chap. 8). Once the paradigm is known, we may assume some model for describing the hemodynamic response to stimulation: the typical form is that of a trapezoid, having smoothed angles and a certain lag, with respect to the stimulus. Then, for each voxel, a correlation of this model function with the measured voxel time course is calculated. The signals of each voxel are treated as two populations, stimulation and rest: the simplest processing approach considers the subtraction of the average of all the images acquired during the rest condition from the average of all the images acquired during the task condition. A t-test is used to assess whether there is a significant difference between the means of the two groups. A statistical threshold is defined, and only the voxels that pass the set statistical threshold are considered. They are usually colored and the color used reflects the statistic value, which, in turn, is a measure of the degree of the signal change. This procedure will provide a map of the activated areas. The color map is then superimposed on a coregistered morphological image to make map localization easier (Fig. 11.4).

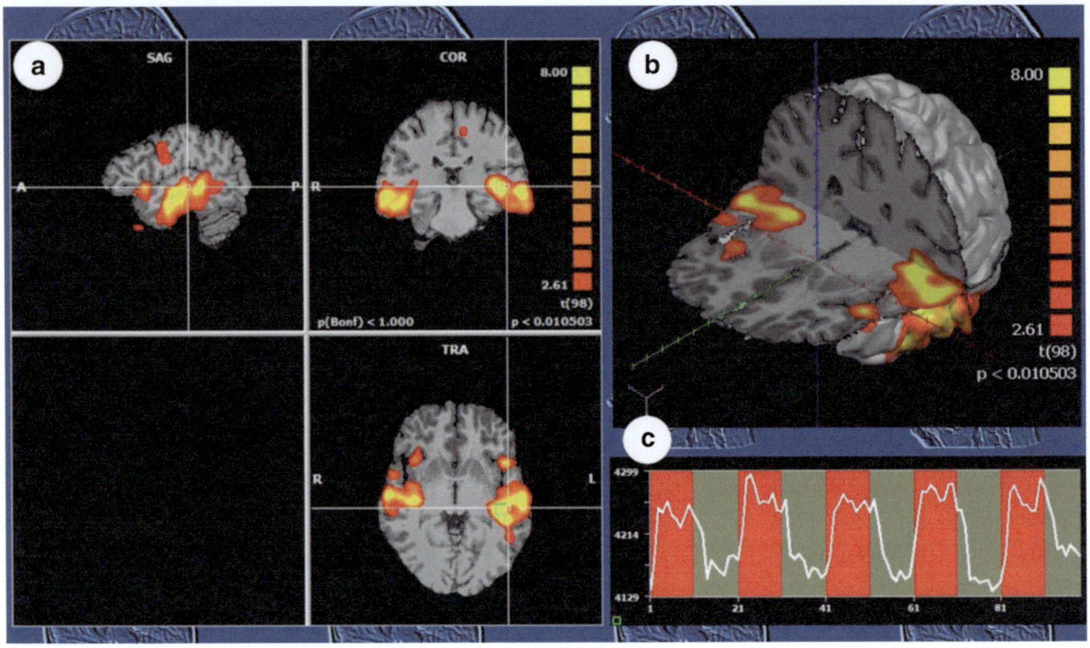


**Fig. 11.4** Summary of the events described in the text. Example of an fMRI block experiment, in which a healthy subject is listening to five different Aesop's fables vs. silence, by nonmagnetic binaural stereophonic earphones. Statistical threshold: $p < 0.001$. (**a**) Multiplanar reconstruction of the activation maps. (**b**) 3D view, with a partial brain removal to show eloquent areas. (**c**) Signal time course of a region of interest, indicated by the cross in (**a**)

## 11.5 Concluding Remarks

Summing up, the localization of the BOLD signal becomes reliable at high MR fields. This allows not only to confirm and deepen many known functional phenomena but also to throw new light in many aspects of the physiology and pathology of the brain.

## References

1. Pauling L, Coryell CD (1936) The magnetic properties and structure of hemoglobin, oxy-hemoglobin and carbonmonoxidhemoglobin. Proc Natl Acad Sci U S A 22:210–216
2. Ogawa S, Lee T-M, Nayak AS, Glynn P (1990) Oxygenation-sensitive contrast in magnetic resonance image of rodent brain at high magnetic fields. Magn Reson Med 14:68–78
3. Mosso A (1884) Applicazione della bilancia allo studio della circolazione sanguigna dell'uomo. Atti R Acad Lincei Mem Cl Sci Fische Mat Nat, Serie 3, Ann 281, 19:531-543
4. Sandrone S, Bacigaluppi M, Galloni MR, Martino G (2012) Angelo Mosso (1846–1910). J Neurol 259:2513–2514
5. James W (1890) The principles of psychology. Henry Holt & Company, New York
6. Field DT, Inman LA (2014) Weighing brain activity with the balance: a contemporary replication of Angelo Mosso's historical experiment. Brain 137:634–639
7. Roy CS, Sherrington CS (1890) On the regulation of the blood- supply of the brain. J Physiol Lond 11:85–108
8. Hill L (1896) The physiology and pathology of the cerebral circulation; an experiment research. J & A Churchill, London
9. Raichle ME (1998) Behind the scenes in functional brains imaging: a historical and physiological perspective. Proc Natl Acad Sci U S A 95:765–772
10. Fulton JF (1928) Observations upon the vascularity of the human occipital lobe during visual activity. Brain 51:310–320
11. Kety S, Schmidt CF (1948) The nitrous oxide method for the quantitative determination of cerebral blood flow in man: theory, procedure and normal values. J Clin Invest 27:476–483
12. Logothetis NK, Pauls J, Augath M, Trinath T, Oeltermann A (2001) Neurophysiological investigation of the basis of the fMRI signal. Nature 412:149–157

13. Iadecola C (1993) Regulation of cerebral microcirculation during neural activity: is nitric oxide the missing link? Trends Neurosci 16:206–214
14. Fox PT, Raichle ME (1986) Focal physiological uncoupling of cerebral blood flow and oxidative metabolism during somatosensory stimulation in human subjects. Proc Natl Acad Sci U S A 83:1140–1144
15. Menon RS, Ogawa S, Hu X, Strupp JP, Anderson P, Uğurbil K (1995) BOLD based functional MRI at 4 Tesla includes a capillary bed contribution: echo-planar imaging correlates with previous optical imaging using intrinsic signals. Magn Reson Med 33:453–459
16. Mandeville JB, Marota JJA, Kosofsky BE, Keltner JR, Weissleder R, Rosen BR, Weisskoff RM (1998) Dynamic functional imaging of relative cerebral blood volume during rat forepaw stimulation. Magn Reson Med 39:615–624

# 3.0 T Brain MRI: A Pictorial Overview of the Most Interesting Sequences

# 12

Teresa Popolizio, Francesca Di Chio, Rosario Francesco Balzano and Tommaso Scarabino

In this chapter, we present a series of 3.0 TMR images of the normal whole brain, illustrating 8 different sequences with 16 slices for each sequence: spin echo (SE) T1 (Fig. 12.1a–p), fast gradient echo (FGE) T1 (Fig. 12.2a–p), inversion recovery (IR) (Fig. 12.3a–p), fluid-attenuated inversion recovery (FLAIR) T1 (Fig. 12.4a–p), fast spin echo (FSE) T2 (Fig. 12.5a–p), FSE T2 with inverted contrast (Fig. 12.6a–p), gradient echo (GE) T2 (Fig. 12.7a–p), and FLAIR T2 (Fig. 12.8a–p). The whole brain is studied by each sequence from base to top in 16 slices (from "a" to "p"). Therefore, for each brain level there are eight images, one for each sequence. Tables 12.1 and 12.2 provide a short description of the technical parameters used.

T. Popolizio (✉) • F. Di Chio • R.F. Balzano
Department of Radiology and Neuroradiology, IRCCS "Casa Sollievo della Sofferenza", San Giovanni Rotondo (Fg), Italy
e-mail: t.popolizio1@gmail.com

T. Scarabino
Department of Radiology and Neuroradiology, PO "L. Bonomo" Hospital, Andria (BT), Italy
e-mail: tscarabino@hotmail.com



T. Scarabino et al. (eds.), *High Field Brain MRI*, DOI 10.1007/978-3-319-44174-0_12

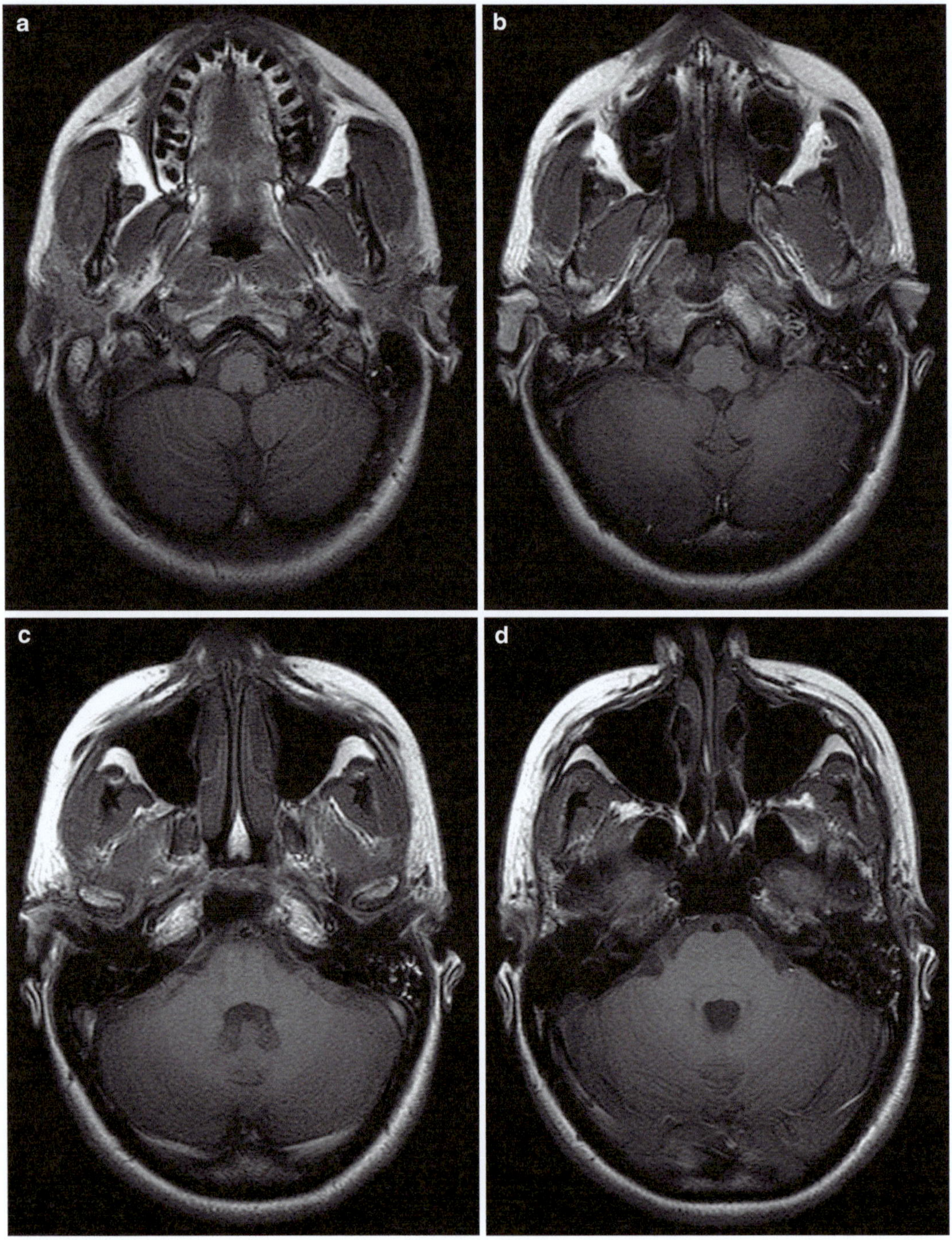


**Fig. 12.1** (**a**) SE, (**b**) SE, (**c**) SE, (**d**) SE, (**e**) SE, (**f**) SE, (**g**) SE, (**h**) SE, (**i**) SE, (**j**) SE, (**k**) SE, (**l**) SE, (**m**) SE, (**n**) SE, (**o**) SE, (**p**) SE

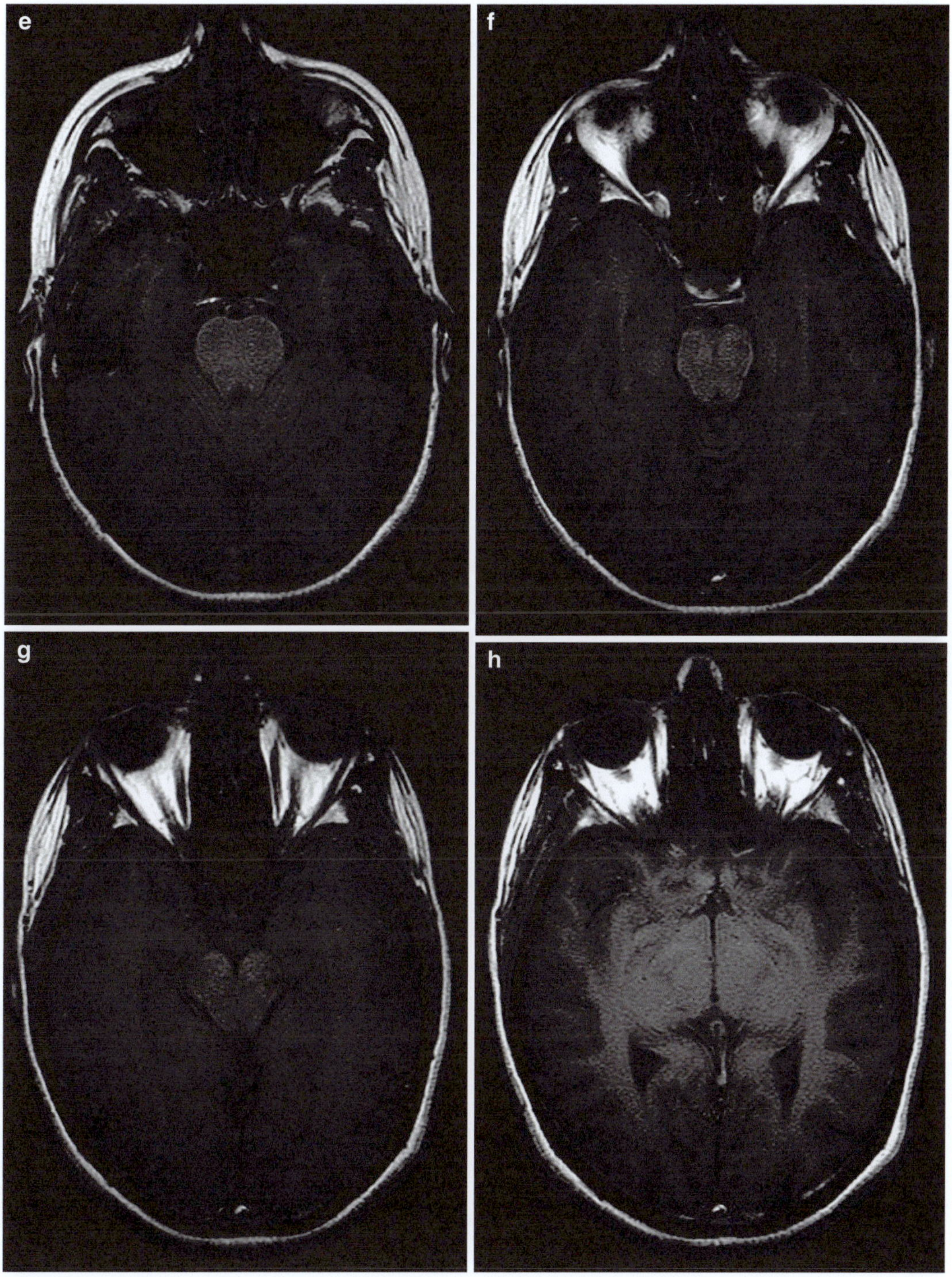


**Fig. 12.1** (continued)

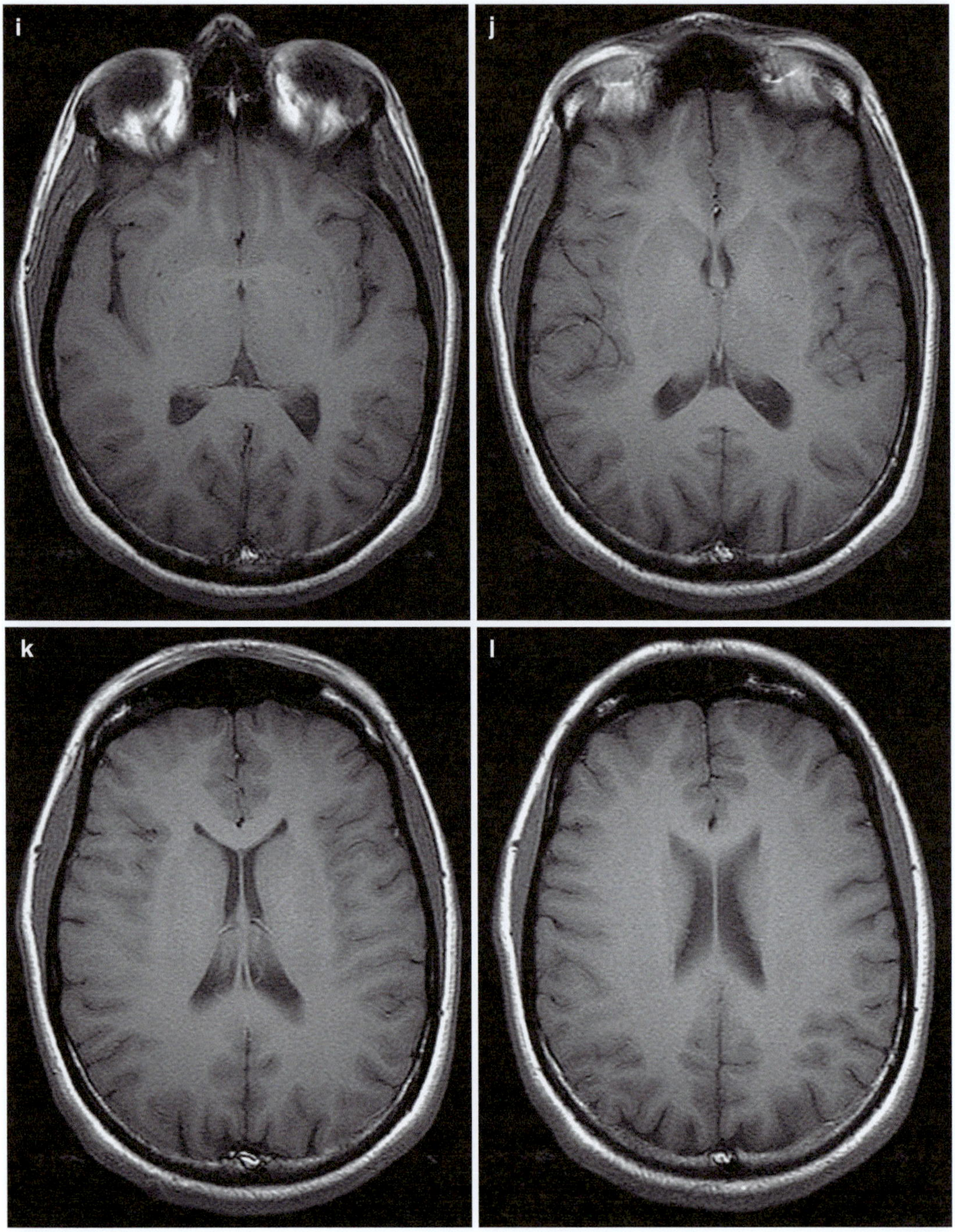


**Fig. 12.1** (continued)

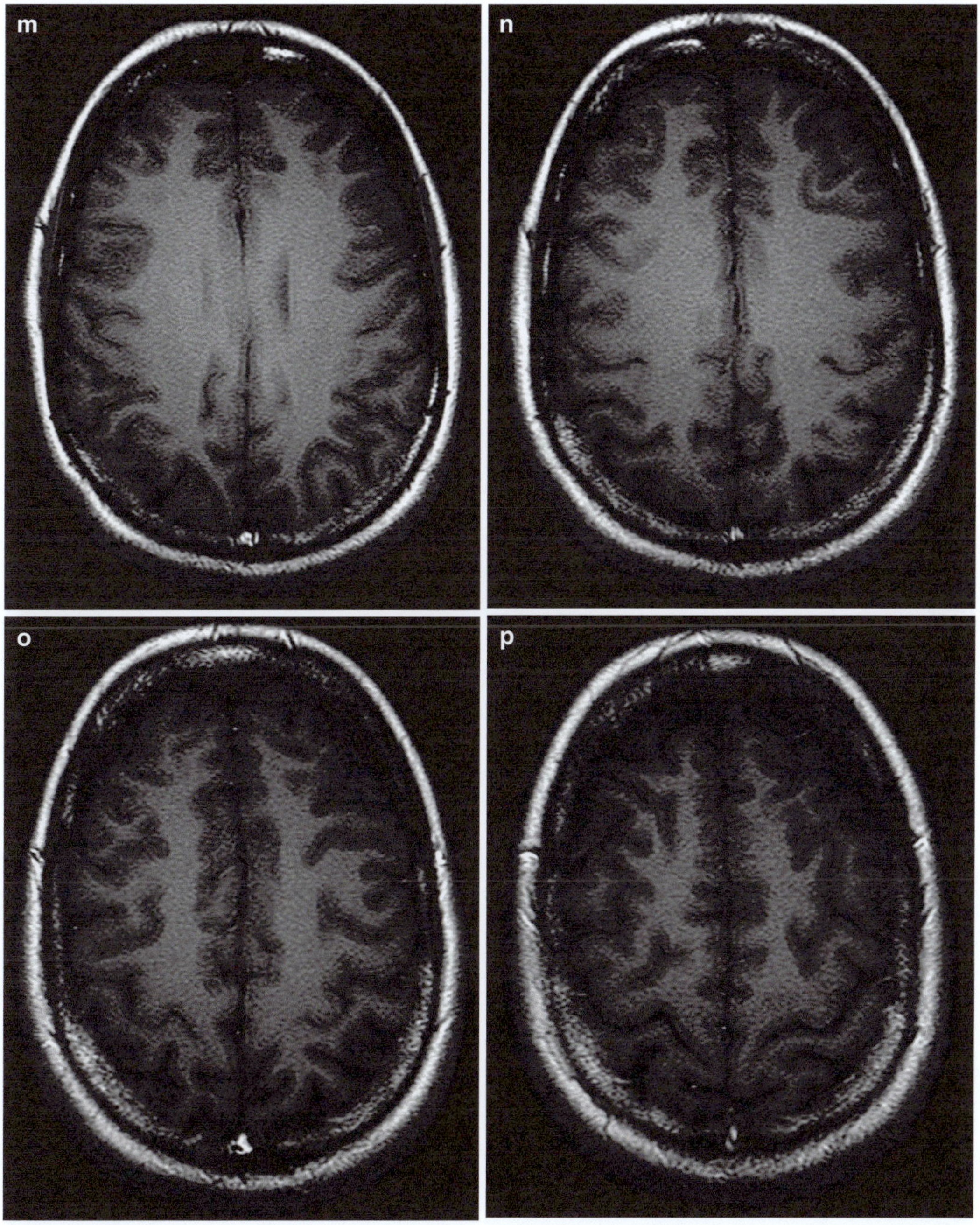


**Fig. 12.1** (continued)

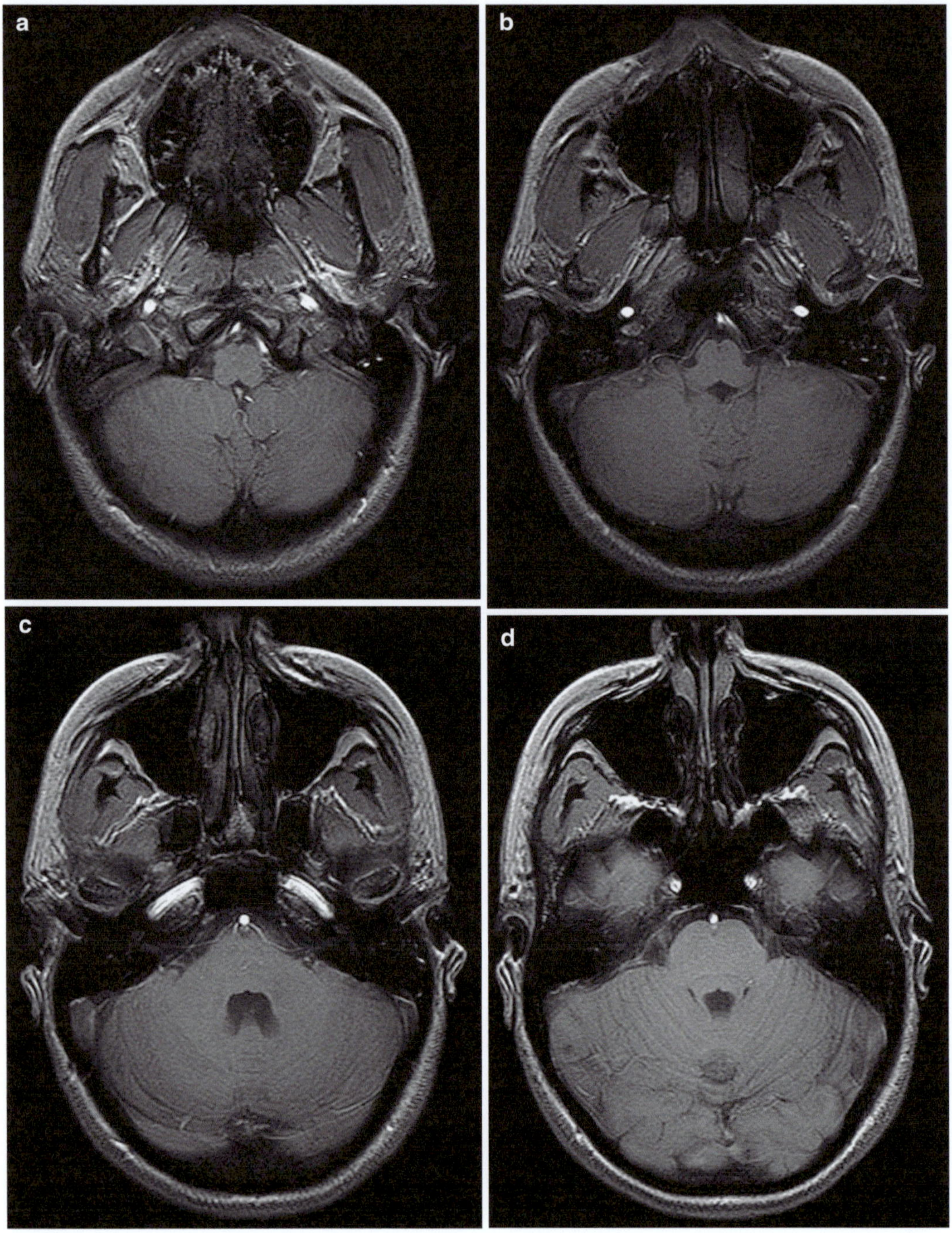


**Fig. 12.2** (**a**) FGE, (**b**) FGE, (**c**) FGE, (**d**) FGE, (**e**) FGE, (**f**) FGE, (**g**) FGE, (**h**) FGE, (**i**) FGE, (**j**) FGE, (**k**) FGE, (**l**) FGE, (**m**) FGE, (**n**) FGE, (**o**) FGE, (**p**) FGE

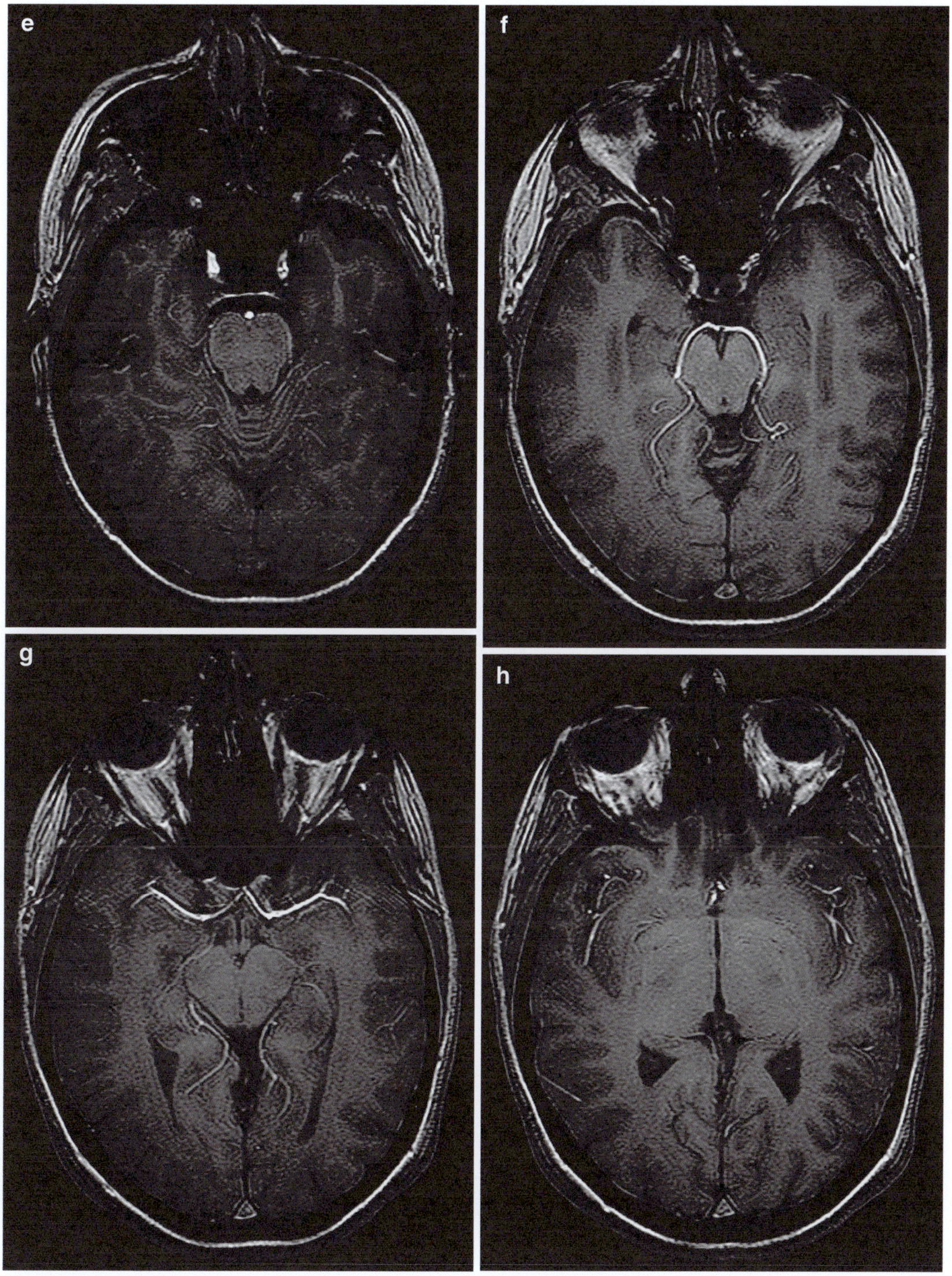


**Fig. 12.2** (continued)

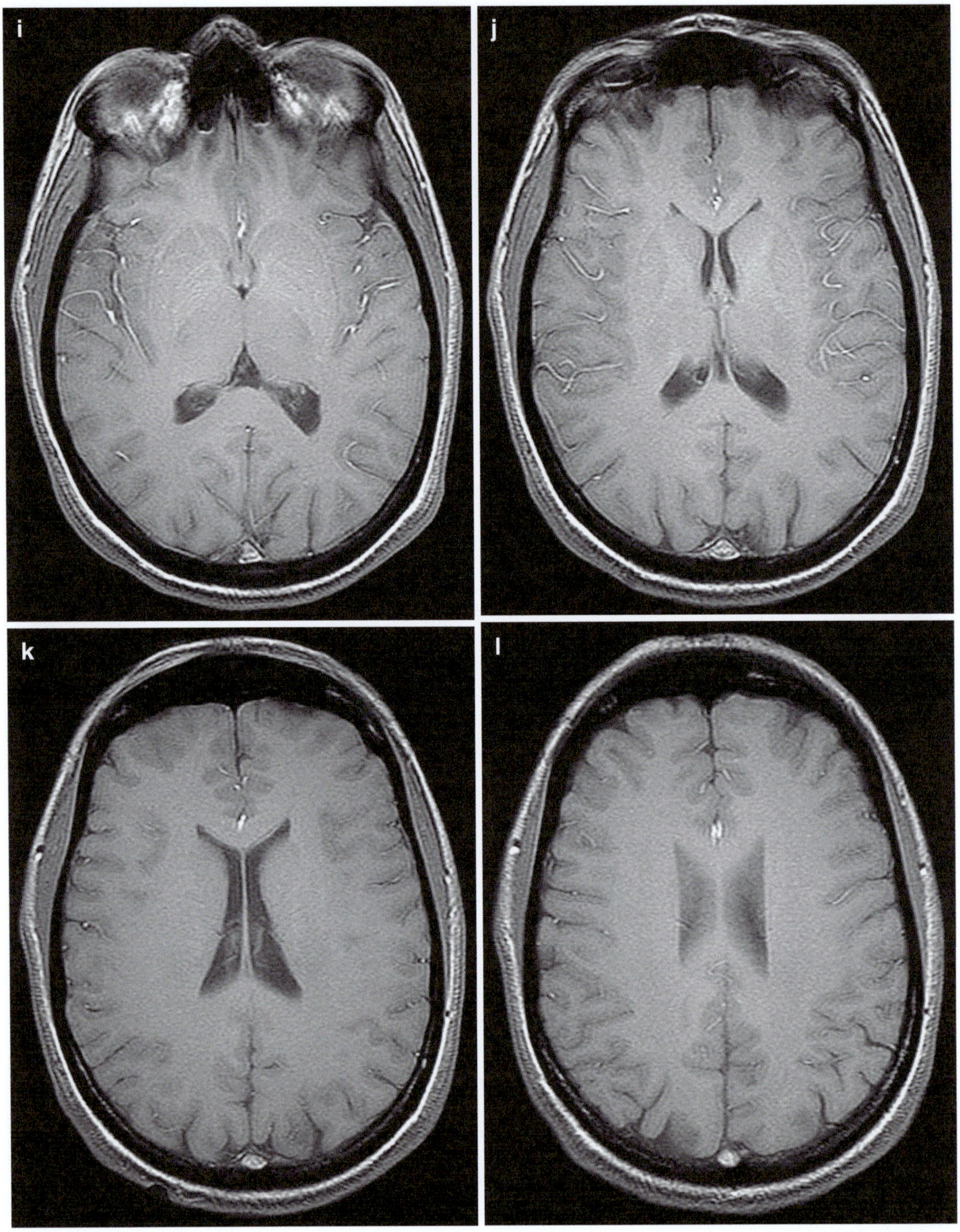


**Fig. 12.2** (continued)

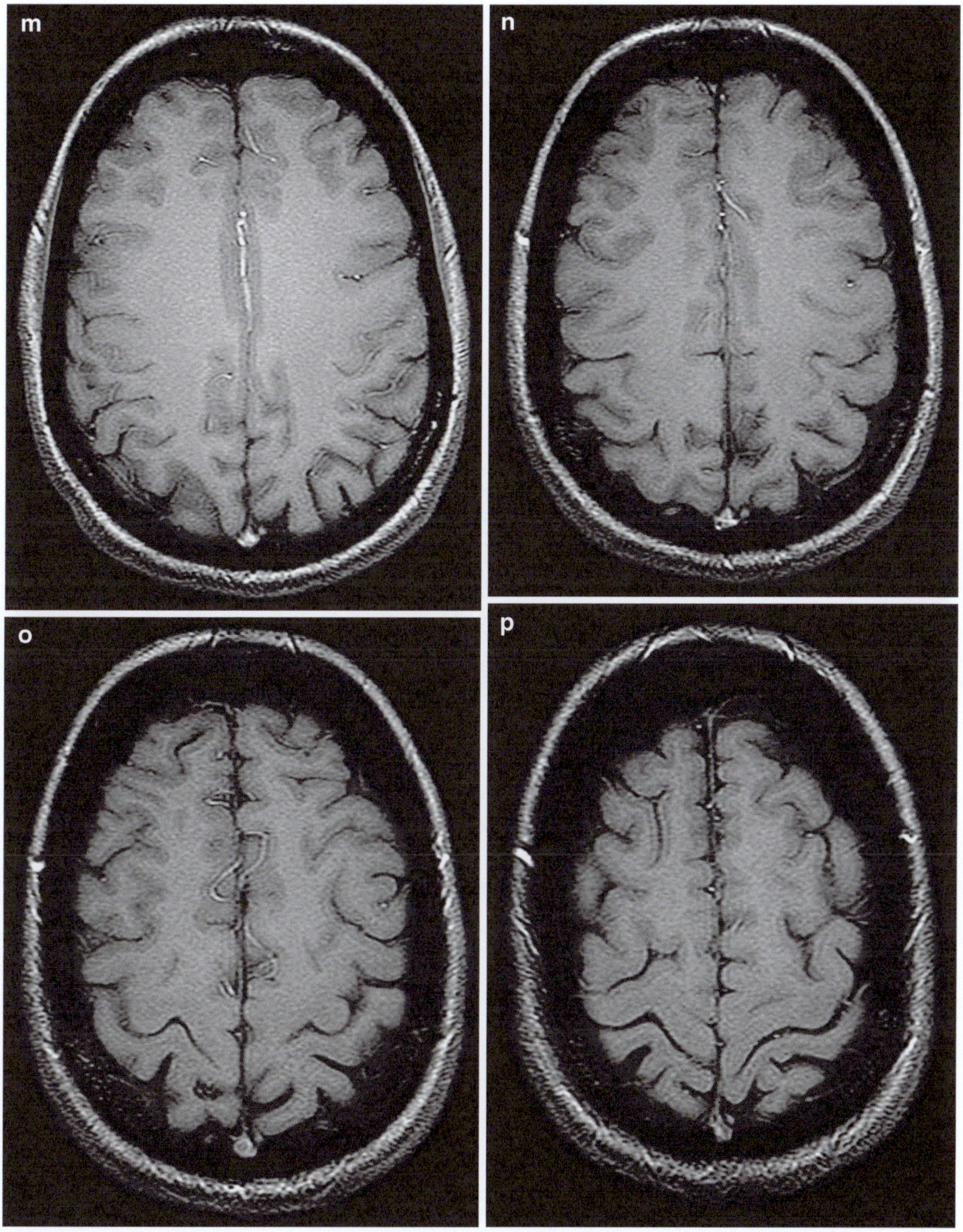


**Fig. 12.2** (continued)

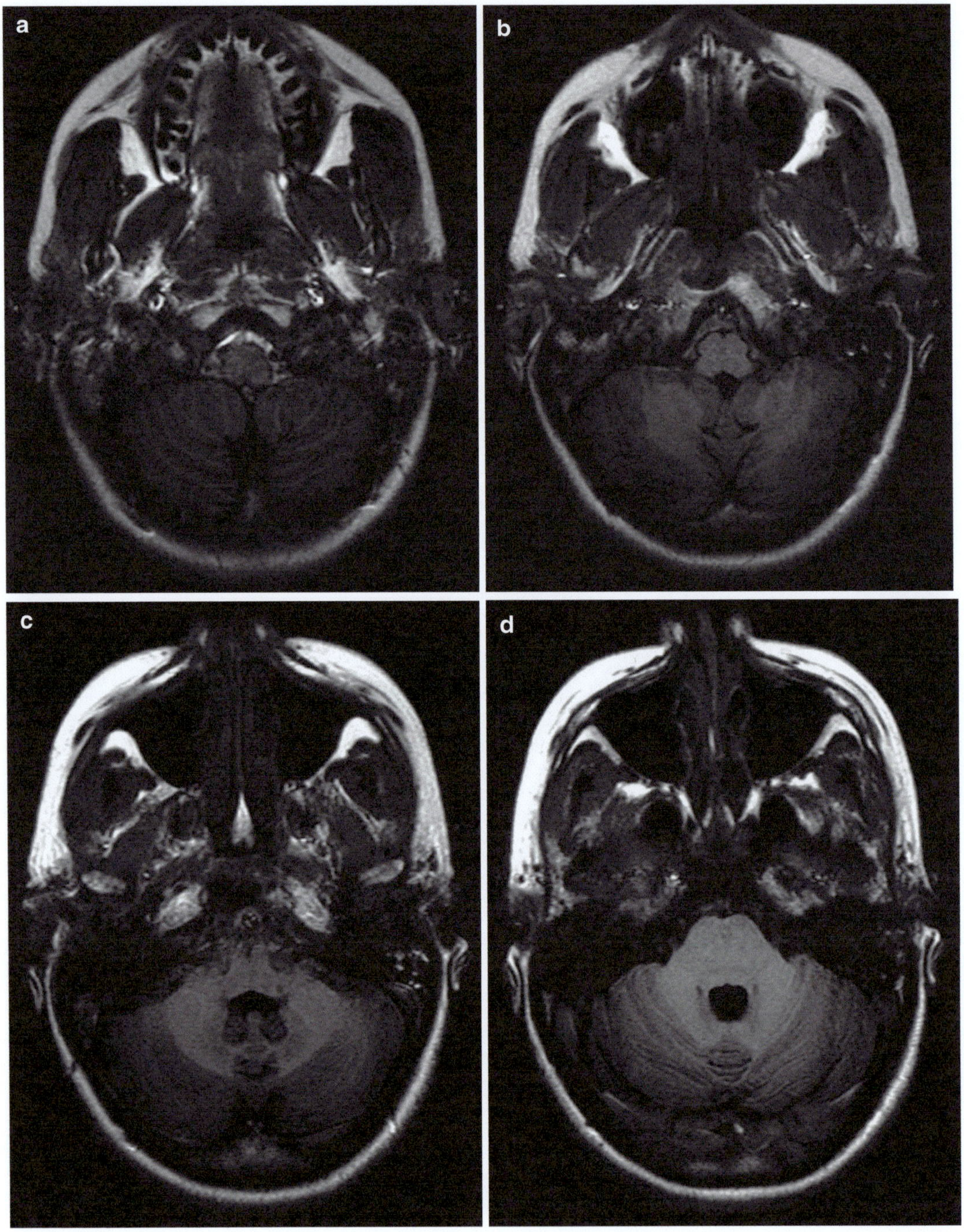


**Fig. 12.3** (**a**) IR, (**b**) IR, (**c**) IR, (**d**) IR, (**e**) IR, (**f**) IR, (**g**) IR, (**h**) IR, (**i**) IR, (**j**) IR, (**k**) IR, (**l**) IR, (**m**) IR, (**n**) IR, (**o**) IR, (**p**) IR

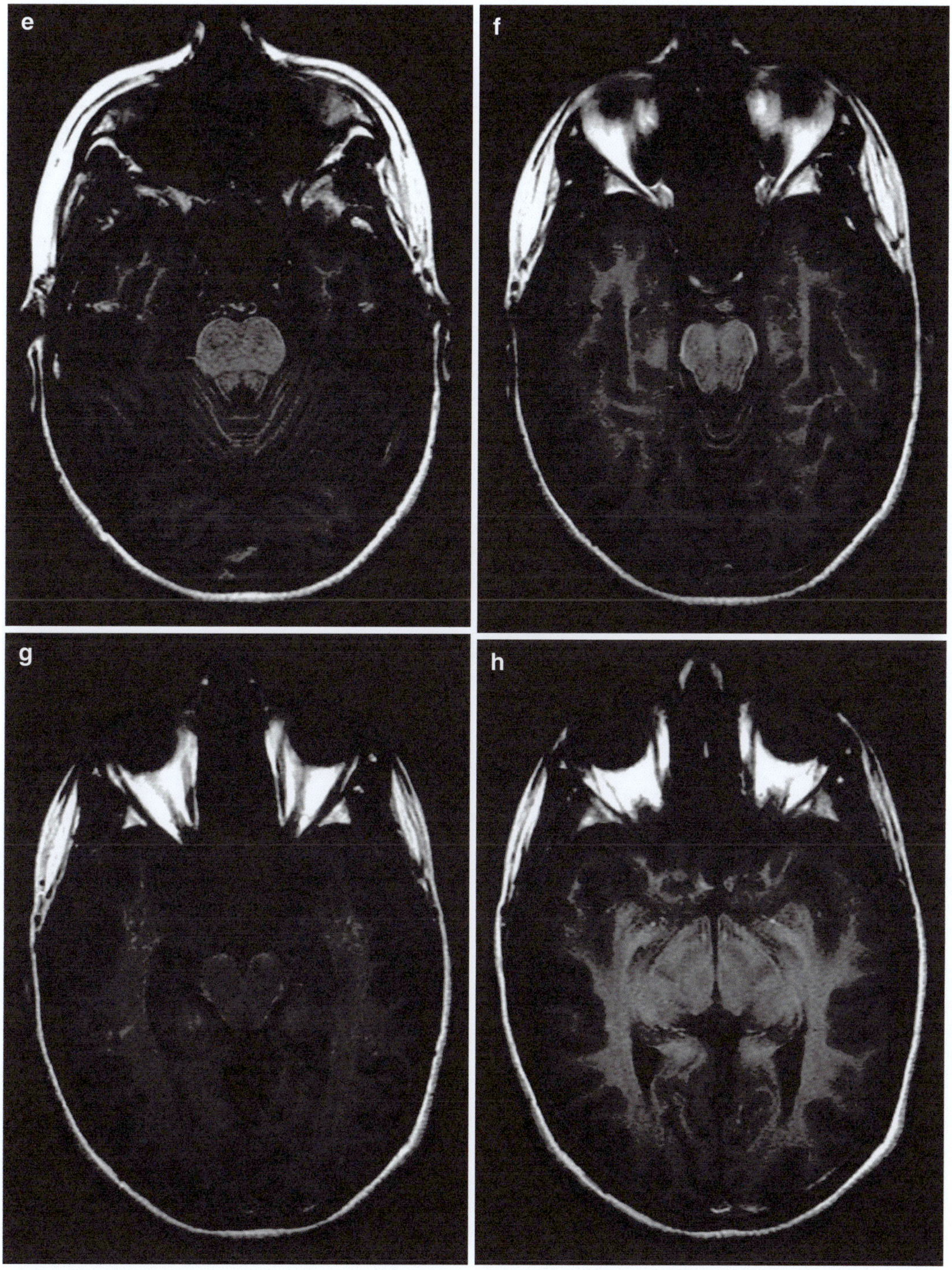


**Fig. 12.3** (continued)

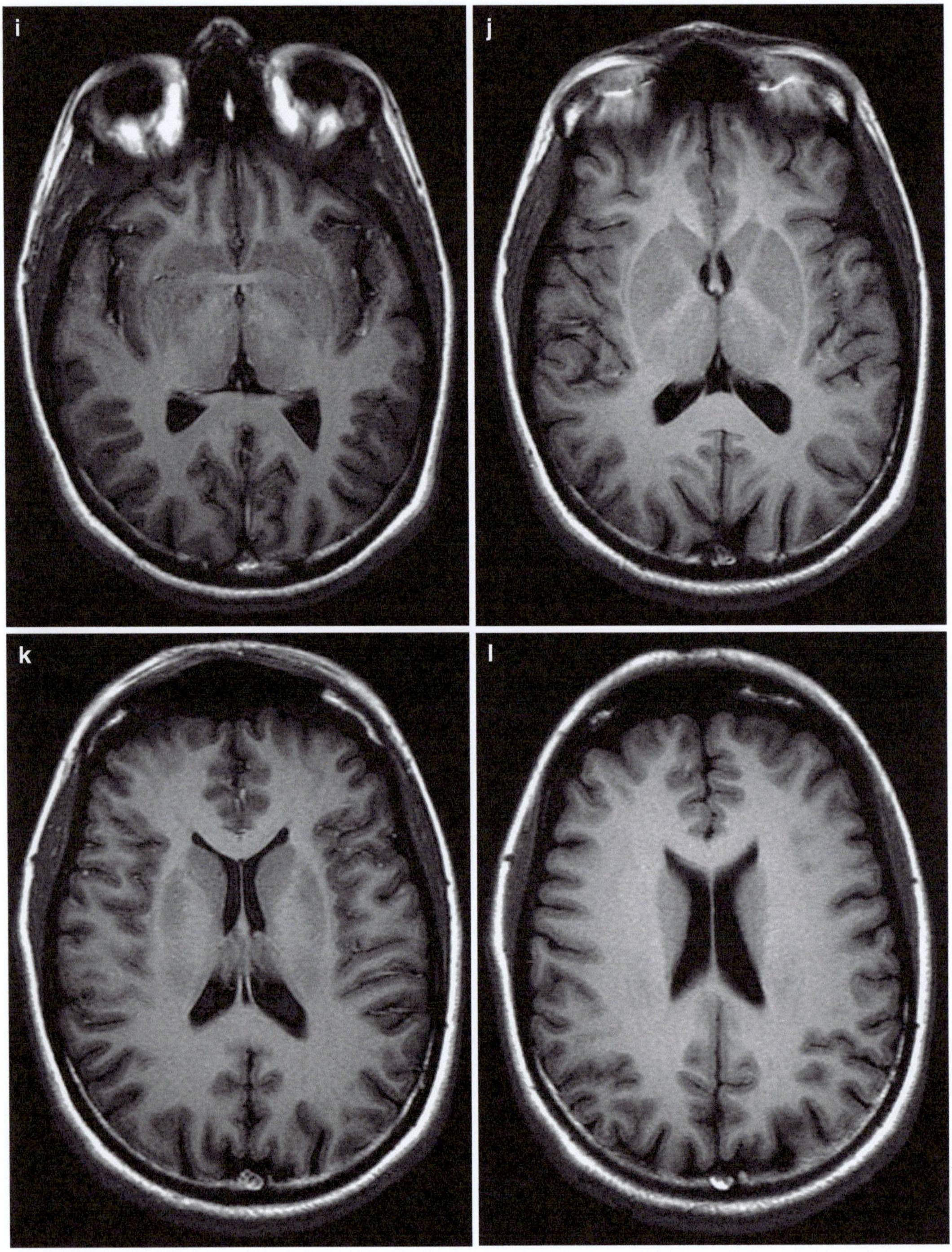


**Fig. 12.3** (continued)

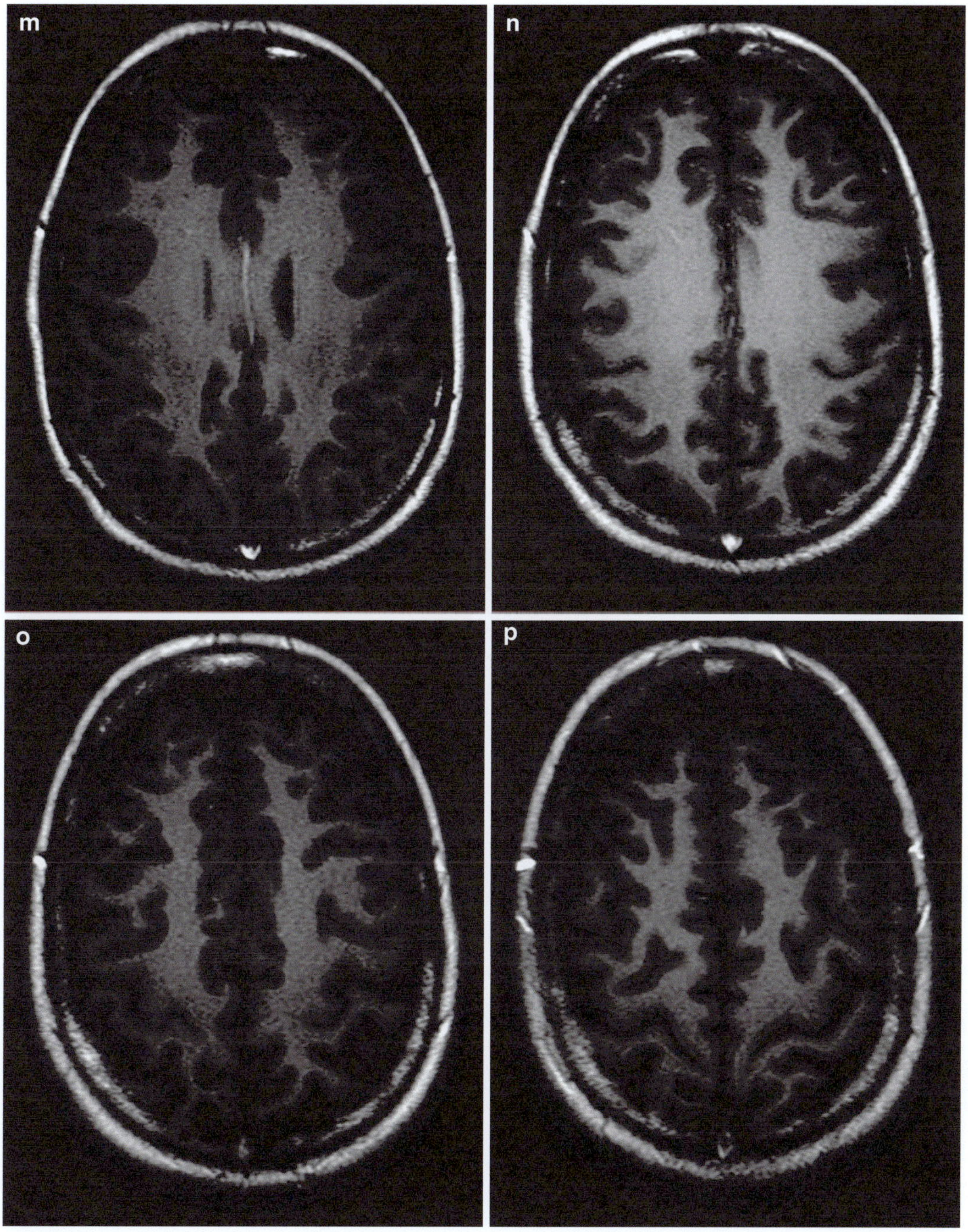


**Fig. 12.3** (continued)

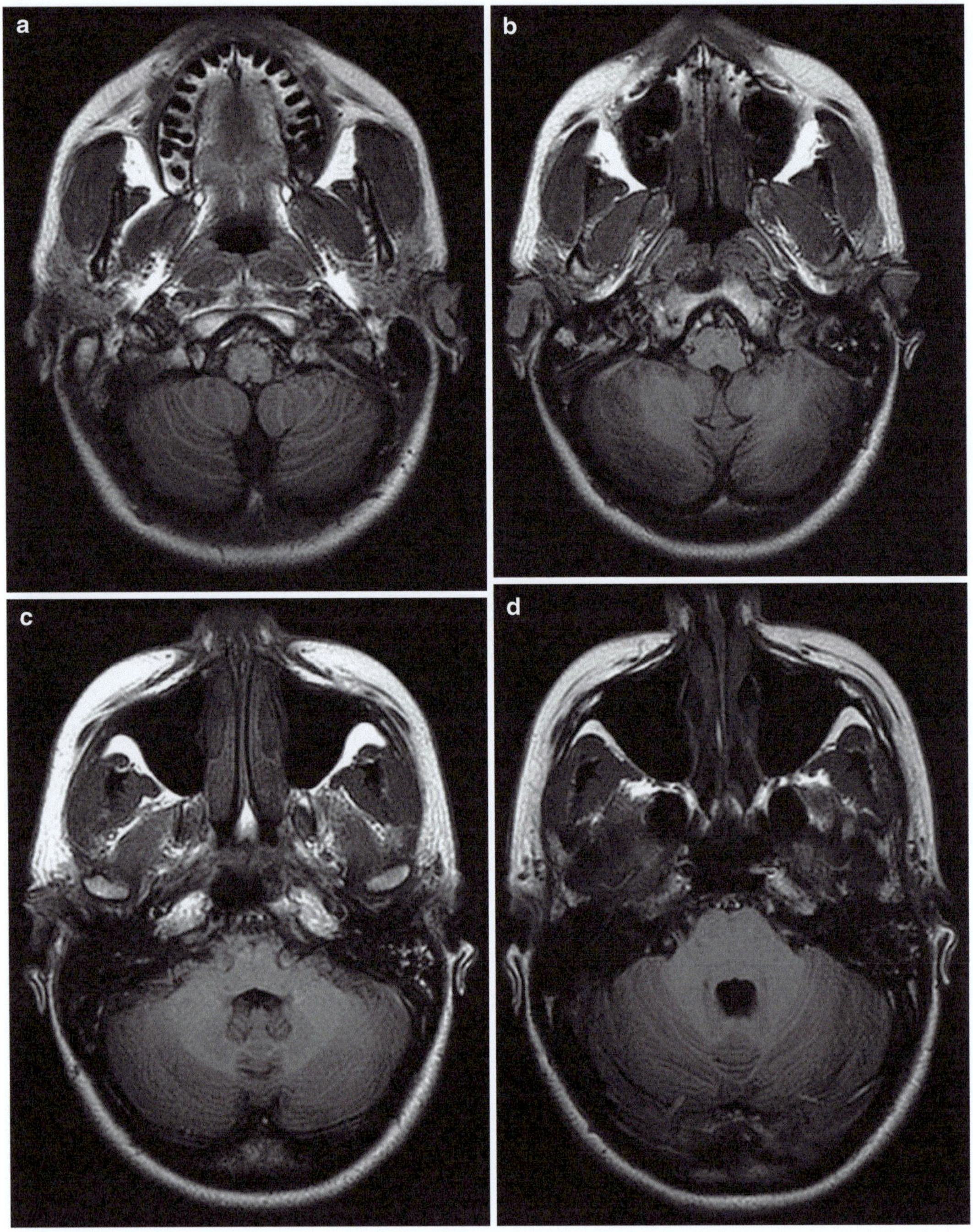


**Fig. 12.4** (**a**) FLAIR, (**b**) FLAIR, (**c**) FLAIR, (**d**) FLAIR, (**e**) FLAIR, (**f**) FLAIR, (**g**) FLAIR, (**h**) FLAIR, (**i**) FLAIR, (**j**) FLAIR, (**k**) FLAIR, (**l**) FLAIR, (**m**) FLAIR, (**n**) FLAIR, (**o**) FLAIR, (**p**) FLAIR

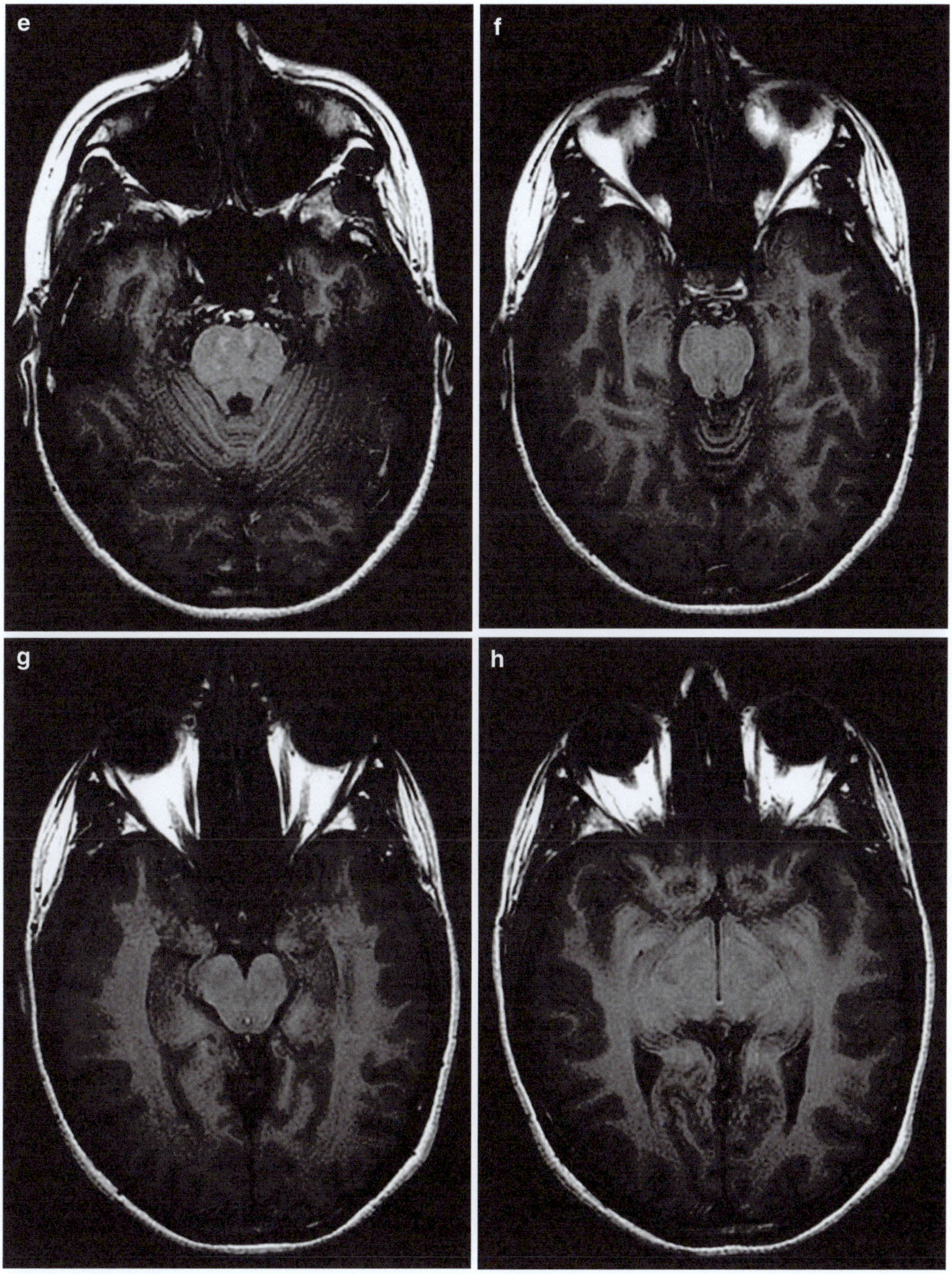

**Fig. 12.4** (continued)

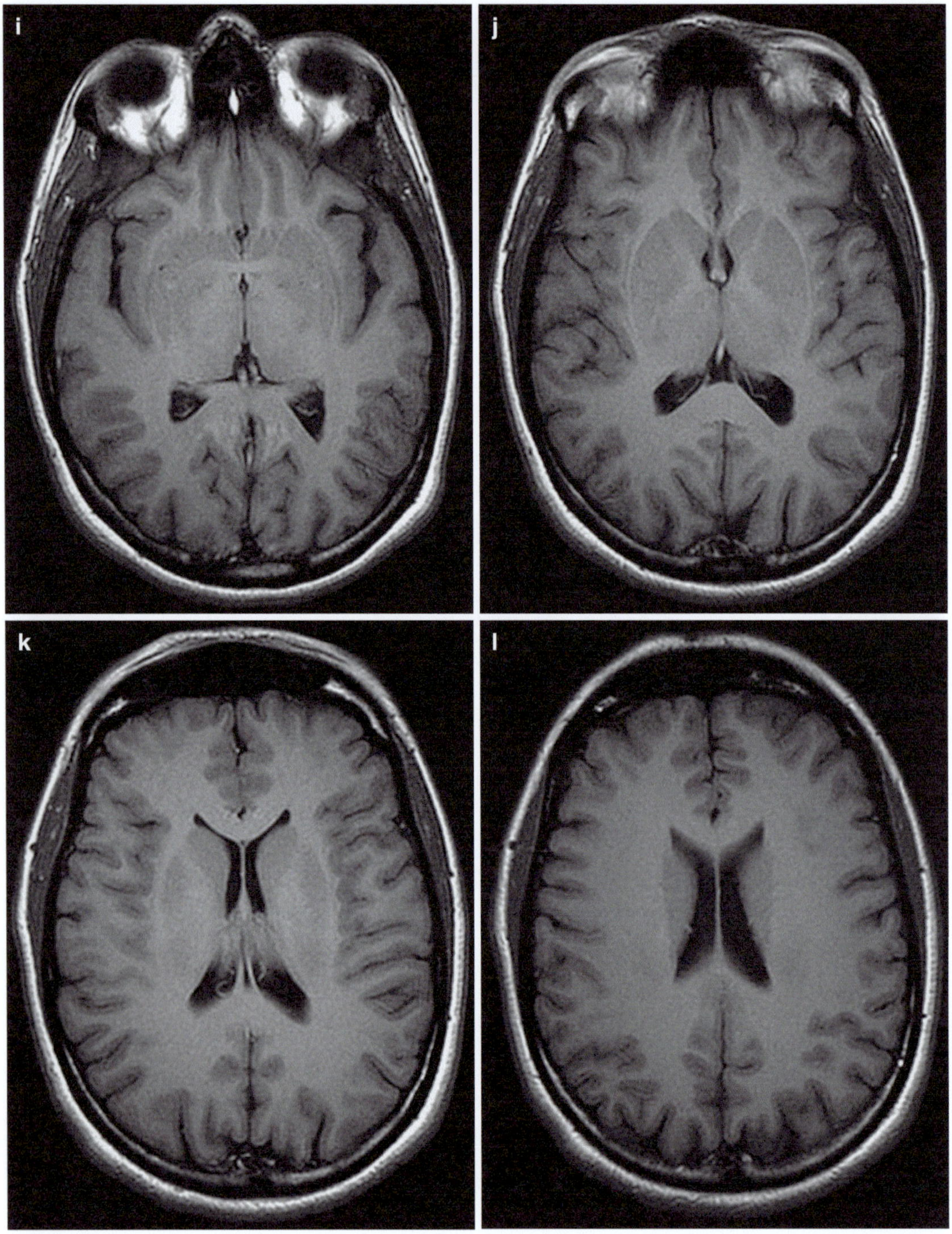


Fig. 12.4 (continued)

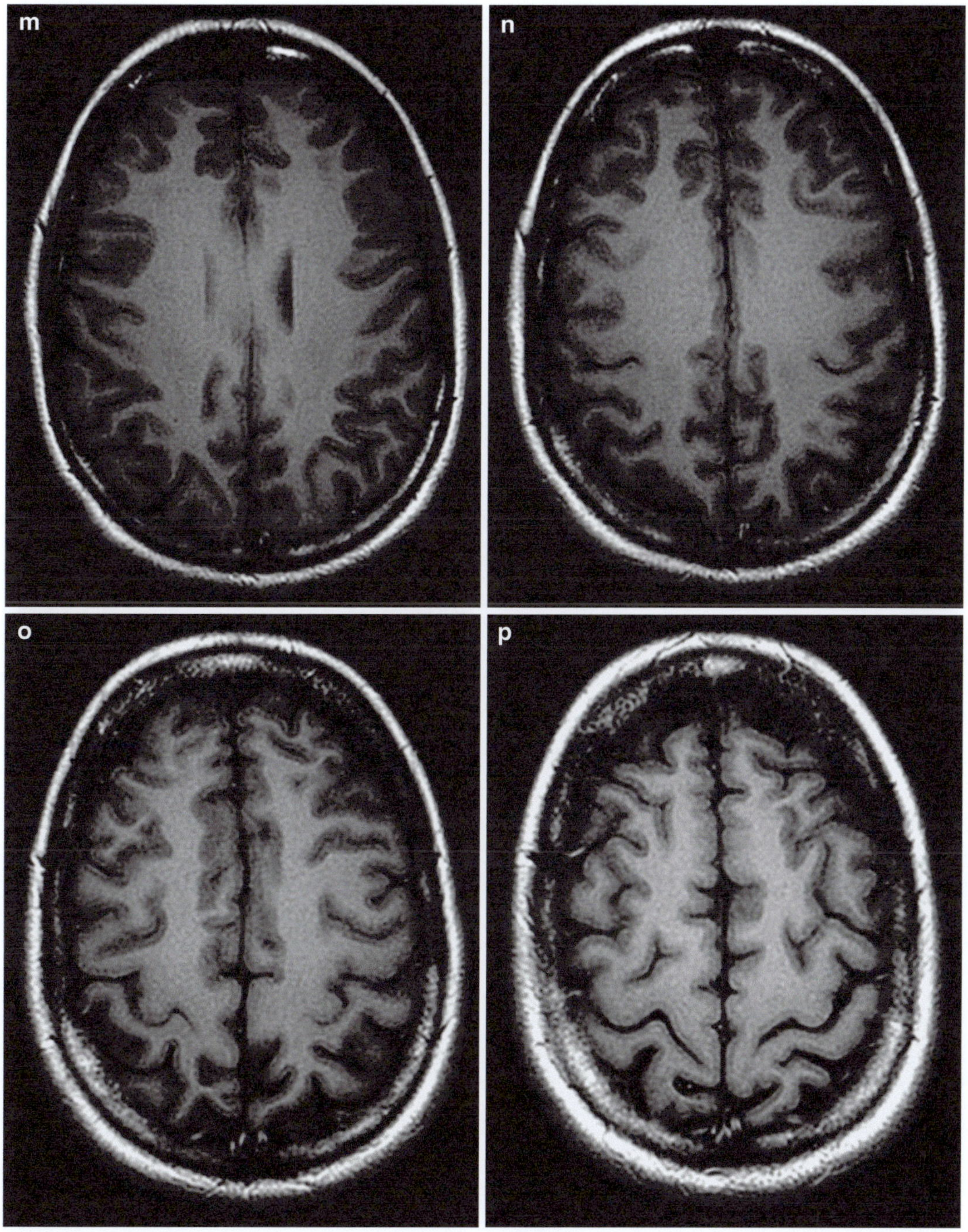


**Fig. 12.4** (continued)

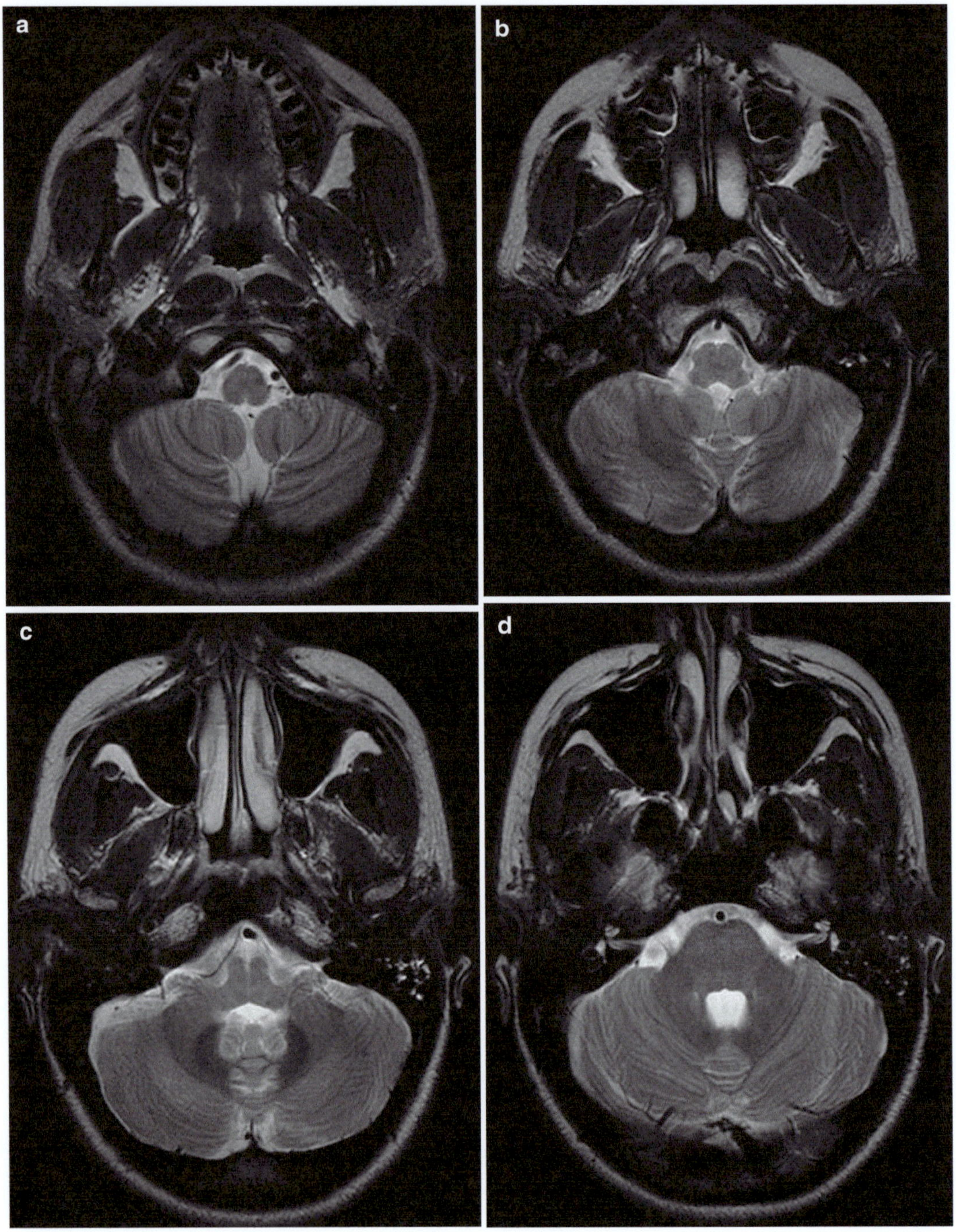


**Fig. 12.5** (**a**) FSE, (**b**) FSE, (**c**) FSE, (**d**) FSE, (**e**) FSE, (**f**) FSE, (**g**) FSE, (**h**) FSE, (**i**) FSE, (**j**) FSE, (**k**) FSE, (**l**) FSE, (**m**) FSE, (**n**) FSE, (**o**) FSE, (**p**) FSE

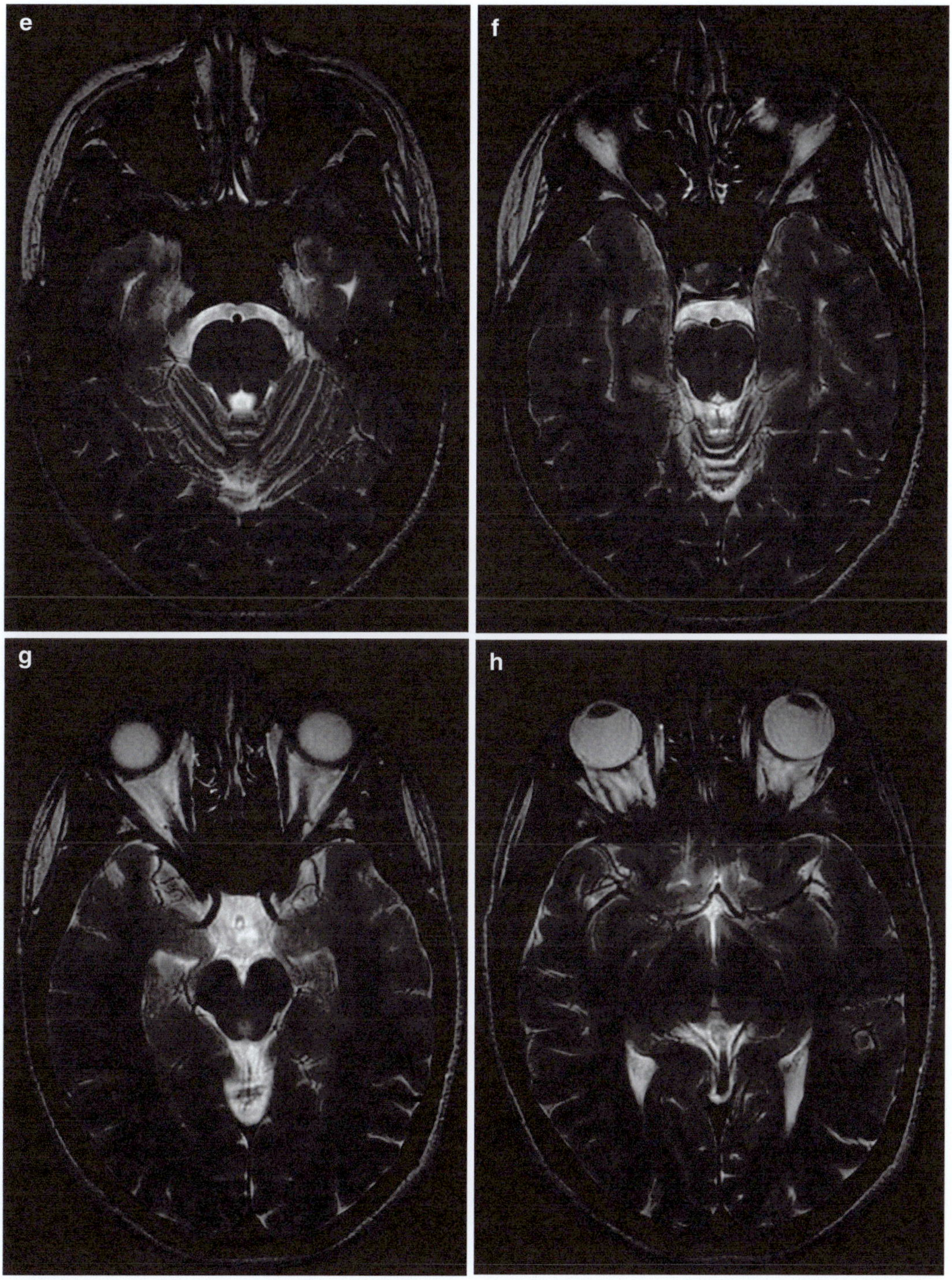


**Fig. 12.5** (continued)

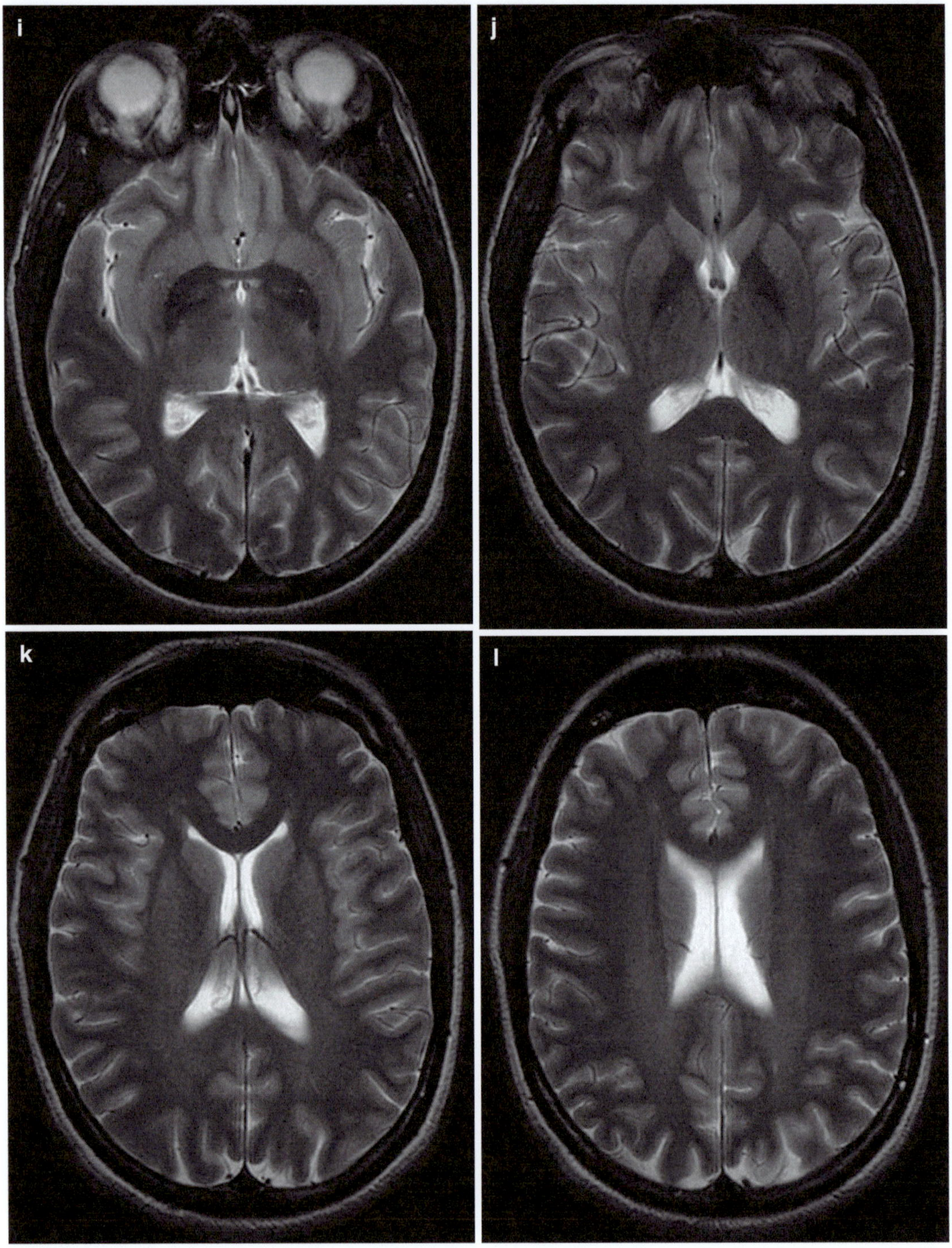


**Fig. 12.5** (continued)

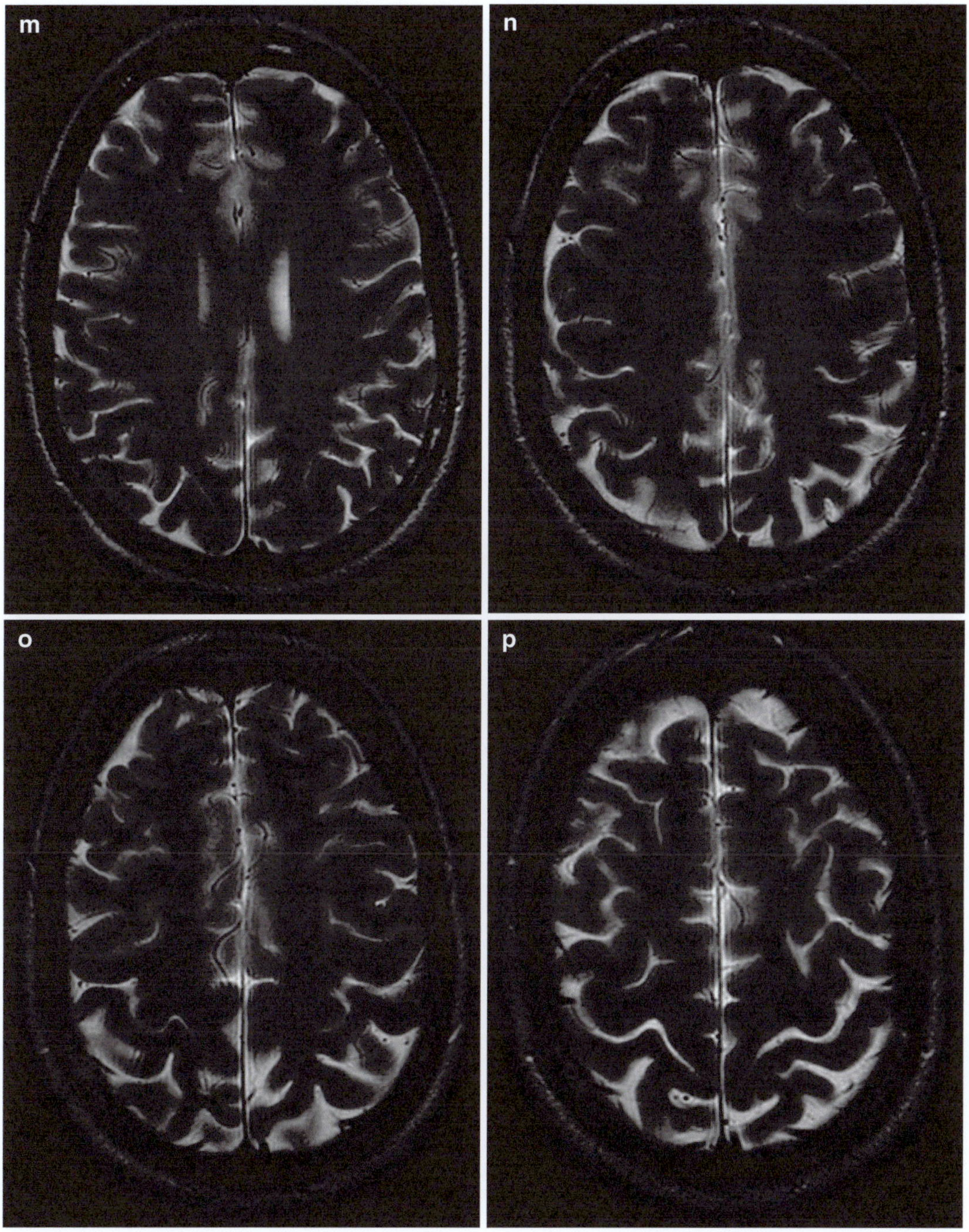


**Fig. 12.5** (continued)

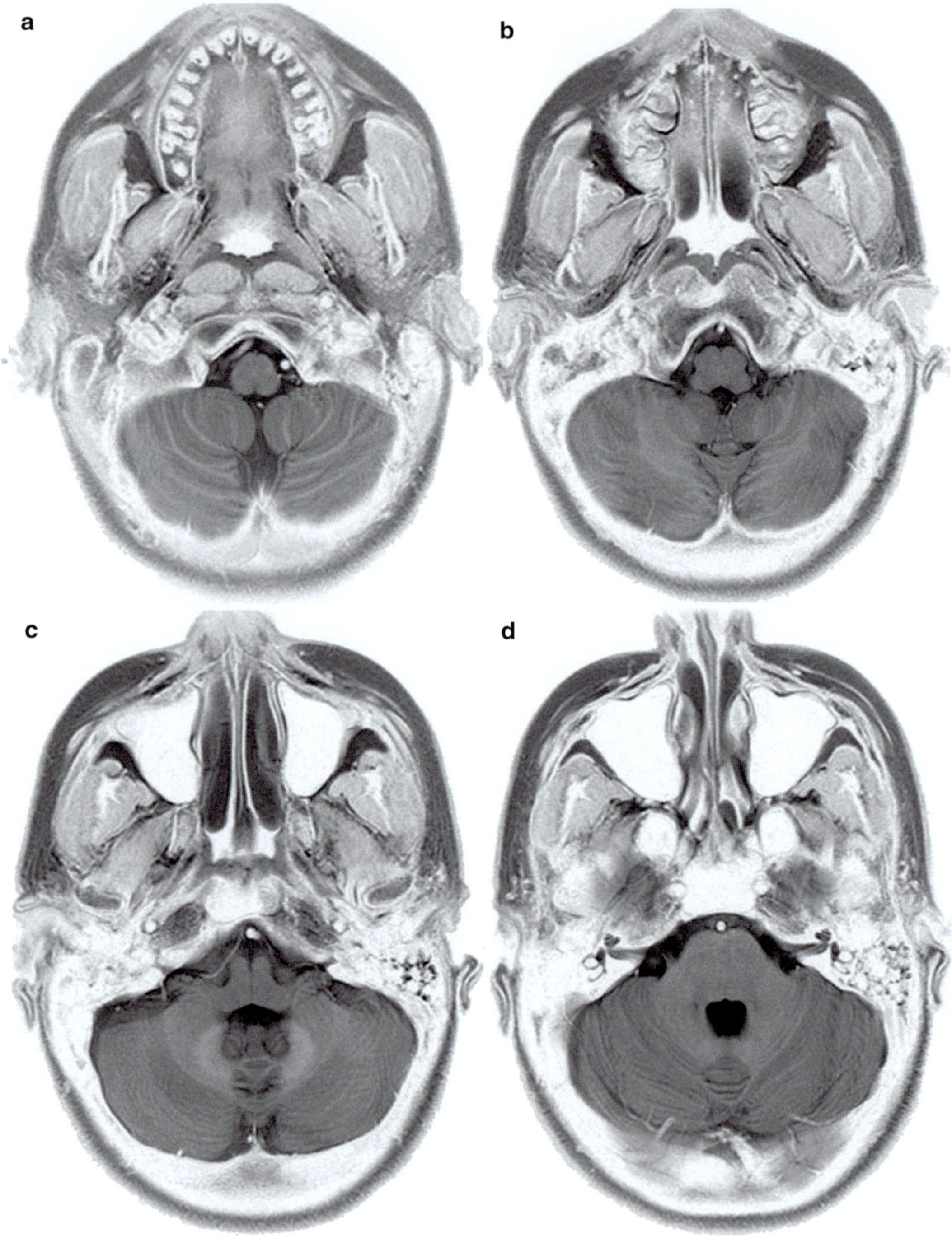


**Fig. 12.6** (**a**) FSE with inverted contrast, (**b**) FSE with inverted contrast, (**c**) FSE with inverted contrast, (**d**) FSE with inverted contrast, (**e**) FSE with inverted contrast, (**f**) FSE with inverted contrast, (**g**) FSE with inverted contrast, (**h**) FSE with inverted contrast, (**i**) FSE with inverted contrast, (**j**) FSE with inverted contrast, (**k**) FSE with inverted contrast, (**l**) FSE with inverted contrast, (**m**) FSE with inverted contrast, (**n**) FSE with inverted contrast, (**o**) FSE with inverted contrast, (**p**) FSE with inverted contrast

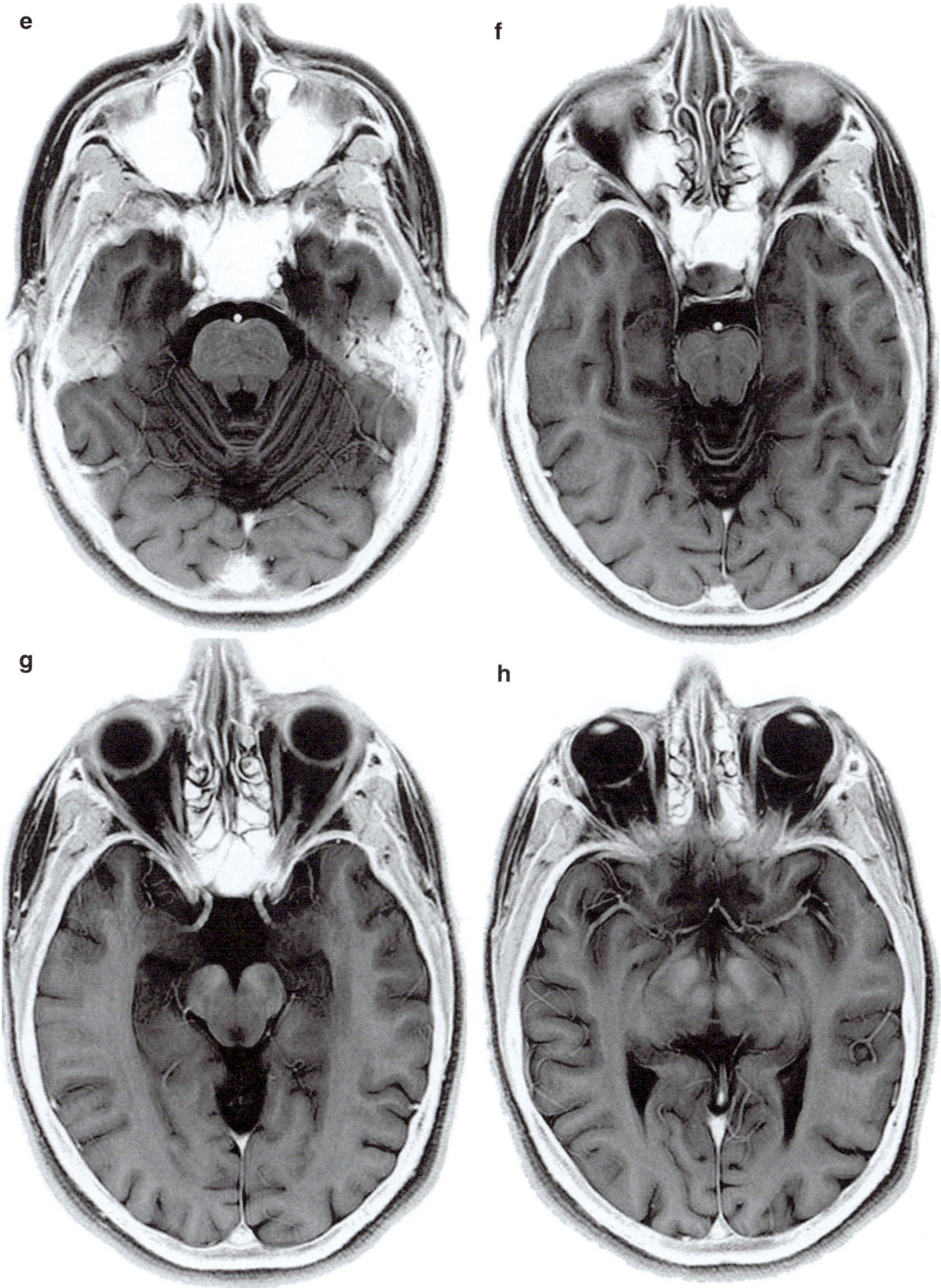


Fig. 12.6 (continued)

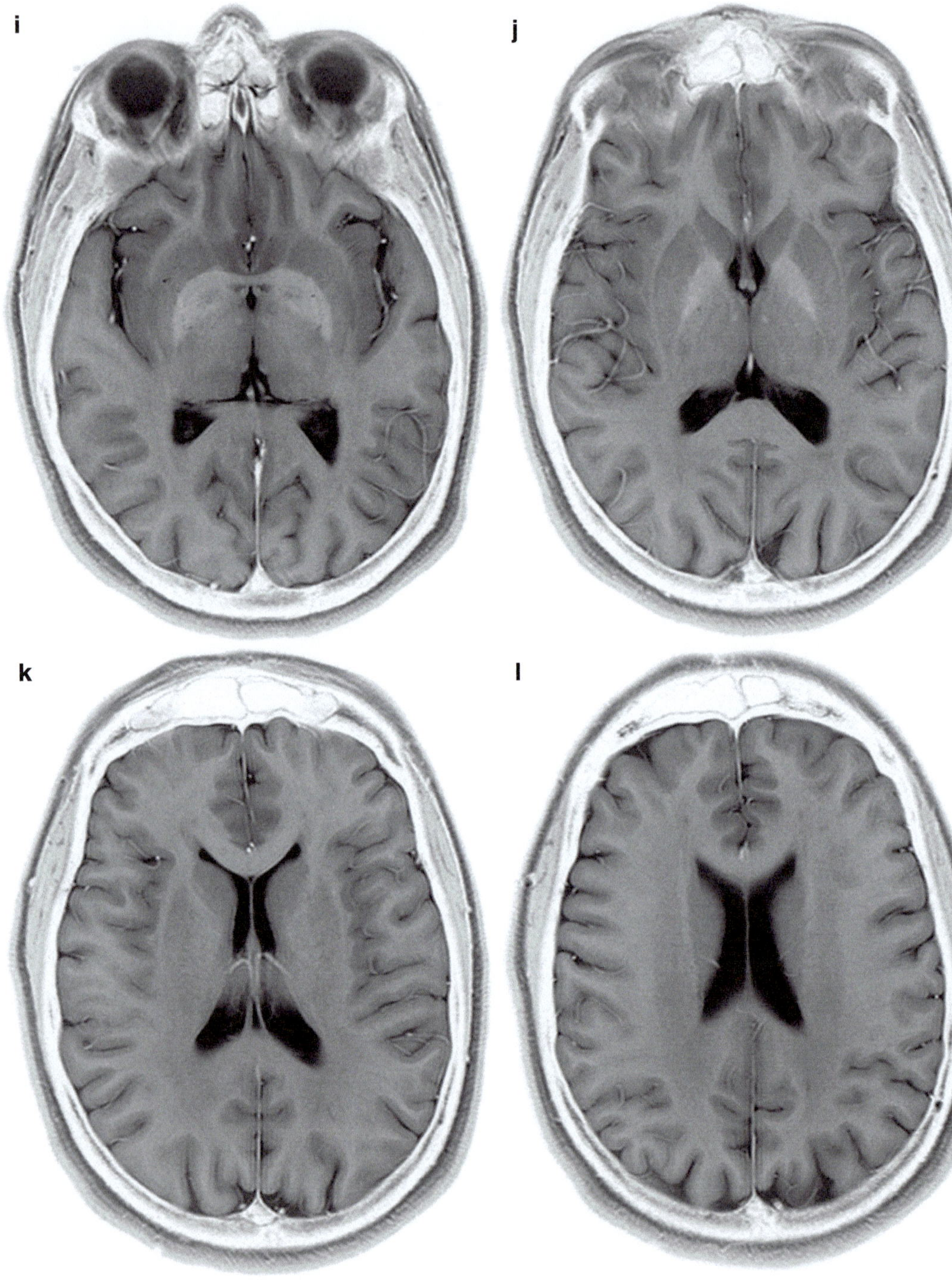


**Fig. 12.6** (continued)

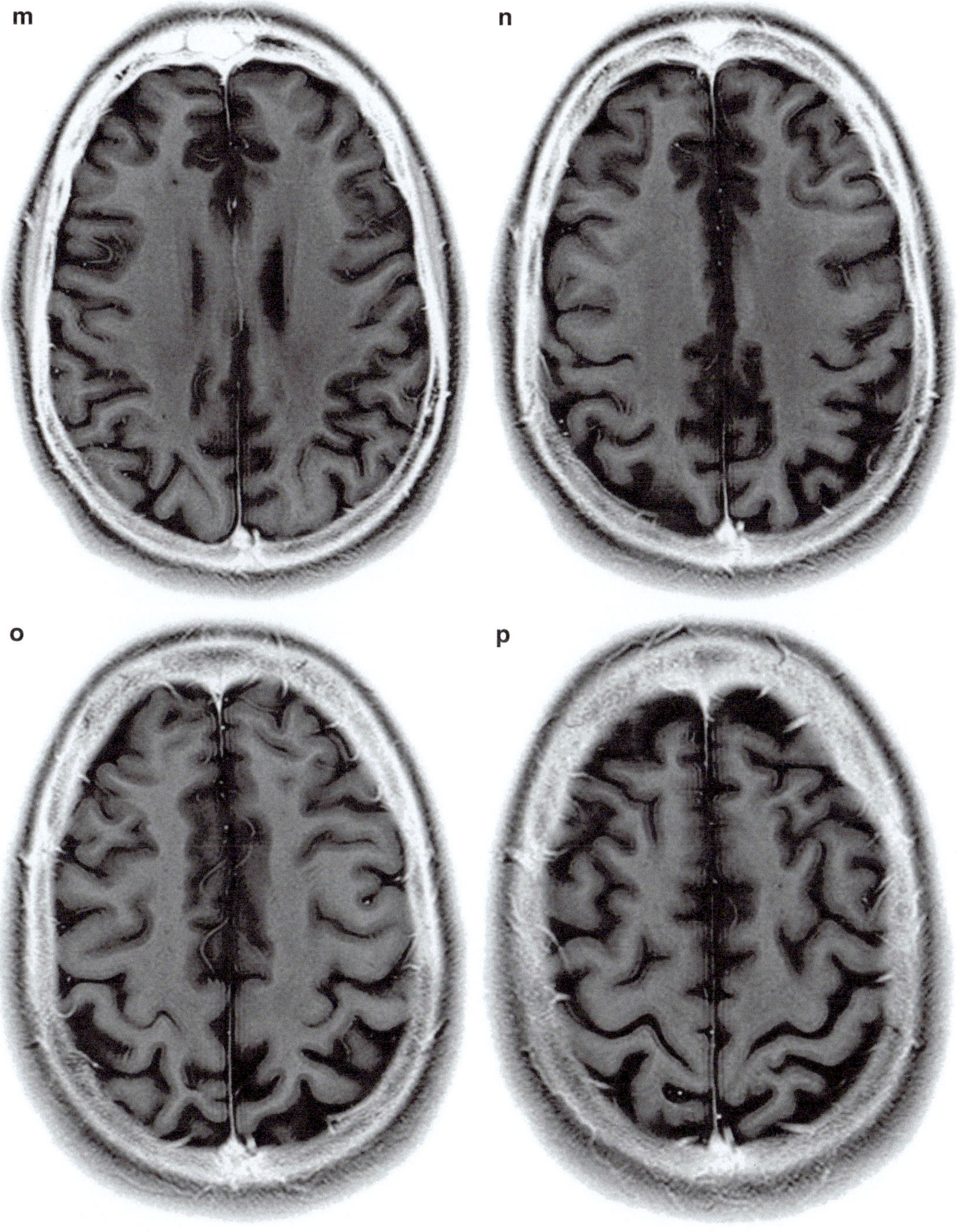


**Fig. 12.6** (continued)

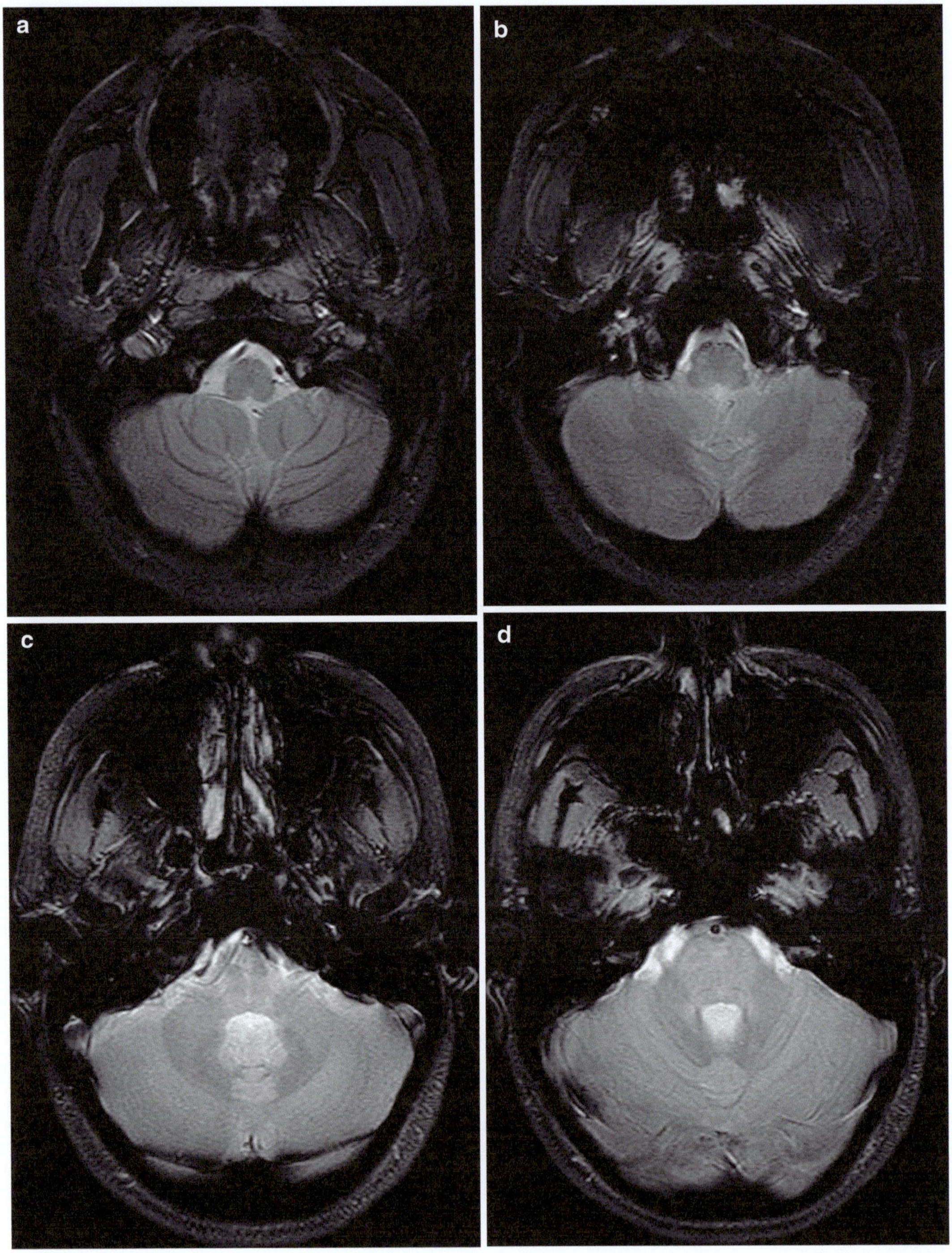


**Fig. 12.7** (**a**) GE, (**b**) GE, (**c**) GE, (**d**) GE, (**e**) GE, (**f**) GE, (**g**) GE, (**h**) GE, (**i**) GE, (**j**) GE, (**k**) GE, (**l**) GE, (**m**) GE, (**n**) GE, (**o**) GE, (**p**) GE

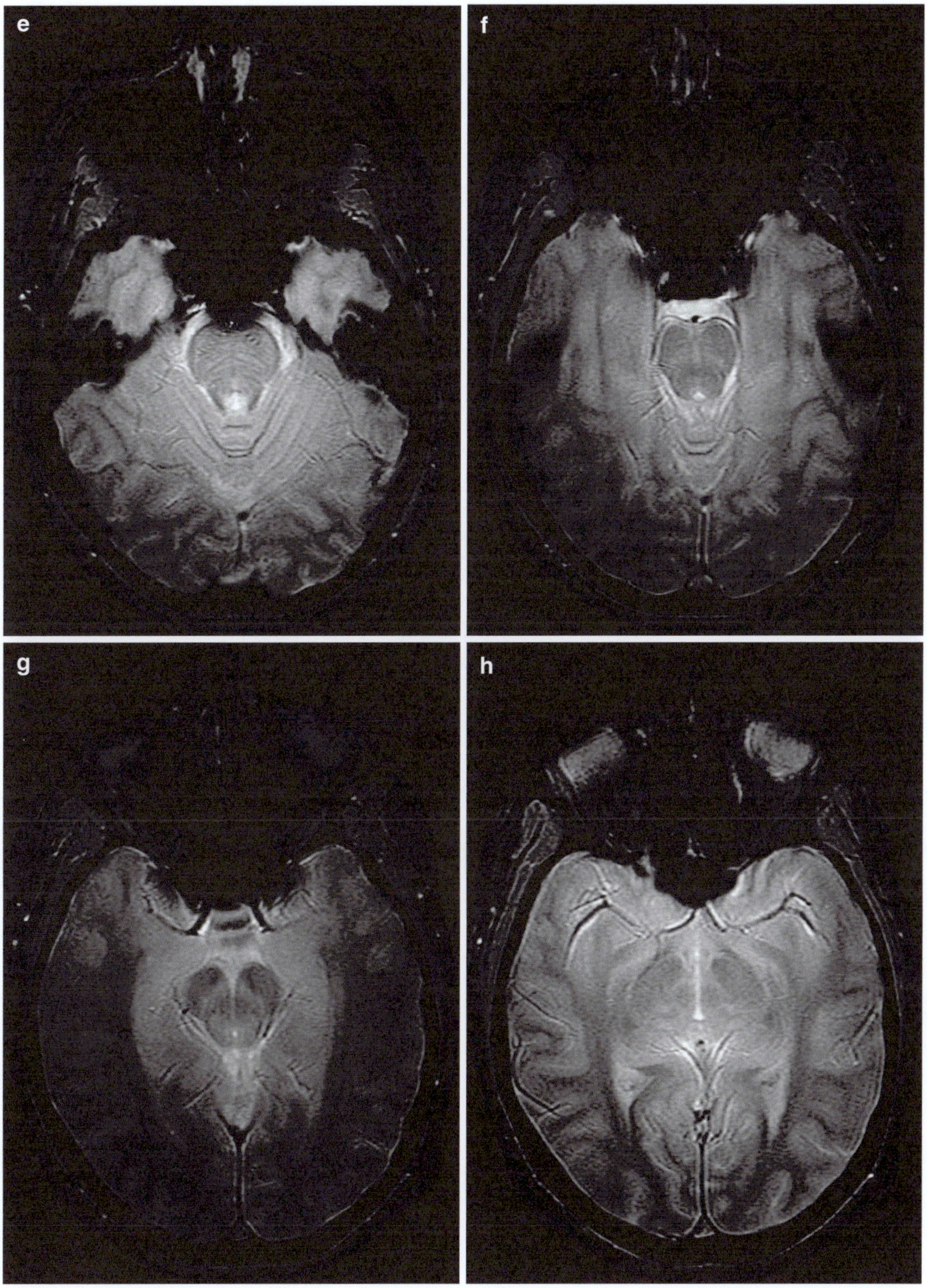


**Fig. 12.7** (continued)

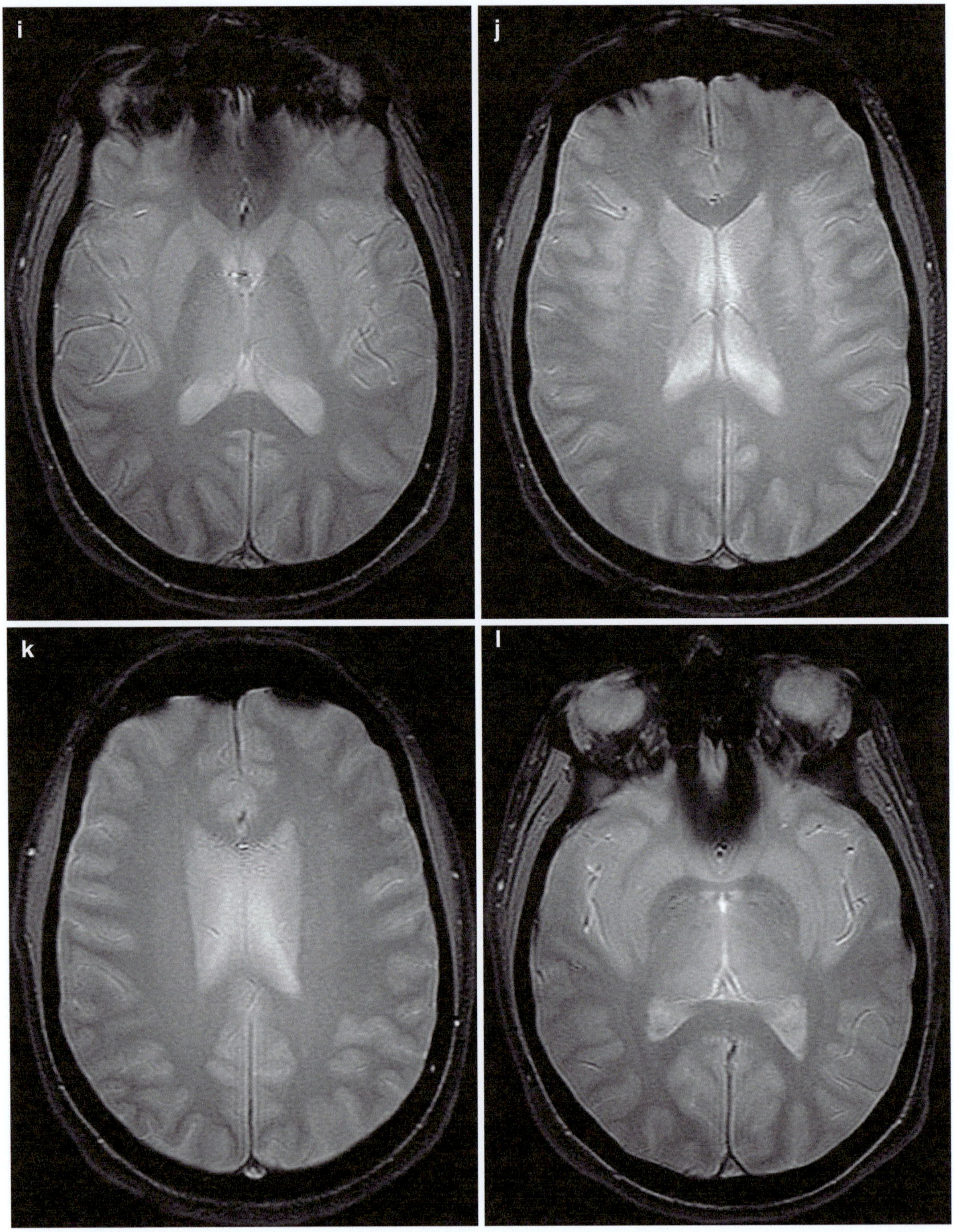


**Fig. 12.7** (continued)

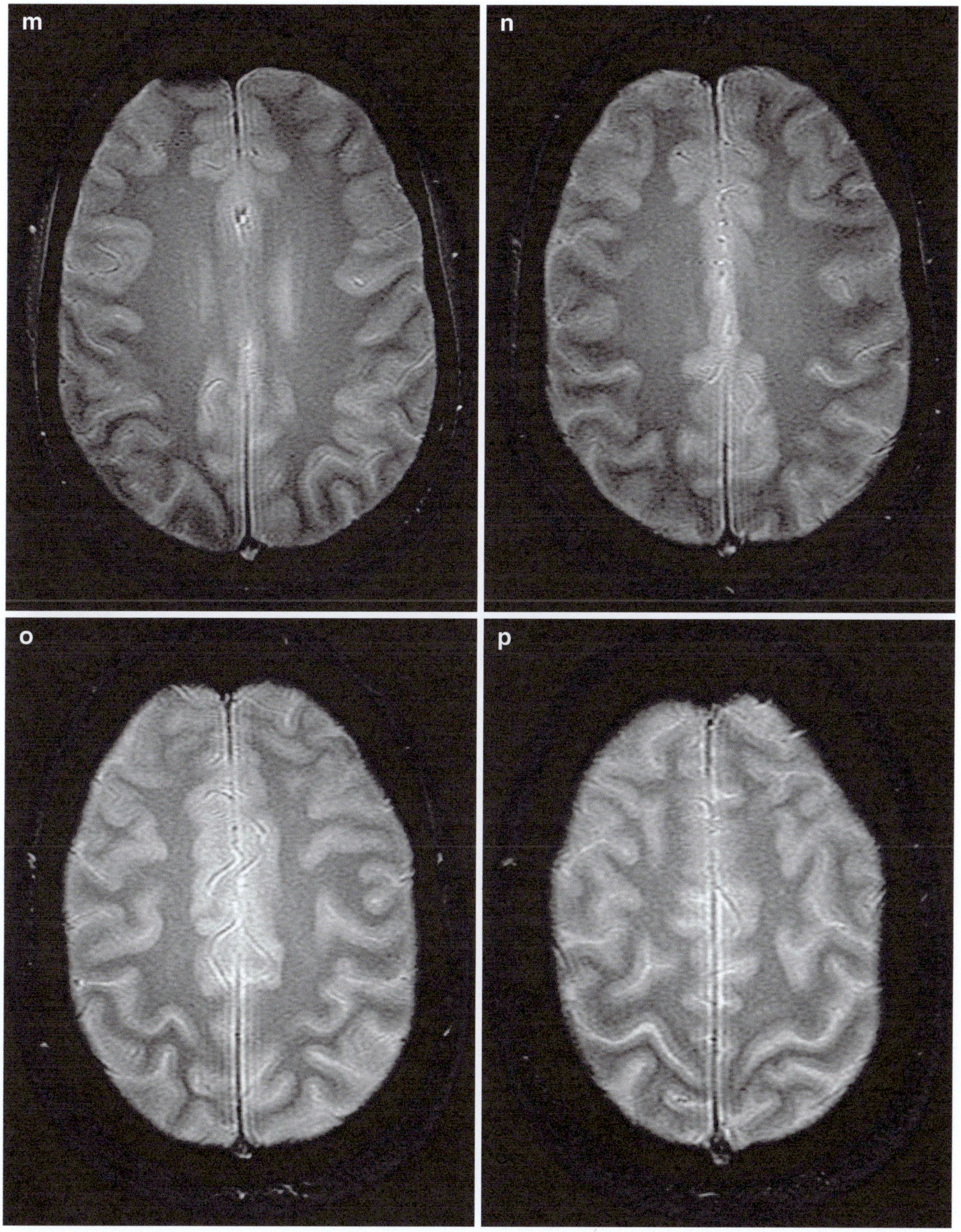


**Fig. 12.7** (continued)

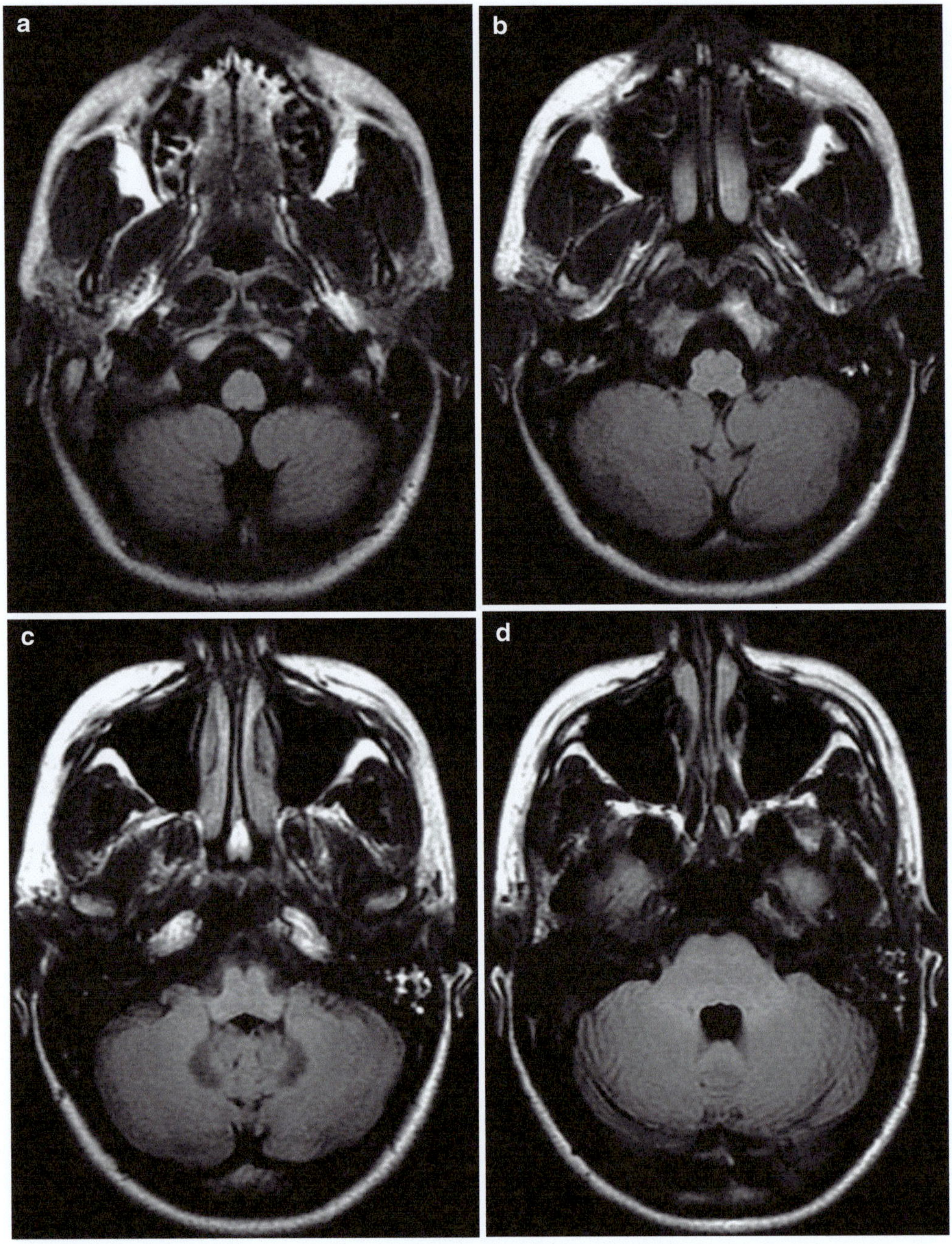


**Fig. 12.8** (**a**) FLAIR, (**b**) FLAIR, (**c**) FLAIR, (**d**) FLAIR, (**e**) FLAIR, (**f**) FLAIR, (**g**) FLAIR, (**h**) FLAIR, (**i**) FLAIR, (**j**) FLAIR, (**k**) FLAIR, (**l**) FLAIR, (**m**) FLAIR, (**n**) FLAIR, (**o**) FLAIR, (**p**) FLAIR

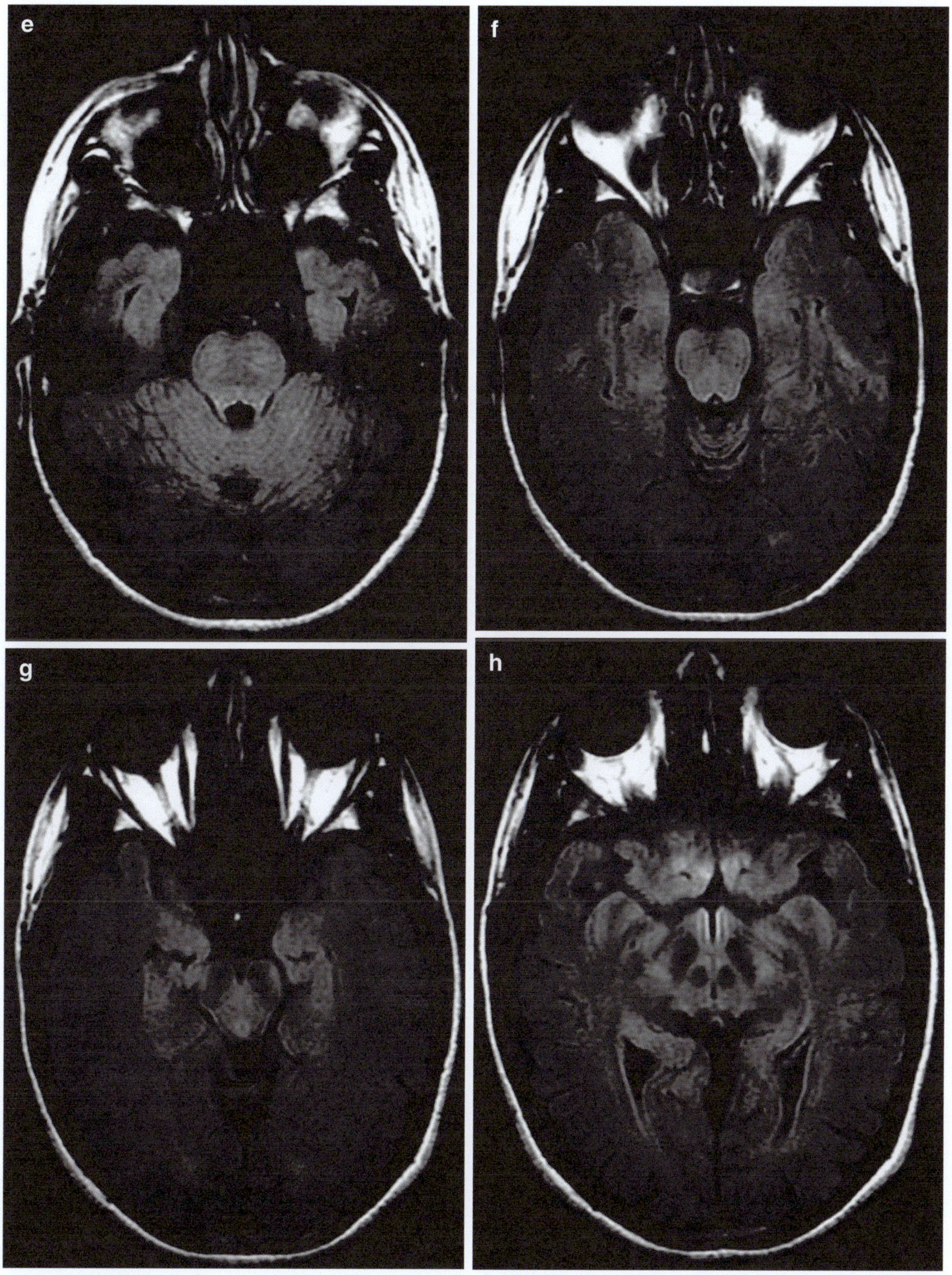


**Fig. 12.8** (continued)

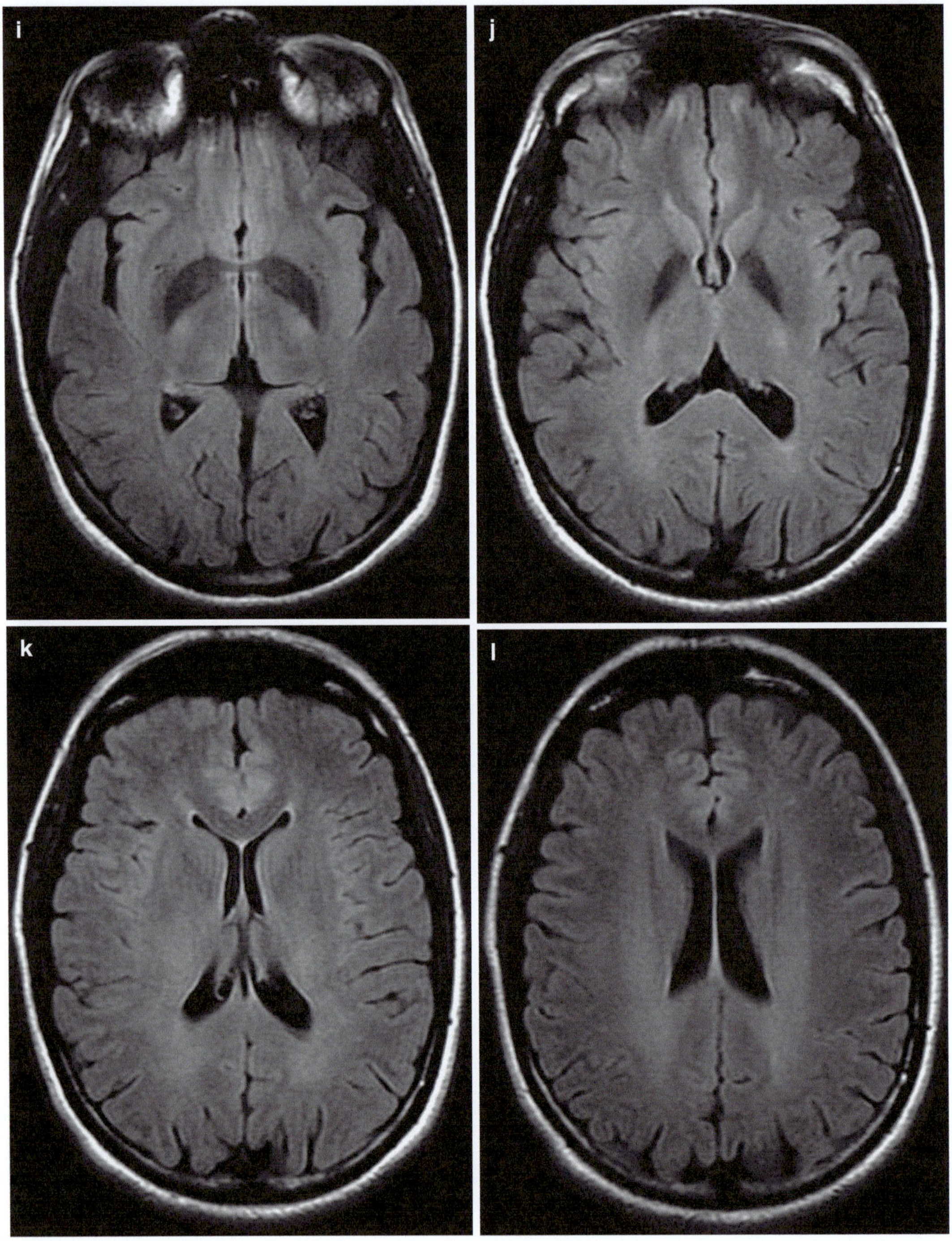


**Fig. 12.8** (continued)

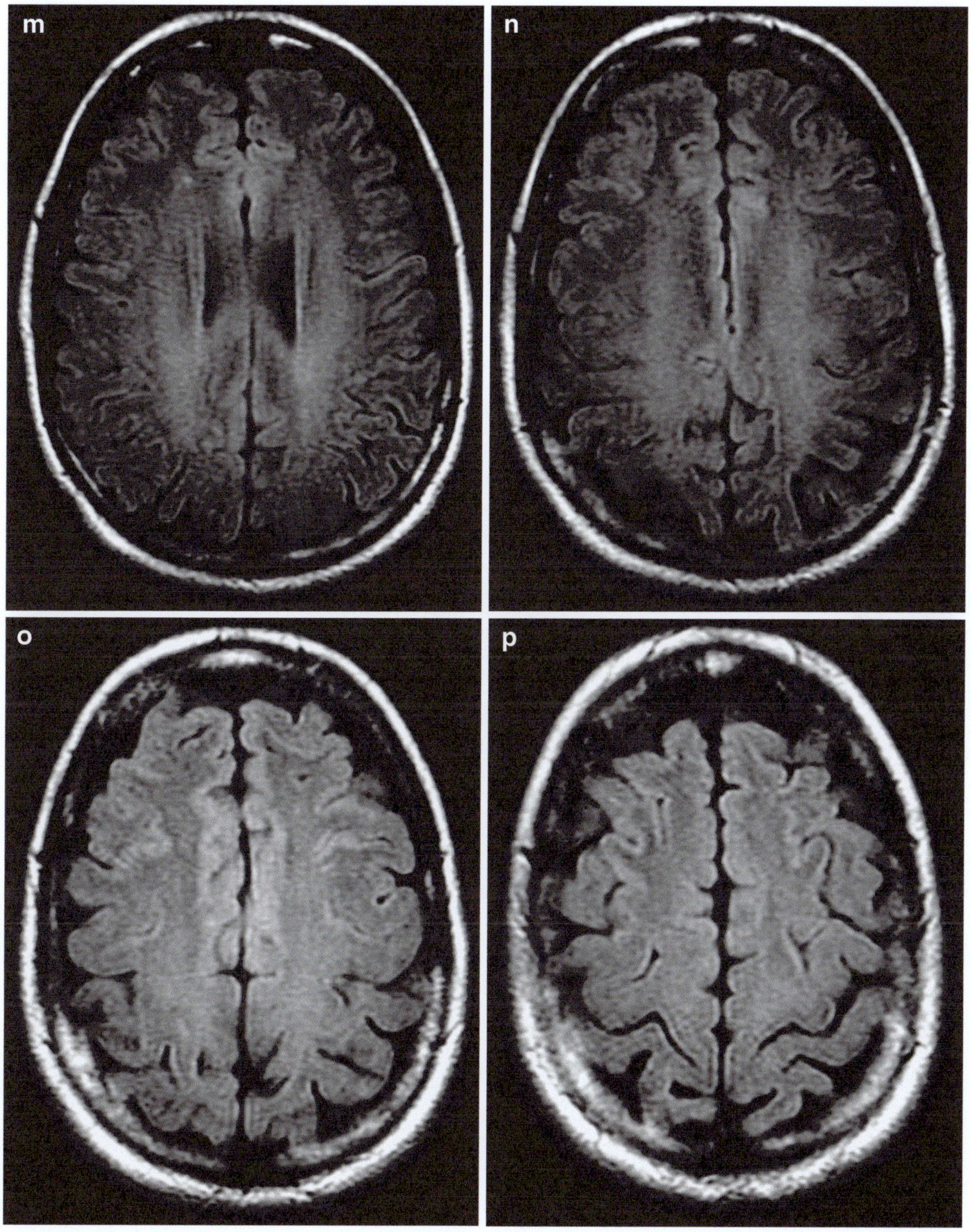


**Fig. 12.8** (continued)

**Table 12.1** T1 images

| | |
|---|---|
| **SE** | **FGE** |
| TR/TE 360/9 | TR/TE/FA 275/2.5/75 |
| 5mmthk | 5mmthk |
| 512×256 | 512×256 |
| FOV 22×22 | FOV 22×22 |
| **IR** | **FLAIR** |
| TR/TE/TI 2,040/28/700 | TR/TE/TI 2,320/27.4/auto |
| 5mmthk | 5mmthk |
| 512×256 | 256×256 |
| FOV 22×22 | FOV 22×22 |

**Table 12.2** T2 images

| | |
|---|---|
| **FSE** | **FSE with inverted contrast** |
| TR/TE/ETL 4,840/75.7/15 | TR/TE/ETL 4,840/75.7/15 |
| 5mm thk | 5mm thk |
| 448×320 | 448×320 |
| FOV 22×22 | FOV 22×22 |
| **GE** | **FLAIR** |
| TR/TE/FA 325/20/20 | TR/TE/TI 11,002/135/2,250 |
| 5mm thk | 5mm thk |
| 256×192 | 288×192 |
| FOV 22×22 | FOV 22×22 |

**Acknowledgments** We would like to thank the following technical staff for their help: C. Bocci, T. Cassano, I. Di Maggio, G. Fraticelli, A. Lombardi, A. Mazza, G. Miscio (Department of Radiology, IRCCS "Casa Sollievo della Sofferenza," San Giovanni Rotondo), and G.W. Antonucci and P. Colasuonno (Department of Radiology and Neuroradiology, "L. Bonomo Hospital", ASL BT, Andria (BT)).

# Setting the Report and Support of the Functional Findings

# 13

Armando Tartaro and Simone Salice

## 13.1 Functional Data in Clinical Practice and Research

Advanced MRI, including functional MRI (fMRI), has become an increasingly useful tool and ever more used, not only in research field but also in clinical practice. Nowadays, MRI is no longer considered just a qualitative diagnostic imaging but also a quantitative tool.

Advanced MRI techniques allow a noninvasive method for investigating normal and pathological tissues. Quantification of metabolite rates, perfusion parameters, and water diffusivity indices opened new scientific applications with a shift from qualitative to quantitative MRI [1, 2].

In the fMRI experiment, data are used to detect, in an indirect way, the changes in specific brain areas of neuronal stimulation-related activity. The fMRI signal is effect related to the local variations in blood flow that follow the changes in neural activity. Although signal intensity varies of only about 1 percent, fMRI allows to recognize brain areas involved in motor, sensorial, and cognitive functions.

A. Tartaro (✉) • S. Salice
Department of Neurosciences, Imaging and Clinical Sciences, Institute of Advanced Biomedical Technologies, University "G. d'Annunzio", Chieti, Pescara, Italy
e-mail: armando.tartaro@gmail.com

Thanks to the greater signal-to-noise ratio, 3 T MRI provides more reliable and more reproducible data than 1.5 T MRI [3]. In clinical practice, combined data, obtained by means of advanced MRI techniques and fMRI, are considered as "potential" biomarkers for the assessment of both microstructural (and/or microvascular) changes and anatomo-functional reorganization of brain connectivity, induced by focal or degenerative brain diseases.

Diffusion-weighted imaging (DWI), diffusion tensor imaging (DTI), magnetic resonance spectroscopy (MRS), and perfusion-weighted imaging (PWI) arterial spin labeling (ASL) provide quantitative, reliable, and reproducible information about microvascularity, neoangiogenesis, metabolism, necrosis, and cellularity of brain masses [4].

Since fMRI began in 1991, the number of people, papers, and abstracts related to fMRI has been increasing. Because fMRI is based on the blood oxygenation level-dependent (BOLD) effect, it does not directly record neural activity. Nevertheless, due to the excellent spatial and time resolution, fMRI is progressing in technology and methodology and increasingly used to investigate human brain function.

Functional connectivity (FC), defined as "temporal correlations between spatially remote neurophysiological events," is the most recent challenge of the fMRI technique. Resting-state fMRI (rs-fMRI), seen as a constant condition



T. Scarabino et al. (eds.), *High Field Brain MRI*, DOI 10.1007/978-3-319-44174-0_13

without sensorial stimuli or significant behaviorally salient events during fMRI recording, may be altered in dementia as well as in aging-related cognitive disorders.

Changes in the brain structure and function are well recognized in Alzheimer's disease (AD). Alterations of FC have been observed in patients affected by AD and mild cognitive impairment (MCI) and in subjects who had subjective cognitive decline (SCD). Among the rs-fMRI observations, the so-called default mode network (DMN), the most active neuronal network at rest and in the absence of a stimuli during fMRI experiment has been particularly studied because alterations to its FC were found in AD and MCI patients [5, 6]. These studies helped to understand the neural substrates in normal and pathological aging brain.

A challenge for clinical application of the advanced and fMRI techniques is closely related to the reliability and reproducibility of the results, which follows a standardization of acquisition techniques and data analysis.

## 13.2 Standardization of Data Handling

### 13.2.1 Image Acquisition

In advanced MRI protocols, brain images are acquired by using different sequences, some of which are critical for structural high-resolution and functional studies.

In general, advanced imaging protocols must include morphological T1-weighted sequences with high spatial resolution and isotropic voxel; currently, for this purpose whole-head 3D gradient-echo (GE) sequences, which though have different owner acronyms, are all of the type GE spoiled (SPGR, mPRAGE, 3D GE, etc.) and can be obtained in 5–6 min. Isotropic high-resolution structural images are used for voxel-based morphometry (VBM) and cortical thickness quantification of the whole brain or specific brain areas in neurodegenerative diseases, such as dementia [7]. These images are also frequently used as anatomical substrate for co-registration of BOLD-fMRI signals and spatially localization of eloquent areas in the presurgical brain mapping.

An ideal and desirable *voxel* spatial resolution for morphological T1-weighted sequences, obtained by using a 3-Tesla MRI system, is 1×1×1 mm or less (e.g. 0.8 × 0.8 × 0.8–1 mm).

T2*-weighted sequences, acquired with echo planar imaging (EPI) technique, are basically used in all BOLD-fMRI, PWI, DWI, and DTI, respectively; functional and microstructural studies, as well as morphological T1-weighted sequences, are used for high-resolution structural quantitative studies (VBM, cortical thickness). When using EPI sequences with a 3-Tesla MR system, in the scan time relative to each TR value (e.g., 1 s), up to 30 gapless, whole-head, 3 mm thickness or less, T2*-weighted images can be acquired.

MRS studies are basically obtained using specific sequences for the acquisition of the spectroscopic signals. Single voxel spectroscopy (SVS) receives spectra from a single voxel only; the signal-to-noise ratio (S/N) is generally high but limited to a circumscribed area. Multivoxel spectroscopy (MVS) explores larger brain regions, but S/N is lower than the SVS for the smaller voxel size. In SVS signal acquisition can be acquired with two different sequences. Basically, in PRESS (Point RESolved Spectroscopy) technique, the signal from the voxel of interest is a spin echo; in STEAM (Stimulated Echo Acquisition Mode) technique, the stimulated echo, corresponding to the S/N from the voxel of interest, is obtained from the cumulated effect of three pulses. The value of time echo (TE) used for PRESS and STEAM sequences determines the number of detectable metabolites on spectroscopic spectrum. When a long TE is selected (e.g., 144 or 288 ms), a more number of metabolites are visible, but S/N is lower than short TE (e.g., 30 ms or less), where a greater number of peaks are visible in the spectrum [8].

Even today, the major limitation is the lack of standardized imaging protocols and sequence parameters (e.g., TR, TE, FA, TI, slice thickness), both in clinical and research studies. Lack of standardization not only affects the reproducibility of the results, but mainly the routinely use of advanced MRI outcomes.

### 13.2.2 Processing of the Stimulus

In fMRI experiments, standardization of the procedures includes also the modalities of stimuli administration, scan paradigms, and data recording. Using standardized fMRI protocols, the starting point is to acquire "some" good advanced MRI data, in both high-resolution structural MRI and fMRI, task or resting state what they are. Before statistical analysis and signal detection is performed, it is necessary to convert and to improve the signal quality by preprocessing the raw data. In the preprocessing, different function must be implemented to obtain reliable data. Slice scan time correction, motion correction, temporal filtering, and spatial smoothing functions must be defined and applied preliminarily when a group analysis is required. Additional preprocessing (e.g., physiological noise correction, storm filtering, band pass) is also recommended before executing group data analysis.

In functional and effective connectivity measures, processing of brain activations is generally based on independent component analysis (ICA) and/or seed-based methods, in order to identify and quantify brain interregional relationships. Both ICA-derived and seed-based connectivity measures are characterized by some advantages and disadvantages, but a direct comparison of the results obtained from the two methods is not trivial. Also different paradigms, designed for brain stimulation, can influence qualitatively brain responses and qualitatively data recording. The major paradigms for fMRI analysis are univariate (hypothesis-driven), multivariate (data-driven), and voxel-based approach. FC networks can be detected from event-related designed paradigm, most often based on trials under stationary condition, or from block design paradigm, considered locally stationary and based on block duration [9].

### 13.2.3 Data Analysis

There are several techniques for interrogation of brain functions and as many available programs for analyzing advanced MRI data, each of which can have a large influence in determining the sensitivity, specificity, reliability, and flexibility of the experimental protocols. There are a large variety of software packages for data analysis, although not all of these single software packages can provide all necessary requirements for both structural and functional processing. fMRI data can be preprocessed and analyzed by using several platform operating systems and a number of software packages, e.g., SPM (statistical parametric mapping), BrainVoyager analysis, AFNI (analyses of functional software neuroimages), FSL (FMRIB Software Library), FreeSurfer, and many others as valuable software [10]. Biomedical image analysis software is a multimodal analysis tool, developed to analyze and visualize the structural and functional brain imaging data recorded from neuroimaging techniques and technologies (fMRI, DTI, EEG, MEG, TMS, PET, etc.). Nowadays, this software allows statistical data analysis based on general linear model (GLM), transformation of anatomical and functional scans into stereotaxic (Talairach-Tournoux) coordinate, automatic co-registration of functional data with high-resolution 3D anatomical data sets, and advanced methods for automatic brain segmentation, surface reconstruction, cortex inflation, and flattening. [11].

After being considered for years, the "future technique," MRS, finally, in the last decade, has become a valuable tool in clinical practice and research, for in vivo analysis of the main brain metabolites. Certainly, it has had great influence on the success of MRS techniques in the progress in signal processing. Currently, different valuable software packages are available for processing and quantitation of MRS data. Automated, proprietary software provided by the scanner manufacturers has the advantage of being fast in the analysis of MRS data, but when the S/N ratio is not high, there may be a lower resolution of the spectra for certain metabolites. A number of semiautomatic dedicated software packages are now available for MRS data generation, either in frequency (e.g., LCModel) or time domain (e.g., jMRUI). Commercially or freely available software packages take longer time for data processing, but S/N ratio is higher than automated software [8]. In general radiologists are more confident with software provided by the scanner manufacturers, because it is easy to use and less time-consuming, and the raw data should not be processed remotely.

As for MRS also PWI and DTI techniques require dedicated software packages for processing the raw data. Most of the radiologists prefer a fast processing of raw data at the end of MRI exam by means of automated software package provided by the scanner manufacturer. But many powerful software packages are freely or commercially available for a more accurate data processing (e.g., FreeSurfer platform and dedicated function included in the package like TRACULA (TRActs Constrained by UnderLying Anatomy)) and for automatic or semiautomatic reconstruction of WM tracts from diffusion-weighted images [12]. Several software packages are also available for calculation of quantitative PWI parameters (CBF, CBV, MTT), but in clinical practice radiologists feel more confident using automatic software provided by the manufacturer of the MRI system, because it is less time-consuming and easy to use even during the clinical activity. More powerful and sophisticated commercially or freely available software packages are fruitfully used for clinical research and require dedicated staff, specifically trained in order to fully exploit their potential. Given the differences of data processing and the wide range of software for data analysis, advanced MRI data, especially from fMRI, still has many limitations for clinical use.

In summary, as for the image acquisition, also for data analysis, there is a lack of standardization, which makes it difficult to compare different results; in some cases it may also notice a variability of the results within the same laboratory, for which it is always recommended the preliminary standardization of procedures and the development of its own database of reference values, both for normal and clinical categories, based on large populations of normal subjects and clinical series, as well as the comparison with scientific literature.

## 13.3 Structured Report

A standardized reporting system for the applications of advanced MRI findings, as a support of a clinical research center, is desirable.

The real-time use of MR images on the console screen and the simultaneous transmission to distance of data and DICOM-structured reports, require the development of remote control interfaces and protocols through workstations that facilitate the transfer rate between radiologist, technician, physicist, and engineer. Written communication, on the basis of the result presentation, should be developed so that researchers are able to work directly on MR protocols, automatically process the data, analyze the results on their own workplace, and write the report. Using as an input the results of advanced MRI and developed software tools, the radiologists can superimpose over anatomical atlas the selected images and create DICOM-structured reports and text files. Even now, compared to the dramatic evolution of neuroimaging technologies, the radiological reporting has remained largely static, both in content and structure. A number of new initiatives and specific technologies have been proposed by the international radiology community, with the unique opportunity to fundamentally change the radiology report from free to structured text supported by images. To this end, the structured report is intended as a computerized document in which various parts of the radiological outcome, accompanied by the most significant images, are coded and structured in a standard format.

The report can be defined as "the document obligatorily drawn up in writing, by which the medical specialist declare conform to the truth the results of diagnostic tests obtained, with the clinical interpretation of the same results, in relation to the clinical findings and the patient's history". The result is a mere outcome of diagnostic tests performed by clinical instruments and is a product free of interpretation or clinical evaluation. A radiology report is the "official record of a diagnostic, interventional, or therapeutic examination or procedure" [13]. This document represents the contribution of the radiologist to the diagnosis and treatment. A standardized lexicon edit in a structured form makes easier and better understood the transmission of radiological results to the referring physicians.

In 2007 the Intersociety Conference deliberated on specific aspects of radiology reports, recommending the use of "structured" reports, subdivided into consequential and systematically ordered sections, drafted in standardized form. More recently, a collaborative initiative for the development of structured radiological report templates was launched in 2013 at the European Congress of Radiology in Vienna, between RSNA and European Society of Radiology.

The increasing use of functional data (e.g., fMRI) in the practice and clinical research requires simple and automated procedures, allowing data "manipulation" (processing of the stimulus, image acquisition, data analysis, and interpretation and reporting of the process of results) [9]. A standardized way for data management is the *structured report*, which should not have additional costs, must be easy to use, include all the potential of the methods and related techniques, and also assist the radiologist in the report drafting.

The *structured report* merges the radiological text with the relevant images in a single report: *report and findings* [14–16].

The clinical *report* includes basic elements, as defined in the guidelines of the American College of Radiology's Practice and the RSNA's Radiology Reporting Committee, divided into clinical indications to the exam, imaging technique descriptions, imaging findings and observations, and summary of the results but also collateral findings, diagnostic hypotheses, or conclusions.

MRI *findings* from advanced techniques include microstructural (from DWI, DTI, MRS) and quantitative microstructural (from VBM and cortical thickness) biomarkers, microvascular parameters (from PWI and ASL), and functional information (from fMRI and rs-fMRI).

The integration *report/findings* must be supported by media (CD, DVD, remote transfer of DICOM images) where, in addition to conventional images, it also shows salient functional images (e.g., in brain mapping).

The first action is to establish a standardized style of reporting for advanced MRI examinations.

Radiological structured reporting allows to use a template of defined checklist based on terms and information, integrated with clinical data, technical parameters, annotations, and key images [17–19].

### 13.3.1 Developing a Report Template for Both Conventional and Functional Exam

A practical guide to implement a structured framework for advanced MRI examination should contain step by step the following items:

Step 1 *Administrative information*

Including referring provider, imaging facility, date of service, and time of service

Step 2 *Patient identification*

Including identification number or medical record number, name, date of birth, and sex

Step 3 *Clinical history and diagnostic appropriateness*

Including medical history, reason of examination and medical necessity, and medical history of allergies.

When we are using experimental tolls or procedures, in a research context, the title of the project and the name of the principal investigator (including his institutional address and phone number for a quick consultation) should be included in the document; moreover, the authorization of the ethics committee (code or number) should be always reported. A focused patient medical history is necessary to evaluate diagnostic appropriateness or meet inclusion criteria when it is running an experimental protocol. As a rule (justification principle and criteria for a good practice), all individual radiological exposures should be justified in advance and always optimized for the patient characteristics and diagnostic purpose.

Step 4 *Imaging techniques*

Including conventional sequences of imaging used for the specific MRI examination (SE, TSE, T-IR, FLAIR, GE, 3D GE); scan parameters (TR, TE, FA, TI) for T1, before and after contrast medium injection, T2-, T2*- and PD-weighted images; and scan planes (sagittal, coronal, axial, or multiple)

Concerning advanced techniques, it is recommended to indicate in DWI/ADC the b values, number of directions in DTI, single or multivoxel and TE values (in millisecond) for MRS, the selected modalities PWI (i.e., EPI-SE, EPI-GE, ASL), and perfusion parameter obtained (CBF, CBV, MTT). In BOLD imaging should be reported the paradigms (i.e., block or single trial) and the modalities of stimuli administration, time of image acquisition, magnetic field strength, contrast materials, and other medications administered (including name, dose, route, way, and time of administration) should be reported.

Step 5 *Data analysis techniques*

Nowadays, MRI and fMRI play an increasingly important role in the investigation of brain structure, function, development, and pathologies. The increasing flexibility and power of MRI and fMRI to answer scientifically interesting and clinically relevant questions have led to a demand for analysis techniques which allow investigators to interrogate their data in as flexible, scientifically informative and convenient a manner as is possible [11].

There are many available programs for analyzing advanced MRI data, each of which can have a large influence in determining the sensitivity, specificity, reliability, and flexibility of the experimental protocols (i.e., MEDx, MATLAB, BrainVoyager, AFNI, FSL, FreeSurfer, SMRUI, etc.)

Step 6 *Findings description*

Narrative description of findings and comparison with previous examinations, findings itemization (or listing). This step includes the simple descriptive outcome, without clinical evaluation or interpretation of the results obtained with the technique used for that exam. The description of the MRI signals and their interpretation serves as a basis for making a decision or formulating a diagnostic hypothesis. Also, it describes the anatomical site of the alteration; the size, shape, and relationships with surrounding anatomical structures; the associated signs such as mass effect or loss of substance; and the presence of edema and gliosis. Measurements, image annotations for highlighting an abnormality, and identification of key images are peculiar of this step.

With the aid of specific software, the outcome of the functional analysis of the advanced MRI findings, without interpretation or clinical assessment, is reported also.

A standardized lexicon developed provides specific or general terms for disease observations or acronyms to indicate imaging procedures.

*Step 7 "Collateral" findings*

Collateral or "incidental" or "occasional" findings, not expected, that can be encountered during an exam run for several reasons that have no direct connection with the clinical question. They may be anatomical variants, be congenital malformations, or be borderline findings (i.e., as in respect to the age of the patient). In other cases they are pathological findings or may potentially become pathological.

It is always appropriate to evaluate accurately all that the image shows, without forgetting the medicolegal implications arising from the failure to report findings that may have an important impact on patient's health.

*Step 8 Observations and conclusions*

Including any recommendations. Report diagnostic hypothesis and collateral findings.

Before reporting the results of functional data, specify that this technique has an experimental value and can only be indicative. Define the anatomic sites where the activations have been located (in case of BOLD imaging)) or the white matter tracts highlighted (DTI).

In summary, the structured report in addition to its clinical function is an instrument of communication, useful for quality improvement, research, and teaching.

### 13.3.2 Support of Functional Findings to the Clinical Report

In the last decade, MRI and fMRI have played an increasingly important role in the investigation of brain structure, function, development, and pathologies. Available techniques for interrogation and analysis of neuroimaging data have had a large influence in determining the flexibility, sensitivity, and scope of neuroimaging experiments.

An advanced functional neuroimaging technique may provide a fundamental tool for differentiating between many disorders such as low- and high-grade brain tumors, aging-related cognitive decline, or neurodegenerative disease, to guide the treatment of ischemic stroke and CNS infectious disease and so on. Despite thousands of scientific papers that have been written on the usefulness of advanced MRI techniques in the study of brain disorders, most of their parts are related to clinical research, hoping it will be as soon as clinical practice.

Growing efforts have been addressed to define advanced MRI data as useful biomarkers for the assessment of brain tumor grading and for better differentiation between benign and malignant brain masses [1, 4]. About the latter, it is known that apparent diffusion coefficient (ADC), derived from DWI technique, and fractional anisotropy (FA), derived from DTI, are, respectively, significantly lower and higher in the central cavity of pyogenic abscesses than in the central cavity of necrotic tumors [20, 21]; biomarkers derived from MRS are usually revealed only in the central cavity of pyogenic abscesses and not in the central cavity of high-grade gliomas or metastases [20]. Cerebral blood volume (CBV), a biomarker derived from PWI, if measured in ring enhancement and perilesional edema, is generally higher in high-grade glioma than in pyogenic abscesses [21, 22].

MRS may provide additional information in cases in which the differential diagnosis of tumors by convectional neuroimaging can be difficult; e.g., a relatively specific finding for meningioma is an unusually high ratio of alanine to creatine detected on [$H^1$]-MRS spectrum.

Nowadays, task and resting-state fMRI is a useful tool for the noninvasive presurgical brain mapping of the cortex for brain tumor and resective epilepsy surgery.

New fields of fMRI for the preclinical and clinical research are concerning dementia and aging-related cognitive disorders, such as subjective cognitive decline (SCD) and mild cognitive impairment (MCI). Despite, diagnosis of dementia remains a clinical prerogative; conventional MRI and fMRI are in vivo, noninvasive modalities to support the diagnosis of different brain pathologies.

Accurate and automated methods for measuring the thickness of human cerebral cortex could provide powerful tools for diagnosing and studying a variety of neurodegenerative and psychiatric disorders [7]. For instance, cerebral atrophy is detected late in the course of the AD, while functional changes in the brain usually appear prior to structural changes. Manual methods for estimating cortical thickness from neuroimaging data are labor intensive, requiring several days of effort by a trained anatomist. VBM of the whole brain (WM+GM) or of specific regions (i.e., hippocampus) can be measured. Nevertheless, folded nature of the cortex is problematic for manual techniques, frequently resulting in measurement errors in regions in which the cortical surface is not perpendicular to any of the cardinal axes. This makes it very difficult to disentangle brain changes in normal aging from the earliest signs of AD.

Resting-state fMRI has recently been highlighted as a new technique for interrogating intrinsic FC network in MCI, AD, cerebrovascular disease, Lewy body disease, or a mixture of these pathologies.

Proton MRS metabolite markers may help identify and track etiologies that typically underlie MCI in the elderly. The role of proton MRS will especially be critical for pathophysiological processes for which a reliable biomarker does not exist such as glial and microglial activation in neurodegenerative dementia.

Dementia with Lewy bodies (DLB) is characterized by fluctuation in cognition and attention. Thalamocortical connectivity and integrity of thalami are central to attentional function. In DLB pathology multimodal techniques including structural MRI, DTI, and 1H-MRS have shown microstructural damage in thalamic regions highlighting the critical role of the thalamus [23].

Major advances have occurred in the development of disease biomarkers in the past two decades. However, the absence of standardized quantitative metric-advanced MRI and FMRI biomarkers constitutes a major deficiency. Failure to move toward a standardized system of quantitative metrics has substantially limited potential diagnostic usefulness advanced neuroimaging in clinical practice.

In summary, advanced and fMRI play an important role on understanding the healthy human brain, but it has much less impact in clinical practice. A reason is in part that data acquisition, paradigm designs, and analysis strategies used are not enough standardized, making comparison of results across single patients, MRI studies, and institutes sometimes not feasible.

## References


1. Caulo M, Panara V, Tortora D, Mattei PA, Briganti C, Salice S, Cotroneo AR, Tartaro A (2014) Data-driven grading of brain gliomas: a multiparametric MR imaging study. Radiology 272(2):494–503
2. Tofts P (2004) Quantitative MRI of the brain: measuring changes caused by disease. John Wiley and Sons, Chichester
3. Wardlaw JM, Brindle W, Casado AM, Shuler K, Henderson M, Thomas B et al (2012) A systematic review of the utility of 1.5 versus 3 Tesla magnetic resonance brain imaging in clinical practice and research. Eur Radiol 22(11):2295–2303
4. Smith ETS (2011) Clinical applications of imaging biomarkers. Part 1. The neuroradiologist's perspective. Br J Radiol 84(Spec Iss 2):S196–S204
5. Wu X, Li R, Fleisher AS, Reiman EM, Guan X, Zhang Y, Chen K, Yao L (2011) Altered default mode network connectivity in alzheimer's disease—a resting functional MRI and bayesian network study. Hum Brain Mapp 32(11):1868–1881
6. Korgaonkar MS, Grieve SM, Etkin A, Koslow SH, Williams LM (2013) Using standardized fMRI protocols to identify patterns of prefrontal circuit dysregulation that are common and specific to cognitive and emotional tasks in major depressive disorder: first wave results from the iSPOT-D study. Neuropsychopharmacology 38:863–871
7. Fischl B, Dale AM (2000) Measuring the thickness of the human cerebral cortex from magnetic resonance images. Proc Natl Acad Sci U S A 97(20):11050–11055
8. Pravat K (2012) Mandal. *In vivo* proton magnetic resonance spectroscopic signal processing for the absolute quantitation of brain metabolites. Eur J Radiol 81(4):e653–e664
9. Soares J, Alves V. Functional magnetic resonance imaging data manipulation – A new approach. IFMBE Proceedings. 2009: 25/V, pp. 36–39.
10. Behroozi M, Daliri MR (2012) Software tools for the analysis of functional magnetic resonance imaging. BCN 3(5):71–83
11. Smith SM, Jenkison M, Woolrich MW et al (2004) Advances in functional and structural MR image analysis and implementation as FSL. Neuroimage 23(suppl 1):S208–S219
12. Glatard T, Lewis LB et al (2015) Reproducibility of neuroimaging analyses across operating systems. Front Neuroinform 9(12):1–14
13. Reed Dunnick N, Langlotz CP (2008) The radiology report of the future: a summary of the 2007 Intersociety Conference. J Am Coll Radiol 5(5):626–229
14. Bosmans JML, Peremans L et al (2012) Structured reporting: if, why, when, how—and at what expense? Results of a focus group meeting of radiology professionals from eight countries. Insights Imaging 3:295–302
15. Bosmans JML, Neri E, Ratib O et al (2015) Structured reporting: a fusion reactor hungry for fuel. Insights Imaging 6(1):129–132
16. Langlotz CP (2009) Structured reporting in radiology: are we there yet? Radiology 253:23–25
17. Cramer J, Elsenmenger L, Pierson N et al (2014) Structured and templated reporting: an overview. Appl Radiol 43(8).

18. Langlotz C P, Burnside E S et al (2008) Towards best practices in radiology reporting. RSNA. Radiol 253(3):852–856
19. Reiner BI, Knight N, Siegel EL (2007) Radiology reporting, past, present and future: the radiologist's perspective. J Am Coll Radiol 4(5):313–319
20. Nath K, Agarwal M, Ramola M, Husain M, Prasad KN, Rathore RK et al (2009) Role of diffusion tensor imaging metrics and in vivo proton magnetic resonance spectroscopy in the differential diagnosis of cystic intracranial mass lesions. Magn Reson Imaging 30:198–206
21. Chiang IC, Hsieh TJ, Chiu ML, Liu GC, Kuo YT, Lin WC (2009) Distinction between pyogenic brain abscess and necrotic brain tumour using 3-tesla MR spectroscopy, diffusion and perfusion imaging. Br J Radiol 82:813–820
22. Reiche W, Schuchardt V, Hagen T, Il'yasov KA, Billmann P, Weber J (2010) Differential diagnosis of intracranial ring enhancing cystic mass lesions–role of diffusion-weighted imaging (DWI) and diffusion-tensor imaging (DTI). Clin Neurol Neurosurg 112(3):218–225
23. Delli Pizzi S, Franciotti R et al (2015) Thalamic involvement in fluctuating cognition in dementia with Lewy bodies: magnetic resonance evidences. Cereb Cortex 25:3682–3689

# Part II

# Applications

# High-Field Neuroimaging in Traumatic Brain Injury and Disorders of Consciousness

# 14

Chiara Falletta Caravasso, Francesco De Pasquale, Rita Formisano, and Umberto Sabatini

## 14.1 Introduction

Traumatic brain injury (TBI) is a debilitating neurological disorder that occurs to the brain as a result of a trauma. It embodies heterogeneous phenomena observed at the moment of impact (in the acute phase) and over time (in the chronic stage) with sequelae potentially seen many years from the onset. The primary parenchymal damage, i.e., the injury sustained at the moment of impact, is followed by a myriad of systemic and local effects such as hypoxia, hypotension, hypercarbia, brain swelling, and compression. All these effects are combined, leading to secondary brain damages. The classification of TBI in terms of severity as mild, moderate, or severe typically relies on the Glasgow Coma Scale (GCS) [1].

Magnetic resonance (MR) is the imaging technique of choice for the study of TBI in clinically stable patients, both in the acute and chronic phases, and it is often comparable to computed tomography (CT) in clinically unstable patients, such as comatose patients [2–5]. However, in this case, the role of MR is still to be established. As a matter of fact, despite the MR high sensitivity to focal traumatic lesions, the relationship between MR parameters and the clinical picture and prognosis is promising but not clear yet. In particular, in patients with TBI and disorder of consciousness (DOC), this technique, in a near future, might provide additional information on the diagnosis and the course of recovery of consciousness to be used for novel therapeutic interventions. This could be partly due to the fact that while there is some evidence that MR parameters might correlate with the prognosis, the typical GCS, used to classify traumatic patients, provides a static picture that is not suitable to predict prognosis in TBI patients, who evolve into a wide range of complex neuropathological conditions [6]. Further, the difficulty of monitoring vital signs in the MR tunnel, suboptimal accuracy in depicting fractures, acquisition times, and costs are additional disadvantages.

Current guidelines consider CT as the imaging technique of choice in unstable patients,

C.F. Caravasso
Department of Radiology, IRCCS Santa Lucia Foundation, Rome, Italy

F. De Pasquale
Faculty of Veterinary Medicine, University of Teramo, Teramo, TE, Italy

R. Formisano
Post-Coma Unit, IRCCS Santa Lucia Foundation, Rome, Italy

U. Sabatini (✉)
Department of Neuroradiology, Magna Graecia University, Catanzaro, Italy
e-mail: u.sabatini@hsantalucia.it



T. Scarabino et al. (eds.), *High Field Brain MRI*, DOI 10.1007/978-3-319-44174-0_14

where the primary goal is rapid detection of hematomas and other lesions requiring surgery [7]. However, the availability of high-field MR, which enables short acquisition times with conventional sequences as well as the use of ultrafast sequences very sensitive to magnetic susceptibility, like echo planar imaging (EPI) [8] and turbo-proton echo planar spectroscopic imaging (t-PEPSI) [9, 10], makes this technique suitable to image clinically unstable patients. Indeed, high-field MR (e.g., $B_0 \geq 3.0$ T) is both more sensitive to focal lesions containing blood components and exhibits an enhanced ability to detect structural, functional, and metabolic changes in apparently intact white and gray matter by the use of advanced techniques such as diffusion tensor imaging (DTI), functional MRI (fMRI), and MR spectroscopy (MRS).

## 14.2 Rationale for MR Imaging of Patients with TBI

In the acute phase of TBI, secondary ischemic injury induced by hypotension and edema or by hemorrhage may be superimposed on the primary, blunt, or penetrating, parenchymal injury. In these patients, the focal injury is studied using T2-weighted and fluid-attenuated inversion recovery (FLAIR) sequences, the ischemic injury with diffusion-weighted sequences (DWI), and hemorrhage using T1- and T2*-weighted and FLAIR sequences: in all cases, the examination time should be as short as possible.

In the chronic phase, patients may exhibit either focal lesions with or without hemoglobin degradation products (diffuse axonal injury, DAI, or mixed features of focal lesions and DAI) and phenomena of anatomical and/or functional deafferentation. The MR protocol for clinically stabilized patients thus aims at detecting focal lesions such as signs of stationary tissue distress and DAI using sequences sensitive to gliosis (T2 weighted and FLAIR) and to hemoglobin degradation products (T2*-weighted sequences) and at evidencing direct or indirect signs of deafferentation.

Current guidelines mandate the use of a number of technical features when imaging patients with TBI, including acquisitions in at least two spatial planes, because structures such as the corpus callosum and brainstem are better appreciated in sagittal and coronal planes; slice thickness not greater than 5 mm; spin echo (SE)-turbo SE (TSE), proton density (PD), and T2 weighted; SE-TSE, T1 weighted; and gradient echo (GE) T2*-weighted and FLAIR sequences.

T2- and PD-weighted sequences afford optimal visualization of edema, which is found in the majority of patients with TBI. T1-weighted sequences are useful to document recent intra- and extra-axial blood extravasation. T2-weighted and FLAIR sequences are very sensitive to thin extracerebral blood collections in brain contusion, DAI, and subarachnoid hemorrhage [11]. T2*-weighted sequences, which are particularly sensitive to the effects of magnetic susceptibility induced by hemoglobin degradation products, are superior to T2-weighted sequences in identifying lesions with a hemorrhagic component, such as contusion and DAI [12–14]. The ultrafast multi-echo planar sequence (time of acquisition 4 s), t-PEPSI [9, 10], is sensitive to static magnetic field inhomogeneities and is optimized for functional neuroimaging as an alternative to T2*-weighted sequences [15, 16]. In this study, these two sequences did not detect a significantly different total number of DAI lesions; the T2*-weighted sequence proved to be significantly superior to t-PEPSI in depicting temporal lesions, as could be expected from the presence in the EPI sequences of geometric distortion and magnetic susceptibility artifacts due to anatomical structures such as the petrous bone in this region. Ultrafast multi-EPI sequences thus dramatically reduce imaging time, and their application should be recommended for the study of clinically unstable or uncooperative patients.

Medium-field magnets like those currently employed in clinical practice (1.5 T) allow the acquisition of a protocol with these features in about 20 min.

## 14.3 High- and Ultrahigh-Field MR in Patients with TBI

The potential advantages of high-field MR in routine clinical practice are the increased spatial contrast and spectral and temporal resolution. In principle, the performance of a 3.0 T (and higher) MR imager should be double than a 1.5 T machine [16, 17]. However, artifacts and technical limitations do not allow to achieve such improvement especially at ultrahigh fields such as 7 T. As a matter of fact, a greater signal/noise ratio (SNR), the main advantage of high-field imaging, can be reduced, among other factors, by local magnetic field variations caused by magnetic field gradient inhomogeneities [16, 18–20].

The reduction in T1 differences among tissue types induces a contrast loss between white and gray matter [5, 21], and it can impair the detection of lesions like contusion and intraparenchymal hematoma, which in the acute stage are difficult to appreciate also at 1.5 T. The MPRAGE sequence has been introduced to address this problem. Volumetric sequences such as MPRAGE have already been performed at 1.5 T to quantify white and gray matter volume in TBI patients with a view to documenting potential correlates between clinical state and atrophy of specific brain lesions (Fig. 14.1) [22].

As far as it regards T2-weighted images, the greater spatial resolution, resulting in better anatomical detail and contrast due to the greater SNR, allows thicker slices and broader matrices to be used and small lesions such as contusions or DAI to be appreciated. A further advantage of high-field T2-weighted sequences is their ability to depict very small deposits of deoxy- or methemoglobin as markedly hypointense areas by virtue of magnetic susceptibility effects, which are amplified by the high field [17, 23].

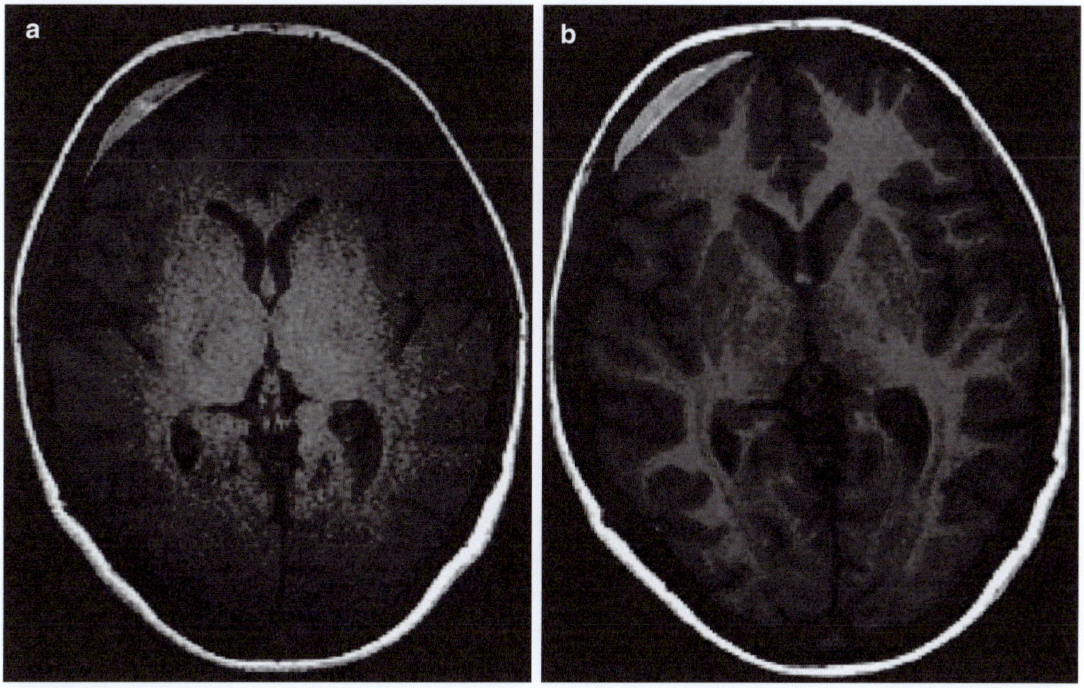


**Fig. 14.1** SE T1: comparison between images acquired in the same patient at 3.0 T (Allegra, Siemens) (**a** *left*) and 1.5 T (Vision, Siemens) (**b** *right*). The thin extra-axial right frontal blood collection, indicating a subacute subdural hematoma, is appreciated in both sequences

High-field GE T2* sequences are more sensitive to the magnetic susceptibility of hemoglobin degradation products and are thus valuable for detecting DAI. A correlation between the number of blood-containing lesions, DAI lesions identified on T2*-weighted sequences, and GCS score was confirmed by Scheid et al. [14], whereas no relationship was documented between focal changes appreciable in T2*-weighted sequences and Glasgow Outcome Scale (GOS) scores [24], suggesting that lesion load may not predict prognosis in these patients (Fig. 14.2).

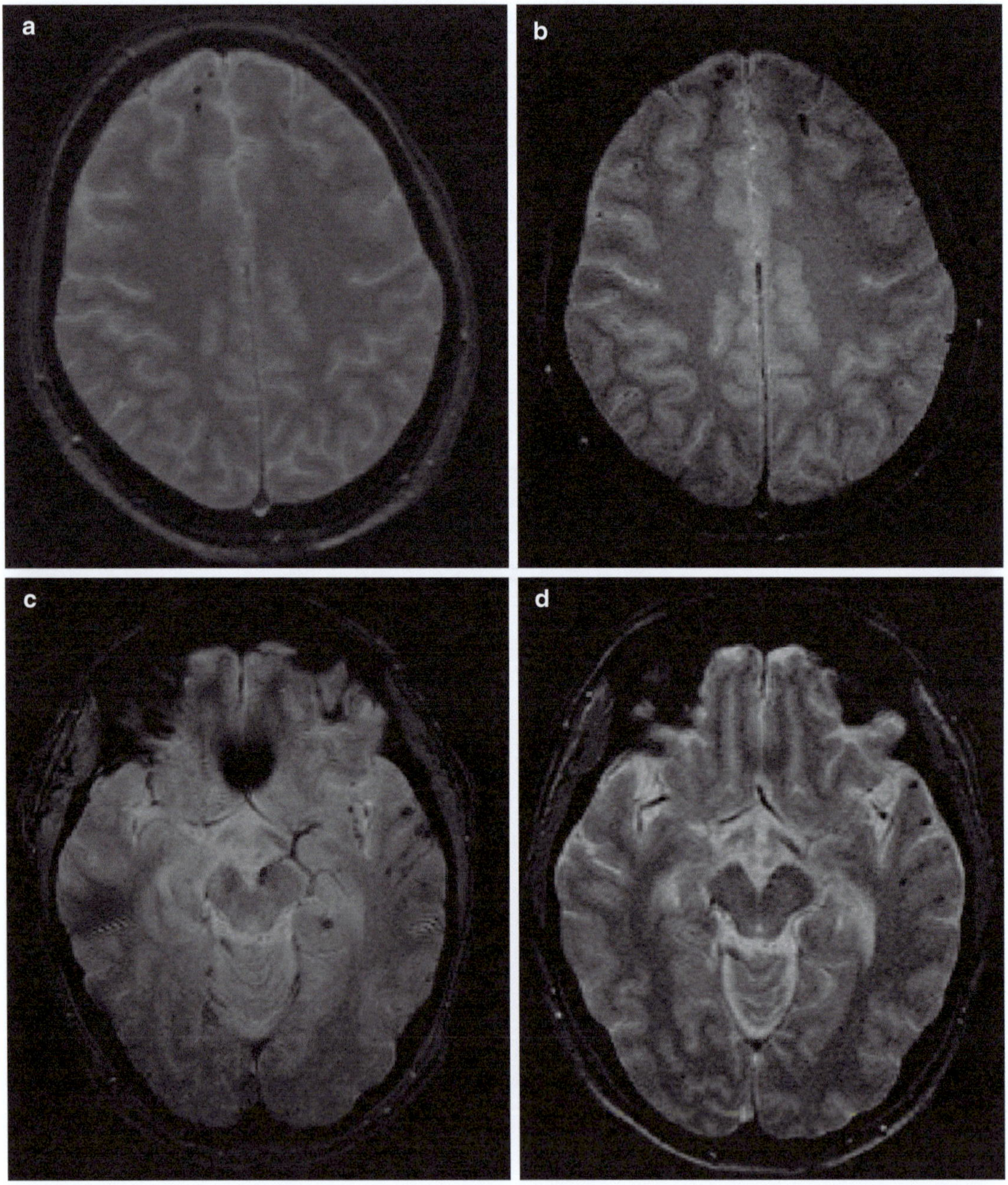


**Fig. 14.2** GE T2*: comparison between images acquired in the same patient at 3.0 T (Allegra, Siemens) (**a**, **c** *left*) and1.5 T (Vision, Siemens) (**b**, **d** *right*). Bilateral frontal subcortical (**a**, **b**) and left temporal and mesencephalic (**c**, **d**) small focal DAI lesions are more numerous and better visualized at 3.0 T

EPI sequences are also more sensitive at 3.0 T than 1.5 T, to the detriment of image geometry. On EPI images, distortion is approximately 30 % greater at 3.0 T than 1.5 T but can be reduced to about 1 % using SSFSE [25]. Furthermore, also the accurate study of intracranial vessels, which is especially useful in patients with TBI and clinically suspected vessel dissection, carotid-cavernous fistula, or dural venous sinus thrombosis, benefits from high-field imaging [26].

Ultrahigh-field systems (>3 T), which are currently under development and validation for clinical imaging, are expected to improve the in vivo imaging of TBI lesions, especially DAI. An improvement in image quality has already been shown at ultrahigh field in ex vivo studies [27]. A recently published in vivo studies at 7 T in a small patient cohort showed for the first time that ultrahigh-field imaging has a much higher potential than assumed in the depiction of small hemorrhagic DAI compared to 3 T [27].

## 14.4 Advanced High-Field Techniques in TBI

It is well established that standard MRI sequences underestimate traumatic brain injury [14, 28–31]. On the other hand, more advanced MRI techniques such as diffusion tensor imaging (DTI), magnetic resonance spectroscopy (MRS), and functional MRI (fMRI) are available at high fields. DTI is able to map fiber tracts and locate pathway disruption; MRS provides information on the altered metabolism, and fMRI can reveal, apart from functional activations, connectivity maps at rest (absence of a specific task). Thus, the combination of these techniques can provide important information regarding the relationship between the structural and functional brain architectures which provide a multivariate prognostic information. In fact, these new MRI techniques have been applied to TBI to gain insights into the mechanisms underlying the patient's clinical condition, predict its evolution and thus prognosis, and optimize therapeutic strategies [32–39].

### 14.4.1 Diffusion Tensor Imaging

DTI is a diffusion-weighted imaging (DWI) technique that paved the way to new possibilities for investigating white matter in vivo as it provides information about white matter anatomy that is not available through any other methods.

DTI provides two essential types of information: a quantitative estimate of anisotropy and its spatial orientation. Tractography uses these microscopic data to track macroscopic axon fibers, and it is capable of noninvasive in vivo imaging of these structures [18, 19, 40]. In DAI, the white matter fibers are typically interrupted; measuring white matter anisotropy with DTI allows the tissue damage to be quantified [41] (Fig. 14.3).

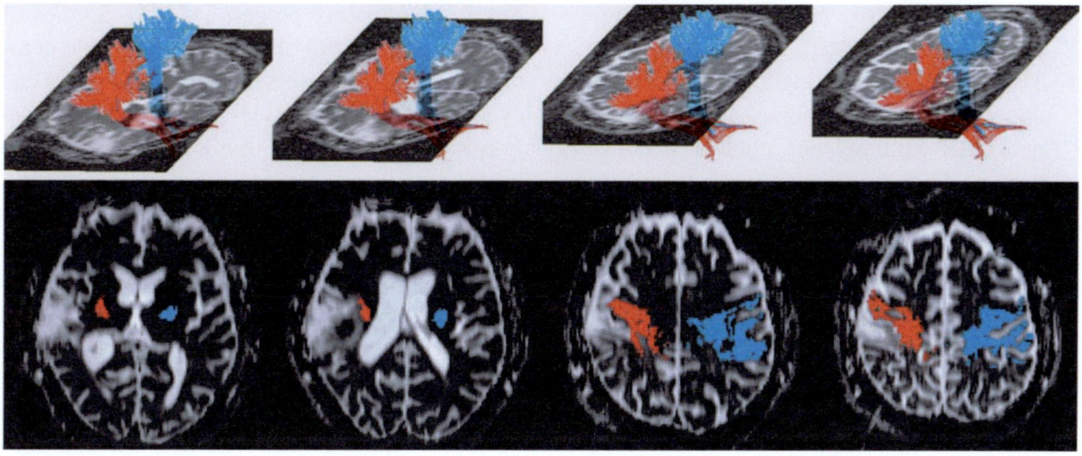

**Fig. 14.3** Tractography at 3.0 T (Allegra, Siemens): visualization of motor areas and pyramidal fibers in an extensive right frontal contusion. The right primary motor area and pyramidal fibers are depicted less clearly than in the contralateral area

Based on these considerations, Huisman et al. [35] proved that DTI can detect structural white matter changes and that these changes correlate with clinical parameters such as GCS score in the acute phase and at discharge. On the other hand, Zheng et al. [42] demonstrated the superior performance of DWI in identifying DAI compared with standard (T2-, T2*-weighted, FLAIR) sequences, but did not address its clinical relevance and thus the potential correlations with prognosis.

The technical characteristics of high-field MR have enhanced the quality of DTI data, particularly the spatial resolution, the spatial deformation induced by magnetic field inhomogeneities, and image SNR, thus improving the accuracy of nerve fiber tracking on mild, moderate, and severe TBI. Furthermore, the advantages of applying DTI to patients with head trauma are:

- An ability to gain information on the microscopic brain damage responsible, alone or in association with the macroscopic damage, for the patient's clinical state.
- An ability to document and quantify the brain plasticity phenomena underpinning clinical recovery, which may be enhanced using pharmacological and rehabilitation therapies.
- The possibility of assessing the therapeutic response even in those patients on whom clinical studies do not provide adequate information; moreover, the quantitative data offered by DTI are not influenced by potential CNS side effects of drug therapy or invasive procedures (e.g., intubation).
- The possibility of using DTI data to predict outcome in trauma patients, since neither standard MR findings nor clinical parameters, such as GCS scores, can predict their future clinical condition.

The potentiality of DTI to map and correlate the disruption in fiber tracts to clinical outcomes led researchers to adopt this technique for the quantification of the primary and secondary damage in DOC patients [43]. Recently, a large literature focused on this topic, i.e., to identify by DTI the different disorder of consciousness [e.g., vegetative state (VS) vs. minimally conscious state (MCS)] [44] or to correlate DTI findings with injury severity and clinical outcome [45–49].

Actually, the use of DTI to determine DOC severity, to aid diagnosis, and to ascertain prognostic outcomes is limited to the research setting. Despite this, DTI has proved a powerful tool as it grants insight into the pathogenesis and specific WM abnormalities underlying different DOC states, casting light on the neural basis of consciousness and the clinical features associated with DOC.

### 14.4.2 MR Spectroscopy

MR spectroscopy is a molecular-based neuroimaging technique that reflects the intracellular metabolic status that can be influenced by the presence of a microscopic injury.

The advantage of using 3.0 T MRS consists of an enhancement of the chemical shift with better separation of the metabolite peaks and high SNR [50]. MRS can document a reduction in the *N*-acetylaspartate (NAA) peak, a neuronal and axonal marker, and in ostensibly normal white matter free of macroscopic focal changes weeks or months after the trauma, and the extent of this reduction significantly correlates with scores on prognostic measures like GOS and Disability Rating Scale (DRS) [36, 37, 50]. Concomitant elevation of the levels of other metabolites, such as *myo*-inositol (Ins) and choline (Cho), is to be ascribed to glial proliferation or an inflammatory process [51–53]. Studies of white matter devoid of focal changes have demonstrated that the levels of these metabolites can eventually revert to normal [52] as well as a progressive reduction in NAA associated with increased Cho [51] or decreased Ins peaks [36]. Shutter et al. [37] studied a group of trauma patients in the subacute phase who underwent MRS within a week of the trauma to detect metabolic changes that could predict clinical outcome. Elevation of metabolite levels such as glutamate/glutamine (Glx) and Cho in apparently normal white and gray matter was found to be highly predictive of long-term adverse outcome with an accuracy of 89 % (Fig. 14.4).

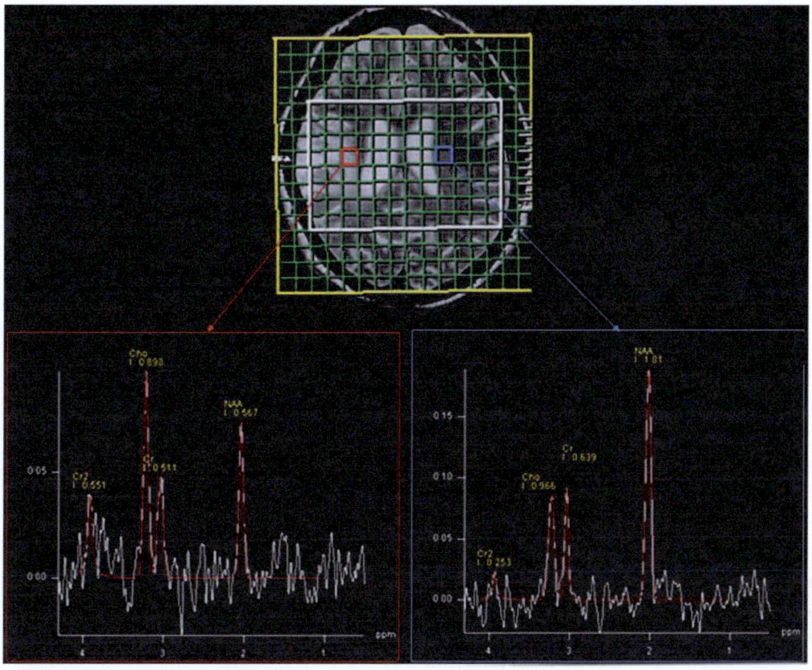

**Fig. 14.4** Magnetic resonance spectroscopy with TE = 135 ms. The left spectrum was obtained from a volume of interest located in the right corona radiata, showing reduced NAA/Cr ratio reflecting neuronal loss. The right spectrum obtained from a VOI positioned contralateral to the lesion is normal

### 14.4.3 Functional MRI

fMRI studies typically measure signal changes induced in the blood volume, flow, and oxygenation when the normal/patient is performing a given task. The resulting acquired signal is hemodynamically coupled to the actual neural activity. In the past decades, fMRI has been used to identify regions specialized in cognitive and/or motor tasks, but more recently, the interest shifted toward a novel fMRI approach, i.e., functional connectivity MRI (fcMRI), which focuses on characterization of the brain's intrinsic functional architecture especially at rest (absence of a specific task) (RS-fMRI) [54]. Therefore, high-field MR, one of whose advantages is a high sensitivity to the BOLD signal, could find applications in the study of the phases of motor and cognitive recovery after TBI, as suggested in the literature [38, 39, 55–57]. In particular, the degree of activation of specific brain areas at fMRI could provide an index of hemodynamic and functional activity in ostensibly healthy tissue in patients with DAI. Longitudinal variations of this index in conjunction with structural parameters and clinical examination could thus assume a prognostic value.

Typically, in task-based fMRI, data are collected with blocked design experiments in which the contrast between two conditions is evaluated in the presence of specific tasks [38, 39, 55–57] . At rest, on the other hand, participants do not perform any active task and are simply instructed to remain still either fixating or with eyes closed.

In a recent study [38], the observed cognitive and behavioral recovery significantly correlated with connectivity changes of resting-state networks (RSNs) in a group of severe TBI patients after a period of intensive neurorehabilitation. In particular, the cognitive recovery was more consistent in patients exhibiting the strongest changes in DMN connectivity (Fig.14.5).

Resting-state connectivity studies are appealing in DOC patients since they do not require the ability to participate in an active task in the scanner and it has been proposed as a prognostic tool in comatose patients [58–60] . The main advantage is that the identified functional systems (or

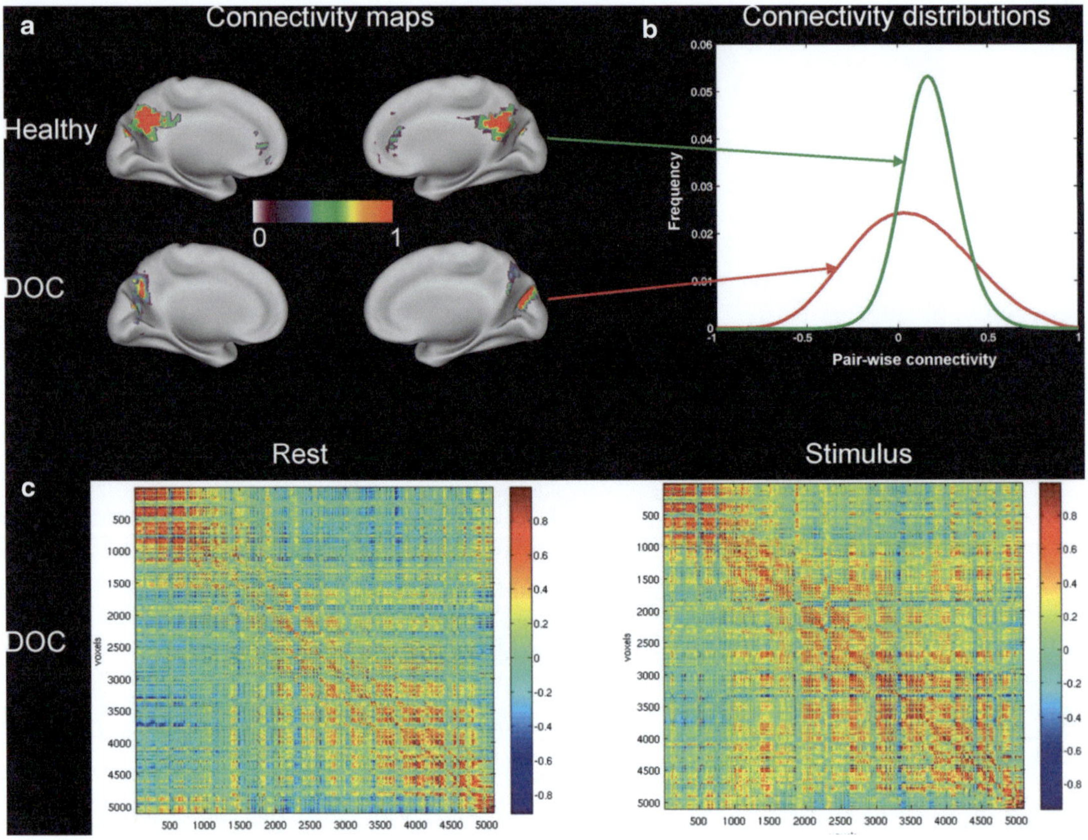


**Fig. 14.5** Functional connectivity in resting DOC patients. (**a**) Connectivity maps in one representative DOC patient and in a healthy subject. Compared to the healthy subject, the DOC patient shows a pattern of increasing disruption in the connectivity maps of the default mode network. (**b**) The distribution of the overall connectivity values at rest shows that the distribution of connectivity in the DOC case shows greater spread than in a healthy subject. In the healthy subjects, the connectivity is stronger on average and also tightly centered around its mean value, i.e., the connectivity dispersion is smaller. (**c**) The cross-correlation matrix estimated at rest before (*REST*) or during an auditory stimulation (STIM) in DOC patient. A 60 % increase in the connectivity can be noted between the two conditions

networks) provide a wide coverage of several functional domains which can be assessed in a single acquisition session [54]. Therefore, there has been renewed interest, throughout the past decade, in the use of functional neuroimaging to distinguish between patients in vegetative state and individuals who are in a minimally conscious state or who exhibit locked-in syndrome [61, 62].

A recent study [59] describes the possibility to extract, from functional connectivity data at rest and during an auditory emotional stimulation, parameters able to characterize important global and local connectivity features, such as the degree of clustering, mean path length, and modularity, in DOC patients and characterize the clinical profile and diagnosis (Fig. 14.6). These results and the existing literature indicate the functional neuroimaging holds considerable promise for indicating valid biomarkers for the recovery and diagnosis in TBI patients. Further, it could generate important insight on the neural basis of consciousness and on the target for therapeutic and neurorehabilitative intervention.

### 14.4.4 Conclusions and Future Prospective

In conclusion, high-field MR has the potential to enhance the accuracy of morphostructural, metabolic, and functional studies of the brain paren-

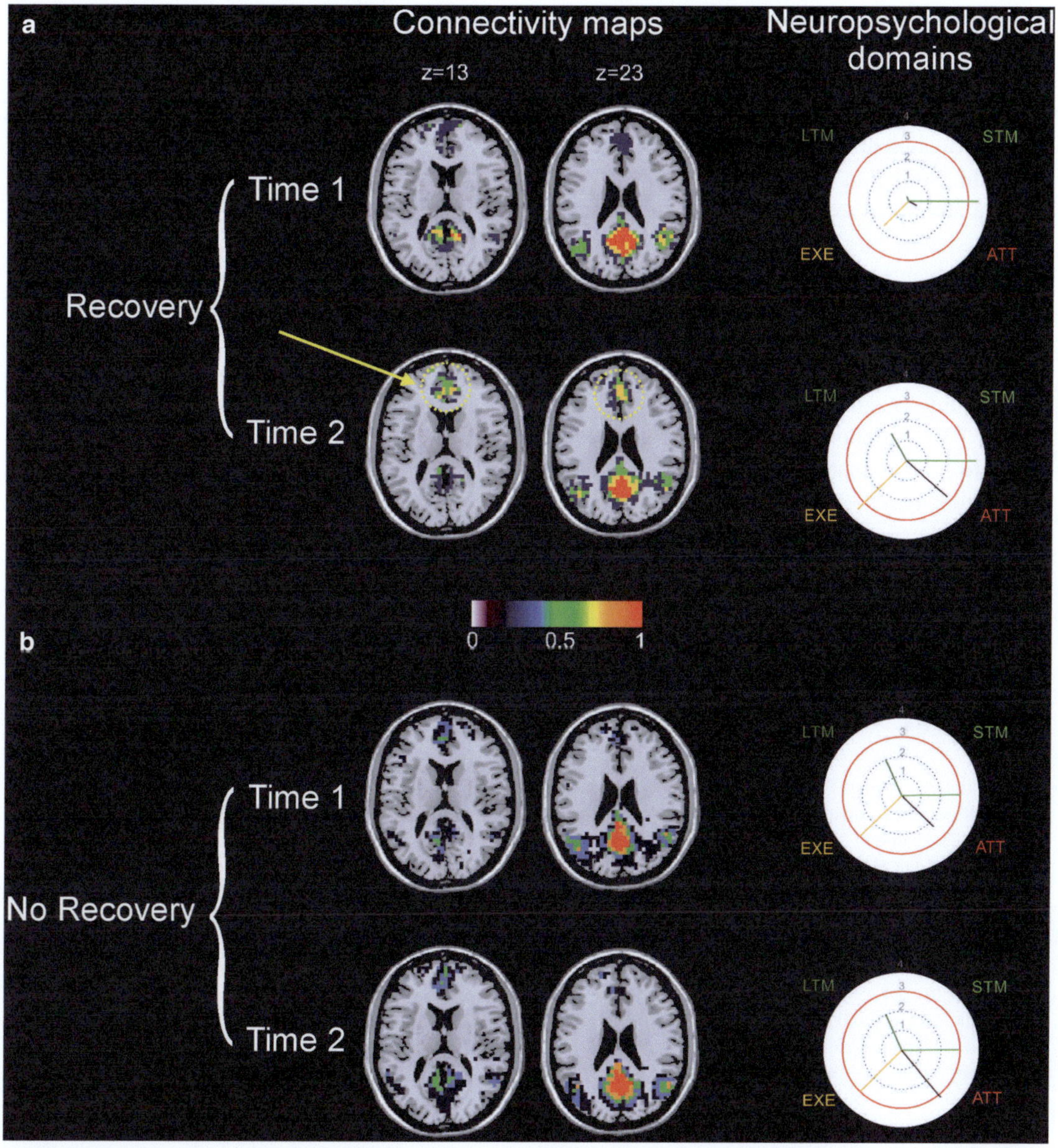


**Fig. 14.6** Connectivity maps and neuropsychological domains of recovery and no recovery groups of acquired brain injury patients over time. (**a**) For the recovery group, the left/right angular gyrus, the precuneus, and regions of the ventromedial prefrontal cortex (vMPFC) show stable connections over time with the posterior cingulate cortex (PCC). The consistency of connections between time 1 and time 2 of the vMPFC (*yellow-dotted circle*) increased from approximately 30 % up to 70 %. Recovery group shows a statistically significant improvement of all neuropsychological domains. (**b**) The consistency maps of no recovery group show an involvement of the main nodes of the default mode network with a stable consistency of approximately 30 % at both times. No significant changes are observed between T1 and T2 in the neuropsychological domains. Long-term memory (LTM, *green*), executive functions (EXE, *yellow*), and attention (ATT, *red*)

chyma in trauma patients, advancing the knowledge of the relationships between changes in nerve fiber ultrastructure and clinical symptoms and allowing the quantification of the brain plasticity phenomena that follow spontaneous clinical recovery or administration of pharmacological and rehabilitation therapies.

Although the actual developments in the high-field MRI hardware and software equipment, the statistical signal analysis, and modeling of brain recordings allow to identify abnormalities in these patients with increasing frequency, additional studies are needed to determine the full significance of these findings, e.g., how they correlate with clinical symptoms in particular for the DOC. In particular, DTI, MRS, and fMRI may provide additional important information regarding coexistent structural and functional brain damage which can be used to further understand the heterogeneity of TBI and may potentially supply prognostic information. Future studies should also focus on the patients' follow-up and on the multimodal integration. For the clinical use on TBI patients, such imaging approaches need to be robustly standardized to allow multicenter-based studies and to be used at the individual level. Such a future development will allow to design ad hoc imaging paradigms for the single patients which will aid the neurorehabilitation and the prognostic accuracy.

## References


1. Teasdale G, Jennett B (1974) Assessment of coma and impaired consciousness. A practical scale. Lancet 2(7872):81–84
2. Parizel PM et al (2005) New developments in the neuroradiological diagnosis of craniocerebral trauma. Eur Radiol 15(3):569–581
3. Newberg AB, Alavi A (2003) Neuroimaging in patients with head injury. Semin Nucl Med 33(2):136–147
4. Harris T et al (2012) Improving outcome in severe trauma: trauma systems and initial management: intubation, ventilation and resuscitation. Postgrad Med J 88(1044):588–594
5. Metting Z et al (2007) Structural and functional neuroimaging in mild-to-moderate head injury. Lancet Neurol 6(8):699–710
6. Giannotta SL, Weiner JM, Karnaze D (1987) Prognosis and outcome in severe head injury. In: Cooper PR (ed) Head injury, 2nd edn. Williams and Wilkins, Baltimore
7. Gentry LR (1994) Imaging of closed head trauma. Radiology 297:1–17
8. Patel MR et al (1999) Echo-planar functional MR imaging of epilepsy with concurrent EEG monitoring. AJNR Am J Neuroradiol 20(10):1916–1919
9. Posse S et al (1999) Enhancement of BOLD-contrast sensitivity by single-shot multi-echo functional MR imaging. Magn Reson Med 42(1):87–97
10. Hagberg GE et al (2002) Real-time quantification of T(2)(*) changes using multiecho planar imaging and numerical methods. Magn Reson Med 48(5):877–882
11. Campbell BG, Zimmerman RD (1998) Emergency magnetic resonance of the brain. Top Magn Reson Imaging 9(4):208–227
12. Kuzma BB, Goodman JM (2000) Improved identification of axonal shear injuries with gradient echo MR technique. Surg Neurol 53(4):400–402
13. Yanagawa Y et al (2000) A quantitative analysis of head injury using T2*-weighted gradient-echo imaging. J Trauma 49(2):272–277
14. Scheid R et al (2003) Diffuse axonal injury associated with chronic traumatic brain injury: evidence from T2*-weighted gradient-echo imaging at 3 T. AJNR Am J Neuroradiol 24(6):1049–1056
15. Giugni E et al (2005) Fast detection of diffuse axonal damage in severe traumatic brain injury: comparison of gradient-recalled echo and turbo proton echo-planar spectroscopic imaging MRI sequences. AJNR Am J Neuroradiol 26(5):1140–1148
16. Basser PJ et al (2000) In vivo fiber tractography using DT-MRI data. Magn Reson Med 44(4):625–632
17. Lucchichenti G et al (2010) 3 Tesla is twice as sensitive as 1.5 Tesla magnetic resonance imaging in the assessment of diffuse axonal injury in traumatic brain injury patients. Funct Neurol 25(2):109–114
18. Mori S, van Zijl PC (2002) Fiber tracking: principles and strategies – a technical review. NMR Biomed 15(7–8):468–480
19. Bammer R, Acar B, Moseley ME (2003) In vivo MR tractography using diffusion imaging. Eur J Radiol 45(3):223–234
20. Habas C (2004) Basic principles of diffusion tensor MR tractography. J Radiol 85(3):281–286
21. Takahashi M, Uematsu H, Hatabu H (2003) MR imaging at high magnetic fields. Eur Radiol 46:45–52
22. Tomaiuolo F et al (2005) Changes in white matter in long-term survivors of severe non-missile traumatic brain injury: a computational analysis of magnetic resonance images. J Neurotrauma 22(1):76–82
23. Scheid R et al (2007) Comparative magnetic resonance imaging at 1.5 and 3 Tesla for the evaluation of traumatic microbleeds. J Neurotrauma 24(12):1811–1816
24. Jennett B, Bond M (1975) Assessment of outcome after severe brain damage. Lancet 1(7905):480–484
25. Conturo TE et al (1999) Tracking neuronal fiber pathways in the living human brain. Proc Natl Acad Sci U S A 96(18):10422–10427
26. Al-Kwifi O, Emery DJ, Wilman AH (2002) Vessel contrast at three Tesla in time-of-flight magnetic resonance angiography of the intracranial and carotid arteries. Magn Reson Imaging 20(2):181–187
27. Moenninghoff C et al (2015) Diffuse axonal injury at ultra-high field MRI. PLoS One 10(3):e0122329

28. Parizel PM et al (1998) Imaging findings in diffuse axonal injury after closed head trauma. Eur Radiol 8(6):960–965
29. Blatter DD et al (1997) MR-based brain and cerebrospinal fluid measurement after traumatic brain injury: correlation with neuropsychological outcome. AJNR Am J Neuroradiol 18(1):1–10
30. Bigler ED, Anderson CV, Blatter DD (2002) Temporal lobe morphology in normal aging and traumatic brain injury. AJNR Am J Neuroradiol 23(2):255–266
31. Tomaiuolo F et al (2004) Gross morphology and morphometric sequelae in the hippocampus, fornix, and corpus callosum of patients with severe non-missile traumatic brain injury without macroscopically detectable lesions: a T1 weighted MRI study. J Neurol Neurosurg Psychiatry 75(9):1314–1322
32. Naganawa S et al (2004) Serial evaluation of diffusion tensor brain fiber tracking in a patient with severe diffuse axonal injury. AJNR Am J Neuroradiol 25(9):1553–1556
33. Arfanakis K et al (2002) Diffusion tensor MR imaging in diffuse axonal injury. AJNR Am J Neuroradiol 23(5):794–802
34. Huisman TA et al (2004) Diffusion tensor imaging as potential biomarker of white matter injury in diffuse axonal injury. AJNR Am J Neuroradiol 25(3):370–376
35. Huisman TA et al (2003) Diffusion-weighted imaging for the evaluation of diffuse axonal injury in closed head injury. J Comput Assist Tomogr 27(1):5–11
36. Garnett MR et al (2000) Early proton magnetic resonance spectroscopy in normal-appearing brain correlates with outcome in patients following traumatic brain injury. Brain 123(Pt 10):2046–2054
37. Shutter L, Tong KA, Holshouser BA (2004) Proton MRS in acute traumatic brain injury: role for glutamate/glutamine and choline for outcome prediction. J Neurotrauma 21(12):1693–1705
38. Falletta Caravasso C et al (2016) The Default Mode Network connectivity predicts cognitive recovery in severe acquired brain injured patients: a longitudinal study. J Neurotrauma 33(13):1247–1262
39. Peran P et al (2014) Supplementary motor area activation is impaired in severe traumatic brain injury parkinsonism. J Neurotrauma 31(7):642–648
40. Hulkower MB et al (2013) A decade of DTI in traumatic brain injury: 10 years and 100 articles later. AJNR Am J Neuroradiol 34(11):2064–2074
41. Strauss S et al (2015) Current clinical applications and future potential of diffusion tensor imaging in traumatic brain injury. Top Magn Reson Imaging 24(6):353–362
42. Zheng WB et al (2007) Prediction of recovery from a post-traumatic coma state by diffusion-weighted imaging (DWI) in patients with diffuse axonal injury. Neuroradiology 49(3):271–279
43. Cherubini A et al (2007) Multimodal fMRI tractography in normal subjects and in clinically recovered traumatic brain injury patients. Neuroimage 34(4):1331–1341
44. Fernandez-Espejo D et al (2011) Diffusion weighted imaging distinguishes the vegetative state from the minimally conscious state. Neuroimage 54(1): 103–112
45. Fernandez-Espejo D et al (2010) Combination of diffusion tensor and functional magnetic resonance imaging during recovery from the vegetative state. BMC Neurol 10:77
46. Fernandez-Espejo D et al (2012) A role for the default mode network in the bases of disorders of consciousness. Ann Neurol 72(3):335–343
47. Perlbarg V et al (2009) Relation between brain lesion location and clinical outcome in patients with severe traumatic brain injury: a diffusion tensor imaging study using voxel-based approaches. Hum Brain Mapp 30(12):3924–3933
48. Newcombe V et al (2011) Mapping traumatic axonal injury using diffusion tensor imaging: correlations with functional outcome. PLoS One 6(5):e19214
49. Cavaliere C et al (2014) Diffusion tensor imaging and white matter abnormalities in patients with disorders of consciousness. Front Hum Neurosci 8:1028
50. Juchem C et al (2004) Region and volume dependencies in spectral line width assessed by 1H 2D MR chemical shift imaging in the monkey brain at 7 T. Magn Reson Imaging 22(10):1373–1383
51. Brooks WM et al (2000) Metabolic and cognitive response to human traumatic brain injury: a quantitative proton magnetic resonance study. J Neurotrauma 17(8):629–640
52. Friedman SD et al (1999) Quantitative proton MRS predicts outcome after traumatic brain injury. Neurology 52(7):1384–1391
53. Maudsley AA et al (2015) Distributions of magnetic resonance diffusion and spectroscopy measures with traumatic brain injury. J Neurotrauma 32(14): 1056–1063
54. Biswal BB, Van Kylen J, Hyde JS (1997) Simultaneous assessment of flow and BOLD signals in resting-state functional connectivity maps. NMR Biomed 10(4–5): 165–170
55. Kasahara M et al (2010) Altered functional connectivity in the motor network after traumatic brain injury. Neurology 75(2):168–176
56. Caeyenberghs K et al (2014) Altered structural networks and executive deficits in traumatic brain injury patients. Brain Struct Funct 219(1):193–209
57. McAllister TW et al (2006) Mechanisms of working memory dysfunction after mild and moderate TBI: evidence from functional MRI and neurogenetics. J Neurotrauma 23(10):1450–1467
58. Silva S et al (2015) Disruption of posteromedial large-scale neural communication predicts recovery from coma. Neurology 85(23):2036–2044
59. De Pasquale F et al (2015) Functional magnetic resonance imaging in disorders of consciousness: preliminary results of an innovative analysis of brain connectivity. Funct Neurol 30(3):193–201

60. Monti MM et al (2010) Willful modulation of brain activity in disorders of consciousness. N Engl J Med 362(7):579–589
61. Owen AM, Coleman MR (2008) Detecting awareness in the vegetative state. Ann N Y Acad Sci 1129: 130–138
62. Vanhaudenhuyse A et al (2010) Default network connectivity reflects the level of consciousness in non-communicative brain-damaged patients. Brain 133(Pt 1):161–171

# 3.0 T Imaging of Ischemic Stroke

# 15

Teresa Popolizio, Giuseppe Guglielmi, Annalisa Simeone, Giuseppe Maria Giannatempo, Marco Perri, Rosario Francesco Balzano, and Tommaso Scarabino

Ischaemic stroke accounts for 70 % of all acute cerebral vasculopathies and is among the leading causes of death and disability in the Western world. It is most often due to brain vessel atherosclerosis and less commonly to infectious arteritis, emboli from the carotid artery or cardiac pump deficits, resulting in systemic hypoperfusion. A significantly reduced blood flow in the vascular territory supplying the affected vessels induces a metabolic tissue imbalance (hypoxia and hypoglycaemia) that gives rise to variably reversible anatomical injury. Four grades of clinical severity can be distinguished on the basis of the duration of symptoms, which are mainly characterized by a focal neurological deficit:

1. TIA (transient ischaemic attack): a sudden-onset, focal, non-convulsive condition that usually resolves within a few minutes and always within 24 h.
2. RIND (reversible ischaemic neurological deficit): symptoms last no more than 48 h and normal conditions are restored within 3 weeks.
3. Progressive stroke: progressive onset of clinical symptoms worsening over the first 24–48 h and leaving a persistent functional deficit.
4. Completed stroke: a stable clinical condition since onset that may improve in time.

This classification is not only useful from a clinical point of view but also from the neuroradiological standpoint, because the duration of parenchymal hypoperfusion, which causes a more or less persistent symptomatology, is related to pathological anatomical characteristics that correspond with distinctive neuroradiological findings. Transient ischaemia damages nerve cells, the elements most sensitive to hypoxia, but not the parenchyma, neither microscopically nor, consequently, "radiologically". In these patients, standard imaging, including high-field MRI, is unable to depict the small hypoperfused area. The cell distress alone can be detected, using functional techniques such as MR diffusion (DWI) and spectroscopic techniques. In ischaemia of longer duration, the glial and mesodermal elements also undergo necrosis and morphostructural changes that can be visualized on standard imaging. In practice, functional DWI, perfusion (PWI) and spectroscopic techniques can identify the affected area in the hours immediately following stroke, whereas

T. Popolizio (✉) • G. Guglielmi • A. Simeone
G.M. Giannatempo • M. Perri • R.F. Balzano
Department of Radiology and Neuroradiology, IRCCS "Casa Sollievo della Sofferenza", San Giovanni Rotondo (FG), Italy
e-mail: t.popolizio1@gmail.com

T. Scarabino
Department of Radiology and Neuroradiology, PO "L. Bonomo" Hospital, Andria (BT), Italy



T. Scarabino et al. (eds.), *High Field Brain MRI*, DOI 10.1007/978-3-319-44174-0_15

conventional techniques enable evaluation of the later phases.

The recent introduction of fibrinolytic therapies [1] capable of inducing the recanalization of occluded vessels before the tissue damage becomes established has made the early identification of the ischaemic focus extremely important. In the hyperacute phase, besides differentiating ischaemia from haemorrhage, the irreversibly injured tissue must be distinguished from that susceptible to functional recovery.

## 15.1 Neuropathological Features

Knowledge of the pathological anatomical changes induced by stroke is essential to understand the basic radiological features that reflect the evolution of cellular and tissue changes. On standard MR, only macroscopic neuropathological alterations give rise to signal changes, whereas the technique is scarcely sensitive to early cellular and subcellular injury. Therefore, hyperacute-phase ischaemia is not depicted on standard, even high-field, images.

The biochemical bases of the ischaemic event are not yet completely clear. It has been demonstrated that the ischaemic area shrinks within a few minutes of the event. The hypoxia-induced disruption of anaerobic glycolysis triggers a histopathological cascade, with alteration of the $Na^+/K^+$ pump and consequent intracellular accumulation of water (cytotoxic oedema). This can be seen microscopically 2 h from the vessel occlusion, during which time the water molecules remain "trapped" in the intracellular space, with a consequent reduction in their diffusion. The cellular injury caused by water accumulation and progressive microvacuolation is reversible over the first 6 h. After this time, the necrotic process becomes established due to accumulation of lactic acid, pH reduction, damage to the microcirculation and an increased concentration of excitatory neurotransmitters. Subsequently, damage to the blood-brain barrier (BBB) causes an accumulation of extracellular water or vasogenic oedema. At 12–24 h, the cytotoxic oedema and related cell degeneration manifest macroscopically as a "pale" area, while the vasogenic oedema can be visualized radiologically. Unlike other organs, in which necrotic tissue is replaced by scar fibrosis, in the brain, it is completely removed by macrophages and replaced by a fluid-filled cavity (porencephaly), whose walls are made up of nerve parenchyma exhibiting an intense proliferation of mesodermal elements (fibroblasts, fibrocytes) with formation of new capillaries. In this phase, defined as gliosis, which can last several weeks, the proliferative phenomena result in increasingly sharp borders of the affected area. Finally, months from the stroke, the ischaemic focus develops as a cavity with more or less regular borders that, due to scar retraction, may undergo deformation together with the adjacent parenchyma [2].

## 15.2 Neuroradiological Protocol

The introduction of thrombolytic therapies capable of reversing the ischaemic injury has changed the neuroimaging protocols, leading to the use of MR also in the emergency workup of these patients. Recent technological advances in hardware (magnet, gradients, coils) and software (ultrafast sequences, post-processing) allow morphological and functional studies to be performed with very short times of acquisition. In clinical practice, functional studies are increasingly being performed in combination with standard MR imaging: DWI and PWI enable identification of the ischaemic area and discrimination of irreversibly damaged tissue from tissue that can respond to treatment instituted in the very first hours from the event [3–6].

After CT has ruled out a haemorrhagic stroke, the current emergency neuroradiological protocol envisages a DWI and PWI study directed mainly at planning treatment. Selection of thrombolysis candidates requires morphological evaluation of the vascular district; this is why in the hyperacute phase the MR study may require angiographic (MRA) sequences for aetiopathogenic investigations. In the chronic phase, when the patient's clinical condition has become stable, the neuroradiological protocol envisages a more detailed standard MR study and an MRA investigation to assess outcome and response to therapy.

The hyperacute-phase MR study consists at least of axial T1 sequences, axial FLAIR, DWI, 2D PC MRA (because it is faster than 3D TOF, which only depicts the large vessels of the circle of Willis) and, if a fibrinolytic treatment is envisaged, PWI sequences.

When the patient's condition has become stable, a spectroscopic study can be performed to establish lesion extension and prognosis, while possible recovery and final lesion extension can be investigated with higher-definition morphological and 3D TOF MRA sequences.

## 15.3 Neuroradiological Diagnostic Imaging

### 15.3.1 Standard MRI

In ischaemic stroke, the diagnostic role of conventional MR is confined to the subacute and chronic phases, since in the very early hours from the event the changes in interstitial water content (free water) induced by $Na^+/K^+$ pump alterations are not yet such as to affect the signal in T2-weighted (FSE or FLAIR) sequences, thus yielding a negative MR examination in the hyperacute phase (Fig. 15.1).

Also in MR studies, one of the first signs of ischaemia secondary to arterial occlusion is a signal change in the lumen of the blocked vessel. Whereas in SE sequences vessels normally present a signal void due to arterial and/or turbulent flow (Fig. 15.2), occluded vessels exhibit a characteristic hyperintensity, especially in FLAIR sequences, with an accuracy that is comparable to that of MRA [7, 8].

Even though the cytotoxic oedema does not give rise to signal changes, it can be indirectly detected in cortical areas through gyral swelling, sulcal effacement and a loss of grey-white matter interface definition. Contrast-enhanced sequences, which are not employed routinely, show vascular enhancement due to the slower flow in the occluded or tributary vessel, sometimes associated with tissue enhancement due to local hyperaemia or extravasation of contrast agent through the disrupted endothelium. MR

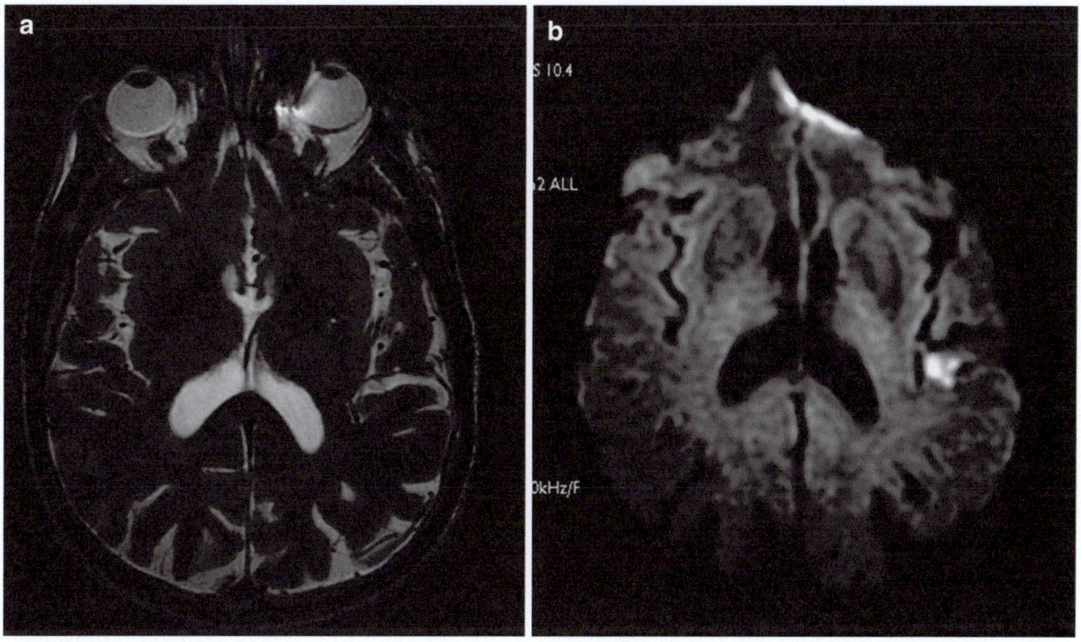


**Fig. 15.1** Small hyperacute stroke. The standard MR study (T2 FSE) is negative (**a**). The DWI image shows a hyperintense left subcortical parietal ischaemic focus (**b**)

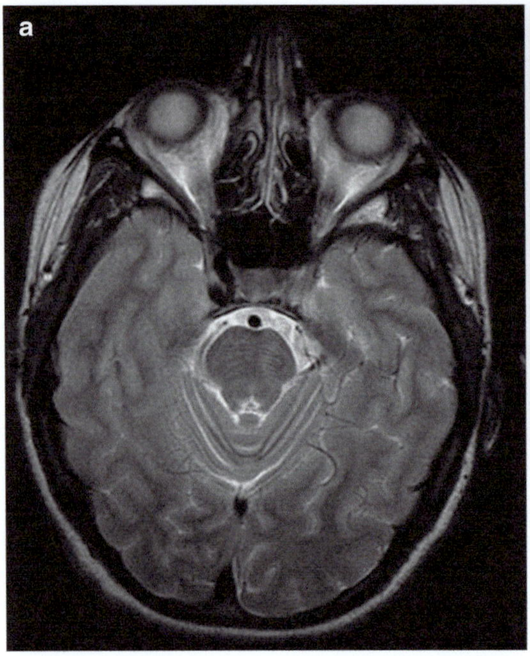


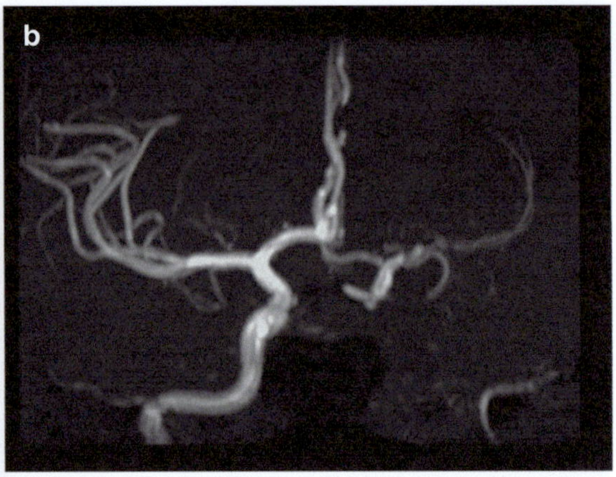


**Fig. 15.2** Combined study with morphological MR sequences in the hyperacute phase. The brain parenchyma does not exhibit ischaemic foci on the standard study (T2 FSE) (**a**); note the flow void in the intracavernous tract of the left internal carotid artery. This finding is confirmed by the 3D TOF MRA study with coronal reconstruction (**b**)

signal changes become evident in the acute phase, when the vasogenic oedema induces hyperintensity in long TR (FSE T2 and FLAIR) sequences (Fig. 15.3) and contrast-enhanced scans may depict a pathological meningeal enhancement [9]. In the subacute phase (3–14 days), the signal changes are more marked due to the increasing mass effect and manifest as a signal increase in T2 FSE and FLAIR sequences and hypointensity in T1 SE. On contrast-enhanced scans, enhancement of the infarcted area, which can persist for more than 2 months, is due to the recanalization of the occluded vessel, the opening of collateral circles (luxury perfusion) and BBB changes. In 20 % of cases, rupture of the vascular endothelium following thrombolysis may result in haemorrhage. This phenomenon appears as hypointense foci in T2 and is best seen in GE sequences [10]. In the chronic phase, a very hypointense "haemosiderin tattoo" due to even slight earlier bleeding is consistently detected in all sequences [2].

Chronic-phase MR findings reflect the morphostructural changes induced by the progressive shrinking of the lacunae, which have a cerebrospinal fluidlike content, while the hyperintensity of the adjacent brain parenchyma (particularly evident in FLAIR sequences) is due to reparative gliosis (Fig. 15.4). In this phase, signs of Wallerian degeneration of axons (and their myelin sheaths) originating from the infarcted area must be sought. Anterograde axon degeneration, which initially induces degradation of the protein component of myelin while comparatively sparing its lipid component (low signal in FSE T2 sequences), and afterwards reparative gliosis, is depicted on standard MR only in very late phases, i.e. when the axon degeneration has become irreversible. Again, earlier detection of these phenomena can be obtained with DWI [10].

### 15.3.2 MR Diffusion

DWI is the most sensitive technique to diagnose hyperacute-phase brain ischaemia (Fig. 15.1). Based on the diffusion of water molecules in the cell compartment, their random movement induced by thermal energy can be measured using conventional SE echo-planar sequences

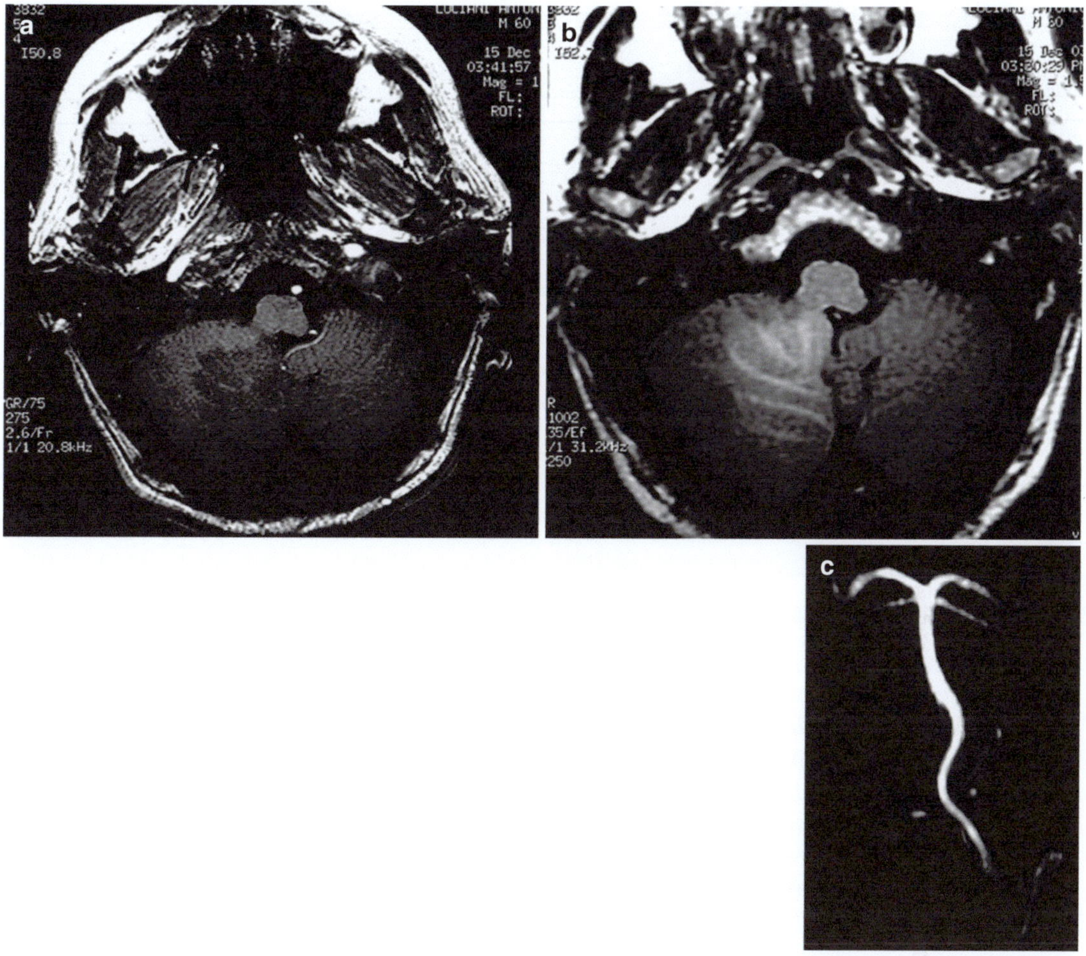


**Fig. 15.3** Combined study with morphological MR sequences in the acute phase. Vast right cerebellar stroke. Right cerebellar hypodense area in T1 FSPGR (**a**); ill-defined right hemicerebellar hyperintense area in T2 FSE (**b**). Occlusion of the right vertebral artery in 3D TOF MRA (**c**)

acquired with specific weighting. These sequences are sensitive to the movement of $H_2O$ molecules and demonstrate the changes in diffusion induced by pathological events in the form of images and numerical values. In hyperacute ischaemia, the histopathological injury is the cytotoxic oedema; the $H_2O$ molecules trapped in the cell thus exhibit an impaired diffusion, which is detected in a few minutes as a signal increase in the pathological tissue [11–13].

DWI techniques are sensitive as well as specific (90 % and 99 %, respectively); these two parameters are directly proportional to the time since disease onset. These techniques show a high predictive value as well. A negative DWI study does not however exclude a diagnosis of ischaemia. Not all patients with a typical picture of stroke also display an altered DWI signal; this may be due to complete recovery from a TIA, to a nonischaemic event or to symptomatic hypoperfusion [14, 15]. Obviously, the DWI study may also have preceded the establishment of an infarcted area, or the lesion may be very small and lie in areas especially difficult to investigate with this method (temporal regions, posterior cranial fossa, medulla); these kinds of lesion may be better detected using elevated *b* values [16].

Unlike standard MR, where the hyperintensity of the ischaemic area in long TR sequences corresponds with the expansion of the vasogenic oedema, DWI enables precise evaluation

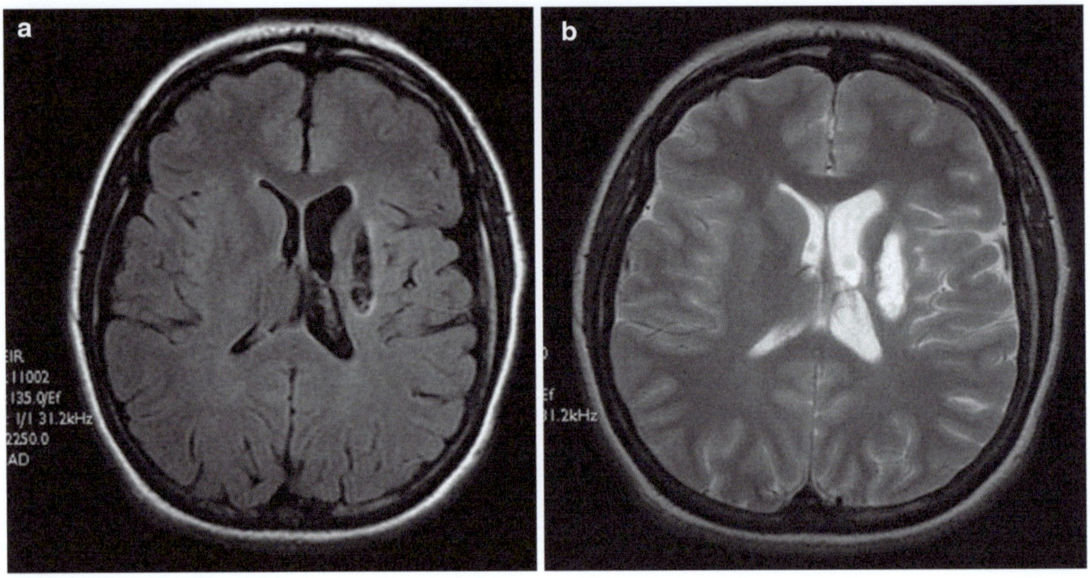


**Fig. 15.4** Lacunar sequelae of a left capsular ischaemic stroke in FLAIR (**a**) and T2 FSE(**b**)

of the injured tissue because the signal hyperintensity peaks within 24 h of clinical onset and never later. In addition, DWI sequences afford separate visualization of the acute ischaemic area, characterized by strongly reduced diffusion, from the peripheral area, where the apparent diffusion coefficient (ADC) is less affected (although PWI techniques are even more informative; see below) and the tissue damage may be reversed [17]. This is the ischaemic penumbra, which has not sustained a stroke proper but exhibits the predisposing physiopathological conditions for a new stroke (energy deficit), making it a high-risk area in the subacute phase. Adequate reperfusion often results in functional recovery of the ischaemic penumbra [13].

Another advantage of DWI over standard MRI is that, in patients with multifocal leukoencephalopathy, it allows the identification of the ischaemic lesions responsible for the active symptoms.

### 15.3.3 MR Perfusion

PWI techniques study changes in blood flow at the level of the microcirculation using ultra-fast sequences with a bolus of paramagnetic contrast medium (gadolinium, Gd) [18]. In normal perfusion and intact BBB conditions, Gd, though remaining confined to the intravascular space, induces a reduction in T2 signal both in vessels and in the brain parenchyma. In a hypoperfused area (for instance, one due to a vascular occlusion), the signal reduction is delayed or attenuated (due to magnetic susceptibility) because of the diminished flow. Since the signal reduction correlates directly with Gd concentration, and thus with cerebral blood volume (CBV), parametric CBV maps of the areas with reduced signal intensity can also be generated.

In stroke patients, the main role of PWI studies is to identify the ischaemic penumbra in the acute phase. Studies of the relationship between cerebral blood flow (CBF) and neuronal disruption have evidenced that there is a short interval related to CBF changes, where neurons, though no longer efficient, are still viable and can be rescued with a suitable therapy. The extension of this area depends both on the duration of the ischaemia and on its entity, because even mild ischaemia, which does not necessarily cause neuronal damage, may induce irreversible injury if protracted.

these gliomas with histone H3 gene mutations, there is great importance for recognition of this distinct glioma entity by pathologists [23].

Imaging genomics, radiogenomics, and radiomics are different names for the something, a field of study focused on understanding the relationship between medical imaging data and molecular feature of disease [25]. In oncology, this approach is being used to combine cancer phenotypes that can be globally assessed by imaging, with relevant molecular data, in order to develop prognostic and predictive biomarkers. Improved diagnostic tests, better clinical decision making, new therapeutic targets, and improved understanding of tumor biology are all potential deliverables. Another promise of this approach is the ability to tailor therapy to enhance treatment effectiveness at the individual patient level. Imaging has the advantage of providing a global assessment of the tumor. In imaging genomics imaging traits obtained from routine imaging studies are being associated with certain gene expression patterns, so these traits can be used as a noninvasive surrogate for providing molecular information about the tumor's genetic profiles [26]. Great interest has been shown in the use of MR imaging for noninvasive genetic profiling of patient with GBM. Aside from being noninvasive, the routine use of MR imaging in the diagnosis, pretreatment planning, and posttreatment follow-up empowers the value of MR imaging as an important tool for genetic profiling [27]. Moreover, it was demonstrated that the intratumoral imaging heterogeneity could also reflect the associated intratumoral genetic heterogeneity in GBM and so MR imaging can give a comprehensive picture of genetic expression of the tumor as a whole [28].

In effect, obtaining tissue samples for histopathological analysis is an invasive procedure which is susceptible to sampling errors, since only a few selected samples can be extracted from what typically is a large heterogeneous tumor volume. To overcome the problem of sampling errors and also provide a much less-invasive alternative, the wide spectrum of magnetic resonance imaging (MRI) techniques has been investigated and shown to offer promising alternatives for the noninvasive characterization of glial brain tumors.

Imaging plays an integral role in detection, diagnosis, and management of the lesions, and advanced imaging, such as perfusion and MR spectroscopy, may help narrow the differential diagnosis and assist in posttreatment follow-up. For AB Smith and coll. [29] however, the limitations of conventional MRI and advanced imaging must be kept in mind when interpreting the results. Conventional MRI is currently limited in its ability to demarcate the exact margins of infiltrative tumors, to accurately grade the neoplasm, and to monitor early changes after treatment. Advanced imaging can be limited too, an example of the limitation is the evaluation of MR spectroscopy when there are no unequivocal cutoff metabolite peaks that clearly differentiate a neoplastic lesion from a nonneoplastic one, and low-grade neoplasms may have spectra that are similar to high-grade neoplasms, lymphoma, and metastases. Tumefactive demyelinating lesions may show the same pattern as well. The possibility to make mistakes is reducted by the integration of data obtained from conventional and advanced MR techniques.

## 19.2 Conventional MRI

MRI is currently the best noninvasive technique available for the overall management of neurooncology patients. The essential reason for the enthusiasm on the part of radiologists and clinicians alike for the use of MR imaging in the search for brain tumors lies in the inherently high sensitivity of this technique for these lesions. MR imaging provides significantly information about intrinsic tissue characterization, discriminates differences in tissue by variations in signal intensities, and parallels findings on gross pathology in most cases. For instance, one of the major pathologic changes in astrocytomas and one of the few prognostically significant factors on histopathology, aside from general tumor cell type and overall grade, is the presence of "necrosis" (Fig. 19.1). The identification of intratumoral necrosis is considered a poor prognostic sign

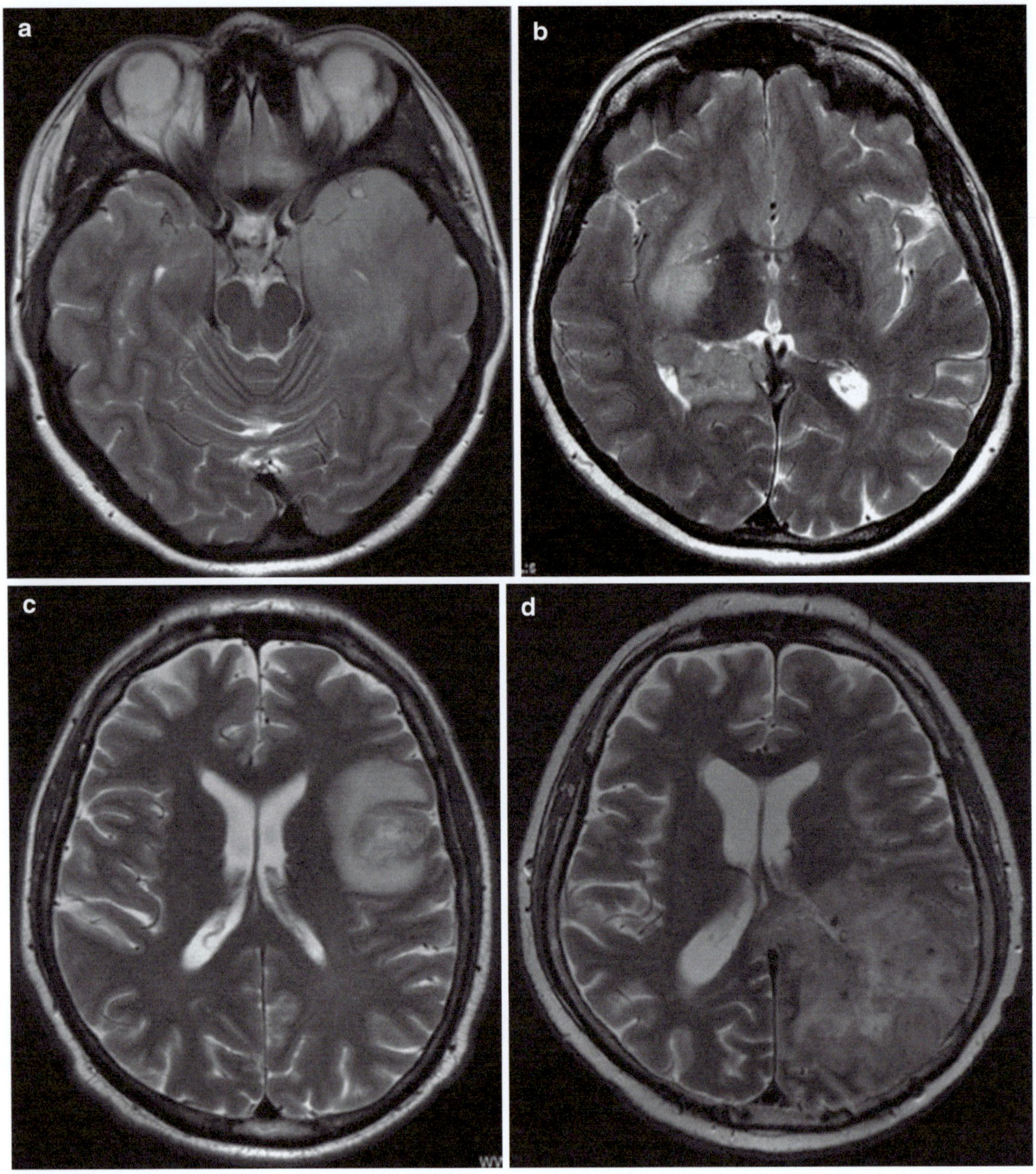


**Fig. 19.1** Axial MR 3T, TSE T2-w images. (**a**) Diffuse infiltrative low-grade glioma. It is ill-defined and tends to blur the normally clear distinction between gray and white matter. (**b**) High-grade glioma with different components, an infiltrative part, and two solid parts with different signal. (**c**) Glioblastoma with heterogeneity of signal, due to the presence of necrotic central part. (**d**) Glioblastoma with heterogeneity of signal, due to solid, necrotic parts, and spots of hypointense signal due to paramagnetic blood breakdown products

found in more aggressive astrocytomas and should be sought by the neuroradiologist interpreting MR of brain tumors [30].

MRI is used in routine clinical practice to establish a differential diagnosis, guide tumor biopsy or resection, plan radiotherapy, and monitor response to treatment and disease progression [31].

When we study a tumor, we have to consider the main properties of the MR sequences [32]:

*Spin echo (SE) and fast/turbo spin echo (F/TSE)* SE has traditionally been considered the mainstay of neuroimaging. T2-weighted SE or FSE/TSE highlights pathologic processes because of its sensitivity to fluid and changes in tissue cellularity. T1-w imaging can be helpful for identifying substances such as fat, melanin, and proteinaceous material, because they appear bright. Intralesional hemorrhages have a variable appearance on T1-w or T2-w images depending on the age of the bleeding.

Gadolinium-based contrast material has to be administrated in a study of a tumor. Gadolinium is a paramagnetic metal that, by itself, is toxic to the human body, so must be tightly chelated to another substance such as diethylenetriaminepentaacetic acid (DPTA) before use. Gadolinium shortens T1 *relaxation* times, causing increased signal on T1-w images wherever the blood barrier has been breached and contrast material is able to enter.

*Gradient echo (GE)* the lack of 180° refocusing pulse and the specific vulnerability to the T2*decay can be exploited to detect intracranial hemorrhage. Paramagnetic blood products create local magnetic field inhomogeneities and induce a characteristic signal loss on GRE sequences. In contrast blood can be more difficult to detect on SE sequences, which are less sensitive to susceptibility effects. The faster imaging time of GRE is particularly useful in 3D imaging, which requires longer scan times than 2D; in particular, 3D-spoiled GRE sequences provide T1-w images and excellent anatomic detail. 3D GRE sequences are useful for characterizing tumor extension in conjunction with gadolinium-based contrast.

*Fluid-attenuated inversion recovery (FLAIR)* is typically a T2-weighted FSE/TSE sequence that uses an inversion pulse to eliminate the signal from CSF. It is useful for highlighting lesions that lie close to ventricles or sulci and are not as conspicuous on T2-w sequences. Suppression of CSF signal allows to distinguish the different components of a neoplastic cystic lesion, for example, the cyst with a content-like CSF are dark and the cyst with protein or fat content are bright. FLAIR imaging is also limited in evaluation of the posterior fossa lesions because of CSF artifacts in the basilar cisterns and third/fourth ventricles. 3D FLAIR is not as susceptible to CSF flow artifact as 2D FLAIR because the inversion pulse is applied to the entire volume imaged and not just a single slice.

*Fat saturation (FS)* is an alternative technique to STIR for eliminating signal from fat. FS exploits the chemical shift between protons in fat and those in water to reduce or remove the signal from the fat. This is clinically useful for diagnosing the fat components of a tumor.

A morphological exam of a tumor has to include T1-weighted precontrast, T2-weighted, DWI, and T1-weighted contrast imaging. FLAIR may be substituted for T2 to save time. PWI, MRS, and other advanced MR imaging techniques may be included in the protocol according to the availability of equipment and clinical scenario.

The standard protocol for brain tumor imaging based on expert panel discussion following the framework of the ACRIN 6686 (American College of Radiology Imaging Network) component of the RTOG 0825 (Radiation Therapy Oncology Group) protocol [33]:

- Three plane localizer/scout in order to acquisition
- T1-weighted precontrast (spin echo)
- T2-weighted axial
- FLAIR (optional to perform after contrast)
- T1 map (quantitation) for DCE MR imaging – 3D gradient echo or 2D TSE/FSE T1
- DWI and/or DTI (can extract DWI data trace/ADC from DTI)
- T2* DSC MR imaging(after presaturation DCE MR imaging sequence)
- T1-weighted postcontrast (spin echo)

These sequences can be used as an adjunct in the clinical brain tumor:

- Functional language, auditory, visual, motor testing, and MRS
- Can do FLAIR before DSC MR imaging
- SWI, gradient echo, additional optional sequences

General parameter recommendations: for section thickness not greater than 5 mm, delay is recommended, which can be built in by performing DWI and/or DTI before acquiring T1-weighted postcontrast sequences. High field strengths provide superior image quality through increased signal intensity. The clinical superiority of 3 T over 1.5 T has been demonstrated in brain imaging [34, 35]. Head coil with ≥32 channels, for use with higher field strengths, offers additional signal intensity-to-noise ratio gains compared with conventional equipment [36, 37]. Delays of up to 20 min postcontrast injection significantly improve lesion detection rates and the assessment of lesion volume [38, 39]. Experimental studies by using a rat glioma model suggested that an 8-min delay postinjection represents a practical compromise between enhanced lesion detection and extended scanning time [40].

When we have to evaluate the morphological imaging of a tumor, we have to consider different aspects:

(a) The side of the lesion: supra or subtentorial, hemispheric or in deep structures
(b) If the lesion is solid, well defined, or diffuse, with ill-defined borders, infiltrating of the structures with distortion of gross morphology
(c) If the signal is homogeneous or dishomogeneous with cystic or necrotic parts
(d) If calcifications are present
(e) The kind of enhancement after contrast administration

The solid lesions are normally well demarcated from surrounding tissue; in general they are low-grade gliomas (pilocytic astrocytoma, ganglioglioma, etc.) (Fig. 19.2). The infiltrative lesions are ill-defined and tend to blur the normally clear distinction between gray and white matter. The signal of the tumor is hypointense on T1-w sequences and hyperintense on T2-w sequences [41].

The heterogeneity of the signal is due to the presence of cystic or necrotic parts of the lesion. Necrosis can be either hemorrhagic or nonhemorrhagic. The effects of necrosis on MR imaging are complex and varied [30], but it can be identified if one uses both T1-weighted and FLAIR sequences. In general necrosis can be either high intensity or low intensity on T1-w images, as well as on T2-w images, due to the presence of paramagnetic cations or free radicals. These substances can shorten relaxation times, whereas regions of cystic necrosis prolong relaxation times [42]. Cystic necrosis has intensities consistent with high water content, and hemorrhagic necrosis parallels the complex intensities relevant

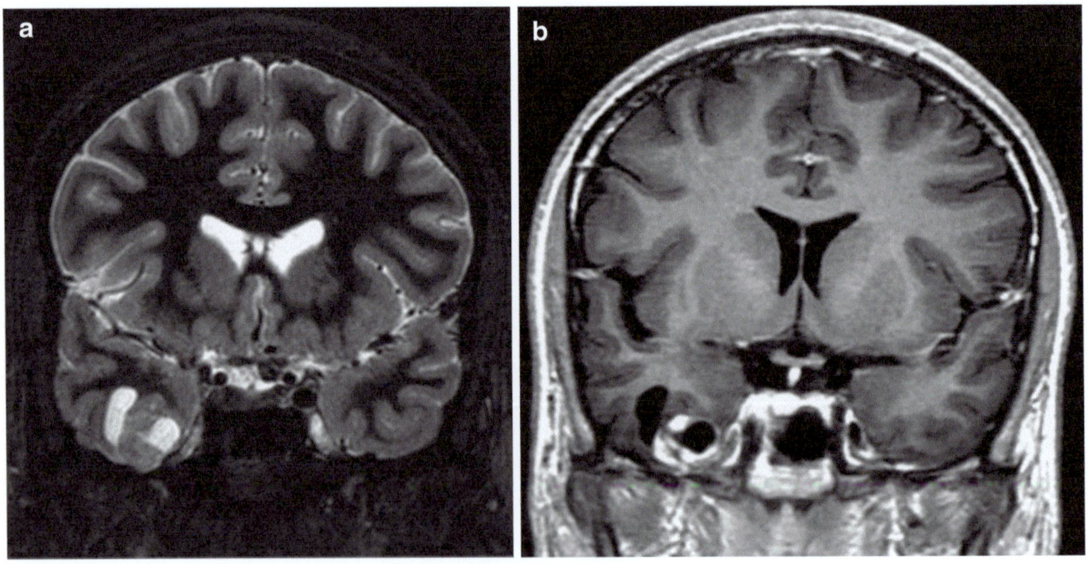


**Fig. 19.2** Coronal MR 3T, (**a**) IR-w image and (**b**) SPGR T1-w, after contrast administration. Gangliocytoma with cystic and solid parts. The solid parts show contrast enhancement

to paramagnetic blood breakdown products. The identification of cystic areas on MR imaging also requires careful scrutiny of lesion intensity relative to CSF on all images. FLAIR can be particularly useful in proving cystic content of a lesion. If a lesion is isointense to CSF on T1-weighted, T2-weighted, and FLAIR images, none can state very confidently that the lesion is cystic, a pattern followed by arachnoid cysts and cysts associated with extra-axial masses. Unfortunately tumor cysts and cystic necrosis within neoplasms are often proteinaceous (Fig. 19.3) or contain dilute

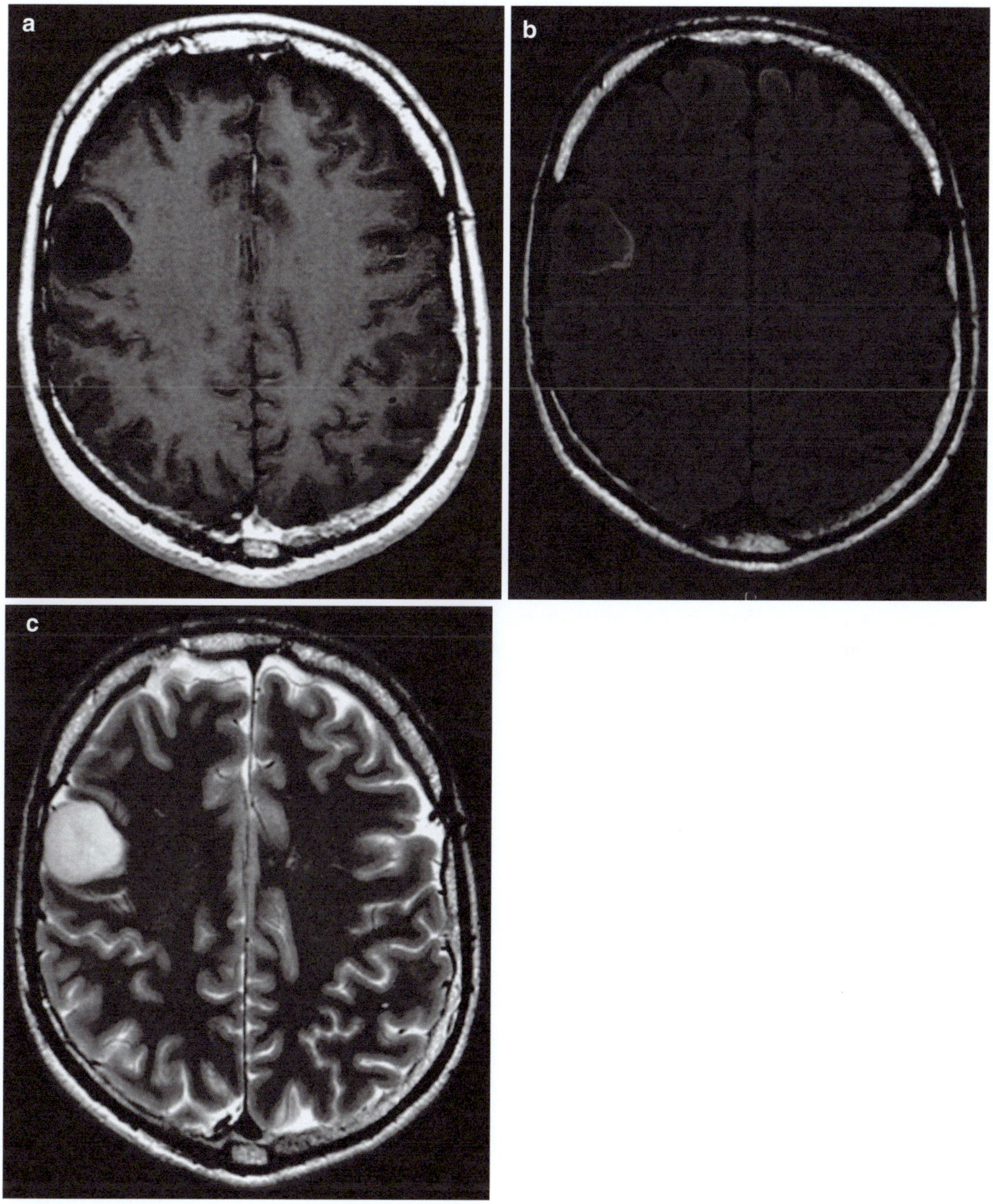


**Fig. 19.3** Axial MR 3T, (**a**) SE T1-w image, (**b**) TSE FLAIR T2-w image, (**c**) TSE T2-w image. Oligodendroglioma with cystic morphology. The cyst is different from CSF in FLAIR sequence in relation to a proteinaceous content

concentration of paramagnetic substances that can shorten T1 enough to alter intensity on these images [43]. Therefore, these regions are hyperintense to normal CSF on FLAIR. Hemorrhage is depicted by MR imaging, because of the paramagnetic properties of the blood breakdown products. On MR imaging, old hemorrhage is easily distinguished from other fluid (like CSF) because of paramagnetic properties of methemoglobin, the major constituents of chronic intracranial hemorrhage [44]. Blood may not evolve as rapidly if it is within tumor tissue, in comparison with evolution of benign hematomas. This delay in evolution may be related to the well-documented intratumoral hypoxia found in human neoplasms [45] or due to repeated episodes of bleeding [46].

Calcifications are more evident on GRE sequences. They appear hypointense with different morphology and are more frequent in low-grade gliomas with slow growing.

### 19.2.1 Tumor Enhancement

Intra-axial enhancement of the brain and spinal cord is never normal. There must be a vascular structure or a breakdown in the blood-brain barrier. In the central nervous system (CNS), contrast enhancement is produced by two related, yet independent, processes: interstitial (extravascular) enhancement and vascular (intravascular) enhancement. The CNS capillaries have a selectively permeable membrane that creates a blood-brain barrier. The normal capillaries are impermeable to intravascularly injected contrast agents. Vascular enhancement is a combinated product of blood volume, blood flow (delivery of contrast agent or "wash in"), and "mean transit time" or time needed for "washout" of contrast agent. In addition to neovascularity, which increases both blood volume and blood flow, vasodilatation of existing normal vessels produces increased intravascular enhancement [47]. Extravascular or interstitial enhancement will also depend on the permeability of these capillaries to contrast agent. On MR imaging only the regions of tissue that lack an intact blood-brain barrier enhance. Interstitial enhancement is related to alterations in the permeability of the blood-brain barrier, whereas intravascular enhancement is proportional to increases in blood flow or blood volume.

The tumor interstitial enhancement is due to accumulation of paramagnetic contrast in the water-containing interstitial space [30]. The contrast agent enhances the relaxation of the water protons nearby, and we visualize the water in the enhancing tissue as high intensity on T1-weighted images. Generally tumors have a tendency to evoke the formation of capillaries within and sometime adjacent to their tissue. Tumor capillaries in gliomas may have near-normal features with functioning blood-brain barriers, so these areas of tumor tissue will not enhance with contrast. In other often more malignant gliomas, on the contrary, formation of capillaries is stimulated whose endothelia are fenestrated; therefore, with no blood barrier, these tumors should theoretically enhance [48]. The formation of tumor capillaries deficient in blood-brain barrier constituents (tight junctions), rather than an active destruction of the blood-brain barrier, is presumed to be the explanation for tumor enhancement. The enhancement may be immediate or delayed, evanescent or persistent, dense and homogeneous, or minimal and irregular. Perhaps one of the most important points for the radiologist to remember is that the lack of enhancement does not necessarily signify lack of tumor. It's not possible to separate tumor from edema in infiltrative gliomas by enhancement, because tumor clearly is often present in area that do not enhance [30].

The low-grade glial tumor can be divided into major group: the infiltrative or diffuse astrocytomas and the localized noninfiltrative astrocytomas. The localized noninfiltrative astrocytomas may become heterogeneous not from necrosis, but through accumulation of serous fluid. The fluid must come from somewhere, so the periphery of the fluid space includes neoplastic tissue.

Almost all "fluid-secreting" gliomas (pilocytic astrocytoma, ganglioglioma, etc.) enhance on MRI. These low-grade lesions may have abnormal capillaries but usually do not show increased blood flow. Most authors believe that the abnormal capillaries in these lesions do not form a blood-brain barrier and that the increased permeability is related to somehow to both fluid production and contrast material [49]. The tumors show the "cyst-with-nodule" appearance, with enhancement of the nodule, but the morphology is varying and can produce the "open-ring sign," an incomplete rim of enhancement (Fig. 19.2).

The well-differentiated astrocytomas show no significant contrast enhancement (Fig. 19.4).

If the lesion has a major grade of malignity (high-grade gliomas), the contrast enhancement is extremely variable and can be focal and nodular, homogeneous, or ringlike. Intraventricular, subarachnoid, or subependymal spread can be seen in this lesions. Vascular endothelial proliferation within and adjacent to the tumor and intratumoral necrosis are characteristics of glioblastoma. Central necrosis within a neoplasm will also produce a ring-enhancing lesion. Remaining residual living tissue surrounds a central zone of necrotic tumor tissue. Enhancement patterns are usually very heterogeneous, often with ringlike enhancement depicted as being thick, irregular, and nodular and surrounding necrotic areas, finding virtually indistinguishable from those seen in metastases and radiation necrosis (Fig. 19.5). The residual/remaining living tumor in the outer rime survives because it maintains a rich blood supply. This hypervascular rim can be several centimeter thick, can be irregular both outside and toward the central necrosis, and often thicker toward the cortical gray matter or basal ganglia. Quite different from an abscess, delayed imaging in a necrotic neoplasm may show progression of enhancement toward the center, from islands of islands of viable tumor that surround remaining patent vessels [49]. However, one study found that up to one third of malignant gliomas did not enhance [50]. Nonenhancing glioblastomas may reflect tumors with only

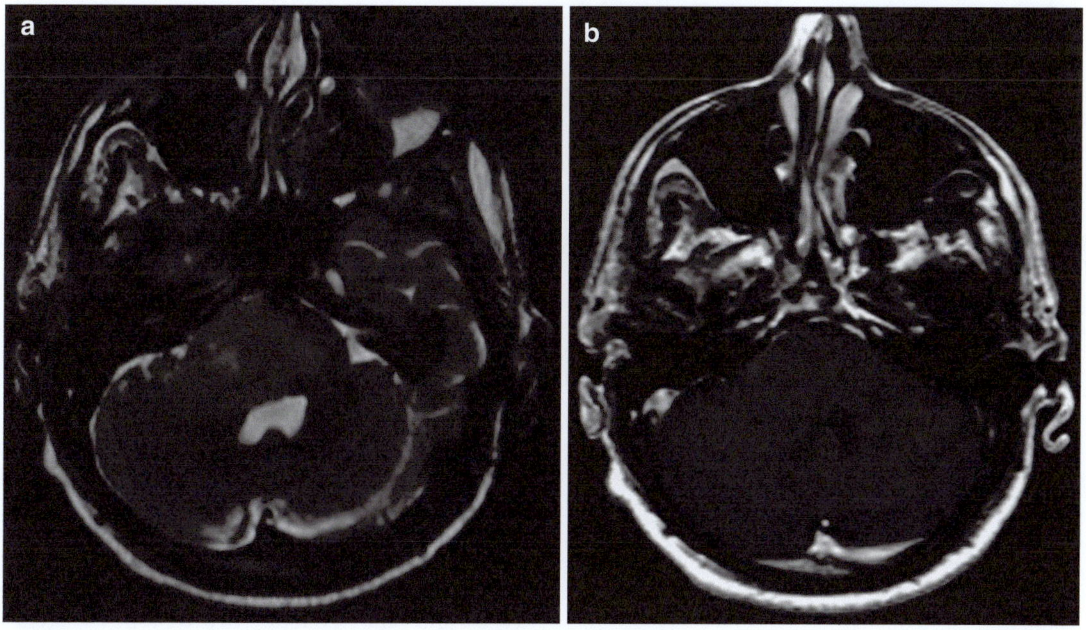


**Fig. 19.4** Axial MR 3T, (**a**) TSE T2-w image, (**b**) SE T1-w image, after contrast administration. Low-grade astrocytoma. The lesion is hyperintense on T2 and doesn't show contrast enhancement

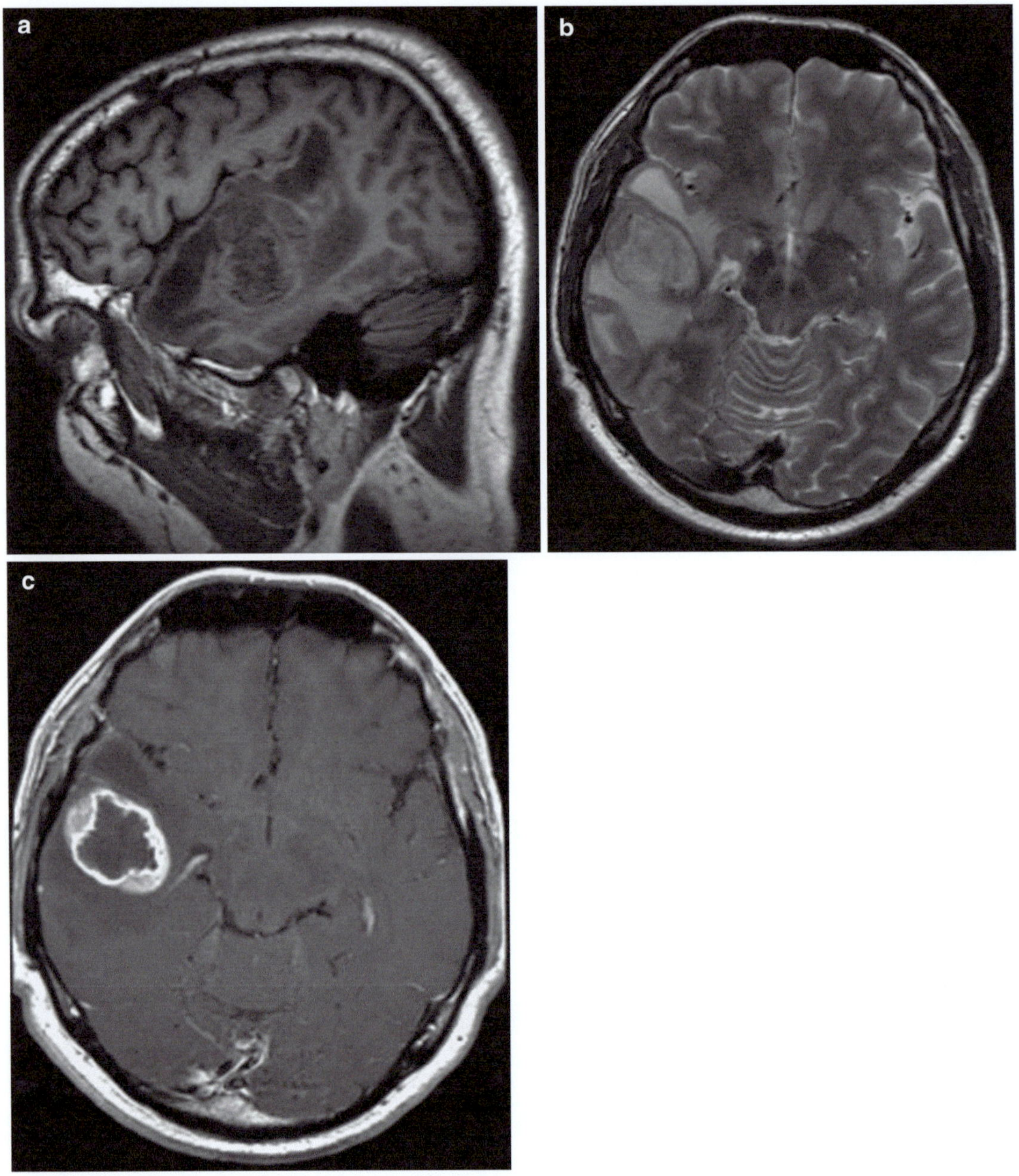


**Fig. 19.5** Sagittal MR 3T, (**a**) SPGR T1-w image, (**b**) axial TSE T2-w image, (**c**) axial SE T1-w image. Glioblastoma with central necrosis and after contrast administration, a ring-enhanced pattern with thick and irregular rim

scattered microscopic changes, including those that arise from and within a lower-grade astrocytoma (Fig. 19.6).

Tumor enhancement characteristics and their correlation with certain genetic expressions in GBM have been the focus of many researchers. Diehn and colleagues [51] described the correlation between contrast-enhanced radiophenotype and the genetic expression of genes involved in tumor hypoxia and angiogenesis (e.g., vascular endothelial growth factor (VEGF)) and found that EGFR (epidermal

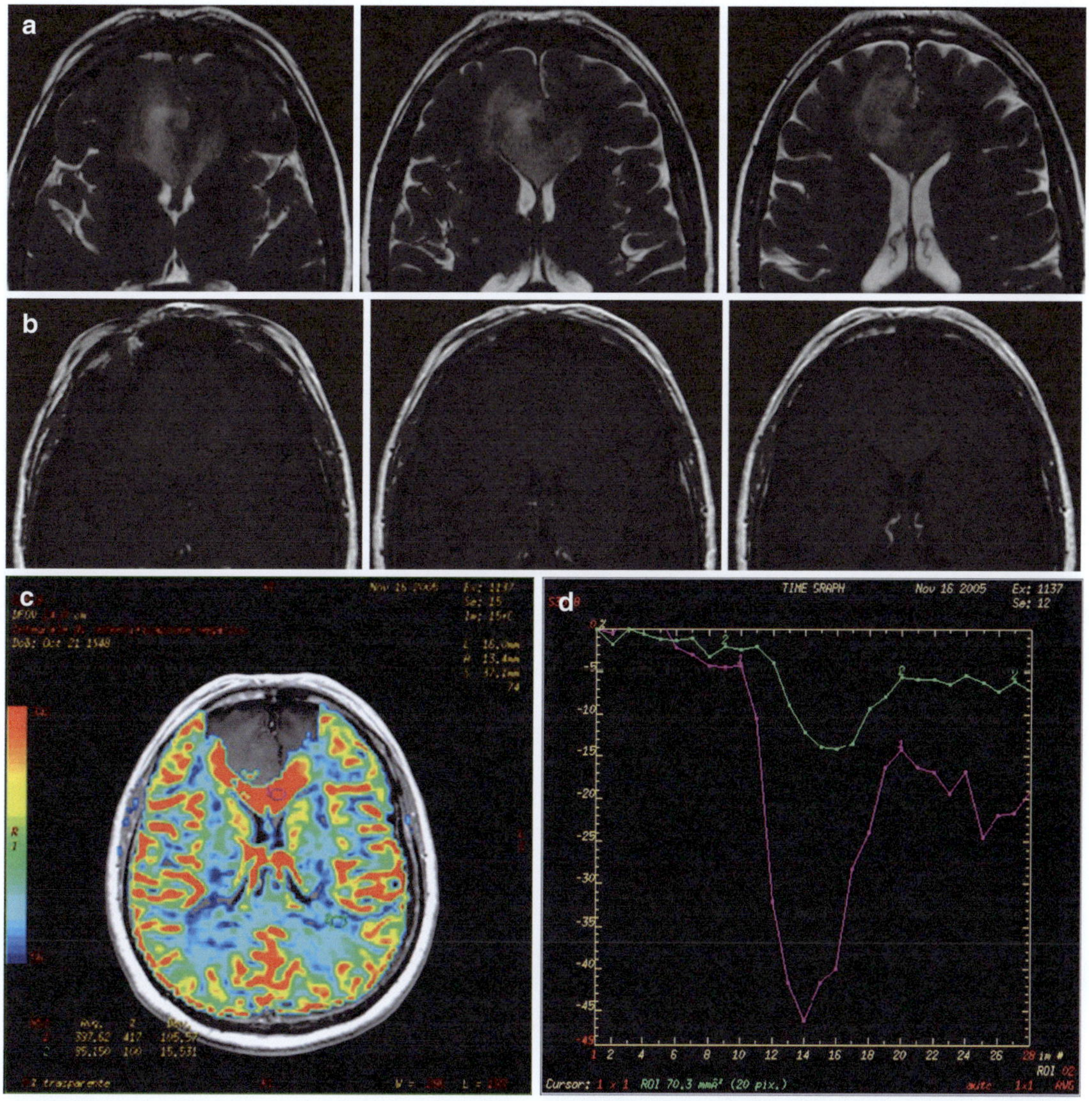


**Fig. 19.6** Axial MR 3T, (**a**) TSE T2-w images, (**b**) SE T1-w images, (**c**) rCBV map, (**d**) rCBV graphic. Infiltrative high-grade glioma, hyperintense on T2-w images and without contrast enhancement. rCBV map shows high value of rCBV (4.17) in confront to normal white matter

growth factor receptor) overexpression was associated with a high ratio of contrast enhancement to necrosis within the same tumor. Pope and colleagues [52] showed that interleukin-8 and VEGF were overexpressed in completely enhancing tumors when compared with incompletely enhancing one. IDH1 mutation proved to be associated with non-contrast-enhancing tumors in a study by Carrillo and colleagues [53] in which they showed that imaging features including larger tumor size and non-contrast-enhancing tumors could be used to determine IDH1 mutational status with 97.5 % accuracy but can poorly predict the MGMT promoter methylation status (Fig. 19.7). However, Drabycz and colleagues [54] found that ring enhancement was associated with unmethylated MGMT-promoter status, whereas irregular and nodular enhancement has been related to methylate and secondary tumor [53].

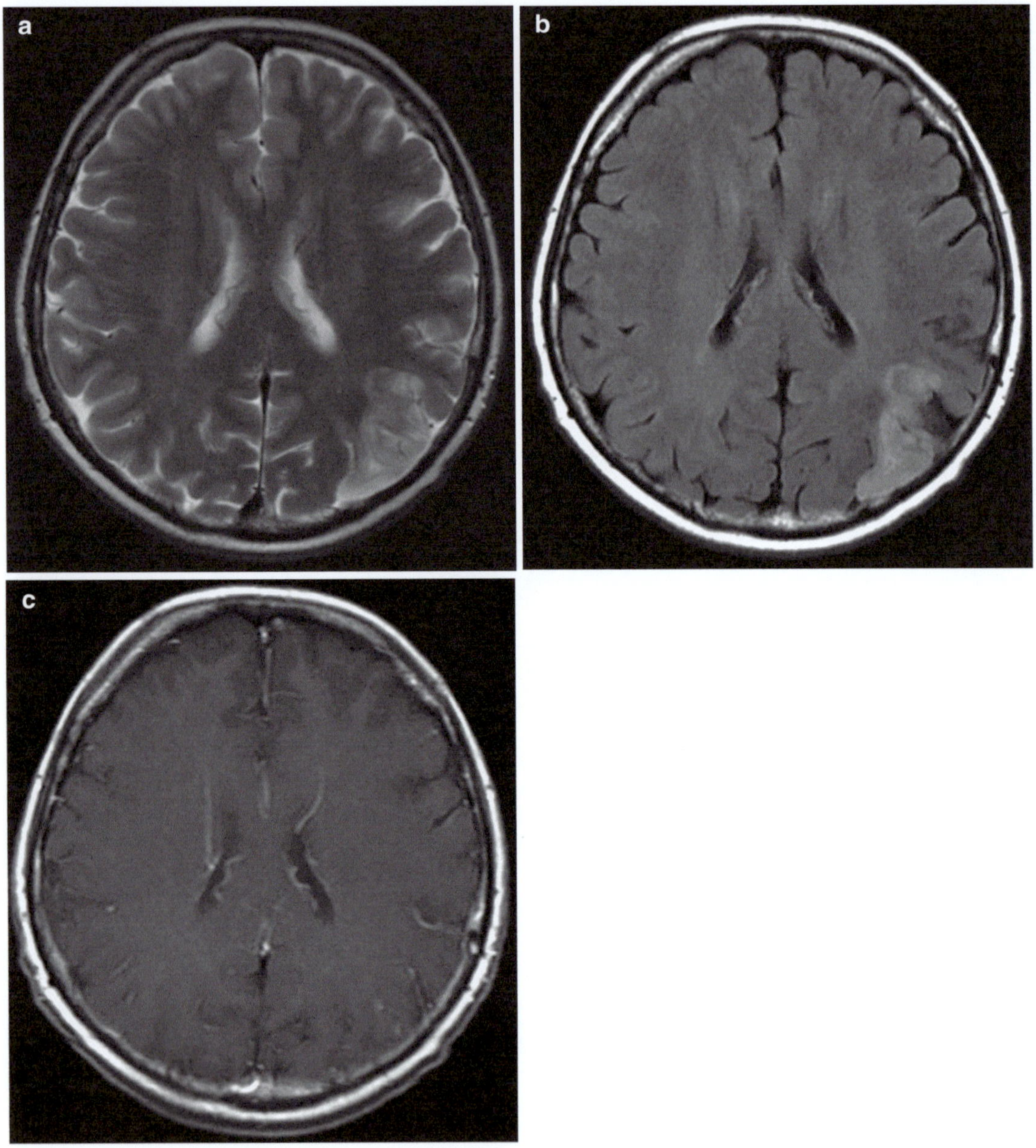


**Fig. 19.7** Axial MR 3T, (**a**) TSE T2-w image, (**b**)TSE FLAIR T2-w image, (**c**) TSE SE T1-w image after contrast administration. Oligodendroglioma with IDH-mutation and 1p/19q codeletion. The lesion doesn't show contrast enhancement

## 19.3 Advanced MRI Techniques

### 19.3.1 Diffusion Imaging (DWI)

The rate of water movement, or diffusion, within the brain and other tissues is believed to be the direct reflection of the local microstructure within the tissue. Anatomic magnetic resonance imaging (MRI) can be modified in a way that makes the images sensitive to the water diffusion within tissues [54]. DWI, which is currently the only MRI technique that provides information on water diffusion, involves the use of phase-defocusing and phase-refocusing gradients to enable the evaluation of the rate of microscopic water diffusion within tissues. This approach has been shown to be sensitive to changing microenvironment such as the increased cell density that typifies growing tumors [56–59]. The gold standard for brain tumor diagnosis is light microscopy analysis of histological tissue samples. Typically definitive diagnosis and differentiation between pathological and normal tissue are achieved by examination of cell-architecture parameters, such as cell arrangement, cell density, cell-size distribution, and nucleus-to-cytoplasm size ratio. MR diffusion imaging probes water molecular diffusion over distances that correspond to typical cell sizes, and this water diffusion is also impeded by membranes, i.e., structures that are an integral part of the cell architecture. With increasing cell density, the impeding effect of membranes is expected to increase. Thus, MR diffusion imaging provides an intriguing access to information that otherwise can only be obtained by invasive light microscopy [60].

DWI has been used to grade or differentiate brain tumors based on cellularity [61]. Because the majority of the translational movement of water occurs in the extracellular space, increased cellularity or swelling should affect the apparent diffusion coefficient (ADC), causing a drop in the values [62] (Fig. 19.8). Several studies have shown that the ADC correlates well with tumor cellularity at histological examination, and calculation of the ADC together with conventional MRI may aid the characterization of cerebral tumors [56, 59, 61]. Simply stated, the higher the cell density, the more boundaries or restriction the water experiences and the lower the apparent diffusion coefficient (ADC), a value that is estimated from the DWIs. In this regard, several reports in the literature have demonstrated an inverse correlation between ADC and cell density in brain tumors [56–59]. Glioma grading and typing are crucial for prognosis, but patients with tumors of the same histopathological characterization and receiving similar treatment may display diverse outcome because of differences in the proliferative potential of disease. Assessment of tumor proliferation has therefore been suggested as an important additional predictor of tumor behavior [63]. In addition, identification of the tumor "hot spot" is important for biopsy guidance. The proliferative activity of each tumor is measured by deriving the Ki-67 proliferation index from immunohistochemical staining of tumor specimens. Neoplasms are associated with increased cellular density, resulting in decreased signal intensity on ADC images. High tumor cellularity has been associated with increased proliferative activity, as assessed by the Ki-67 index [64]. Several studies have shown that lower ADCs suggest malignant glioma, whereas higher ADCs suggest low-grade astrocytomas findings reflecting more restricted diffusion with increasing cellularity [59–65] (Fig. 19.9). The median minimum ADC of the high-grade astrocytomas is significantly lower than that of the low-grade astrocytomas [66]. Higher ADC values in intracranial tumors are attributed to low tumor cellularity, necrosis, or cysts, and lower values are attributed to attenuated highly cellular tumors [67]. These higher ADC values in lower grade gliomas may reflect an increase in the water content of the interstitial spaces [66].

The commonly used *b*-factor is around 1000/s $mm^2$ for the diffusion-weighted images. With this *b*-factor and with the typical magnetic field gradient and echo time employed on clinical MR systems, the average water molecule has several tens of milliseconds to diffuse and may migrate up to 10 micrometers in a random direction and is therefore likely to be hindered by the cell membrane or intracellular membranes [60]. Unlike normal white and gray matter, which for a normal *b*-factor range exhibit very similar ADC values, diffusion values observed in different tumor types are dissimilar and cover a wide range. In general, brain tumor ADC values measured over a normal *b*-factor range, clearly exceed ADC values of normal gray and white matter. This difference in diffusion, however, can rarely be gainfully applied to determine the extent of tumor growth within normal tissue, since tumors are often surrounded by edematous tissue, where diffusion is also elevated and thus difficult to distinguish from diffusion values representative for tumor

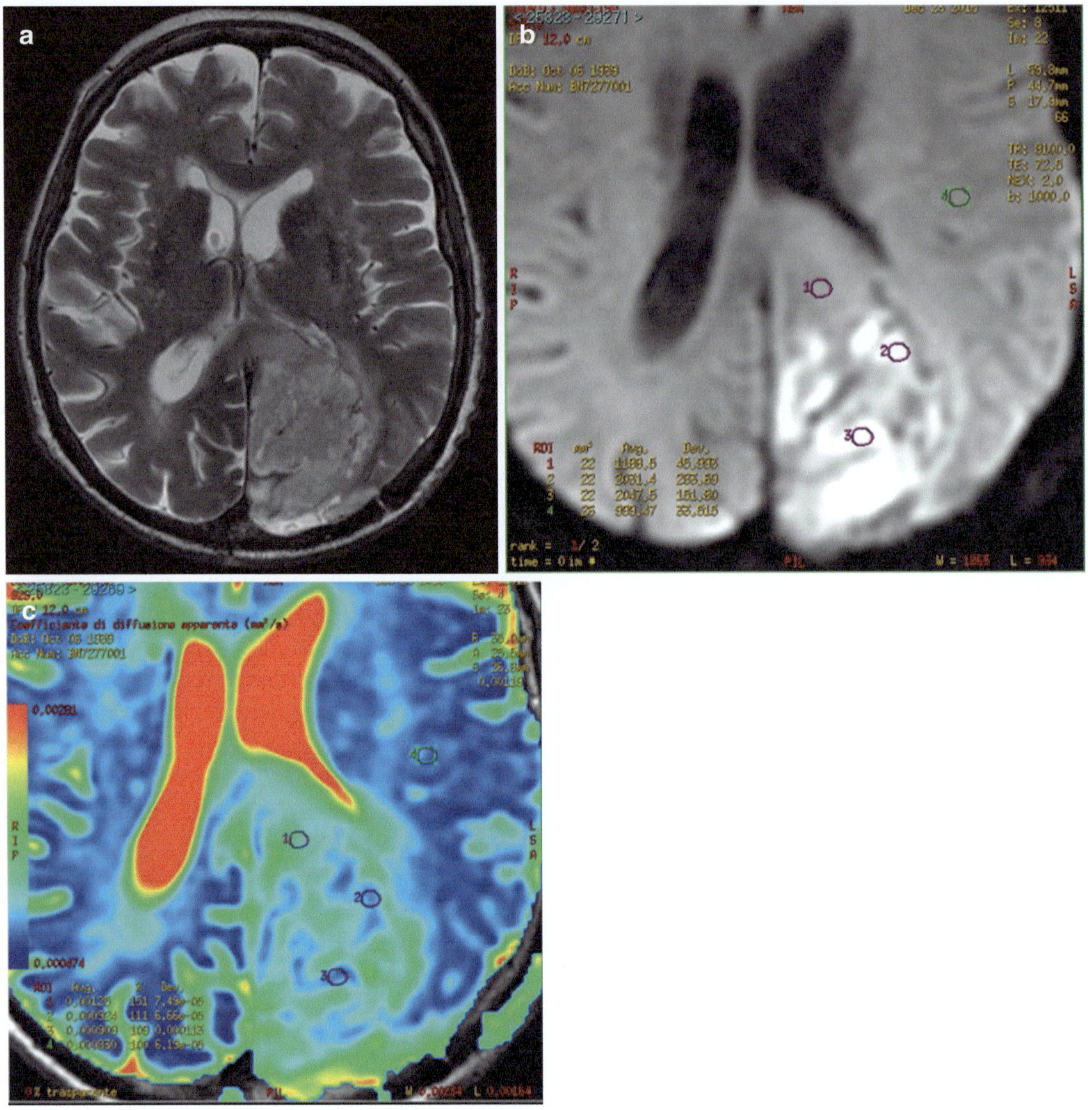


**Fig. 19.8** Axial MR 3T, (**a**) TSE T2-w image, (**b**) DWI image, (**c**) ADC map. MGMT-methylated glioblastoma. The lesion presents dishomogeneity in diffusion sequence with areas with increased ADC values, in relation to the normal white matter, and areas with low ADC, due to increasing cell density

[60]. Very high diffusion values in peritumoral edema of high-grade gliomas may reflect the destruction of the extracellular matrix ultrastructure by malignant cell infiltration [68]. On the other hand, the elevated values of diffusion coefficients in a tumor may to some extent also be the result of edema that arises inside the tumor. The brain tumor edema is vasogenic, but may also be related to failure of membrane pump systems (cytotoxic) or to transependymal movement fluid from the ventricles.

The complete absence of cell membranes in cystic lesions and the destruction of cell membranes in necrotic brain lesions create an environment where diffusion is virtually unhindered. Consequently, the diffusion constant is very high and easily distinguished from the diffusion constant of any other tissue, including tumor tissue.

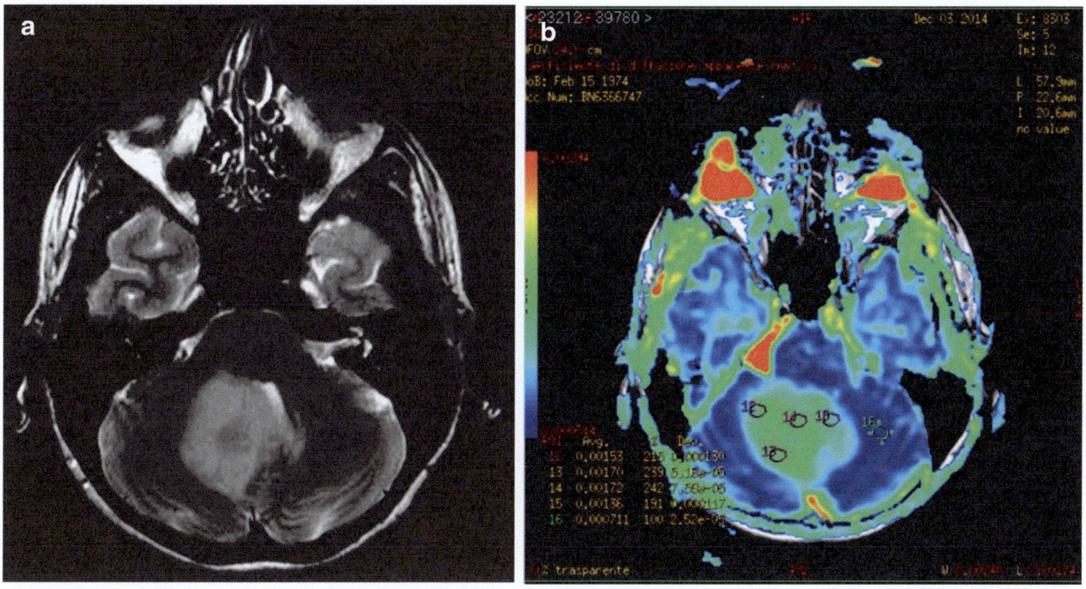


**Fig. 19.9** Axial MR 3T, (**a**) TSE T2-w image, (**b**) ADC map. Low-grade astrocytoma with MGMT methylation, no IDH-mutation and very low Ki 67 (5 %). The ADC of the lesion is higher (1.9–2.4) of contralateral cerebellar hemisphere

Large areas of necrosis can be well detected and delineated based on elevated ADC within the tumor lesion [69].

Diffusion imaging is also useful to document characteristic fluid volume changes in the intra- and extracellular compartments that occur during nonsurgical therapy of brain tumors. For gliomas, studies have shown that ADC values increase during successful cytotoxic therapy and decrease during tumor growth [70], suggesting ADC values can be used as a biomarker for brain cellularity. Tumor areas at initial stage of treatment response present transient cell swelling or ischemia with decreased diffusion values. Tissue experiencing successful response with cell lysis or apoptosis displays a characteristic increase of diffusion, meanwhile tumor areas resistant to therapy exhibit unaltered diffusion values [71]. It has also been demonstrated that changes observed during the first stage of therapy are an early indicator of the final treatment response [72]. The correct interpretation about an unresponsive to therapy tumor may facilitate a timely decision for protocol adjustment or alternative therapy.

Diffusion-weighted brain images with very high *b*-factors of 5000 s/mm$^2$ or higher, which clearly depict tissue structures above the noise threshold, can readily be obtained on clinical scanners. The residual signal at very high *b*-values is distinctly higher. Of course, compared to images acquired at *b*-factors of 1000 s/mm$^2$, there is an increased signal loss of up 90 % or more, which typically has to be compensated with a decrease in spatial resolution [60]. However, the acquisition of image data at multiple *b*-factors permits a more detailed analysis of the diffusion-related signal decay. Without diffusion weighting, tumor and edema cannot be distinguished and exhibit higher signal than normal white matter. With increasing diffusion weighting, the signal of the edematous tissue decreases more rapidly than the signal of the other tissue and approaches the signal level of normal white matter. Tumor tissue exhibits the slowest signal decay and shows the highest residual signal at very high *b*-factors. High *b*-diffusion-weighted imaging, although currently purely experimental, seems to provide a good differentiation in normal tissues and in different pathologies, in relation to the different diffusion signal decay observed in tissues. Serious limitations for clinical studies are currently the long scan times, low SNR, and lower resolution [60].

### 19.3.2 Diffusion Tensor Imaging (DTI)

Diffusion tensor imaging (DTI) is an MRI-based technique that can demonstrate white matter anatomy by measuring the directional anisotropy of water. Diffusion MRI is the first noninvasive technique for measuring white matter fiber structure in vivo [73]. In DTI analysis, a tensor model is used to represent the orientation of white matter fibers, in relation to the preferential diffusion of water in brain tissue, which decreases perpendicular to the myelin sheaths and cell membranes of white matter axons. Computation of the diffusion tensor yields for each voxel three diffusion coefficients (diffusion eigenvalues) along three orthogonal principal direction (diffusion eigenvectors). In white matter (WM), the eigenvector associated with the largest eigenvalue (principal eigenvector) defines the tissue's fiber tract axis [74]. In voxels where one white matter fiber population is predominant, the principal diffusion direction is aligned with the white matter fiber tract direction [75]. By following principal directions of diffusion, a process called tractography [76, 77] estimates the trajectories of white matter fiber tracts. These reconstructions may then be displayed in three dimensions providing a detailed map of the configuration of the tracts and their relationship to other structures. Increasingly color code maps are used for a combined and easy to interpret visualization of anisotropy and principal eigenvector direction [78].

The most useful application of the directional dependence of the diffusion-related signal decay lies not inside the main tumor lesion, but rather within the surrounding highly structured white matter.

In patients with brain tumors, DTI can demonstrate displacement, interruption, or infiltration of white matter tracts by the tumor [79–84]. The distinction of these situations is often not possible to organize. A useful tool to understand the various scenarios is the paper by Fields et al. [85] who described four basic categories of tumor growth-related white matter changes in relation to anisotropy maps and principal eigenvector direction:

(a) *Dislocation* caused by the mass effect of the tumor and edema is showed by the loss of symmetry, the distorted appearance, and the abnormal location of tracts on the anisotropy maps. Principal eigenvector within the tract remains aligned with the tract orientation. In the absence of edema, the anisotropy within the tract is unchanged (Fig. 19.10a, b, c).
(b) *Edema* within the fiber structures is characterized by uniformly reduced white matter anisotropy, increased lateral tract dimensions, and absence of localized areas with very low anisotropy. Principal eigenvectors within the tract remain aligned with the tract orientation (Fig. 19.10d, e, f).
(c) *Tumor infiltration or invasion* is characterized by a variable degree of anisotropy reduction and principal eigenvectors that remain aligned with the tract orientation. Differentiation from edema may be difficult, but localization close to the primary tumor and evidence of high malignancy or the absence of edema on corresponding T2-weighted maps may be indicative of infiltration or invasion (Fig. 19.10g, h, i).
(d) *Complete tract destruction* by tumor tissue replacing the original white matter produces a significant loss in anisotropy and lack in coherence of the principal eigenvector directions. The tract destruction may also impress by the abrupt change of anisotropy and eigenvector directions along the tracts (Fig. 19.10j, k, l).

A clear differentiation is not often possible because more than one of these characteristics can be present and it has to be considered the confounding effect of edema. Due to these and other pathological changes throughout the brain, the identification of known neuroanatomy is often not straightforward in tumor patient. For Golby et al. [86] in order to define relevant anatomy, it would be useful to identify those fibers that pass within a certain distance of the tumor or which run through the tumor, as well as those associated with particular, patient specific, cortical areas such as fMRI activation or magnetoencephalography (MEG) findings. This can provide a preoperative functional brain map defining both the critical cortical functional areas and the WM tracts leading to and from these areas.

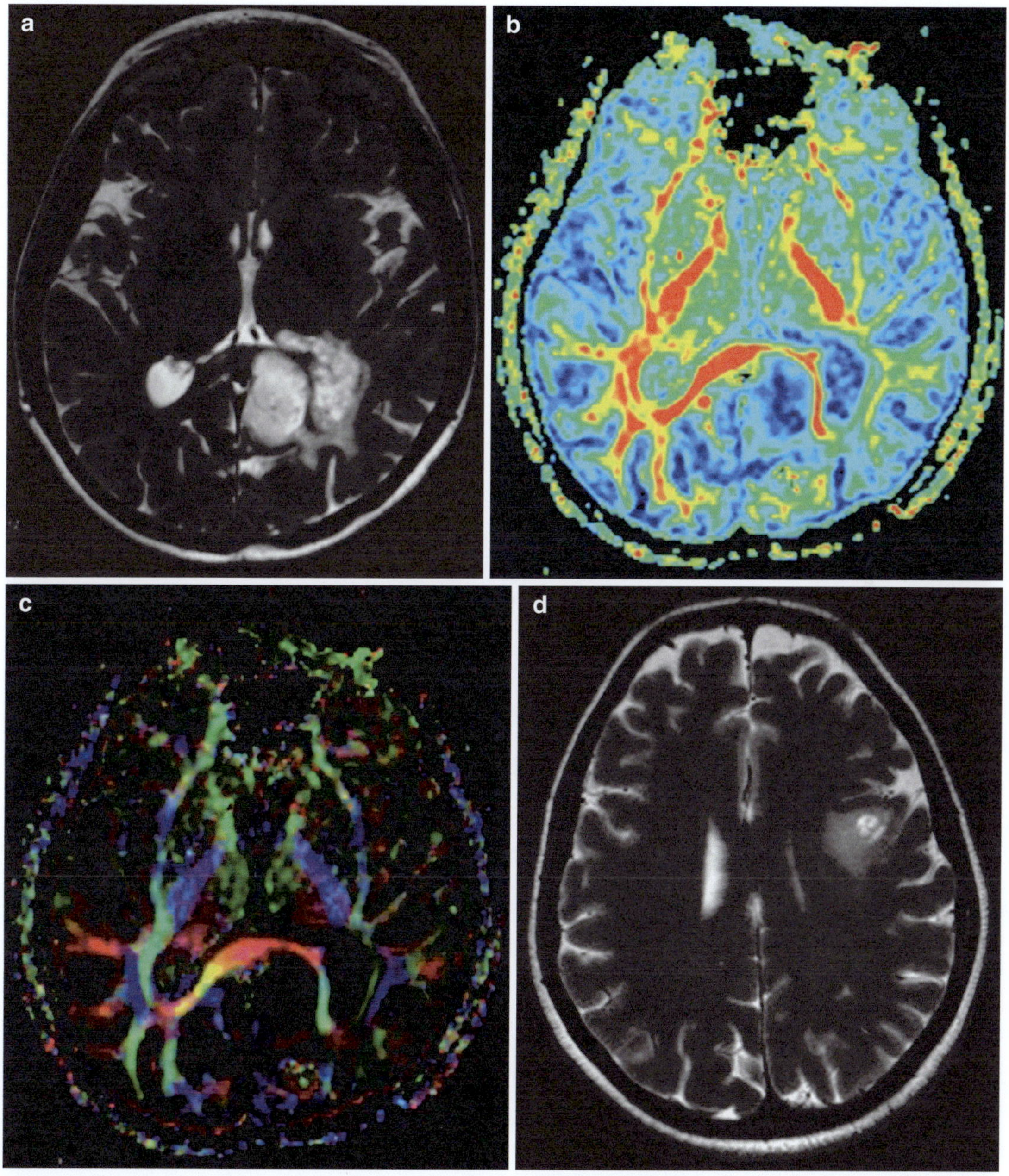


**Fig. 19.10** Axial MR 3T, (**a**, **d**, **g**, **h**) TSE T2-w images; (**b**, **e**, **h**, **m**) FA map; (**c**, **f**, **i**, **n**) color-coded map. Possible DTI patterns in case of *dislocation* (**a–c**): distorted appearance and abnormal location of tracts on the anisotropy maps. The tract remain aligned with the tract orientation in color-coded map. *Edema* (**d–f**): uniformly reduced white matter anisotropy, increased lateral tract dimensions, and absence of localized areas with very low anisotropy. The tract remain aligned with the tract orientation. *Tumor infiltration or invasion* (**g–i**): variable degree of anisotropy reduction and principal eigenvectors that remain aligned with the tract orientation. *Complete tract destruction* (**j–l**): tumor tissue replacing the original white matter produces a significant loss in anisotropy and lack in coherence of the principal eigenvector directions

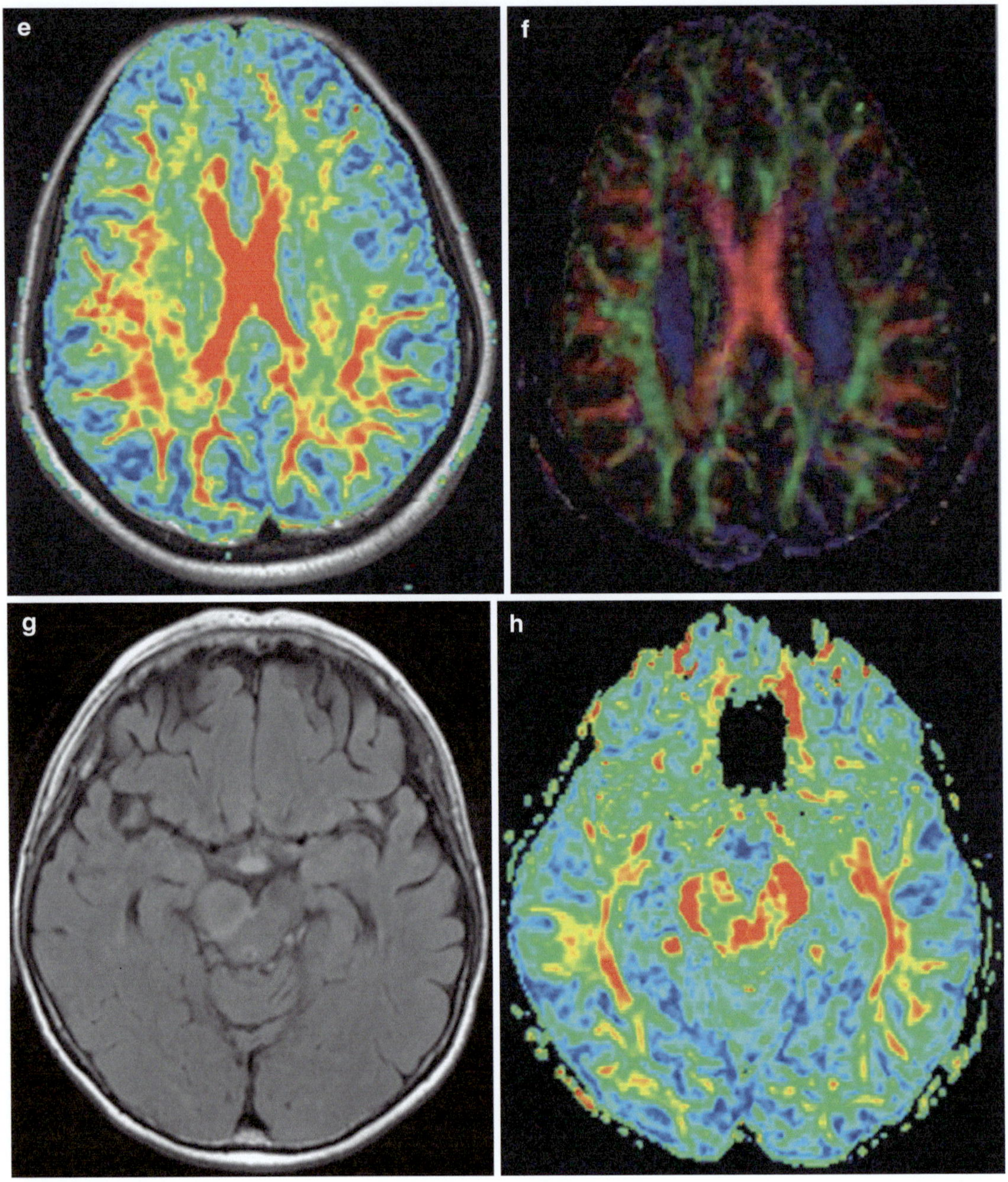


**Fig. 19.10** (continued)

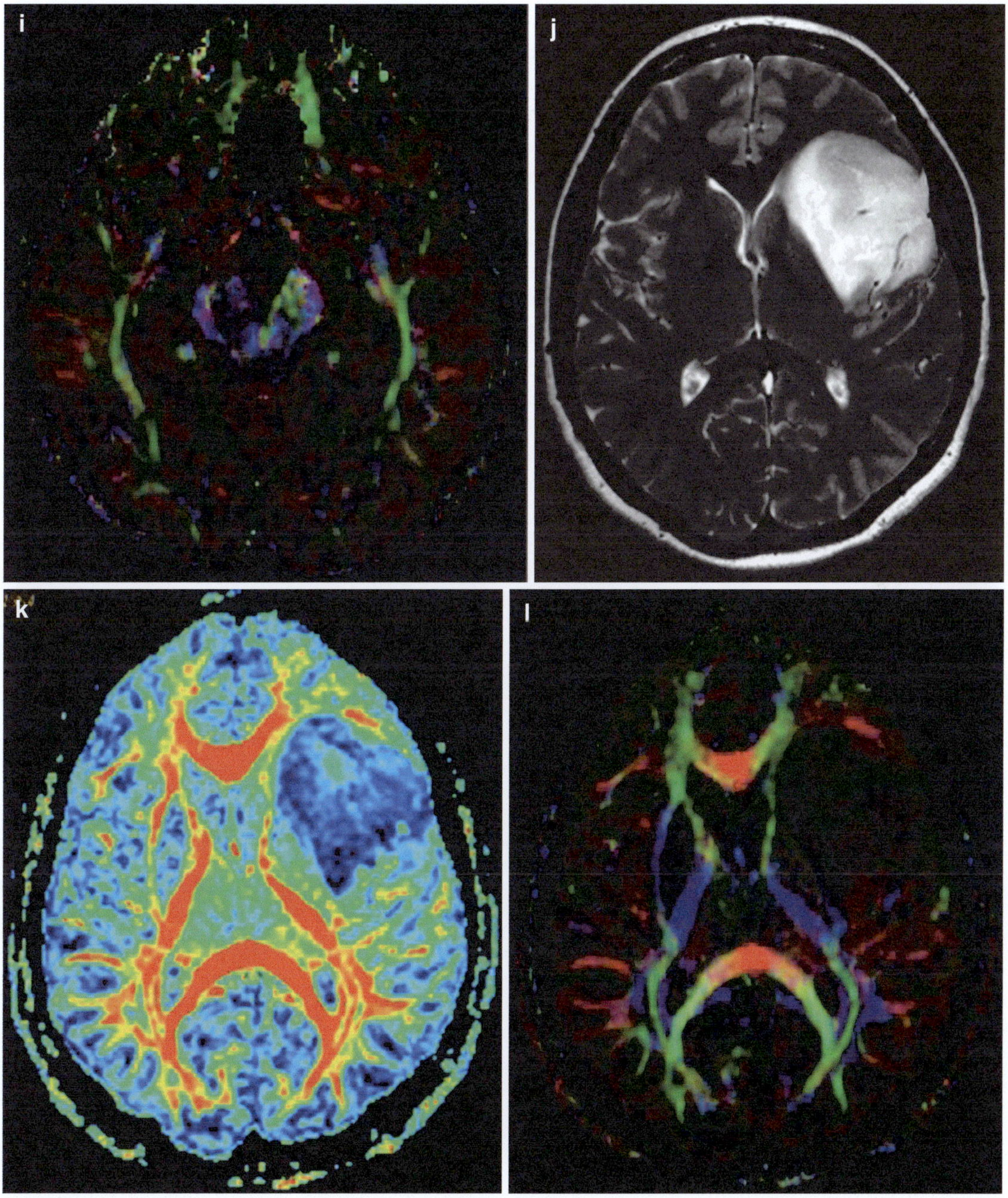


**Fig. 19.10** (continued)

If clinically it is critically important to distinguish between cases where the lesion infiltrates the white matter and cases where the fibers are displaced by the lesion, this also determines the extent of resectability of the lesion. DTI and fiber tractography can demonstrate the orientation and integrity of white matter fibers in vivo. The metrics commonly used include the mean diffusivity (MD) and fractional anisotropy (FA). MD represents a measure of the overall magnitude of diffusion, independent of tissue orientation, similar to the ADC. FA, which is a measure of the directionality of molecular motion, is thought to reflect white matter fiber integrity [87, 88]. Normal white matter appears brighter than tumors on FA image maps due to the directional movement along white matter structures in normal brain that are often disrupted or absent in tumors. FA in brain tumors has been found to be influenced by histological characteristic and correlates with cellularity, vascularity, cell density, neuronal and axonal structures, and fiber tracts [89–91]. The decrease in FA values within brain tumors can be explained as a loss of structural organization, and a strong correlation was observed between the FA and Ki-67 index, although a clear physiological basis linking FA values with the Ki-67 labeling index remains to be determined [92]. For this reason, the DTI has been used in the attempt at differentiating tumor-infiltrated edema from purely vasogenic edema. It has been demonstrated [62] as significantly higher MD in the peritumoral edema, which surrounds metastatic tumors when compared with that in the edema surrounding high-grade gliomas. Increases in the peritumoral MD for malignant gliomas are tempered by the infiltrative rather than expansive growth patterns with the presence of tumor cells in the peritumoral abnormality. At the same way, a reduced FA in the peritumoral region of malignant glioma reflects the presence of infiltrating tumor cells, which may destroy rather than simply displace the white matter tracts [87]. Nevertheless it has been observed [93] that FA values in the tumor marginal area, but not in tumor core, differed significantly between low-grade and high-grade gliomas. This could be consequence of more extensive fiber tract destruction and accordingly lower anisotropy in high-grade gliomas than in low-grade gliomas, whereas in the center of the lesions, the fiber destruction was assumed to be more or less complete, irrespective of tumor grade.

In a recent study [94], it has demonstrated that DTI tractography could be a useful tool in predicting surgical outcome in patients with gliomas located near eloquent areas (Fig. 19.11). By establishing the presence of intact, displaced, or infiltrated fascicles, it was possible to estimate the chance of performing a total resection. Unchanged reconstructed tracts showed normal anisotropy, location, and orientation, compared with homologous contralateral tracts. Displaced tracts had a normal or only slightly decreased anisotropy and showed abnormal location or trajectories when compared with those of contralateral unaffected hemisphere. Infiltrated tracts showed substantially decreased FA with abnormal hues on directional color maps, because infiltrating tumor disrupts the directional organization of fiber tracts causing altered color patterns on directional maps (Fig. 19.10).

Other commonly derived DTI parameters are axial (AD) and radial (RD) diffusivity that represent diffusion properties along the axial and radial directions, respectively. Server et al. [95] have investigated the value of AD coefficient and RD coefficient in grading tumor. They have demonstrated that ADC, RD, and AD are useful DTI metrics for the differentiation between low-grade and high-grade gliomas with a diagnostic accuracy of more than 90 % and can be used as noninvasive reliable biomarkers in the grading of gliomas. There was a significant difference in the minimum ADC values between low-grade and high-grade gliomas. The AD coefficient and RD coefficient values were significantly higher in low-grade gliomas compared with high-grade gliomas, according to Yuan et al. [96]. In their study it was revealed a good inverse correlation between ADC, RD, AD and WHO grade II–IV astrocytic tumors. Findings related to AD and RD within tumor groups may be an indirect manifestation of the combined effects of axonal damage, demyelination, and tumor mass within the cranial compartment. ADC describes microscopic water

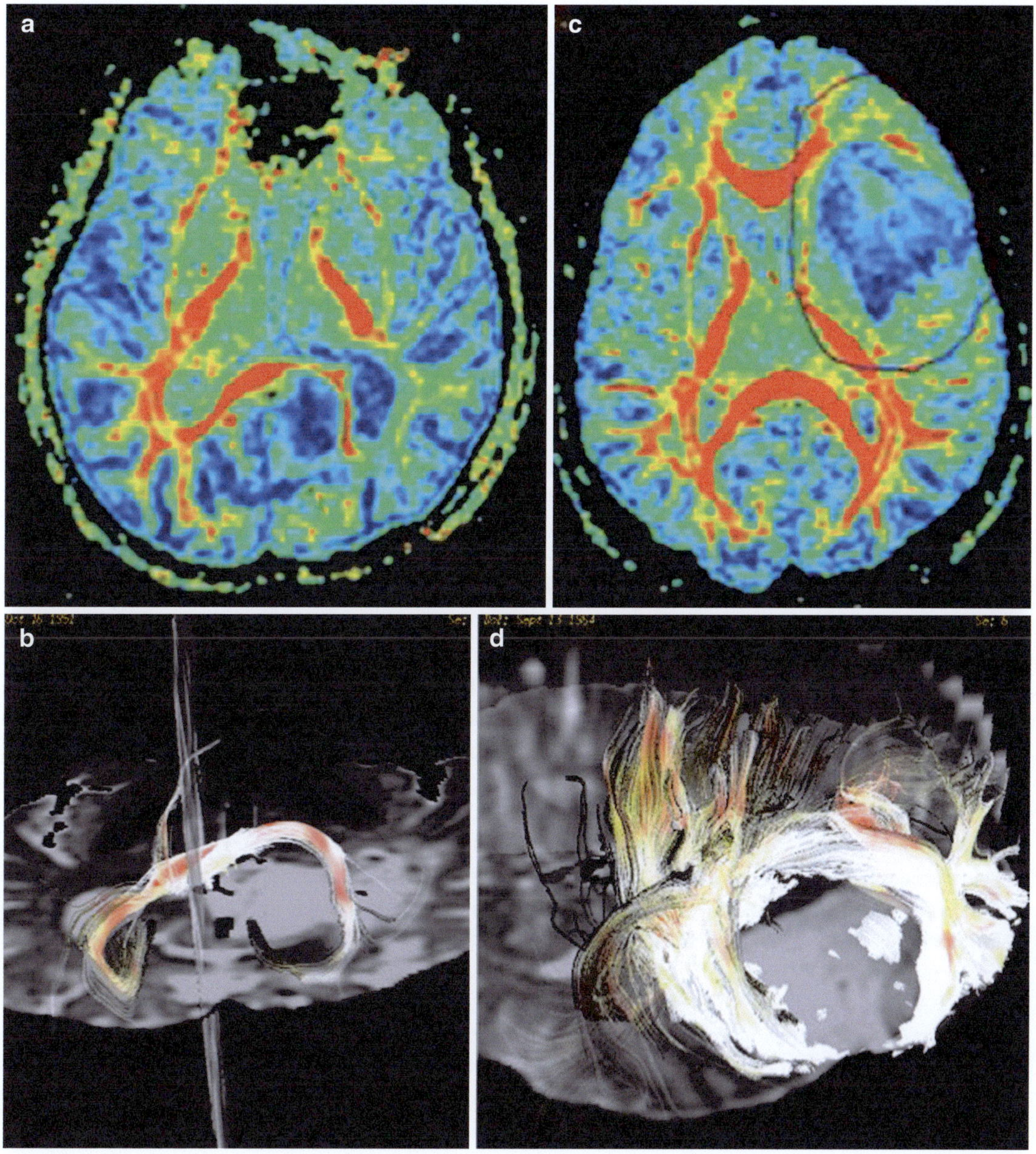


**Fig. 19.11** MR 3T, (**a**, **c**) FA map, (**b**, **d**) DTI tractography. The FA maps show reduction of FA by the left temporo-occipital and left frontal lesions. In tractography reconstruction the fascicles have been displaced by the lesions

movement parallel to axonal tracts and has been associated with axonal damage [97]. In a recent study [98], the association of RD with both demyelination and axonal damage was reported. Inano et al. [99] have developed a new method using multiple DTI-based parameters for voxel-based clustered images in a supervised manner that can be used to visually grade gliomas. By algorithms applied to DTI data, they can noninvasively predict the grade of gliomas with accuracy and may perform regional grading of glioma, which is useful for targeting biopsy, because gliomas are heterogeneous tumors. In this way the regional grading of the tumor can preoperatively be predicted, and it's possible to establish which region must be resected, including peritumoral edematous lesions. We know that LGGs develop into HGGs and >10 % of gliomas differentiate into more malignant grades [100] but we cannot know when tumor grade progresses. By using regional grading based with the Inano et al. methods, the authors can clarify when LGGs progress into HGGs during follow-up and provide an appropriate adjuvant treatment at the optimum time.

Most diffusion tensor imaging studies that measure the directional dependence of diffusion employ *b*-factors up to 1000 s/mm$^2$. Diffusion imaging at higher *b*-factors increases the dynamic range of directionally dependent signal variations, which can be gainfully applied to detect fibers crossing at high angular resolution. Typically, a prohibitive large number of around 250 directions or more are required to achieve a good level of confidence in measuring fiber orientations within crossings [101]. Scan time, at the moment, exceeds 1 h and volume coverage is limited. The potential for diagnostic imaging in brain tumors and improved detection of crossing nerve fiber tracts are interesting. However, further technical development is required to reduce the excessive scan times and limitation in spatial resolution.

More recently, diffusion tensor MR imaging has been used to noninvasively detect genetic characteristics of gliomas, especially the IDH1 R132H mutation [102]. High fractional anisotropic (FA) values and low apparent diffusion coefficient (ADC) values were shown in a wild-type IDH1 group when compared with a mutation group in grade II and III gliomas. The authors found that, although FA and ADC values can detect IDH1 mutation, the ratio of minimal ADC is the best measurement for this proposal.

### 19.3.3 Intravoxel Incoherent Motion Diffusion-Weighted MR Imaging (IVIM)

Diffusion-weighted imaging is considered very sensitive for early pathological changes of a lesion and can potentially be useful in evaluating the feature of gliomas. To overcome a limitation of DWI, in which perfusion can substantially confound diffusion measurement because of the incoherent motion of the blood, a new MR technique, intravoxel incoherent motion (IVIM) based on DWI, has been proposed in differentiating the histologic grade among human gliomas [103, 104]. The major advantages of IVIM MR imaging are as follows: it allows the simultaneous acquisition of diffusion and perfusion parameters.

The IVIM model generated parametric images for apparent diffusion coefficient ADC, slow diffusion coefficient D (or D slow), fast diffusion coefficient D* (or D fast), and fractional perfusion-related volume *f*. Hu et al. [104] assess the relationship between ADC, D, D*, and *f*, based on IVIM models and the glioma grades, and determine the cutoff values of suggested parameters for differentiating high- from low-grade gliomas. They evaluated whether the IVIM MRI could be used preoperatively to grade gliomas. There were significant differences in parameters ADC, D, D*, and *f* between low- and high-grade gliomas. The ADC and D are correlates with cellularity and nuclear atypia [105, 106], and their values were significantly lower in high-grade gliomas compared with low-grade gliomas, according to Iima et al. [107]. The degree of neovascularization is critical in assessing tumor grade and malignancy [108]. Malignant gliomas are characterized by increased angiogenesis, which is a marker of the histological grading system [109]. The parameter D* from the IVIM model is influenced by microvessel density within the tumor, which is associated with an average length of capillaries and blood flow velocities [110]. Several study have suggested that the relative cerebral blood volume (rCBV) value is correlated with the grade and vascularity in gliomas [111, 112], low-grade gliomas show no increase in tumor rCBV, whereas high-grade gliomas demonstrate high rCBV that in some cases even extends outside the contrast-enhancing portions of the tumor [113]. The parameter *f* represents the fraction of the fast diffusion component and is affected by abundance of capillaries (Fig. 19.12). In the Hu

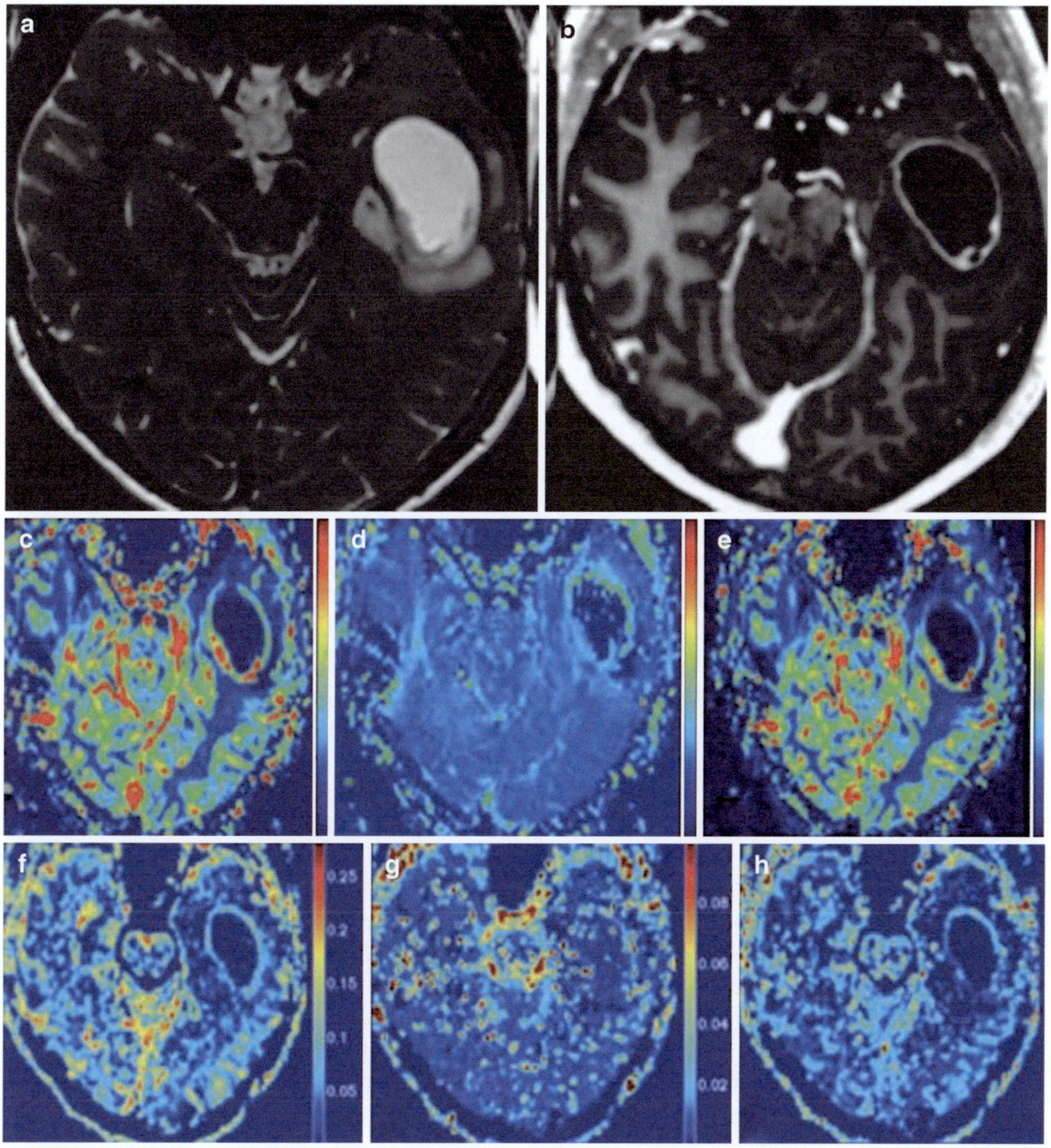


**Fig. 19.12** Axial MR 3T. (**a**)TSE T2-w image; (**b**) SE T1-w image after contrast administration, DSC MR perfusion; (**c**) the CBV map; (**d**) the MTT map; (**e**) the CBF map; IVIM (**f**) the *f* map; (**g**) the D*map; (**h**) the *f*D*map. Necrotic contrast-enhancing high-grade glioma. The CBV and *f* maps demonstrate a higher perfusion fraction region in the corresponding areas of contrast-enhancing compared to the healthy white matter. The D* map shows a slightly decreased fast diffusion values in the tumor tissue compared to the healthy white matter

et al. [104] study, the diagnostic efficacy of IVIM parameters in differentiating glioma grades was shown.

Also for Bisas et al. [103], D, D*, and *f* in the high-grade gliomas demonstrated significant differences compared to the healthy white matter. D* and *f* showed a significant difference between low- and high-grade gliomas. D tended to be slightly lower in the WHO grade II compared to WHO grade III–IV tumors. *f* and D* demonstrated higher coefficients of variation than the ADC and D in tumor.

In conclusion the IVIM-fitted post-processing of DWI signal decay in human gliomas could show significantly different values of fractional perfusion-related volume and fast diffusion coefficient between low- and high-grade tumors, which might enable a noninvasive WHO grading in vivo.

### 19.3.4 Perfusion

Perfusion is physiologically defined as the steady-state delivery of blood to an element of tissue. The term "perfusion" is also used to emphasize contact with the tissue or, in other words, capillary blood flow [114].

There are two major approaches to measure cerebral perfusion with MRI. The first is application of an exogenous, intravascular, nondiffusible contrast agent, usually a gadolinium-based contrast agent that emphasizes either the susceptibility effects of gadolinium-based contrast agents on the signal echo, namely, first-pass dynamic susceptibility contrast-enhanced (DSC) MR perfusion or the relaxivity effects of gadolinium-based contrast agents on the signal echo, namely, dynamic contrast-enhanced (DCE) MR perfusion. The second is application of an endogenous contrast agent using magnetically labeled arterial blood water as a diffusible flow tracer in arterial spin labeling (ASL) MR perfusion.

*Dynamic susceptibility contrast-enhanced MR perfusion* (DSC MR perfusion) is a technique in which the first pass of a bolus of gadolinium-based contrast agent through brain tissue is monitored by a series of T2-or T2*-weighted MR images. The susceptibility effect of the paramagnetic contrast agent leads to a signal loss in the intensity-time curve. Using the principles of the indicator dilution theory, the signal information can then be converted into a contrast medium concentration-time curve on a pixel-by-pixel basis. From these data, parametric maps of cerebral blood volume (CBV) and flow (CBF) can be obtained. Regional CBF and CBV values can be measured by region of interest analysis (Fig. 19.13e, f).

*Dynamic contrast-enhanced MR perfusion* (DCE MR perfusion) is based on the acquisition of serial T1-weighted images before, during, and after administration of extracellular low-molecular-weight MR contrast media, such as gadolinium-based contrast agent. The resulting signal intensity-time curve reflects a composite of tissue perfusion, vessel permeability, and extravascular-extracellular space [115]. DCE MR perfusion imaging depicts the wash-in, plateau, and washout contrast kinetics of the tissue, providing insight into nature of the bulk tissue properties at the microvascular level. With pharmacokinetic modeling of DCE MR perfusion data, several metrics are commonly derived: the transfer constant ($k^{trans}$), the fractional volume of the extravascular-extracellular space ($v_e$), the rate constant ($k_{ep}$), and the fractional volume of the plasma ($v_p$).

*Arterial spin-labeling MR perfusion* (ASL MR perfusion) is a method that uses magnetically labeled blood as an endogenous tracer. There are two main types of ASL technique: continuous ASL and pulsed ASL [116, 117]. In continuous ASL, there is a prolonged radio frequency pulse that continuously labels arterial blood water below the imaging slab until a steady state of tissue magnetization is reached [118]. In pulsed ASL, a short radio frequency pulse is used to label a thick slab of arterial blood at a single point in time, and imaging is performed after a period of time to allow distribution in the tissue of interest [119]. A new technique, called "pseudocontinuous ASL," represents a compromise between pulsed ASL and continuous ASL. This technique may provide improved balance between labeling efficiency and signal-to-noise ratio (SNR) compared with conventional ASL methods [120]. This method is considered completely noninvasive, and it allows the determination of absolute quantitative values of CBF, in contrast with DSC MR perfusion (Fig. 19.13c, d). It is also insensitive to permeability.

In general DSC and DCE MR perfusion achieve a substantially higher SNR that allows imaging at a higher temporal and spatial resolution, and DSC MR perfusion allows the visualization and quantification of the whole brain in less than a minute of acquisition time. ASL has a limited SNR and much longer scanning time.

Clinically, established methods for quantitative perfusion measurement usually include normalization of the mean or maximum perfusion values in the tumor region in relation to mean values in normal appearing white matter. Normalized rCBV measurements are considered to be the clinical standard [121]. However, white matter is often affected by treatment and/or

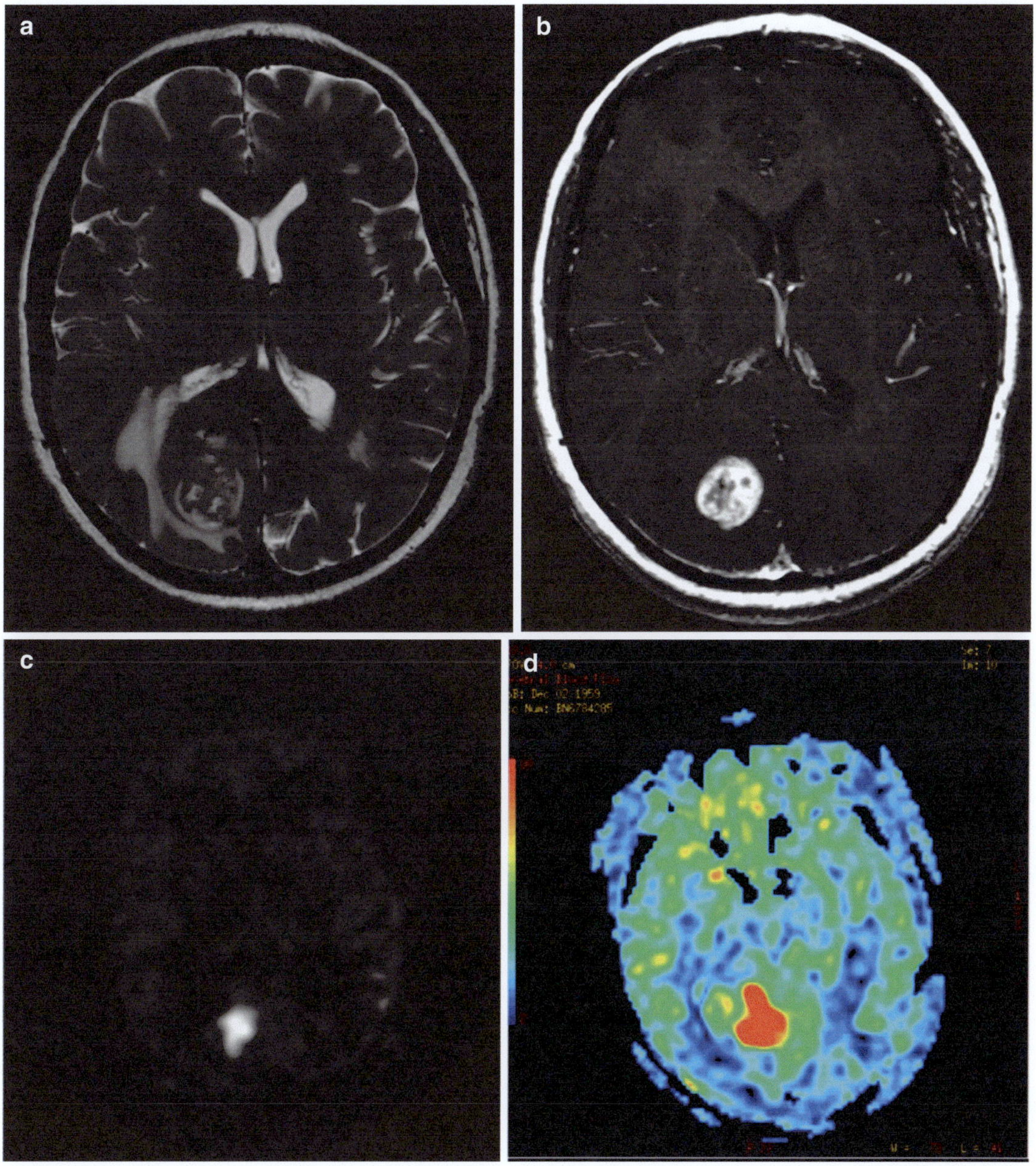


**Fig. 19.13** Axial MR 3T, (**a**) TSE T2-w image, (**b**) SE T1-w image after contrast administration, (**c**, **d**)ASL images, (**e**, **f**) rCBV map and graphic derived from GE-DSC perfusion, (**g**, **h**) $K^2$ map and rCBV map corrected in function to permeability. MGMT-methylated glioblastoma. The lesion is hyperperfused in all images. The hyperperfused area in rCBV map corrected is larger than the same area in rCBV map uncorrected

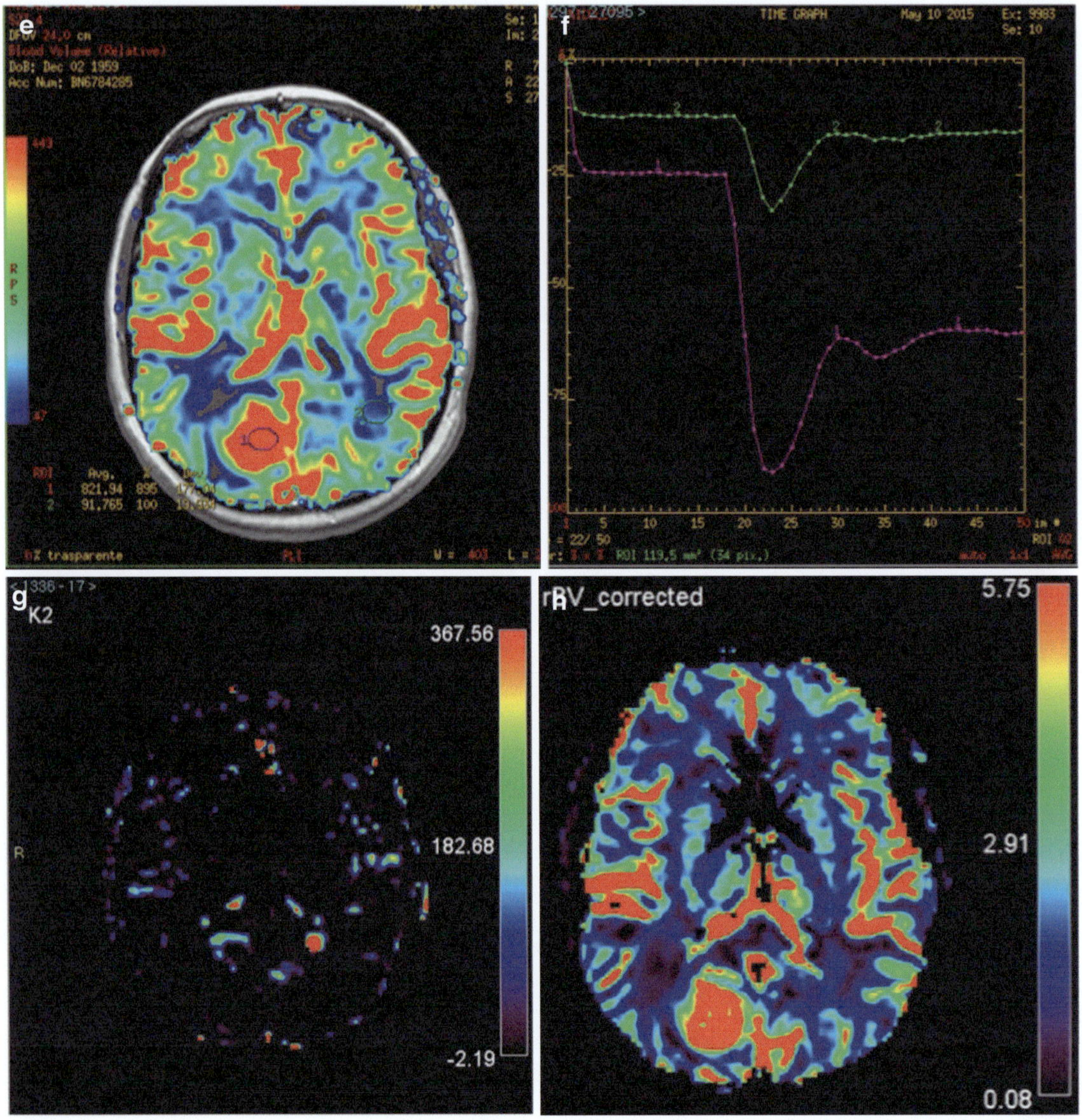


**Fig. 19.13** (continued)

edema or may invaded by diffuse tumor growth. In these cases the cerebellum could be used as a reference region [122].

One of the characteristics of brain tumors, irrespective of grade, is to produce a mass effect, which compresses the microcirculation in the normal tissue around the lesion and alters the permeability properties of vessels, including those that feed the tumor. In addition, high-grade gliomas also generate new blood vessels, which have very abnormal physiologic properties, including the peculiarity of allowing fluid from the intravascular compartment to seep through them. This occur indiscriminately within and around the tumor [60].

Hypoxic tumors tend to grow and metastasize faster than well-oxygenated tumors, and to be more resistant to radio- and chemotherapy [123]. In high-grade gliomas, the extent of tumor hypoxia is correlated with time to progression and overall survival [124]. Tumor secures their supply of oxygen and other nutrients by stimulating tissue angiogenesis, and the extent of vessel formation is closely related to tumor development and is in indirect marker of high malignancy and aggressiveness. The effects of vascular endothelial growth factor/vascular permeability factor (VEGF/VPF) and other growth factors on vascular perfusion and permeability have studied since Folkman J. (1971) first described the association of tumoral growth with angiogenesis [125]. Perfusion and permeability magnetic resonance (MR) imaging can now measure parameters such as CBV e $K^{trans}$, which can be directly correlated with these histopathologic changes as well as molecular markers such as VEGF [126, 127]. rCBV have been shown to correlate reliably with tumor grade and histologic findings of increased tumor vascularity [128, 131]. The degree of vascular proliferation, or angiogenesis, is one of the most important histologic criteria for determination of the degree of malignancy of a glioma. Vascular networks are not only the principal route for delivery of oxygen and nutrients to the neoplastic cells but also serve as paths for tumor infiltration along perivascular spaces. The cerebral capillary endothelium, site of blood-brain barrier, is frequently destroyed by malignant tumor cells. A hypermeable blood barrier associated with or without immature angiogenic vessels allows for contrast agent enhancement, extravasation, and, hence, measurement of vascular permeability [132]. These pathophysiologic changes have been shown to provide good correlation between tumor biology and rCBV, CBF, CBV $K^{trans}$, and $V_p$ measurement. Due to an increase in CBV from microvascular density, as well as many collateral and tortuous vessels, from angiogenesis, it is felt that the mean transit time (MTT) should be prolonged. However, because of the immense heterogeneity of the tumor microvasculature in some regions, MTT may also decrease due to increased CBF, particularly at the tumor margins, where there is rapid shunting of blood flow [133]. There have been numerous publications demonstrating a good correlation between the value of rCBV and tumor biology. Comparison of rCBV measurements between LGG and HGG has demonstrated LGG to have maximal rCBV values of between 1.11 and 2.14 and HGG to have maximal rCBV values of between 3.54 and 7.32 [67, 129, 130, 134]. A larger study demonstrated LGG to have rCBV values of 2.14 and HGG to have rCBV values of 5.18 [129]. DSC MR imaging increases the sensitivity and predictive value in predicting glioma grade compared with conventional contrast-enhancement MR imaging.

In clinical practice, 95–100 % sensitivity has been reported for differentiating HGGs from LGGs using threshold of 1.75 and 1.5 for rCBV, respectively [129, 135].

The role of VEGF, also known as VPF, as a mediator of tumor growth and angiogenesis has also resulted in several investigators demonstrating a good correlation between vascular permeability and glioma grade. It seems clear, however, in part due to the heterogeneity of glioma vasculature that the regions of increased rCBV are spatially heterogeneous and different to areas of increased permeability [136, 137].

Previous studies have demonstrated no correlation between rCBV and low- versus high-grade gliomas [138] and no statistical difference in rCBV between grade I and II, grade II and III, and grade III and IV gliomas [139]. The disparity of these findings suggests that careful attention must be paid to the rCBV computation process, and one point of differing methodology involves contamination of derived concentration-time data by contrast agent extravasation [140]. When confined to intravascular space, paramagnetic contrast agents (Gd-DTPA) produce signal intensity loss in the extravascular space on T2-weighted scan, and susceptibility contrast-based rCBV maps are computed by integrating the resulting transverse relaxivity changes that occur over a dynamic first-pass injection. However, because Gd-DTPA is also an effective enhancer, the susceptibility-contrast signal intensity loss can be masked by signal intensity increase in region where T1 effects are significant. This occurs in enhancing tumors, where Gd-DTPA extravasates into the interstitial space of lesions with significant blood-brain barrier breakdown. In such instances, rCBV will be underestimated, which may affect tumor grade prediction (Fig. 19.14).

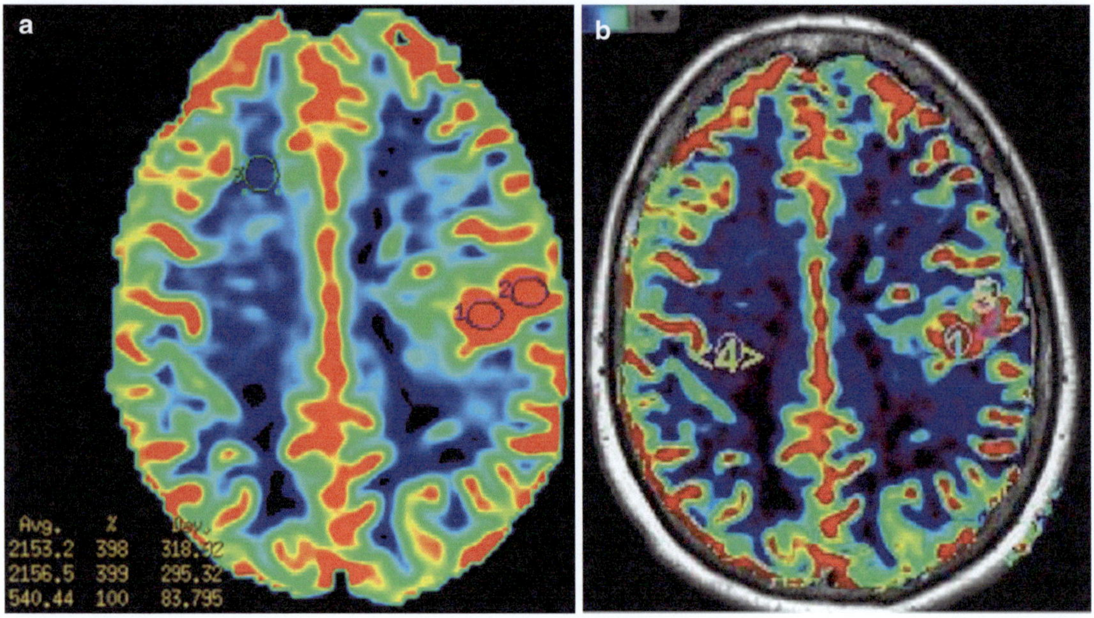


**Fig. 19.14** MR 3T, (**a**) rCBV map and (**b**) corrected rCBV map, derived from GE-DSC perfusion. The values of regions of interest (*blue* and *white circles*) placed in the lesion are in uncorrected rCBV map 3.98–3.99, compared to the healthy white matter, in the corrected map they are 5.7–6.1

Boxerman et al. [140] use a linear fitting to estimate the T1 contamination due to agent extravasation and, by removing the leakage term, allow generation of both corrected rCBV maps and first-order estimate of vascular permeability. In this way they show that rCBV corrected for contrast agent leakage correlates significantly with histopathologic tumor grade, whereas uncorrected rCBV does not (Fig. 19.15).

Another problem is the kind of sequence to use. GE-EPI acquisition is sensitive to vessels of all size, as opposed to SE acquisition, which has peak sensitivity to capillary-sized microvessels [141]. Although early reports documented significant correlation between SE rCBV and tumor grade [134], this has been refuted subsequently by Donahue et al. [142] and Schmainda et al. [143], who demonstrated that GE- but not SE-derived rCBV maps significantly correlate with tumor grade. This would seem to underscore the fact that the neovascularity characteristic of aggressive, high-grade tumors often consists of disorganized, large-scale microvessels that do not have feature typical of capillaries and would therefore be best interrogated with GE acquisition possessing wide-range microvascular sensitivity that can distinguish tumor angiogenesis from normal capillary beds. For these reasons, GE acquisition should be used for tumor perfusion studies because GE-based rCBV will be a statistically significant predictor of tumor grade [140]. Of course, GE acquisition are also sensitive to macrovessels, which must carefully excluded from the regions of interest used to compute rCBV and estimate tumor grade.

The dynamic nature of CNS tumors is well known and the follow-up is long enough; all low-grade tumors progress to high-grade tumors. What is still unknown is how, when, and why a dormant (silent) tumor becomes aggressive. A very important concept related to the tumoral progression is the “angiogenic switch” [136, 137]. This concept refers to the transition of an avascular tumor to an angiogenic one and represents a distinct step in the malignant transformation of gliomas [144]. Overexpression of angiogenic factors or hypoxia results in the production of certain growth factors and cytokines that ultimately

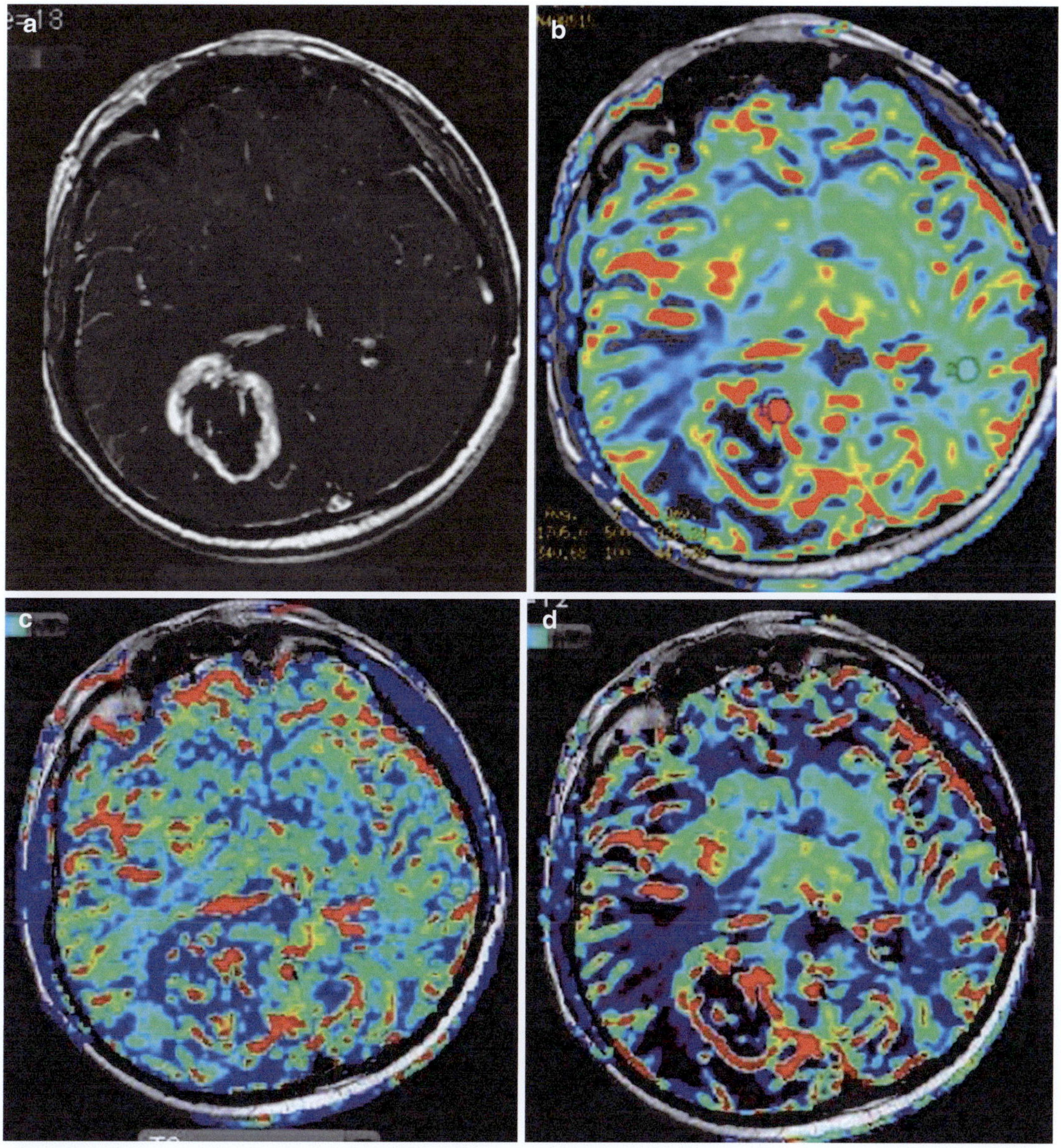

**Fig. 19.15** MR 3T. (**a**) Axial SE T1-w image after contrast administration; (**b**) uncorrected CBV map, derived from GE-DSC perfusion; (**c**) CBV corrected in function to AIF (arterial input function); (**d**) CBV map corrected in function to permeability. Glioblastoma with central necrosis. CBV is higher (*red color*) around the necrotic area in rCBV corrected map

induce angiogenesis in gliomas. Danchaivijitr et al. [145] demonstrated that in transforming LGG, DSC perfusion imaging can demonstrate significant increases in rCBV up to 12 months before contrast enhancement is apparent on T1-weighted MR images. This result indicates that an increase in microvascular density occurs well in advance of blood-brain barrier leakage reflected by pathologic contrast enhancement. rCBV is therefore likely to provide an earlier noninvasive indicator of malignant progression and may likely indicate this "angiogenic switch" [132]. Contrast enhancement as a marker of anaplastic transformation presents some disadvantages and poses limitations. It appears late and its appearance proves that anaplastic transformation has already occurred [146]. Additionally, it is a nonspecific feature, resulting from the blood-brain barrier breakdown due to, e.g., inflammatory and ischemic changes, radiotherapy, as well as lack of normal BBB in vasculature formed by angiogenesis. The extent of contrast enhancement also depends on the dose of glucocorticoids and even the examination technique. Although contrast enhancement is considered to be typical of HGGs, it should be remembered that about 40 % of high-grade tumors do not show contrast enhancement [129, 131–133, 147] whereas 10–39 % of LGGs do [148, 149]. However, PWI gives access to information on the capillary microcirculation of tissues and reflects tissue microvascularity density, prior to the occurrence of contrast enhancement. The normalized rCBV = 1.75 is the most frequently accepted cut-off value differentiating LGGs from HGGs as well as LGGs with short and long transformation time [133, 150].

An expected relationship between molecular markers of angiogenesis and increase of tumor perfusion parameters has been shown by Batchelor et al. [151]. Jain and colleagues [152], on the other side, reported a lack of significant difference in CBV among the molecular classes of GBM, which is surprising, given the relative overexpression of proangiogenic molecules in some of the subclasses compared with others. Although CBV appears to be unrelated to molecular class of GBM, proneural tumors have been found to have significantly lower levels of contrast enhancement, while mesenchymal tumors lacked of nonenhancing tumor (nCET) areas. These data support Pope and colleagues' previous findings suggesting that the presence of nCET is associated with genes that are overexpressed in the proneural class of GBM [52]. In another study Pope and colleagues also found imaging features associated with mesenchymal GBMs [153]. Thus there is mounting evidence that, while some perfusion metrics such as CBV may be similar between molecular classes of GBM (Figs. 19.16e and 19.17), there are inter-class differences in imaging features that can be derived from standard MRI sequences [53].

## 19.3.5 Spectroscopy

Since its discovery over 50 years ago, the field of magnetic resonance spectroscopy (MRS) has become an invaluable means for the analysis of molecular structure. The power in the approach lies both in its nondestructive nature and in its sensitivity to the molecular environment of an individual atom.

In a clinical setting, this method has evolved into MR imaging, a technique for spatial localization of tissue, water and fat. The MR signals from the water and fat hydrogen atoms are mapped according to their location within the patient. The other application of MR is the technique known as MR spectroscopy (MRS). MRS has become one of the major techniques used in chemistry and physics laboratories for the analysis of molecular interactions and for the identification of chemical compounds [154]. MR spectroscopy in the brain can be performed in vivo with a preselected volume of interest placed entirely in the lesion, ex vivo on excised tissue (HR-MAS), and in vitro on solutions obtained from multiple samples of the lesions. It provides information content on neuronal/axonal viability, energetics of the cellular structures, and status of the cellular membranes [155]. However, one of the most powerful aspects of MR spectroscopy, the ability to perform chemical identification, is lost in the imaging process.

In recent years, improvements in hardware and software have made it possible to merge the two techniques. In vivo MR spectroscopy combines the localization features of imaging with the ability for chemical analysis to provide a non-invasive method for the study of biochemical processes in a patient.

MR spectra may be obtained from different nuclei, but *protons* (*$^{1}H$*) are more commonly used for spectroscopy because of their natural abundance in organic structures and their magnetic sensitivity when compared with other nuclei, such as *phosphorus*, *sodium*, *carbon*, *fluorine*, and *lithium*, which require specialized coils and amplifiers for observation. For this reason it's

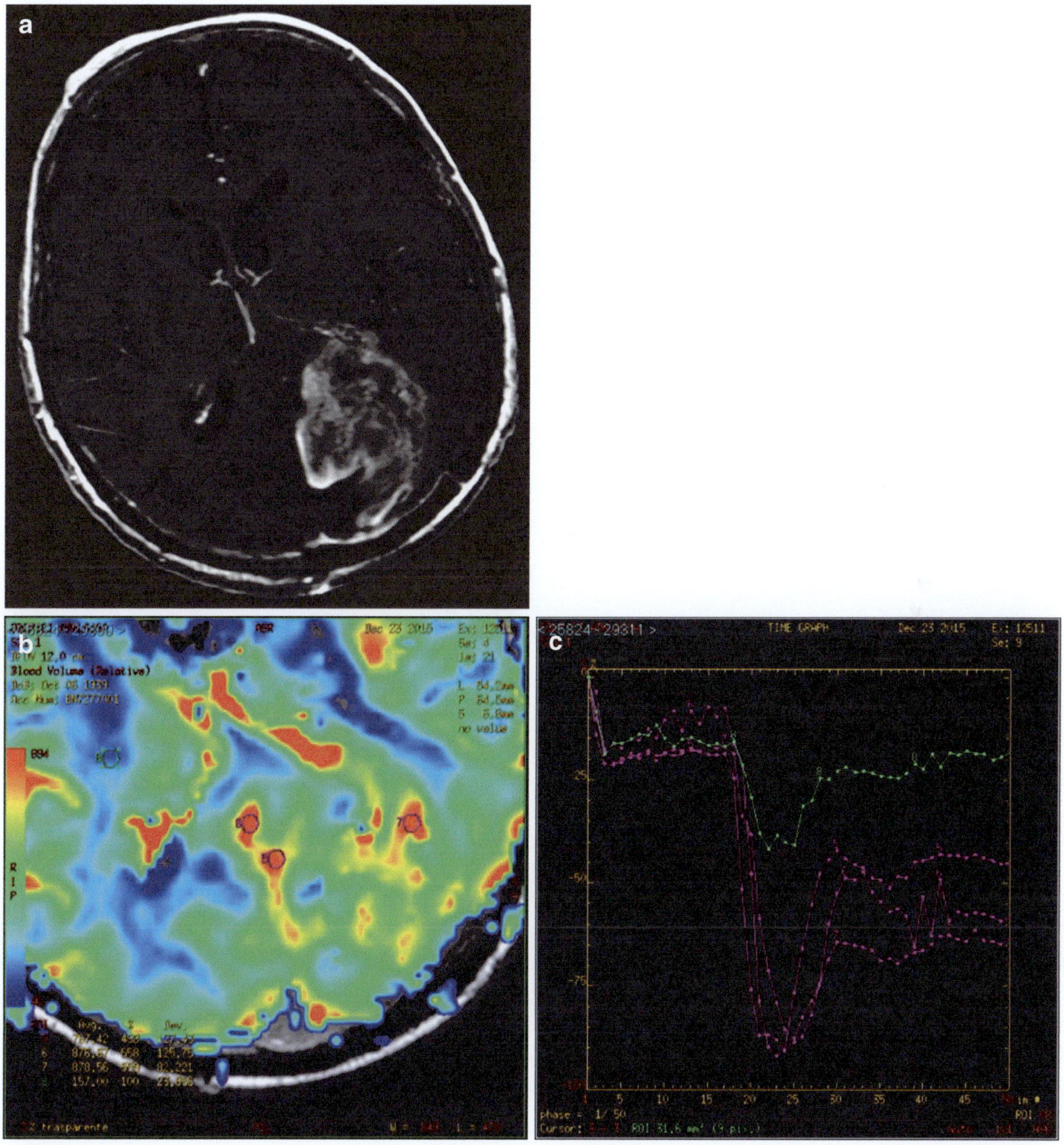


**Fig. 19.16** MR 3T. (**a**) Axial SE T1-w image after contrast administration, (**b**, **c**) rCBV map and graphic derived from GE-DSC perfusion. MGMT-methylated glioblastoma with rCBV max 5.6, compared to the healthy white matter

possible to use the same hardware as standard MRI.

In the same moment, the system detects the $^1$H signal, and the main difference between standard MRI and MRS is that the frequency of the MR signal is used to encode different types of information. MRI uses high spatial resolution to generate anatomical images. MRS provides chemical information about the tissues.

Spatial location determines the frequency with MRI, whereas the tissue's chemical environment determines the frequency in MRS.

However, spectroscopy differs from conventional MR imaging in that spectra provide physiologic and chemical information instead of anatomy. Rather than images, MRS data are usually presented as a line spectra. The shift of peaks in their relationship to one another on the

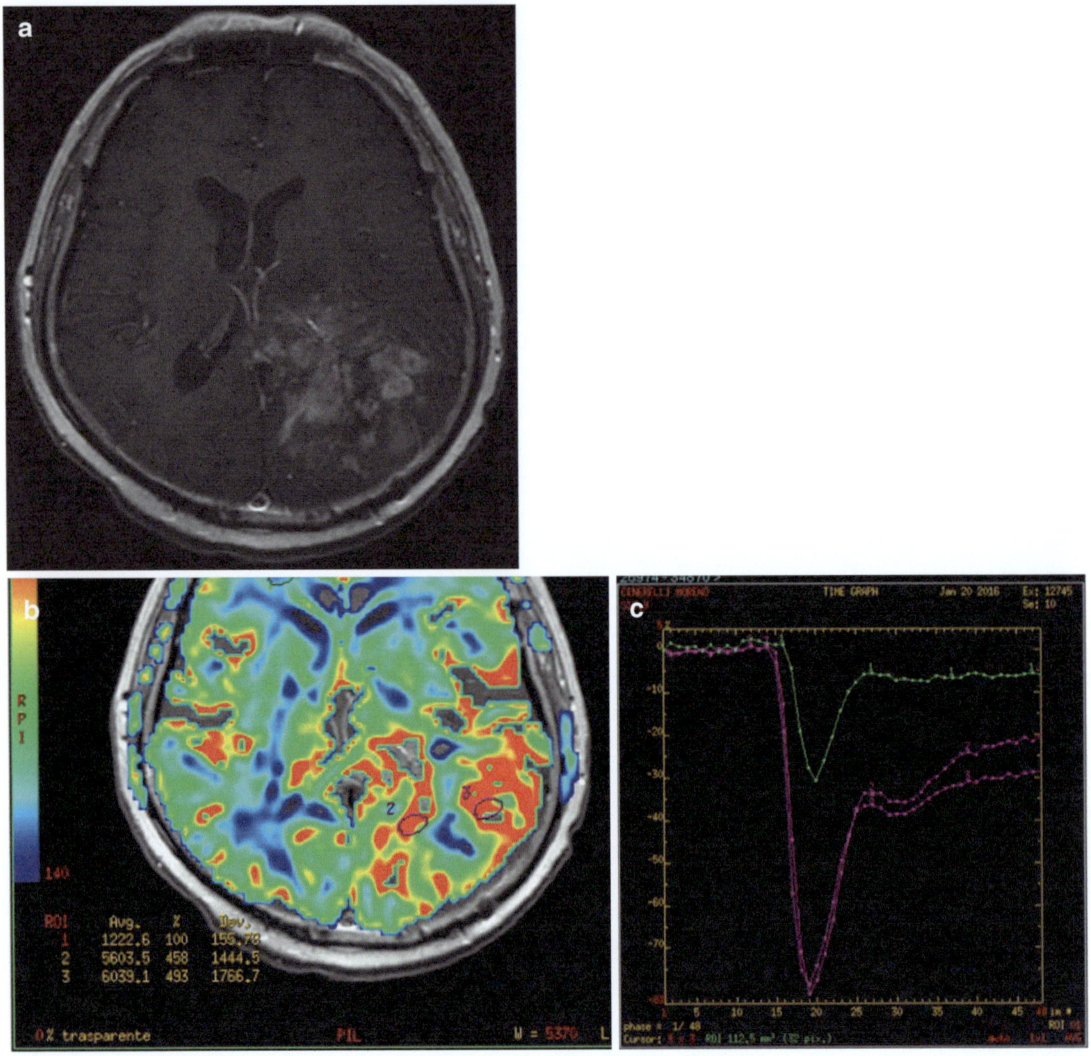


**Fig. 19.17** MR 3T. (**a**) Axial SE T1-w image after contrast administration, (**b**, **c**) rCBV map and graphic derived from GE-DSC perfusion. No-methylated glioblastoma IDH wild-type with rCBV max 4.9 compared to the healthy white matter

frequency axis is known as chemical shift. Instead of a frequency scale which is dependent on magnetic field strength, a "part per million" or "ppm" scale is commonly used to describe the position of the spectral peaks on the x-axis. Each metabolite has a characteristic set of the chemical shift values in its signals [156].

The area under each peak representing the relative concentration of nuclei is detected for a given chemical species.

While imaging systems are available using low-field magnets, the small net magnetization generated by these systems makes them impractical for spectroscopic studies: the reduced signal necessitates an enormous number of acquisitions producing long measurement times. While clinical spectroscopic studies have been performed at 1.0 T or lower field strengths, most in vivo studies are performed at 1.5 T or higher providing improved spectral separation of resonances as well as increased SNR (signal/noise ratio).

$^{1}$H MRS 3 T has higher SNR and shorter acquisition time than 1.5 T and better resolution. The better spatial resolution increases the

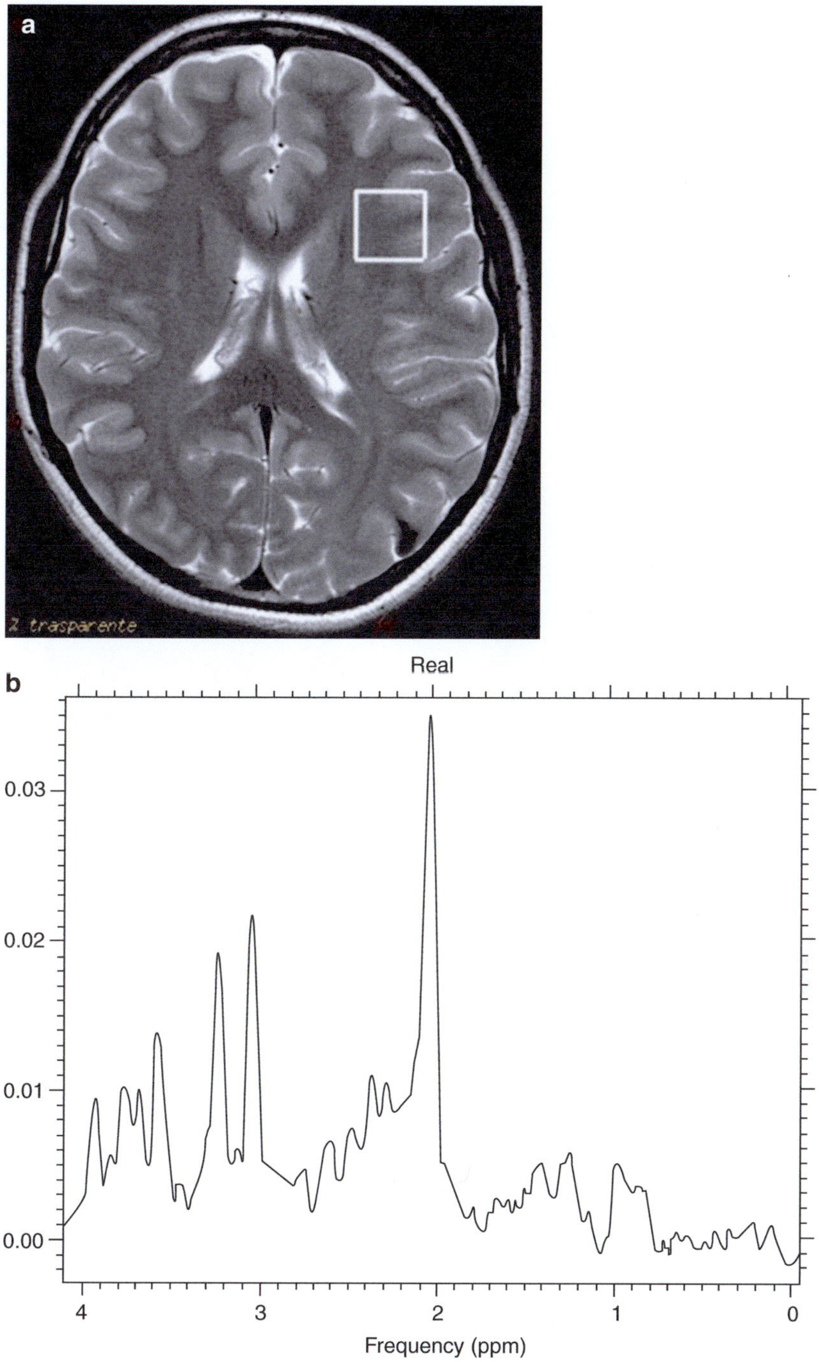


**Fig. 19.18** SV spectroscopy MR 3 T, (**a**) axial TSE T2-w image with volume of interest, (**b**) reference of $^{1}$H MR spectrum obtained from a 2 × 2 × 2 cm VOI in the left frontal cortex in a healthy 30-year-old subject (TR 2000, TE 35)

distance between peaks, making it easier to distinguish each other.

The $^{1}$H MRS acquisition starts with anatomic images, which are used to select a volume of interest (VOI), where the spectrum will be acquired.

The techniques for spectrum acquisition may be single voxel spectroscopy (SVS) (Fig. 19.18) or multivoxel spectroscopy (MRS) (Fig. 19.19) using both long and short echo times (TE) [157].

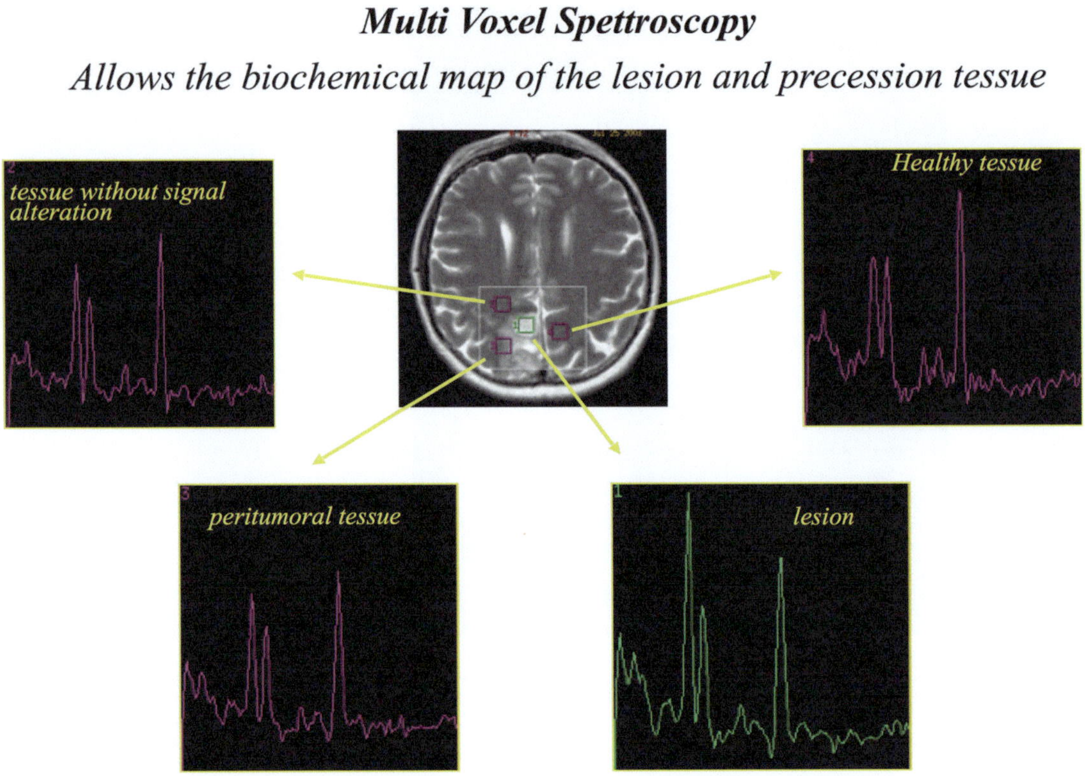


**Fig. 19.19** MV spectroscopy MR 3T, axial TSE T2-w image with volume of interest (VOI) and reference of $^{1}$H MR spectra in different parts of a lesion and healthy tissue around (TR 2000, TE 144)

Short TE (20–40 ms) allows for recognition of more metabolites than long TE, which is important for differential diagnosis of brain masses and grading tumors. For example, myoinositol, a marker for low-grade gliomas, is only seen on short TE acquisition [158].

MV $^{1}$H MRS simultaneously records spectra from multiple regions and therefore maps the spatial distribution of metabolites [159]. MV $^{1}$H MRS provides smaller volumes of interest compared with single voxel (SV), avoiding sampling error. It can be used to determine spatial heterogeneity of the lesions [158, 160]. The advantages of SV $^{1}$H MRS is that it is quicker and easier to obtain in standard clinical setting [161]. SV H MRS provides better quality spectra compared with MRS imaging. It is used to obtain an accurate quantification of the metabolites.

One of two techniques is used for acquisition of SV $^{1}$H MRS spectra: pointed resolved spectroscopy (PRESS) and stimulated echo acquisition mode (STEAM). In the PRESS sequences, the spectrum is acquired using 1 of 90° pulse followed by 2 of 180° pulses. In the STEAM all 3 pulses applied are 90° pulses. The most used SVS technique is PRESS, where SNR is 50 % higher than in STEAM [157].

MV $^{1}$H MRS/CSI (chemical shift imaging) is a method for collecting spectroscopic data from multiple adjacent voxels covering a large VOI in a single measurement:

However, SV $^{1}$H MRS provides better quality spectra compared with MV $^{1}$H MRS, so it could be recommendable that both techniques be used in the evaluation of brain lesions.

### 19.3.6 Spectra Analysis

$^{1}$H MRS allows the detection of brain metabolites and their pathological alterations. To detect these spectral alterations, it is fundamental to know the normal brain spectra and their variations according to the applied technique, patient's age, and brain region. Metabolite peaks may differ slightly according to the brain region studied. Nevertheless, no significant asymmetries of metabolite spectra between the left and right hemispheres or between genders have been found.

In clinical setting, metabolite ratios are often used both for SVS or MRSI rather than obtaining absolute metabolite concentrations due to variations in magnetic field homogeneity, radio frequency coil homogeneity, and susceptibility of patient tissues. Internal Cr signal is used as the reference metabolite.

The interpretation of MR spectrum arises from variation in chemical ratio and/or concentrations, which alter the peak area for endogenous metabolites and the appearance of pathological metabolites. Only few of the metabolites can be commonly quantified in clinical MRS and have a clinical significance in diagnosis of gliomas.

The key metabolites are discussed according to their spectral locations, relative to water located at 4.7 ppm.

*N-Acetylaspartate (NAA).* Assigned at 2.02 ppm NAA is synthesized in the mitochondria of neurons. NAA is exclusively found in the nervous system, and it is a marker of neuronal and axonal viability and density. NAA plays a role as cerebral osmolyte. The absence or decreased concentration of NAA is a sign of neuronal loss or degradation like in high-volume lesions, dementia, hypoxia, or multiple sclerosis. Due to the relationship between the decline in NAA concentration and increasing glioma grade connected with decrease in neuronal density, it is possible to use NAA as a substantial diagnostic marker [162]. Thus, the high level of NAA is associated with a good prognosis of brain tumor [163]. NAA is also a useful marker for differentiation of primary brain tumors from metastasis and nonneuronal tumors where the metabolite is lacking in the spectra. An exception to this is glioblastoma because this extremely malignant tumor of glial origin also has a very low level of NAA [164].

*Choline-containing compounds (Cho), Free Choline (fCho), Phosphorylcholine (PCho), and Glycerophosphorylcholine (GPCho).* Assigned at 3.22 ppm. Its signal is considered as one of the most important for glioma examination. Only PCho, a precursor of cell membranes synthesis, is associated with oncogenic and malignant transformation of cells because high expression of choline kinase, which is the enzyme that converts Cho in PCho, is required for cancer cell growth [165]. By contrast, fCho is a degradation product of cell membranes that can be utilized again for membrane synthesis. The protein Ki-67 is a cellular marker for proliferation; thus, the higher rate of Ki-67 positive cells corresponds with greater malignancy of gliomas [166, 167]. Because a correlation between Ki-67 positivity and Cho level in gliomas has been proven, high-grade gliomas with increased cell density show an increase in the level of Cho [168].

*Creatine (Cr) and Phosphocreatine.* Assigned at 3.02 ppm. Cr is a marker of energetic systems and intracellular metabolism. The concentration of Cr is relatively constant, and it is considered as a stable metabolite. It is an internal reference for calculating metabolite ratio. Decrease in Cr may occur, representing energy failure in aggressive malignant neoplasms.

*Myoinositol (mIns).* Assigned at 3.56 ppm. mIns is considered as a glial marker because it is synthesized in glial cells (astrocytes) and participates in their osmoregulatory system. mIns is elevated in proliferation of glial cells or with increased glial cell size, as found in inflammation. The Myo/Cr ratio is usually higher in lower-grade than in higher-grade tumors [159]. A high level of mIns is present mainly in low-grade gliomas with better prognosis, while its progressive decrease is noted in gliomas with higher level of lactate as product of insufficient energy metabolism of glial cell, i.e., in gliomas of grade III and mainly grade IV [170]. Thus, the mIns level has implication in the grading of cerebral astrocytomas, and it plays also an important role in glioma invasion.

*Lactate (Lac).* The peak of lactate is a doublet at 1.33 ppm. Lac is a product of anaerobic glycolysis and is not detected in healthy brain tissue. Its concentration increases under anaerobic metabolism: hypoxia, ischemia, seizures, and metabolic disorders (especially mitochondrial ones). Lactate is directly related to tumor grade in adult brain tumors, with higher peaks seen in higher-grade tumors. Malignant transformation of the glial tumors is accompanied by an increase in cell density with their relative ischemia resulting in higher level of Lac. However, lactate is found in essentially all pediatric brain tumors regardless of histologic grade [171] (Fig. 19.20).

*Lipids (Lip).* There are two peaks of lipids at 1.3 ppm and at 0.9 ppm. Lipids are components of cell membranes and they are absent in the normal brain. Increased levels of lipids are caused by necrosis and membrane breakdown, such as metastasis and malignant tumors. A prominent lipid peak is also a characteristic for radiation necrosis. Thus, the level of Lip detected by MRS appears to reflect the severity of tissue damage.

*Glutamate-Glutamine (Glx).* Glx has complex peaks, assigned at 2.05–2.50 ppm. Glutamate is an excitatory neurotransmitter. Glutamine is an

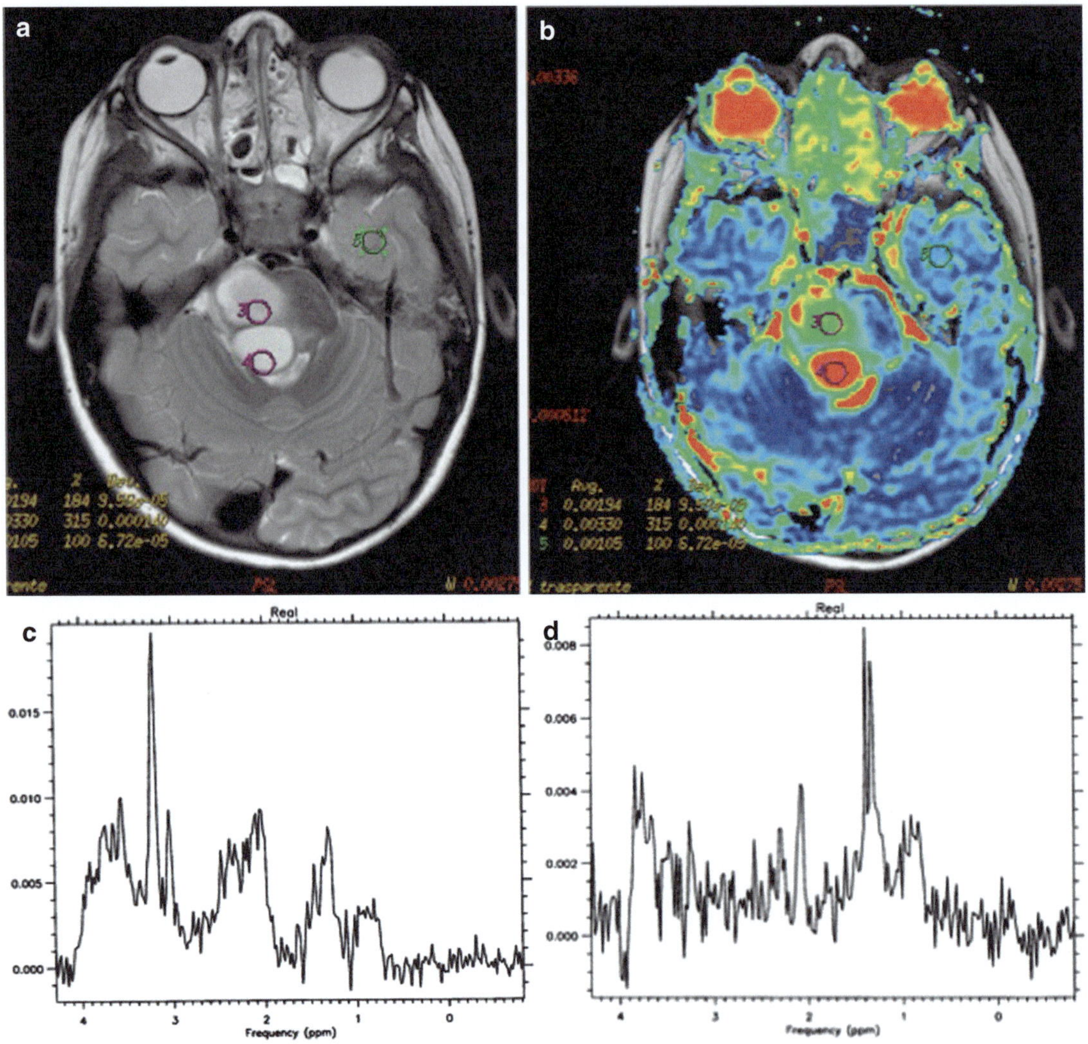


**Fig. 19.20** MR 3T. (**a**)Axial TSE T2-w image, (**b**) ADC map, (**c**) reference of $^{1}$H MR spectrum (TR2000, TE 35) obtained from a VOI placed the solid part of the lesion (pilocytic astrocytoma) and in the cystic part (**d**). ADC in cystic part is similar to ADC of CSF and the spectrum shows a double peak of lactate at 1.34 and 1.39 ppm. The peak of Cho-containing compounds (3.22) is very high in solid part of the lesion, and the peak of mIns is elevated too; NAA is reduced (**d**)

inhibitory neurotransmitter. Elevated concentration of glutamine is found in oligodendrogliomas (Fig. 19.21), hepatic encephalopathy, and demyelinating lesions.

*2-Hydroxyglutarate* (*2-HG*). 2-HG has complex peaks, assigned at 2.25 ppm. IDH1 mutations are associated with alterations in DNA methylation of isocitrate, resulting in overproduction and accumulation of the putative oncometabolite 2-HG. IDH1 appears to function as a tumor suppressor that, when mutationally inactivated, contributes to tumorigenesis partially through induction of the angiogenesis pathway [17]. 2-HG in gliomas may serve as a potential biomarker for identifying patients with IDH1-mutant brain tumors. Detection of 2-HG could be a potential tool used to differentiate primary from secondary GBMs and may provide insights into tumor progression and help monitor treatment effects [17, 172–174].

Radiological grading of gliomas by conventional MR imaging has a sensitivity ranging from 55 to 83 % [129]. Despite a low specificity, detection of significant differences in levels of metabolite by MRS can increase sensitivity in determining glioma grade, which can have important implications for treatment planning and prognosis (Fig. 19.22). We consider to simplify, according to WHO classification system dated 2007, a four-tiered system (grade I–grade IV) of brain glial tumors.

*WHO grade I gliomas.* It refers to well-circumscribed glial lesions with low proliferative potential (e.g., pilocytic astrocytoma) that may be cured by surgical extirpation alone. Previous reports of MRS performed on the solid portions of pilocytic astrocytoma have documented elevation in Cho/NAA and Cho/Cr ratios [175, 176]. Nevertheless, the higher values of tCho in pilocytic astrocytoma do not reflect its malignity. In vivo and in vitro studies have proved that GPCho is the dominant choline-containing metabolite in pilocytic astrocytoma, whereas the main biomarker of tumor malignancy, i.e., PCho, is relatively low [177]. The higher value of mIns is the next MRS feature of grade I gliomas [178]. Despite the benign histology of the tumor, which

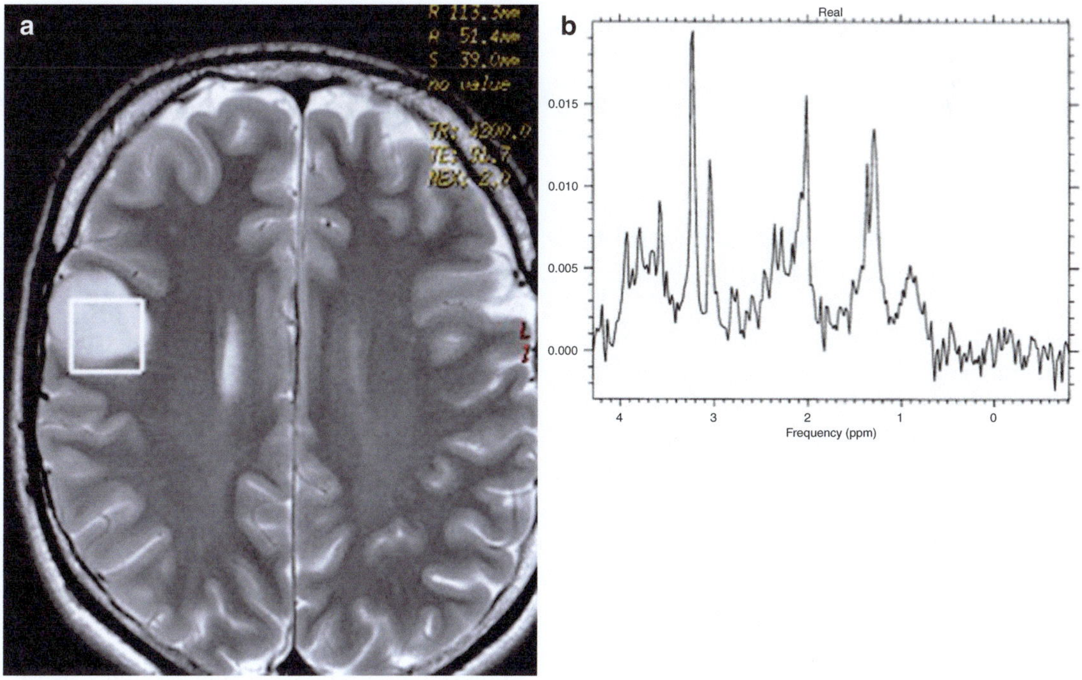


**Fig. 19.21** MR 3T. (**a**) Axial TSE T2-w image with volume of interest, (**b**)$^1$H MR spectrum (TR2000, TE 35) obtained from a VOI placed in oligodendroglioma. Glx at 2.05–2.50 ppm is higher than normal

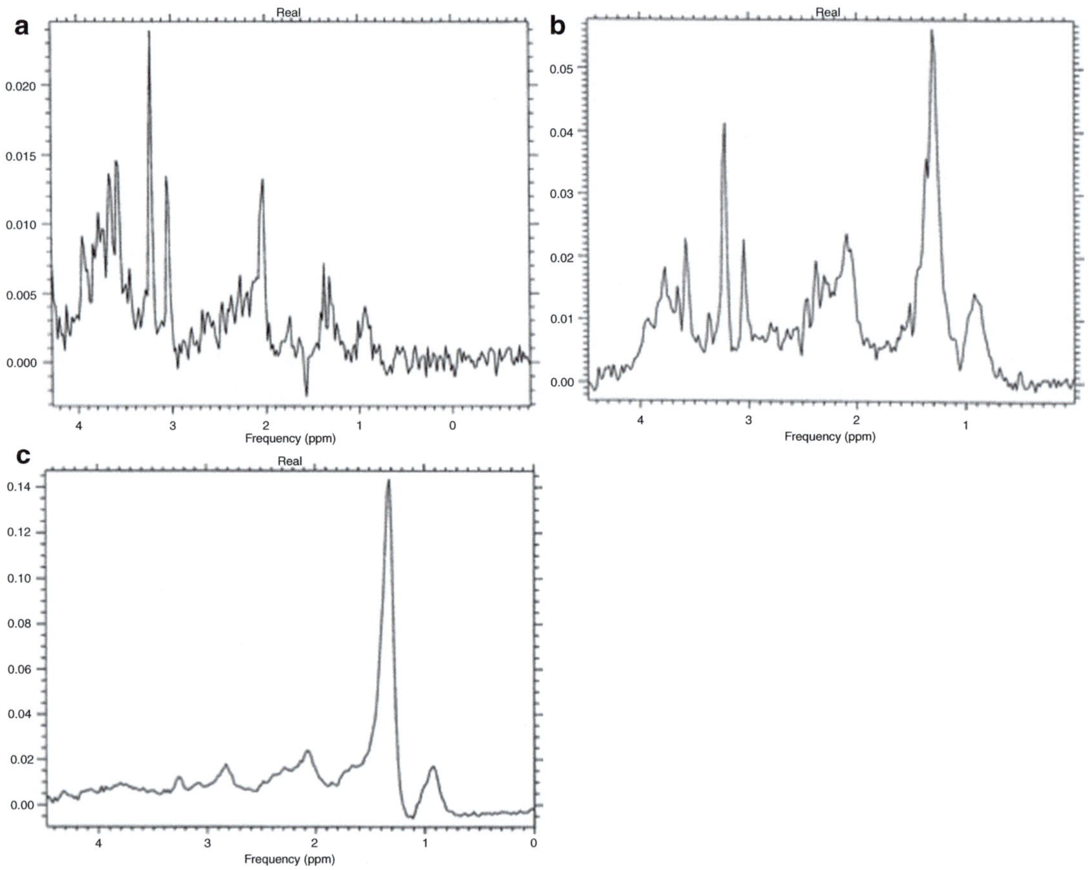


**Fig. 19.22** MR 3T. Spectra (TR2000, TE 35) obtained in (**a**) II° glioma, (**b**) III° glioma, (**c**) glioblastoma. The peak of Cho-containing compounds is usually higher in solid part of II° and III° gliomas. The peak of Cho-containing compounds is low in necrotic areas. NAA is decreased in brain tumors (destruction of normal tissue). mIns is elevated in low-grade gliomas and reducted in high-grade gliomas. Lipids and lactate are observed in high-grade lesions, and they are correlated with necrosis. In glioblastoma lipids and lactate represent the main characteristic of the spectrum

generally lacks necrosis, a lactate signal has been detected in some studies [175] (Fig. 19.20).

*WHO grade II gliomas* Grade II gliomas are generally infiltrative in their nature. Despite low-level proliferative activity, they often recur because a diffuse infiltration of the surrounding brain. It renders them incurable by surgery, and there is no improvement in local control or survival despite high-dose radiotherapy. Although grade II gliomas are generally considered as low-grade gliomas, they have a progressive tendency to higher grades of malignancy; thus, they considerably differ from grade I gliomas. About 70 % of grade gliomas transform to grade III and IV disease within 5–10 years after diagnosis [179]. Continuous growth and infiltration of brain parenchyma preferentially along the white matter fiber tracts, basement membranes of blood vessels, or other basement membrane-like structures are characteristic features of grade II gliomas. This tumor invasion causes destruction of both neurons and their axons organized in tracts. Because NAA reflects the integrity of neuronal component of nervous tissue, there is a decrease in peak of NAA on the MR spectra that represents the decrease in NAA concentration within the grade II gliomas compared to that in grade I gliomas. Generally, the increase cellular density of glioma due to proliferation of tumorous cell is connected with higher MRS peak of Cho-containing compounds (Fig. 19.22a). However, glial neoplasms with variable mass effect and a lack of contrast enhancement on MR images, thus typically grade II gliomas, can show no elevation of Cho or Cho/Cr ratio compared to values in a healthy brain [180]. This unusual MR spectroscopic pattern of some gliomas is connected with a marked increase in mIns [181]. Nevertheless, the correlation of the relative levels of Cho and NAA with the proliferation index Ki-67 of the tumor makes MRS helpful for detection of grade II glioma region with aggressive growth that are suitable targets for biopsy [182].

*WHO grade III gliomas* They are anaplastic astrocytomas that exhibit distinct hypercellularity with readily identifiable nuclear irregularities. Cell density is significantly higher than in low-grade infiltrating astrocytomas, but a critical microscopic feature of anaplastic astrocytoma, the main representative of the grade III gliomas, is the presence of mitotic figures [183]. Compared to the grade II gliomas, a progressive increase in the higher cell density of III gliomas reflects the fact that there is an additional increase in Cho concentration. Due to an infiltrative growth of grade III gliomas, these tumors consist of a core mass and a penumbra of invasive cells decreasing in number toward the periphery [184]. This histopathological feature of the anaplastic glioma results in a continuous decline in the NAA level from surrounding tissue toward the center of the tumor. On the other hand, there is a trend toward lower mIns levels in anaplastic astrocytomas compared with low-grade astrocytomas [170]. Although the lipid levels correlate with necrosis which is a histopathological feature of IV gliomas, there is an increase in mobile lipids within grade III gliomas caused by hypoxic stress of some tumor cells prior to necrosis [185, 186]. Inadequate blood supply leads to hypoxic stress of many quickly dividing cells following malignant transformation; thus, the increase in lipid MRS signals may be an early marker of malignant transformation prior to necrosis [156] (Fig. 19.22b).

*WHO grade IV gliomas* Glioblastoma is the most malignant glioma tumor with uncontrolled cellular proliferation and diffuse infiltration. Despite a prominent microvascular proliferation, blood supply is limited due to increasing tumor volume and presence of a microthrombotic process; thus, foci of necrosis surrounded by broad hypercellular zones are the most typical feature of glioblastoma allowing differentiation between the grade III and the grade IV gliomas [187, 188]. Tumorous cells under hypoxic stress can either develop an adaptive response that includes anaerobic glycolysis and angiogenesis or undergo cell death by promoting apoptosis and/or necrosis [189]. Cellular breakdown and necrosis is associated with the presence of lipids on the spectra, while lactate as a by-product of anaerobic glycolysis indicates hypoxic tumor metabolism, tumor infiltration, and growth. Thus, the typical MRS feature of glioblastoma is a high value of Lac and Lip (Fig. 19.22c). Since necrosis may comprise more than 80 % of the total glioblastoma volume, there is a significant decrease in the volume of the viable tumor tissue accompanied by a variable depression in the levels of Cho and other metabolites that are dependent on viable cells [190]. This fact leads to a decrease in commonly used metabolite ratios (NAA/Cho, Cho/Cr) measured by MRS despite the progression of glioma grade from III to IV. Progress in glioma grading is connected with a decrease in mIns level that has the lowest value in glioblastoma. An increase in concentration of the mIns level has been described in the contralateral normal-appearing white matter of patients with glioblastoma that is consistent with mild astrocytosis suspected of early infiltration by glial neoplastic cells [191].

At the end, it is important to understand that MRS is very sensitive to abnormal metabolic changes, but the specificity is relatively low. Gonzalez-Bonet [192] has stated that sensitivity, specificity, positive predictive value, and negative predictive value for identifying high-grade gliomas by MR spectroscopy are 89.9 %, 88.2 %, 95.3 %, and 79.7 %, respectively. Moreover, combining different advanced MR techniques has the potential to increase diagnostic accuracy [129]. The application of a comprehensive multiparametric MR protocol enables grading of gliomas with almost

100 % accuracy. This is likely to be due to complementary information provided from perfusion- and diffusion-weighted imaging and spectroscopic parameters [193]. The best performing MR modality, when considering the techniques separately, is DSC-MRI. However, a combination of the parameters of perfusion, diffusion, and Lips/tCho could still provide a better differentiation between high- and low-grade gliomas, possibly providing diagnosis on the individual patient level [194].

### 19.3.7 Treatment Response

MRI is a valid noninvasive tool for monitoring growth and response to therapy of gliomas. Several imaging features have been shown to have potential prognostic value.

The Macdonald criteria are based on bidimensional measurements of enhancing lesions in conjunction with clinical evaluation and corticosteroid use and have been used to assess the posttherapeutic response of high-grade gliomas [195]. These criteria define tumor progression as an increase in the size of the contrast-enhancing lesion or the appearance of new enhancing lesions. However, there are significant recognized limitations to these criteria, like the difficulty in measuring irregularly shaped tumors and multifocal lesions and the lack of assessment of nonenhancing portion of the neoplasm. Thus, tumor changes observed on FLAIR imaging characterized by the nonenhancing portion of the lesion are not assessed. Contrast enhancement in posttreatment brain neoplasms is a nonspecific finding and may not be considered a true surrogate marker for tumor response, because some treatment-related changes may be observed as a new area of contrast enhancement (Figs. 19.23e, 19.24, and 19.25).

Another possibility to assess the response to therapy is by the Response Assessment in Neuro-oncology (RANO) criteria, more recently published updated guidelines [196]. Based on prior observation after brain tumor therapy, these response criteria suggest that the nonenhancing component of the tumor should also be taken into account when making assessments about progression or response. The major modification proposed by the RANO guidelines is the assessment of the

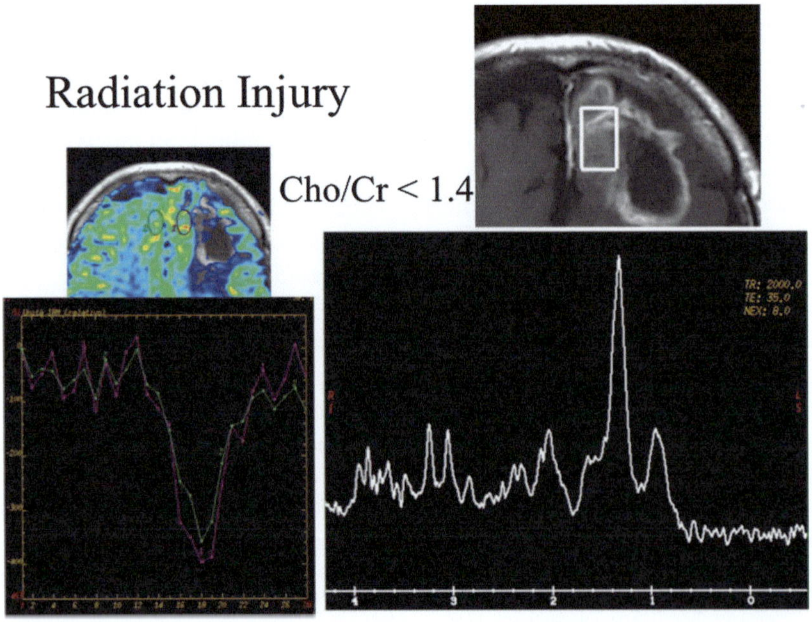


**Fig. 19.23** Radiation injury. The left frontal enhanced lesion shows rCBV similar to the healthy contralateral white matter, and the peak of Cho-containing compounds is in normal range. Lipids at 1.3 and 0.9 ppm are due to the radiation therapy

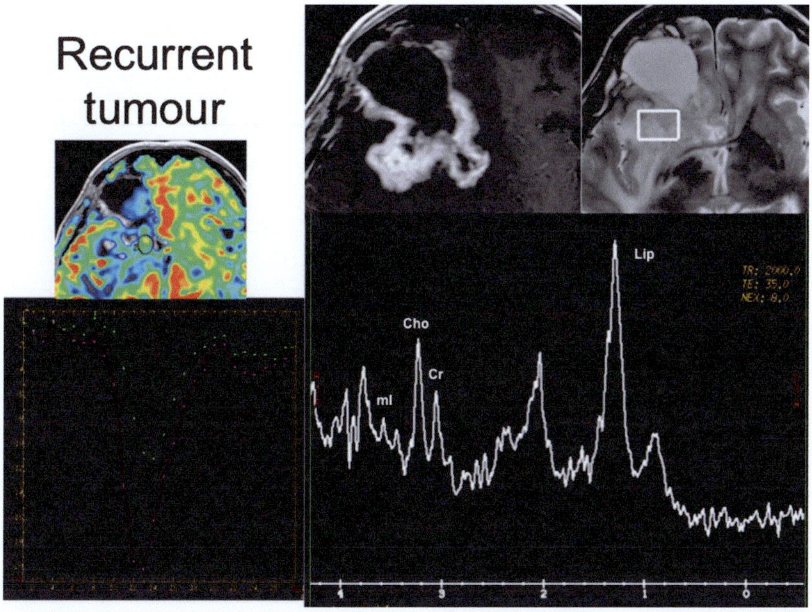


**Fig. 19.24** Recurrent tumor. The right frontal-enhanced lesion shows rCBV increased compared with the healthy contralateral white matter, and the peak of Cho-containing compounds is higher than the Cr peak. Lipids at 1.3 and 0.9 ppm are due to neoplastic necrosis and effect of the radiation therapy

nonenhancing area and the signal intensity changes on FLAIR imaging as evidence of tumor progression. The inclusion of nonenhancing tumor in the determination of overall tumor burden improves the accuracy of determining tumor progression in the setting of antiangiogenic therapy.

*Pseudoprogression* is defined as an increase in a contrast-enhancing lesion size just after completion of radiation therapy plus concomitant chemotherapy with TMZ in patients with high-grade tumors, followed by subsequent improvement or stabilization without any further treatment. It has been described in about 10–30 % of high-grade gliomas. The RANO criteria proposed that within the first 12 weeks of completion of radiation therapy, when pseudoprogression is most prevalent, tumor progression can only be determined if most of the new enhancement is outside the radiation field or if there is pathologic confirmation [197]. A high association between pseudoprogression and MGMT promoter status has been described. Pseudoprogression has been demonstrated in more than 90 % of high-grade gliomas with MGMT promoter methylation, while only 40 % of unmethylate MGMT patients have developed. Therefore, the MGMT methylation status is related to a high incidence of pseudoprogression as a consequence of higher sensitivity to treatment [196]. Pathologically, pseudoprogression is characterized as reactive radiation-induced changes, increased blood-brain barrier permeability, necrosis, edema, and gliosis. No single imaging technique has been validated to recognize and adequately establish a diagnosis of pseudoprogression. More recent publications have suggested that rCBV obtained from a DSC perfusion sequence may better predict a distinction between pseudoprogression and true tumor progression [198–200].

*Pseudoresponse* is caused by antiangiogenic agents used as second-line therapy for unresponsive or recurrent high-grade gliomas. These agents produce a rapid decrease in contrast enhancement, within hours, secondary to an antipermeability effect, with a pseudonormalization of the blood-brain barrier, rather than tumor reduction [196]. Thus, tumors appear to respond to treatment, and tumor progression is more difficult to detect. This phenomenon is denominated pseudoresponse. The pseudonormalization of the

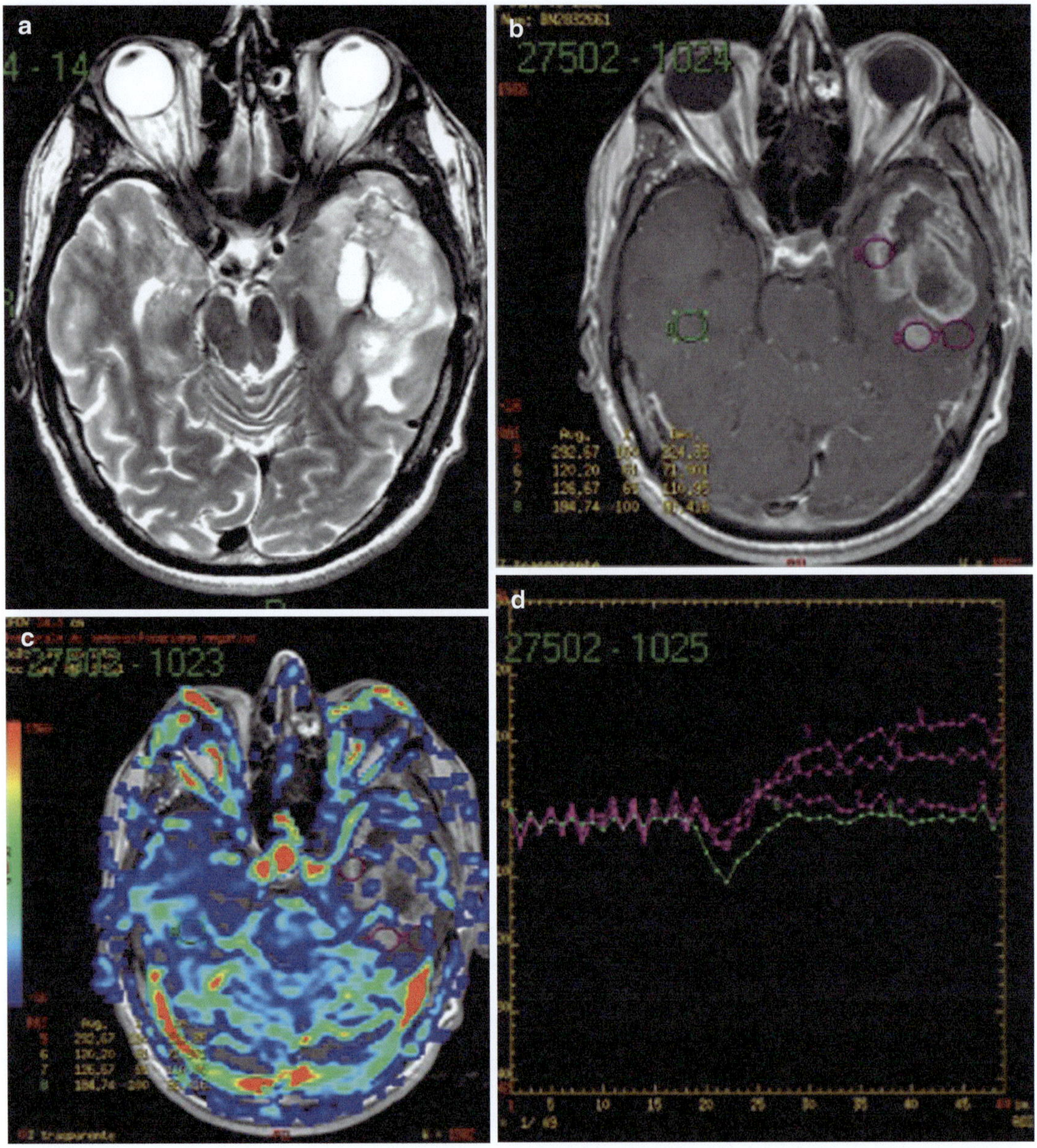


**Fig. 19.25** Axial MR 3T. (**a**) TSE T2-w image, (**b**) SE T1-w image after contrast administration and references of ROI rCBV, (**c**, **d**) rCBV map, and graphic. Pseudoprogression: a lesion with dishomogeneous signal and enhancement. rCBV is similar to the healthy contralateral white matter

blood-brain barrier leads to a reduction in the vasogenic edema, which may improve the clinical symptoms and brain function. Although some patients display clinical improvement with a high response rate and progression-free survival, only modest effects on overall survival were noted. Patients may present with an enlargement of the nonenhancing portion of the lesion on T2-weighted and FLAIR sequences in follow-up MR imaging examinations, corresponding to tumor progression [201]. During antiangiogenic treatment, areas with restricted diffusion may be seen within the lesion and even outside the confines of an enhancing tumor. Although some investigations suggest that these lesions reflect hypercellular and aggressive tumor [202], other studies suggest that these lesions represent chronic hypoxia and atypical gelatinous necrotic tissue [203]. These findings have implications for the management of patients with recurrent malignant gliomas.

## Bibliography


1. Vigneswaran K, Neill S, Hadjipanayis CG (2015) Beyond the World Health Organization grading of infiltrating gliomas: advances in the molecular genetics of glioma classification. Ann Transl Med 3(7):95
2. Ohgaki H (2009) Epidemiology of brain tumors. Methods Mol Biol Cancer Epidemiol 472(14):323–342
3. Nygaard R et al (1991) Second malignant neoplasms in patients treated for childhood leukemia. A population-based cohort study from Nordic countries. The nordic Society of Pediatric Oncology and Hematology (NOPHO). Acta Paediatr Scand 80:1220–1228
4. Little MP et al (1998) Risks of brain tumor following treatment for cancer in childhood: modification by genetic factors, radiotherapy and chemotherapy. Int. J Cancer 78:269–275
5. Walter AW et al (1998) Secondary brain tumors in children treated for acute lymphoblastic leukemia at St Jude Children's Research Hospital. J Clin Oncol 16:3761–3767
6. Brustle O et al (1992) Primitive neuroectodermal tumors after prophylactic central nervous system irradiation in children. Association with an activated K-ras gene. Cancer 69:2385–2392
7. Louis DN, Ohgaki H, Wiestler OD et al (2007) The 2007 WHO classification of tumors of the central nervous system. Acta Neuropathol 114:97–109
8. Van den Bent MJ (2010) Interobserver variation of the histopathological diagnosis in clinical trials on glioma: a clinician's perspective. Acta Neuropathol 120:297–304
9. Pollo B (2011) Neuropathological diagnosis of brain tumours. Neurol Sci 32(Suppl 2):S209–S211
10. Sun Y, Wei Z, Chen D et al (2014) A glioma classification scheme based on coexpression modules of EGFR and PDGFRA. PNAS 111(9):3539–3543
11. Hegi ME, Diserens AC, Gorlia T et al (2005) MGMT gene silencing and benefit from temozolomide in glioblastoma. N Engl J Med 352:997–1003
12. Stupp R, Hegi ME, Mason WP et al (2009) Effects of radiotherapy with concomitant and adjuvant temozolomide versus radiotherapy alone on survival in glioblastoma in a randomised phase III study: 5-year analysis of the EORTC-NCIC trial. Lancet Oncol 10(5):459–466
13. Brandes AA, Franceschi E, Ermani M et al (2014) Pattern of care and effectiveness of treatment for glioblastoma patients in the real world: results from a prospective population-based registry. Could survival differ in a high-volume center? Neurooncol Pract 1(4):166–171
14. Ceccarelli M, Barthel FP, Malta TM et al (2016) Molecular profiling reveals biologically discrete subsets and pathways of progression in diffuse glioma. Cell 164(3):550–563
15. Louis DN, Perry A, Burger P (2014) International Society of Neuropathology-Haarlem Consensus. Guidelines for nervous system tumor classification and grading. Brain Pathol 24:429–435
16. The Cancer Genome Atlas Research Network (2015) Comprehensive, integrative genomic analysis of diffuse lower-grade gliomas. N Engl J Med 372(26):2481–2498
17. Yan H, Parsons DW, Jin G et al (2009) IDH1 and IDH2 mutations in gliomas. N Engl J Med 360(8):765–773
18. Cairncross G, Wang M, Shaw E et al (2013) Phase III trial of chemoradiotherapy for anaplastic oligodendroglioma: long-term results of RTOG 9402. J Clin Oncol 31:337–343
19. Liu XY, Gerges N, Korshunov A et al (2012) Frequent ATRX mutations and loss of expression in adult diffuse astrocytic tumors carrying IDH1/IDH2 and TP53 mutations. Acta Neuropathol 124: 615–625
20. Eckel-Passow JE, Lachance DH, Molinaro AM (2015) Glioma groups based on 1p/19q, IDH, and TERT promoter mutations in tumors. N Engl J Med 372(26):2499–2508
21. Sahm F, Reuss D, Koelsche C, Capper D, Schittenhelm J, Heim S, Jones DT, Pfister SM, Herold-Mende C, Wick W, Mueller W, Hartmann C, Paulus W, von Deimling A (2014) Farewell to oligoastrocytoma: in situ molecular genetics favor classification as either oligodendroglioma or astrocytoma. Acta Neuropathol 128(4):551–559
22. Hinrichs BH, Newman S, Appin CL, Dunn W, Cooper L, Pauly R, Kowalski J, Rossi MR, Brat DJ (2016) Farewell to GBM-O: genomic and transcriptomic profiling of glioblastoma with oligodendroglioma component reveals distinct molecular subgroups. Acta Neuropathol Commun 4(1):4
23. Solomon DA, Wood MD, Tihan T, Bollen AW, Gupta N, Phillips JJ, Perry A (2015) Diffuse Midline Gliomas with histoneH3-K27M mutation: a series of 47 cases assessing the spectrum of morphologic variation and associated genetic alterations. Brain Pathol. doi:10.1111/bpa.12336
24. Buczkowicz P, Bartels U, Bouffet E, Becher O, Hawkins C (2014) Histopathologic spectrum of paediatric diffuse intrinsic pontine glioma: diagnostic and therapeutic implications. Acta Neuropathol 128:573–581
25. Pope WB (2015) Genomics of brain tumor. Neuroimag Clin N Am 25:105–119

26. Rutman AM, Kuo MD (2009) Radiogenomics creating a link between molecular diagnostics and diagnostic imaging. Eur J Radiol 70(2):232–241
27. Elbanan MG, Ahmed MA et al (2015) Imaging genomics of glioblastoma. State of the art bridge between genomics and neuroradiology. Neuroimag Clin N Am 25:141–153
28. Liang Y, Diehn M et al (2005) Gene expression profiling reveals molecularly and clinically distinct subtypes of glioblastoma multiforme. Proc Natl Acad Sci U S A 102(16):5814–5819
29. Smith AB, Smirniotopoulos JG (2013) Intra-axial neoplasms. Imaging Brain 32:692–727, Saunders Elsevier
30. Atlas SW, Lavi E, Fisher PG (2002) Intraaxial brain tumors. Magn Res Brain I(14):565–693
31. Jenkinson MD, Du Plessis DG et al (2007) Advanced MRI in the management of adult gliomas. Br J Neurosurg 21(6):550–561
32. Kim JJ, Mukherjee S (2013) Static anatomic techniques. Imaging Brain 1:3–22, Saunders Elsevier
33. RTOG Study Chairs (Coordinanting Group) PHASE III double-blind placebo-controlled trial of conventional concurrent chemoradiation and adjuvant temozolamide plus bevacizumab versus conventional concurrent chemoradiation and adjuvant temozolamide in patients with newly diagnosted glioblastoma. ACRIN: American College of Radiology Imaging Network 2009.aspx. Accessed 14 Jan 2011
34. Attenberger UI, Runge VM, Morelli JN et al (2010) Evaluation of gadobutrol, a macrocyclic, nonionic gadolinium chelate in a brain glioma model: comparison with gadoterate meglumine and gadopentetate dimeglumine 1.5T, combined with an assessment of field strength dependence, specifically 1.5 versus 3T. J Magn Reson Imaging 31:549–555
35. Biswas J, Nelson CB, Runge VM et al (2005) Brain tumor enhancement in a magnetic resonance imaging: comparison of signal-noise-ratio (SNR) and contrast-to-noise-ratio (CNR) at 1.5 versus 3 Tesla. Invest Radiol 40:792–797
36. Wiggins GC, Triantafyllou C, Potthast A et al (2006) 32-channels 3 Tesla receive only phase array head coil with soccer ball element geometry. Magn Reson Med 56:216–223
37. Wiggins GC, Polimeni JR, Potthast A et al (2009) 96-channel-receive only head coil for 3 Tesla: design optimization and evaluation. Magn Reson Med 62:754–762
38. Ba-Salamah A, Nobauer-Huhmann IM, Pinker K et al (2003) Effect of contrast dose and field strength in the magnetic resonance detection of brain metastases. Invest Radiol 38:415–422
39. Schneider G, Kirchin MA, Pirovano G et al (2001) Gadobenate dimeglumine-enhanced magnetic resonance imaging of intracranial metastases: effect of dose on lesion detection and delineation. J Magn Reson Imaging 14:525–539
40. Engelhorn T, Schwartz MA, Eyupoglu IY et al (2010) Dynamic contrast enhancement of experimental glioma an intra-individual comparative study to assess the optimal time delay. Acad Radiol 17:188–193
41. Burger PC, Scheithauer BW (1994) Atlas of tumor pathology, 3rd series, fascicle 10: Tumors of the central nervous system. Armed Forces Institute of Pathology, Washington, DC
42. Kovalikova Z, Hoehn-Berlage MH et al (1987) Age-dependent variation of T1 and T2-relaxation times of adenocarcinoma in mice. Radiology 164:543–548
43. Hackney DB, Grossman RI et al (1987) Low sensitivity of clinical MR imaging to small changes in the concentration of non-paramagnetic protein. AJNR Am J Neuroradiol 8:1003–1008
44. Bradley WG, Schmidt PG (1985) Effect of methemoglobin formation on the MR appearance of subarachnoid hemorrhage. Radiology 156:99–103
45. Gatenby RA, Coia LR et al (1985) Oxygen tension in human tumors: in vivo mapping using CT-guided probes. Radiology 156:211–214
46. Sze G, Krol G et al (1987) Hemorrhagic neoplasms: MR imaging mimics of occult vascular malformations. AJR Am J Roentgenol 149:1223–1230
47. Smirniotopoulos JG, Smith A et al (2013) Pattern of contrast enhancement. Imaging Brain 5:79–95, Saunders Elsevier
48. Sage MR (1982) Blood-brain barrier: phenomenon of increasing importance to the imaging clinician. AJR Am J Roentgenol 138:887–898
49. Takeuki H, Kubota T et al (2004) Ultrastructure of capillary endothelium in pilocytic astrocytomas. Brain Tumor Pathol 21:23–26
50. Scott JN, Pm B et al (2002) How often are nonenhancing supratentorial gliomas malignant? A population study. Neurology 59:947–949
51. Diehn M, Nardini C et al (2008) Identification of noninvasive imaging surrogates for brain tumor gene-expression modules. Proc Natl Acad Sci U S A 105(13):5213–5218
52. Pope WB, Chen JH et al (2008) Relationship between gene-expression and enhancement in glioblastoma multiforme: exploratory DNA microarray analysis. Radiology 249(1):268–277
53. Carrillo JA, Lai A et al (2012) Relationship between tumor enhancement, edema, IDH1 mutational status, MGMT promoter methylation, and survival in glioblastoma. AJNR Am J Neurorad 33(7):1349–1355
54. Drabycz S, Roldan G et al (2010) An analysis of image texture, tumor location, and MGMT promoter methylation in glioblastoma using magnetic resonance imaging. Neuroimage 49(2):1398–1405
55. Ellingson MB, LaViolette PS et al (2011) Spatially quantifying microscopic tumor invasion and proliferation using a Voxel-Wise solution to a glioma growth model and serial diffusion MRI. Magn Reson Med 65(4):1131–1143
56. Sugahara T, Korogi Y et al (1999) Usefulness of diffusion-weighted MRI with echo-planar technique in the evaluation of cellularity in gliomas. J Magn Reson Imaging 9:53–60
57. Hayashida Y, Hirai T et al (2006) Diffusion-weighted imaging of metastatic brain tumors: comparison

with histologic type and tumor cellularity. AJNR Am J Neurorad 27(7):1419–1425
58. Kinoshita M, Hashimoto N et al (2008) Fractional anisotropy and tumor cell density of the tumor core show positive correlation in diffusion tensor magnetic resonance imaging of malignant tumors. Neuroimage 43(1):29–35
59. Kono K, Inoue Y et al (2001) The role of diffusion-weighted imaging in patients with brain tumors. AJNR Am J Neuroradiol 22(6):1081–1088
60. Maier SE, Sun Y, Mulkern R (2010) Diffusion imaging of brain tumors. NMR Biomed 23(7):849–864
61. Yamasaki F, Kurisu K et al (2005) Apparent diffusion coefficient of human brain 232 tumors at MR imaging. Radiology 235:985–991
62. Lee EJ, Ahn KJ et al (2013) Potential role of advanced MRI techniques for the peritumoral region in differentiating glioblastoma multiforme and solitary metastatic lesions. Clin Radiol 68:689–697
63. Alexiou GA, Tsiouris S et al (2010) Assessment of glioma proliferation using imaging modalities. J Clin Neurosci 17:1233–1238
64. Kiss R, Dewitte O et al (1997) The combined determination of proliferative activity and cell density in the prognosis of adult patients with supratentorial high-grade astrocytic tumors. Am J Clin Pathol 107:321–331
65. Muarakami R, Hirai T et al (2009) Grading astrocytic tumor by using apparent diffusion coefficient parameters: superiority of one-versus two parameters pilot method. Radiology 251:838–845
66. Lee EJ, Lee SK et al (2008) Preoperative grading of presumptive low-grade astrocytomas on MR imaging: diagnostic value of minimum apparent diffusion coefficient. Am J Neuroradiol 29:1872–1877
67. Yang D, Korogi Y et al (2002) Cerebral gliomas: prospective comparison of multivoxel 2D chemical-shift proton MR spectroscopy, echoplanar perfusion and diffusion-weighted MRI. Neuroradiology 44:656–666
68. Morita K, Matsuzawa H et al (2005) Diffusion tensor analysis of peritumoral edema using lambda chart analysis indicative of the heterogeneity of the microstructure within edema. J Neurosurg 102(2):336–341
69. Lying H, Haraldseth O et al (2000) Measurement of cell density and necrotic fraction in human melanoma xenografts by diffusion weighted magnetic resonance imaging. Magn Reson Med 43(6):828–836
70. Chenevert TL, McKeever PE, Ross BD (1997) Monitoring early response of experimental brain tumors to therapy using diffusion magnetic resonance imaging. Clin Cancer Res 3:1457–1466
71. Chan YL, Yeug DK et al (2003) Diffusion weighted magnetic resonance imaging in radiation-induced cerebral necrosis. Apparent diffusion coefficient in lesion component. J Comput Assist Tomogr 27(5):674–680
72. Mardor Y, Roth Y et al (2004) Pre-treatment prediction of brain tumors response to radiation therapy using high b-value diffusion-weighted MRI. Neoplasia 6(2):136–142
73. Basser PJ, Mattiello J, LeBihan D (1994) Estimation of the effective self-diffusion tensor from the NMR spin echo. J Magn Reson B 103(3):247–254
74. Lin CP, Tseng WY et al (2001) Validation of diffusion tensor magnetic resonance axonal fiber imaging with registered manganese-enhanced optic tracts. Neuroimage 14(5):1035–1047
75. Beaulieu C (2002) The basis of anisotropic water diffusion in the nervous system-a technical review. NMR Biomed 15(7–8):435–455
76. Mori S, Barker PB (1999) Diffusion magnetic resonance imaging: its principle and applications. Anat Rec 257(3):102–109
77. Mori S, van Zijl PC (2002) Fiber tracking: principles and strategies – a technical review. NMR Biomed 15(7–8):468–480
78. Pajevic S, Pierpaoli C (1999) Color schemes to represent the orientation of the anisotropic tissue from diffusion tensor data: application to white matter fiber tract mapping in the human brain. Magn Reson Med 42(3):526–540
79. Witwer BP, Moftakhar R et al (2002) Diffusion-tensor imaging of white matter tracts in patients with cerebral neoplasm. J Neurosurg 97(3):568–575
80. Bello L, Gambini A, Castellano A et al (2008) Motor and language DTI fiber tracking combined with intraoperative sub cortical mapping for surgical removal of gliomas. Neuroimage 39(1): 369–382
81. Lu S, Ahn D et al (2003) Peritumoral diffusion tensor imaging of high grade gliomas and metastatic brain tumors. AJNR Am J Neuroradiol 58(6):937–994
82. Smits M, Vernooij MW et al (2007) Incorporating functional MR imaging into diffusion tensor tractography in the preoperative assessment of the corticospinal tract in patients with brain tumors. AJNR Am J Neuroradiol 28(7):1354–1361
83. Wieshmann UC, Symms MR et al (2000) Diffusion tensor imaging demonstrates deviation of fibres in normal appearing white matter adjacent to a brain tumour. J Neurol Neurosurg Psychiatry 68(4):501–503
84. Yamada K, Kizu O, Mori S et al (2003) Brain fiber tracking with clinically feasible diffusion-tensor MR imaging: initial experience. Radiology 227(1): 295–301
85. Field AS, Alexander AL et al (2004) Diffusion tension eigenvector directional color imaging patterns in the evaluation of cerebral white matter tracts altered by tumor. J Magn Reson Imaging 20(4):555–562
86. Golby AJ, Kindlmann G et al (2011) Interactive diffusion tensor tractography visualization for neurosurgical planning. Neurosurgery 68(2):496–505
87. Gupta A, Shah A et al (2010) Imaging of brain tumors: functional magnetic resonance imaging and diffusion tensor imaging. Neuroimaging Clin N Am 20:379–400
88. Byrnes TJ, Barrick TR et al (2011) Diffusion tensor imaging discriminates between glioblastoma and cerebral metastases in vivo. NMR Biomed 24:54–60

89. Sinha S, Bastin ME et al (2002) Diffusion tensor imaging of high-grade cerebral gliomas. AJNR Am J Neuroradiol 23:520–527
90. Beppu T, Inoue T et al (2003) Measurement of fractional anisotropy using diffusion tensor MRI in supratentorial astrocytic tumors. J Neurooncol 6:109–116
91. White ML, Zhang Y et al (2011) Diffusion tensor MR imaging of cerebral gliomas: evaluation fractional anisotropy characteristics. AJNR Am J Neuroradiol 32:374–381
92. Alexiou GA, Zikou A et al (2014) Correlation of diffusion tensor, dynamic susceptibility contrast MRI and $^{99m}$Tc-Tetrofosmin brain SPECT with tumour grade and Ki-67 immunohistochemistry in glioma. Clin Neurol Neurosurg 116:41–45
93. Goebell E, Paustenbach S et al (2006) Low-grade and anaplastic gliomas: differences in architecture evaluated with diffusion-tensor MR imaging. Radiology 239(1):217–222
94. Castellano A, Bello L et al (2012) Role of diffusion tensor magnetic resonance tractography in predicting the extent of resection in glioma surgery. Neuro Oncol 14(2):192–202
95. Server A, Graff BA et al (2014) Analysis of diffusion tensor imaging metrics for gliomas grading at 3 T. Eur J Radiol 83:156–165
96. Yuan W, Holland SK et al (2008) Characterization of abnormal diffusion properties of supratentorial brain tumors: a preliminary diffusion tensor imaging study. J Neurosurg Pediatr 1(4):263–269
97. Budde MD, Xie M et al (2009) Axial diffusivity is the primary correlate of axonal injury in the experimental autoimmune encephalomyelitis spinal cord: a quantitative pixelwise analysis. J Neurosci 29(9):2805–2813
98. Klawiter EC, Schmidt RE et al (2011) Radial diffusivity predicts demyelination in ex vivo multiple sclerosis spinal cords. Neuroimage 55(4):1454–1460
99. Inano R, Oishi N et al (2014) Voxel-based clustered imaging by multiparameter diffusion tensor images for glioma grading. Neuroimage Clin 5:396–407
100. Law M, Babb S et al (2006) Low-grade gliomas: dynamic susceptibility-weighted contrast enhanced perfusion MR imaging – prediction of patient clinical response. Radiology 238:658–667
101. Tuch DS (2004) Q-ball imaging. Magn Reson Med 52(6):1358–1372
102. Tan WL, Huang WY et al (2014) Can diffusion tensor imaging noninvasively detect IDH1 gene mutations in astrogliomas? A retrospective study of 112 cases. AJNR Am J Neuroradiol 35:920–927
103. Bisdas S et al (2013) Intravoxel incoherent motion diffusion-weighted MR imaging of gliomas; feasibility of the method and initial results. Neuroradiology 55:1189–1196
104. Hu Y-C, L-F Y et al (2014) Intravoxel incoherent motion diffusion-weighted MR imaging of gliomas: efficacy in preoperative grading. Sci Rep 4:7208
105. Higano S et al (2006) Malignant astrocytic tumors: clinical importance of apparent diffusion coefficient in prediction of grade and prognosis. Radiology 241:839–846
106. Wen PY, Kesari S (2008) Malignant gliomas in adults. N Engl J Med 359:492–507
107. Iima M et al (2014) Characterization of glioma microcirculation and tissue features using intravoxel incoherent motion magnetic resonance imaging in a rat brain model. Invest Radiol 49:485–490
108. Kang Y et al (2011) Gliomas: histogram analysis of apparent diffusion coefficient maps with standard- or high-b-value diffusion-weighted MR imaging–correlation with tumor grade. Radiology 261:882–890
109. Plate KH, Breier G, Weich HA, Risau W (1992) Vascular endothelial growth factor is a potential tumour angiogenesis factor in human gliomas in vivo. Nature 359:845–848
110. Luciani A et al (2008) Liver cirrhosis: intravoxel incoherent motion MR imaging–pilot study. Radiology 249:891–899
111. Thompson G, Mills SJ, Coope DJ, O'Connor JP, Jackson A (2011) Imaging biomarkers of angiogenesis and the microvascular environment in cerebral tumours. Br J Radiol 84 Spec No 2:S127–S144
112. Shin JH et al (2002) Using relative cerebral blood flow and volume to evaluate the histopathologic grade of cerebral gliomas: preliminary results. AJR Am J Roentgenol 179:783–789
113. Hu LS et al (2012) Correlations between perfusion MR imaging cerebral blood volume, microvessel quantification, and clinical outcome using stereotactic analysis in recurrent high-grade glioma. AJNR Am J Neuroradiol 33:69–76
114. Essig M, Shiroishi MS et al (2013) Perfusion MRI: the five most frequently asked technical questions. AJR Am J Roentgenol 200(1):24–34
115. Brix G, Semmler W et al (1991) Pharmacokinetic parameters in CNS Gd-DTPA enhanced MR imaging. J Comput Assist Tomogr 15:621–628
116. Kim HS, Kim SY (2007) A prospective study on the added value of pulsed arterial spin labeling and apparent diffusion coefficients in the grading of gliomas. AJNR Am J Neuroradiol 28:1693–1699
117. Kwong KK, Chesler DA et al (1995) MR perfusion studies with T1-weighted echo planar imaging. Magn Reson Med 34:878–887
118. Petersen ET, Zimine I et al (2006) Non-invasive measurement of perfusion: a critical review of arterial spin labelling techniques. Br J Radiol 79:688–701
119. Golay X, Hendrikse J, Lim TC (2004) Perfusion imaging using arterial spin labelling. Top Magn Reson Imaging 15:10–27
120. Wu WC, Jiang SC, Lien SH (2011) Pseudocontinuous arterial spin labelling perfusion magnetic resonance imaging: a normative study of reproducibility in the human brain. Neuroimage 56:1244–1250
121. Jenkinson MD, Smith TS, Joyce KA et al (2006) Cerebral Blood volume, genotype and chemosensitivity in oligodendroglial tumours. Neuroradiology 48:703–713

122. Jarnum H, Stefferson EG et al (2010) Perfusion MRI of brain tumours: a comparative study of pseudocontinuous arterial spin labeling and dynamic susceptibility contrast imaging. Neuroradiology 52:307–317
123. Vaupel P, Mayer A (2007) Hypoxia in cancer: significance and impact on clinical outcome. Cancer Metastasis Rev 26:225–239
124. Bar EE (2011) Glioblastoma, cancer stem cells and hypoxia. Brain Pathol 21:119–129
125. Folkman J (1971) Tumor angiogenesis: therapeutic implications. N Engl J Med 285:1182–1186
126. Provenzale JM, Wang GR et al (2002) Comparison of permeability in high-grade and low-grade brain tumors using dynamic susceptibility contrast MR imaging. AJR Am J Roentgenol 178(3):711–716
127. Maia ACM Jr, Malheiros SMF et al (2005) MR cerebral Blood volume maps correlated with vascular endothelial growth factor expression and tumor grade in nonenhancing gliomas. AJNR Am J Neuroradiol 26(4):777–783
128. Aronen HJ, Perkio J (2002) Dynamic susceptibility contrast MRI of gliomas. Neuroimaging Clin N Am 12:501–523
129. Law M, Yang S et al (2003) Glioma grading: sensitivity, specificity and predictive values of perfusion MR imaging and proton MR spectroscopic imaging compared with conventional MR imaging. AJNR Am J Neuroradiol 24(10):1989–1998
130. Shin JH, Lee HK et al (2002) Using relative cerebral blood flow and volume to evaluate the histopathologic grade of cerebral gliomas: preliminary results. Am J Roentgenol 179(3):783–789
131. Wong JC, Provenzale JM, Petrella JR (2000) Perfusion MR imaging of rain neoplasms. Am J Roentgenol 174(4):1147–1157
132. Lacerda S, Law M (2009) Magnetic resonance perfusion and permeability imaging in brain tumors. Neuroimag Clin N Am 19:527–557
133. Law M, Young R et al (2006) Comparing perfusion metrics obtained from a single compartment versus pharmacokinetic modeling methods using dynamic susceptibility contrast-enhanced perfusion MR imaging with glioma grade. AJNR Am J Neuroradiol 27(9):1975–1982
134. Aronen HJ, Gazit IE et al (1994) Cerebral blood volume maps of gliomas: comparison with tumor grade and histologic findings. Radiology 191(1):41–51
135. Lev MH, Rosen BR (1999) Clinical applications of intracranial perfusion MR imaging. Neuroimaging Clin N Am 9(2):309–331
136. Law M, Yang S et al (2004) Comparison of cerebral blood volume and vascular permeability from dynamic susceptibility contrast-enhanced perfusion MR imaging with glioma grade. AJNR Am J Neuroradiol 25(5):746–755
137. Lupo JM, Cha S et al (2005) Dynamic susceptibility-weighted perfusion imaging of high-grade gliomas: characterization of spatial heterogeneity. AJNR Am J Neuroradiol 26(6):1446–1454
138. Hacklander T, Hofer M et al (1995) Possibilities of the use of MR tomography-based cerebral blood volume maps in the diagnosis of brain tumors. Rofo 163:484–489
139. Lam WW, Chan KW et al (2001) Pre-operative grading of intracranial glioma. Acta Radiol 42:548–554
140. Boxerman JL, Schmainda KM et al (2006) Relative cerebral blood volume maps corrected for contrast agent extravasation significantly correlate with glioma tumor grade, whereas uncorrected maps do not. AJNR Am J Neuroradiol 27(4):859–867
141. Boxerman JL, Hamberg LM et al (1995) MR contrast due to intravascular magnetic susceptibility perturbations. Magn Reson Med 34:555–566
142. Donahue KM, HG K et al (2000) Utility of simultaneously acquired gradient-echo and spin-echo cerebral blood volume and morphology maps in brain tumor patients. Magn Reson Med 43:845–853
143. Schmainda KM, Rand SD et al (2004) Characterization of a first-pass gradient-echo spin-echo method to predict brain tumor grade and angiogenesis. AJNR Am J Neuroradiol 25:1524–1532
144. Kerbel RS (2008) Tumor angiogenesis. N Engl J Med 358(19):2039–2049
145. Danchaivijitr N, Waldman AD et al (2008) Low-grade gliomas: do changes in rCBV measurements at longitudinal perfusion-weighted MR imaging predict malignant transformation? Radiology 247(1):170–178
146. Bobek Billewicz B, Stasik-Pres G et al (2014) Anaplastic transformation of low-grade glioma (WHO II) on magnetic resonance imaging. Folia Neuropathol 52(2):128–140
147. Henson JW, Ulmer S et al (2008) Brain tumor imaging in clinical trials. AJNR Am J Neuroradiol 29:419–424
148. Liu X, Tian W et al (2011) MR diffusion tensor and perfusion weighted imaging in preoperative grading of supratentorial nonenhancing gliomas. Neuro Oncol 13:447–455
149. Quant EC, Wen PY (2011) Response assessment in neuro-oncology. Curr Oncol Rep 13:50–56
150. Law M, Young RJ et al (2008) Gliomas: predicting time to progression or survival with cerebral blood volume measurement at dynamic susceptibility-weighted contrast-enhancement perfusion MR imaging. Radiology 247:490–498
151. Batchelor TT, Sorensen AG et al (2007) AZD2171, a pan-VEGF receptor tyrosine kinase inhibitor normalizes tumor vasculature and alleviates edema in glioblastoma patients. Cancer Cell 11(1):83–95
152. Jain R, Poisson L et al (2013) Genomic mapping and survival prediction in glioblastoma: molecular subclassification strengthened by hemodynamic imaging biomarkers. Radiology 267(1):212–220
153. Naeini KM, Pope WB et al (2013) Identifying the mesenchymal molecular subtype of glioblastoma

using quantitative volumetric analysis of anatomic magnetic resonance images. Neuro Oncol 15(5):626–634
154. Salibi N, Brown MA (1998) Clinical MR spectroscopy: first principles, vol 1, pp 1–4
155. Cecil Kim M (2013) Proton magnetic resonance spectroscopy. Technique for the neuroradiologist. Neuroimag Clin N Am 23:381–392
156. Bulik M, Jancalek R et al (2013) Potential of MR spectroscopy for assessment of glioma grading. Clin Neurol Neurosurg 115:146–153
157. Bertholdo D, Watcharakorn A, Castillo M (2013) Brain proton magnetic resonance spectroscopy. introduction and overview. Neuroimag Clin N Am 23:359–380
158. Fayed N, Olmos S et al (2006) Physical basis of magnetic resonance spectroscopy and its application to central nervous system diseases. Am J Appl Sci 3:1836–1845
159. Nagae-Poetscher LM, Bonekamp D et al (2004) Asymmetry and gender effect in functionally lateralized cortical regions: a proton MRS imaging study. J Magn Reson Imaging 19(1):27–33
160. Hetherington HP, Mason GF et al (1994) Evaluation of cerebral gray and white matter metabolite difference by spectroscopic imaging at 4.1T. Magn Reson Med 32:565–571
161. Kreis R, Ernst T et al (1993) Absolute quantitation of water and metabolites in the human brain. II. Metabolite concentrations. J Magn Reson B 102:9–19
162. Moller-Hartmann W, Hermighaus S et al (2002) Clinical application of proton magnetic resonance spectroscopy in the diagnosis of intracranial mass lesions. Neuroradiology 44:371–381
163. Warren KE, Frank JA et al (2000) Proton magnetic resonance spectroscopic imaging in children with recurrent primary brain tumors. J Clin Oncol 18:1020–1026
164. Young GS (2007) Advanced MRI of adult brain tumors. Neurol Clin 25:947–973
165. Hernandez-Alcoceba R, Saninger L et al (1997) Choline kinase inhibitors as a novel approach for antiproliferative drug design. Oncogene 15:2289–2301
166. Scholzen T, Gerdes J (2000) The Ki-67 protein: from the known and the unknown. J Cell Physiol 182:311–322
167. Barbarella G, Ricci R et al (1998) In vivo single voxel [1]HMRS of glial brain tumor: correlation with tissue histology and in vitro MRS. Int J Oncol 12: 461–468
168. Shimizu H, Kumabe T et al (2000) Correlation between choline level measured by proton MR spectroscopy and Ki-67 labeling index in gliomas. AJNR Am J Neuroradiol 21:659–665
169. Kreis R, Ernst T, Ross BD (1993) Development of the human brain: in vivo quantification of metabolite and water content with proton magnetic resonance spectroscopy. Magn Reson Med 30: 424–437
170. Castillo M, Smith JK et al (2000) Correlation of myo-inositol levels and grading of cerebral astrocytomas. AJNR Am J Neuroradiol 21:1645–1649
171. Brandao LA, Castillo M (2013) Adult brain tumors. Clinical applications of magnetic resonance spectroscopy. Neuroimaging Clin N Am 23:527–555
172. Esmaeili M, Vettukattil R, Bathen TF (2013) 2-Hydroxyglutarate as a magnetic resonance biomarker for glioma subtyping. Trans Oncol 6(2):92–98
173. Andronesi OC, Kim GS et al (2012) Detection of 2-Hydroxyglutarate in iDH-mutated glioma patients by in vivo spectral-editing and 2D correlation magnetic resonance spectroscopy. Sci Transl Med 4(116):116ra4
174. Lazovic J, Soto H et al (2012) Detection of 2-Hydroxyglutaric acid in vivo by proton magnetic resonance spectroscopy in U87 glioma cells overexpressing isocitrate dehydrogenase-1 mutation. Neuro Oncol 14(12):1465–1472
175. Hwang JH, Egnaczyk GF et al (1998) Proton MR spectroscopic characteristic of pediatric pilocytic astrocytomas. AJNR Am J Neuroradiol 19:535–540
176. Sutton LN, Wang Z et al (1992) Proton magnetic resonance spectroscopy of pediatric brain tumors. Neurosurgery 31:195–202
177. Davies NP, Wilson M et al (2008) Identification and characterisation of childhood cerebellar tumours by in vivo proton MRS. NMR Biomed 21:908–918
178. Harris LN, Davies NP et al (2008) Magnetic resonance spectroscopy in the assessment of pilocytic astrocytomas. Eur J Cancer 44:2640–2647
179. Furnari FB, Fenton T et al (2007) Malignant astrocytic glioma: genetics, biology, and paths to treatment. Genes Dev 21:2683–2710
180. Londono A, Castillo M et al (2003) Unusual MR spectro-myo-inositol and glycine levels. AJNR Am J Neuroradiol 24:942–945
181. Saraf-Lavi E, Bowen BC et al (2003) Proton MR spectroscopy of gliomatosis cerebri: case report of elevated myoinositol with normal choline levels. AJNR Am J Neuroradiol 24:946–951
182. McKnight TR, Lamborn KR et al (2007) Correlation of magnetic resonance spectroscopic and growth characteristics within Grades II and III gliomas. J Neurosurg 106:660–666
183. Burger PC, Vogel FS et al (1985) Glioblastoma multiforme and anaplastic astrocytoma. Pathologic criteria and prognostic implications. Cancer 56:1106–1111
184. Giese A, Bjerkvig R et al (2003) Cost of migration: invasion of malignant gliomas and implications for treatment. J Clin Oncol 21:1624–1636
185. Howe FA, Barton SJ et al (2003) Metabolic profiles of human brain tumors using quantitative in vivo 1H magnetic resonance spectroscopy. Magn Reson Med 49:223–232
186. Remy C, Fouilhe N et al (1997) Evidence that mobile lipids detected in rat brain glioma by 1 H nuclear

magnetic resonance correspond to lipid droplets. Cancer Res 57:407–414
187. Raza SM, Lang FF et al (2002) Necrosis and glioblastoma: a friend or a foe? A review and a hypothesis. Neurosurgery 51:2–12 , discussion 12–13
188. Brat DJ, Van Meir EG (2004) Vaso-occlusive and prothrombotic mechanism associated with tumor hypoxia, necrosis, and accelerated growth in glioblastoma. Laboratory investigation. J Tech Methods Pathol 84:397–405
189. Olivier L, Olivier C et al (2009) Hypoxia and the malignant glioma microenvironment: regulation and implications for therapy. Curr Mol Pharmacol 2:263–284
190. Kleihues P (2000) Pathology and genetics of tumours of the nervous system. In: Kleihues P, WK C (eds) World Health Organization classification of tumors. IARC Press, Lyon
191. Kallenberg K, Bock HC et al (2009) Untreated glioblastoma multiforme: increased myo-inositol and glutamine levels in the contralateral cerebral hemisphere at proton MR spectroscopy. Radiology 253:805–812
192. Gonzalez-Bonet LG (2008) Stereotactic biopsy versus spectroscopy in cases of gliomas with a high degree of malignancy. A review of the literature. Rev Neurol 47:310–314
193. Roy B, Gupta KR et al (2013) Utility of multiparametric 3-T MRI for glioma characterization. Neuroradiology 55:603–613
194. Van Cauter S, De Keyzer F et al (2014) Integrating diffusion kurtosis imaging, dynamic susceptibility-weighted contrast-enhanced MRI, and short echo time chemical shift imaging for grading gliomas. Neurooncology 16(7):1010–1021
195. Macdonald DR, Cascino T et al (1990) Response criteria for phase II studies of supretentorial malignant glioma. J Clin Oncol 8:1277–1280
196. Hygino da Cruz LC Jr, Rodriguez I et al (2011) Pseudoprogression and pseudoresponse: imaging challenges in the assessment of posttreatment glioma. AJNR Am J Neuroradiol 32(11):1978–1985
197. Wen PY, Macdonald DR et al (2010) Updated response assessment criteria for high-grade gliomas: response assessment in neuro-oncology working group. J Clin Oncol 28:1963–1972
198. Cha J, Kim ST et al (2004) Differentiation of tumor progression from pseudoprogression in patients with posttreatment glioblastoma using multiparametric histogram analysis. AJNR Am J Neuroradiol 35(7):1309–1317
199. Kong DS, Kim ST et al (2011) Diagnostic dilemma of pseudoprogression in the treatment of newly diagnosed glioblastoma the role of assessing relative cerebral blood flow volume and oxygen-6-methylguanine-DNA methyltransferase promoter methylation status. AJNR Am J Neuroradiol 32:382–387
200. Tsien C, Galban CJ et al (2010) Parametric response map as an imaging biomarker to distinguish progression from pseudoprogression in high-grade glioma. J Clin Oncol 28(13):2293–2299
201. Norden AD, Young GS et al (2008) Bevacizumab for recurrent malignant gliomas: efficacy, toxicity and patterns of recurrence. Neurology 70:779–787
202. Gupta A, Young RJ, Karimi S (2011) Isolated diffusion restriction precedes the development of enhancing tumor in a subset of patients with glioblastoma. AJNR Am J Neuroradiol 32:1301–1306
203. Mong S, Elligson BM et al (2012) Persistent diffusion-restricted lesions in bevacizumab-treated malignant gliomas are associated with improved survival compared with matched controls. AJNR Am J Neuroradiol 33:1763–1770

# 3.0 Tesla of Advanced Neuroimaging of CNS Infection: A Pictorial Essay

# 20

Simone Salice, Piero Chiacchiaretta, Antonio Ferretti, and Armando Tartaro

## 20.1 Introduction

Central nervous system infectious diseases include acute and chronic nosologic entities with various etiologies (viral, bacterial, mycobacterial, fungal, parasitic) that can affect brain, spinal cord, and/or meninges.

Viral infection of the brain is referred as encephalitis, whereas focal bacterial, fungal, or parasitic brain infections are classified as either cerebritis or abscess, on the basis of the presence or not of an external capsule. Spinal cord inflammation is referred as myelitis, while encephalomyelitis refers to both spinal cord and brain involvement. Inflammation of the meninges by microbiological causes can be due to bacteria, viruses, parasites, or fungi. Frequently, brain and meninges are involved in the infective process at the same time, and this is referred as meningoencephalitis.

In many of these cases, early diagnosis and effective treatment can be lifesaving, and imaging plays an important role in the diagnostic process because symptoms may be nonspecific. Indeed, initial clinical presentation with fever and headache is not rare, while more specific symptoms like altered consciousness, focal neurologic deficits, and seizures can occur only in the later stages of the disease. Moreover, even when neurologic signs and symptoms are typical for infection, imaging is necessary to identify the site of brain or spinal cord involvement, to define the entity of the pathologic process, to hypothesize the etiology, or to exclude complications such as cerebral edema, vasculitis, hydrocephalus, cranial nerve involvement, or subdural empyema.

### 20.1.1 Advanced Neuroimaging

Computed tomography (CT) is usually performed at first instance in uncooperative patients presenting with altered consciousness, focal neurologic deficits, and seizures, and it is useful to rule out hydrocephalus before lumbar puncture. However, MRI remains the method of choice when central nervous system infection is suspected.

3 Tesla MRI allows higher spatial resolution and contrast resolution with respect to 1.5 Tesla. Furthermore, very high field permits to significantly reduce exam acquisition duration that is particularly desirable in uncooperative patients. Then, several advantages derive from advanced MRI techniques at 3 T with respect to 1.5 T.

S. Salice • P. Chiacchiaretta • A. Ferretti • A. Tartaro (✉)
Institute of Advanced Biomedical Technologies
Department of Neurosciences, Imaging and Clinical Sciences, "G. d'Annunzio" University,
Chieti (PE), Italy
e-mail: armando.tartaro@gmail.com



T. Scarabino et al. (eds.), *High Field Brain MRI*, DOI 10.1007/978-3-319-44174-0_20

Advanced MRI techniques include magnetic resonance spectroscopy (MRS), perfusion-weighted imaging (PWI), diffusion-weighted imaging (DWI), and diffusion tensor imaging (DTI).

MRS-derived semiquantitative parameters are metabolite peaks and areas, usually expressed as ratios of each other, from which it is possible to assume relative metabolite concentration. 3 T MRS permits to exploit advantages due to higher signal-to-noise ratio and higher chemical shift with respect to 1.5 T. Higher signal-to-noise ratio is desirable to better estimate concentration of metabolites, which peaks are several times smaller than water's, even after water peak suppression. Higher chemical shift improves separation among metabolites, with a consequent improvement of spectral resolution.

Cerebral blood volume (CBV), cerebral blood flow (CBF), and mean transit time (MTT) are PWI-derived semiquantitative parameters that describe microcirculation kinetics of a tracer passing through a voxel. Tracers can be endogenous, like in arterial spin labeling (ASL) technique, or exogenous, like in dynamic susceptibility contrast (DSC) and dynamic contrast-enhanced (DCE) techniques. The MR perfusion technique usually performed in patients with suspected CNS infectious disease is DSC. 3 T permits a proportional increase of the susceptibility effects caused by the rapid passage of the contrast media bolus in the capillary bed with respect to 1.5 T. The consequent advantages are increase of SNR, higher spatial resolution, and opportunity to work with half the dose of contrast material reducing issues coming from blood-brain barrier disruption.

Advantages of 3 T magnetic field with respect to 1.5 T are not obvious because diffusion-weighted imaging (DWI) is a technique sensitive to Brownian motion, and magnetic field magnitude does not influence water molecule diffusion properties. Moreover, artifacts in areas like the skull base are higher at 3 T with respect to 1.5 T. Nevertheless, it has been showed that DWI performed at 3 T can have a greater diagnostic accuracy with respect to 1.5 T in the detection of infectious diseases [1]. The main reason is that thinner slices and higher b-values are achievable at 3 T.

Finally, in DTI studies, very high field permits more gradient directions within reasonable duration of the exam with respect to 1.5 T.

## 20.2 Meningitis

Meningitides are classified as acute, subacute, or chronic on the basis of clinical course. Often, bacterial and viral acute meningitides have similar clinical presentation; the most common pathogens of community acquired bacterial meningitis are *Streptococcus pneumoniae* (~50 %), *N. meningitidis* (~25 %), group B streptococci (~15 %), and *Listeria monocytogenes* (~10 %) [2, 3], while the most common viruses causing meningitides in adults are *Enteroviruses* and HSV-1 [4]. In patients with a weakened immune system, several bacterial or fungal microorganisms (*M. tuberculosis*, *C. neoformans*, *H. capsulatum*, *C. immitis*, *Borrelia burgdorferi*, and *T. pallidum*) can cause a subacute or chronic meningitis lasting more than 2 weeks; less frequently the causative pathogens can be viruses or parasites (*T. gondii*, *Enterovirus*, HIV) [5].

Lumbar puncture is diagnostic (lymphocytic pleocytosis and normal glucose concentration for viral meningitis vs polymorphonuclear pleocytosis and hypoglycorrhachia for bacterial meningitis), and it should be performed before any neuroimaging study in immunocompetent patients, with normal level of consciousness, no recent head trauma, no papilledema, and no focal neurologic deficits [6]. Anyway CT is recommended before lumbar puncture to rule out conditions that might lead to brain herniation.

Leptomeningeal enhancement, subarachnoid hyperintense signal in fluid-attenuated inversion recovery (FLAIR) sequences, and arterial narrowing or occlusion in angiography sequences are aspecific MRI signs of both viral and bacterial acute meningitides [7] (Fig. 20.1).

MRI also plays an important role in the diagnosis and monitoring of meningitis complications such as hydrocephalus, cerebritis, abscess, cranial nerves inflammation, venous thrombosis, vasculitis, infarct, ventriculitis, and subdural empyema [8].

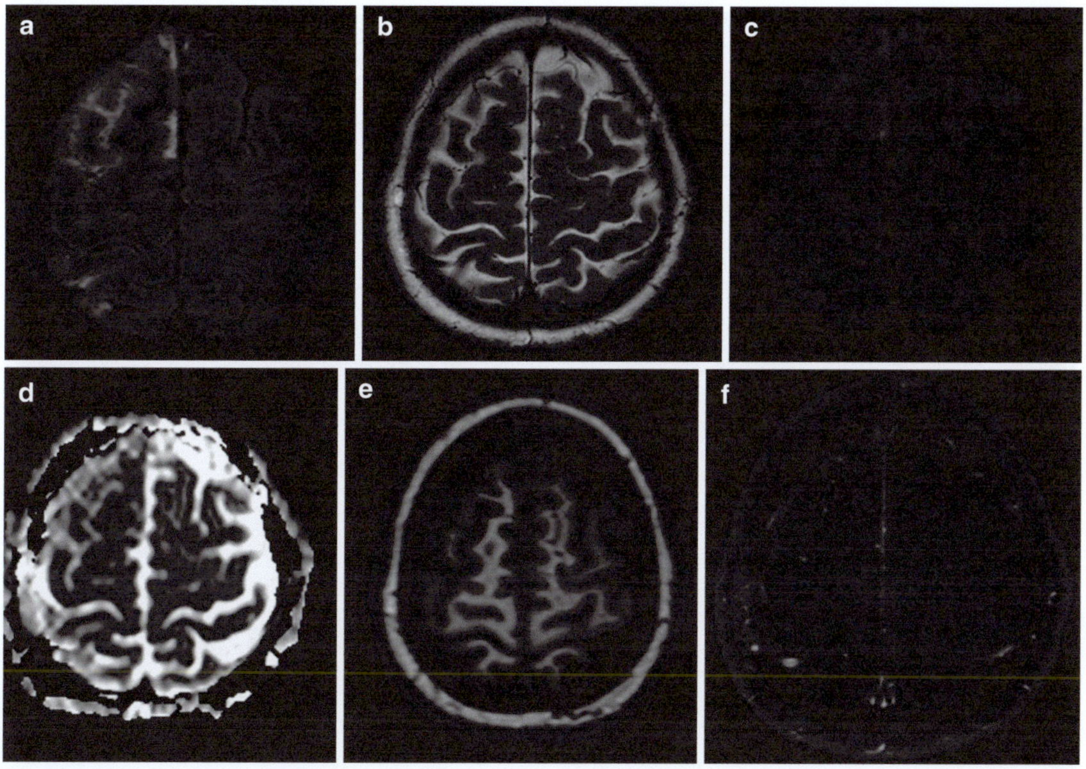


**Fig. 20.1** Pneumococcal meningoencephalitis in a 57-year-old patient. (**a**) Axial FLAIR and (**b**) axial T2 TSE images show hyperintensity of right frontoparietal gray matter and leptomeningeal spaces. (**c**) b1000 DWI and (**d**) ADC map show restricted diffusivity of leptomeninges and subarachnoid space, as compared to the contralateral side. (**e**, **f**) axial T1-weighted TSE images, respectively, without and with fat suppression technique, before and after contrast agent administration, show diffuse right leptomeningeal and cortical frontoparietal enhancement

In a recent study [9], differences of DTI indices in several limbic regions and in the white matter close to the globus pallidus were found in patients with chronic neuropsychological sequelae of chronic meningitis with respect to healthy subjects. Authors argued that their results suggest that white matter alterations may be involved in the psychopathology and pathophysiology of chronic meningitis. To our knowledge, there are no other studies investigating the utility of advanced MRI techniques in the diagnosis and monitoring of meningitis.

## 20.3 Encephalitis

Encephalitis is an acute inflammation of the brain. The etiology is most frequently viral. Childhood and adult herpes simplex virus (HSV) encephalitis is usually due to HSV-1 (90 %). Reactivation of dormant HSV-1 in the trigeminal ganglion precipitated by various factors (trauma, immunosuppression, hormonal fluctuations, stress) causes necrotizing and hemorrhagic involvement of white and gray matter that primarily affect the limbic system. Frontal, parietal, and occipital cortex can also be involved, while basal ganglia are usually spared. Lesions are usually asymmetric and bilateral.

Conventional MRI signs include gray and subcortical white matter hyperintensity on T2-weighted sequence with corresponding signal decrease on T1-weighted sequence, loss of gray-white matter junction, sulci effacement, and focal hypointensities on T2* images. Enhancement is best seen 1 week after initial symptoms; it may be gyral, leptomeningeal, ring, or diffuse.

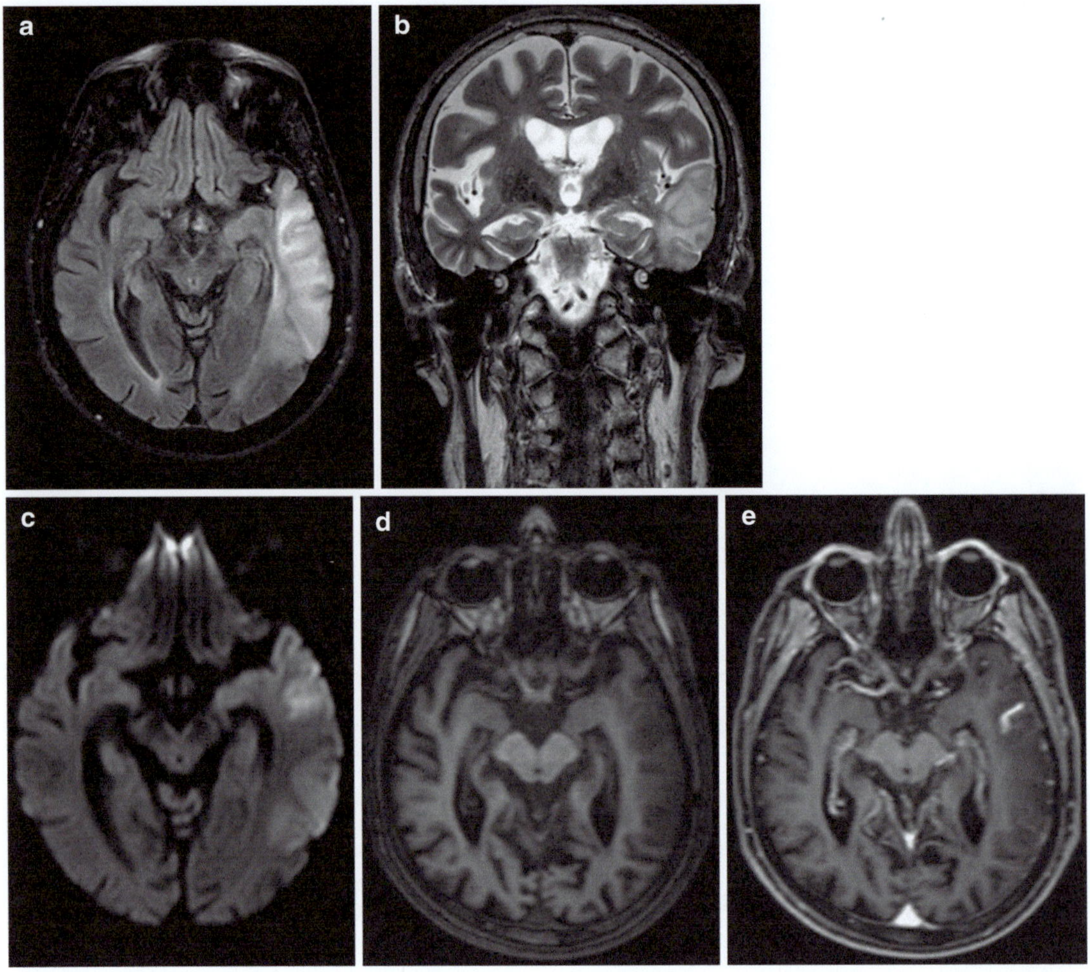


**Fig. 20.2** HSV encephalitis in a 64-year-old patient. (**a**) Axial FLAIR and (**b**) coronal T2 TSE image show left temporal lobe gray and subcortical white matter hyperintensity, with brain swelling and sulci effacement. (**c**) b1000 DWI showing restricted diffusivity of left temporal cortex. (**d**, **e**) axial T1-weighted TSE images before and after contrast agent administration show cortical enhancement

Restricted diffusivity of the affected cortex is a more sensitive sign of HSV encephalitis with respect to other conventional imaging signs. However, 14 days after symptom onset, diffusivity in the cerebral cortex is no longer restricted, while T2WI and FLAIR abnormalities persist (Fig. 20.2).

## 20.4 Cerebritis, Abscesses, and Granulomas

Infective focal brain lesions include abscesses and granulomas. A pyogenic infection of the brain can cause the formation of an abscess, through the activation of a purulent inflammatory process evolving through four stages: early cerebritis, late cerebritis, early capsule formation, and late capsule formation. Contrarily, chronic granulomatous inflammation mediated by cells of the mononuclear phagocyte system leads to the formation of well-demarcated focal lesions, containing cellular debris, macrophages, lymphocytes, plasma cells, and fibroblasts. Parasitic and fungal granulomas contain also eosinophils.

### 20.4.1 Bacterial

Most frequent pathogens responsible of abscesses formation are *Streptococcus* spp.,

*Enterobacteriaceae*, anaerobes, and staphylococci. Brain involvement can be direct from a contiguous site of infection (otitis media, mastoiditis, paranasal sinusitis, dental infection, head trauma, neurosurgical procedure) or indirect by hematogenous dissemination from distant sites of infection.

In the early cerebritis stage (days 1–3), a central core of coagulative necrosis is surrounded by a perivascular infiltration of inflammatory cells and marked edema; conventional MRI shows an ill-defined mass, hyperintense on T2-weighted sequence, and isointense-hypointense on T1-weighted sequence with a patchy enhancement after contrast agent administration.

In the late cerebritis stage (days 4–9), the necrotic purulent center and the surrounding inflammatory infiltrate of macrophages and fibroblasts are divided by a thin capsule of fibroblasts; conventional MRI shows a central core hypointense/hyperintense on T1-/T2-weighted sequences, a peripheral rim mildly hyperintense/hypointense on T1-/T2-weighted sequences, and a marked but irregular rim enhancement after contrast agent administration.

In the early capsule formation stage (days 10–13), a well-demarcated capsule is surrounded by marked edema; conventional MRI shows a ring-enhancing lesion with a typical smooth inner margin of the ring, a hypointense signal of the rim on T2-weighted images, and a markedly restricted diffusivity of the central core (Fig. 20.3).

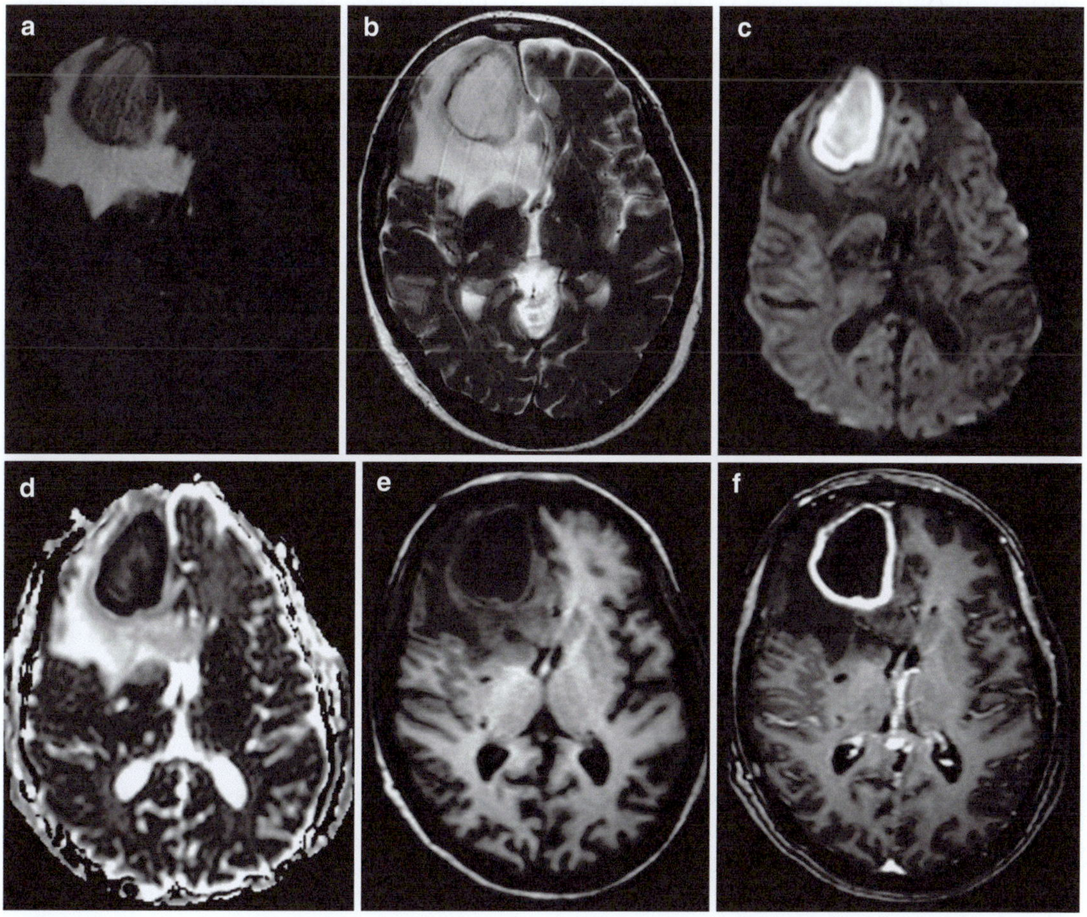


**Fig. 20.3** Pyogenic abscess in a 71-year-old patient. (**a**) Axial FLAIR and (**b**) axial T2 TSE images show a right frontal expanding lesion surrounded by large edema. Note the hypointense ring. (**c**) b1000 DWI and (**d**) ADC map show a markedly restricted diffusivity of the internal cavity. (**e, f**) Axial T1-weighted TSE images before and after contrast agent administration show smooth margins of the inner and outer layers of the enhanced ring

In the late capsule formation stage (more than 14 days), a well-formed necrotic core and surrounding marked gliosis with large numbers of reactive astrocytes are divided by a dense collagenous capsule; conventional MRI shows thickening of the enhancing rim and reduction of edema signs with respect to the previous stage.

Restricted diffusivity in the central core of a ring-enhancing lesion is by far the most specific advanced MRI technique sign for pyogenic brain abscess [10] opposite to non-pyogenic lesions that show hypointense or mixed signal on b1000 DWI images. However, as exceptions to the rule, histologically proven pyogenic brain abscesses that didn't show restricted diffusivity of their central core were reported [11, 12]. Furthermore, metastases and glioblastomas with ring enhancement and restricted diffusivity of their central core were also reported [11].

In unclear cases, additional information can be gathered from other advanced MRI techniques (Fig. 20.4).

Fractional anisotropy (FA) in the central cavity of a ring-enhancing lesion is higher in pyogenic abscesses with respect to glioblastomas and metastases [13–14]. MRS reveals amino acids only in the central cavity of pyogenic abscesses and not in the central cavity of necrotic tumors [15]. Lactate cytosolic amino acids with/without succinate, acetate, alanine, and glycine peaks are markers of abscess [15]. Cerebral blood volume (CBV), if measured in the areas of ring enhancement and perilesional edema, is generally higher in malignant lesions than in pyogenic abscesses [16, 17].

### 20.4.2 Fungal

Fungal brain infection are rare in subjects with an intact immune system and are usually secondary to primus focus elsewhere. The most frequent fungal microorganisms causing encephalitis in immunocompromised patients are *Cryptococcus*, *Aspergillus*, and *Candida*. Imaging findings are typically aspecific because of the inadequate immune response.

Sinusitis or pulmonitis caused by inhalation of *Aspergillus fumigatus* spores constitutes the most frequent sites of primary infection for the subsequent cerebral localization. Pathological manifestations of cerebral aspergillosis include meningitides, granulomas, infarctions, and aneurysm formation. Initially, fungal hyphae grow in the vessels causing hemorrhagic strokes; consequent purulent abscesses and chronic granulomas formation give the final MRI pattern (Fig. 20.5).

### 20.4.3 Parasitic

Toxoplasmosis is a parasitic disease caused by *T. gondii*, transmitted through undercooked meat or by handling objects contaminated by cat feces. In immunocompetent subjects *T. gondii* infection is subclinical. The reactivation of a latent previous infection is one of the most common complications in patients affected by acquired immune deficiency syndrome (AIDS) and with a CD4+ T-cell counts $<200/\mu L$. However, nowadays the incidence is decreasing thanks to highly active antiretroviral therapy (HAART). Clinically manifested toxoplasmosis occurs also in the other conditions of immune system depression or in case of transplacental transmission of the parasite.

In the earlier phase of cerebral toxoplasmosis, a vacuolated area with numerous tachyzoites is surrounded by cysts at different stages. In the absence of an effective treatment, necrotic lesions surrounded by abundant tachyzoites increase in number and size. In the final stage, the necrotic lesions are surrounded by late cysts; parasites are absent.

Multiple ring-enhancing lesions of different sizes surrounded by edema give the typical MRI pattern. Also a T2 ring sign was described [18]; it consists of a central hypointense region due to necrosis and cellular debris heavily infiltrated with neutrophils and histiocytes; an intermediate hyperintense region due to vascular congestion and proliferating tachyzoites; and an outer

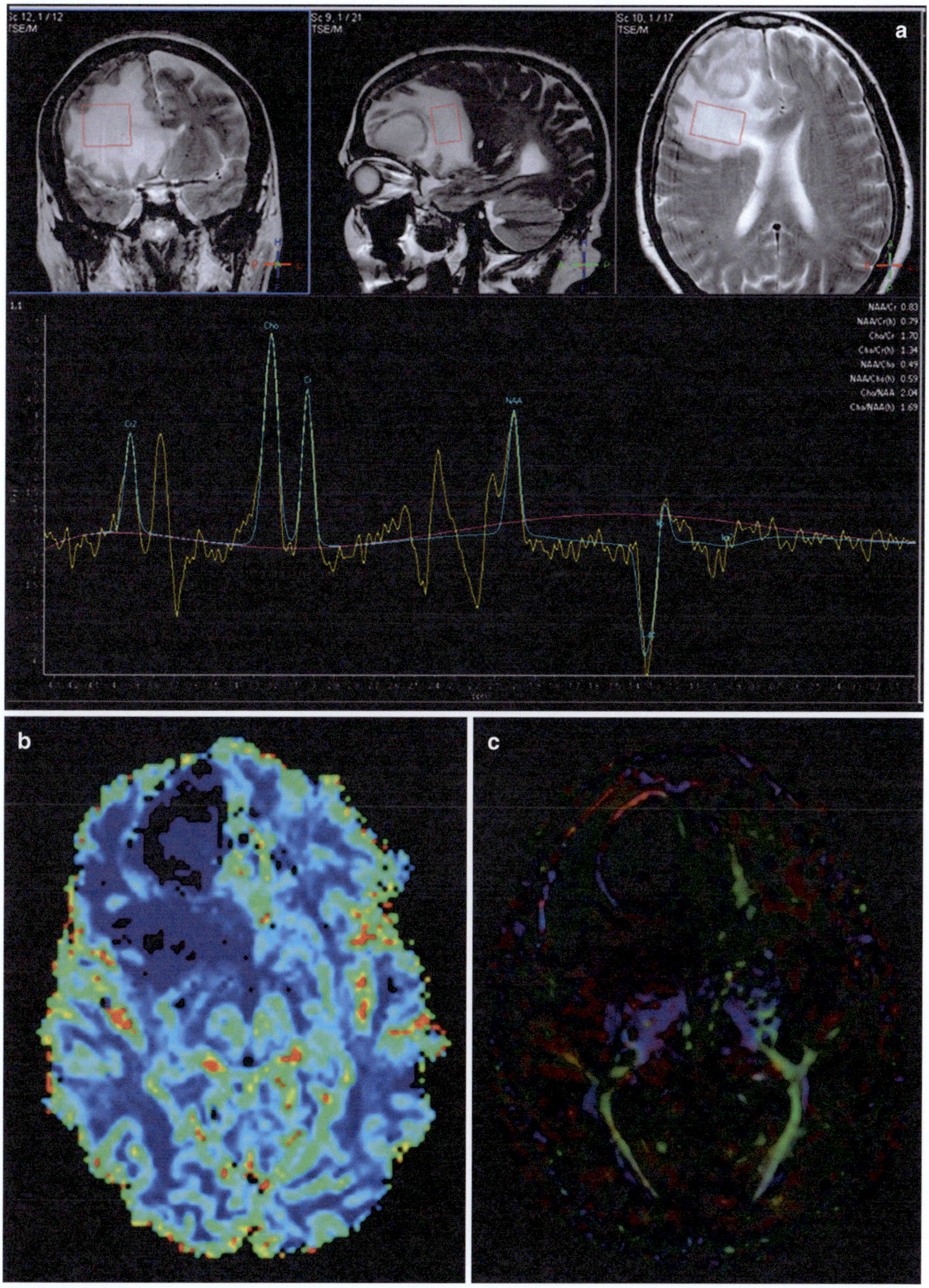


**Fig. 20.4** Same case as in Fig. 20.3. (**a**) 3 T single-voxel long-echo time (TE = 144 ms) water-suppressed *1H*-MRS spectrum shows lactate and lipid peaks not only in the internal cavity but also in the perilesional edema. (**b**) 3 T dynamic susceptibility contrast-enhanced cerebral blood volume color map shows low CBV values in the ring and in the perilesional edema. (**c**) 3 T DTI color map shows that frontal forceps fibers are not interrupted

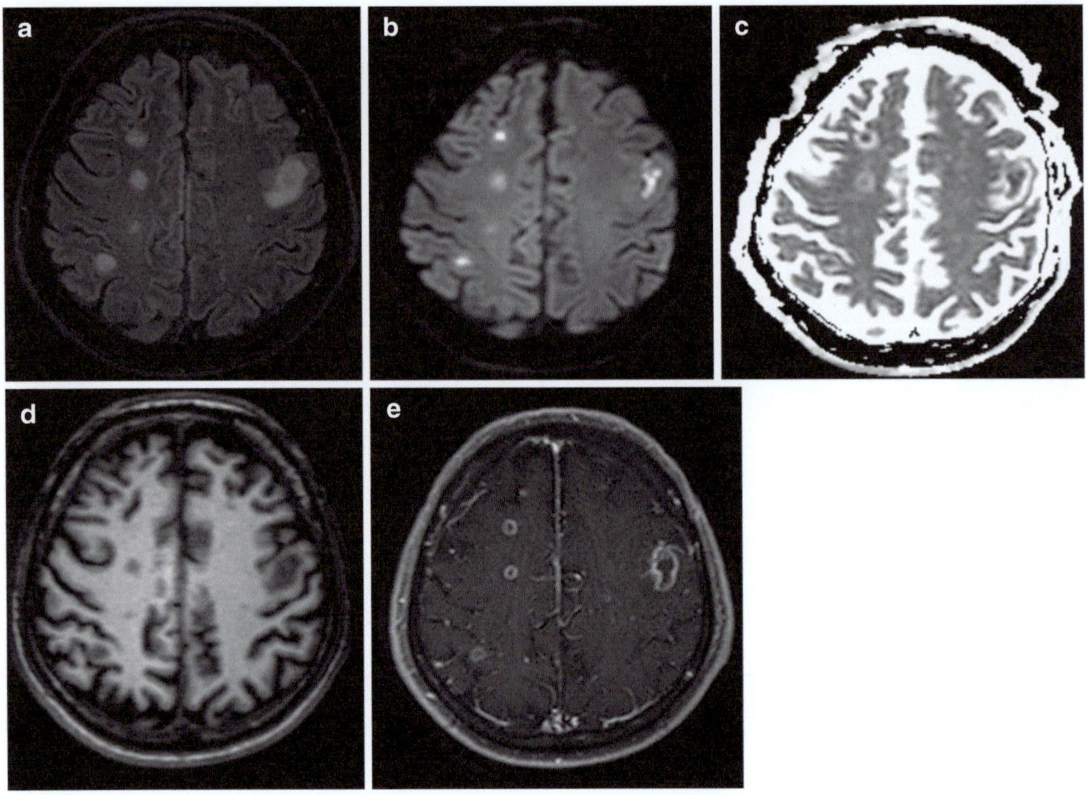


**Fig. 20.5** Cerebral Aspergillosis in a 50-year-old patient. (**a**) Axial FLAIR image shows bilateral subcortical fronto-parietal expanding lesions surrounded by low edema. (**b**) b1000 DWI and (**c**) ADC map show restricted diffusivity of the internal cavity of the lesions. (**d**, **e**) axial T1-weighted TSE images, respectively, without and with fat suppression technique, before and after contrast agent administration, show ring enhancement and smooth margins of the inner and outer layers of the ring

hypointense region due to less inflammation, less vascular changes, and fewer tachyzoites (Fig. 20.6).

However, in patients with severe immunodepression, MRI findings can be completely aspecific, and differential diagnosis with other opportunistic diseases can be a challenge. For instance, in fulminant encephalitic variant, MRI can show widespread T2-weighted lesions and no contrast enhancement; also solitary large lesions with marked contrast enhancement are described.

The main differential diagnosis is primary central nervous system lymphoma (PCNSL), while tubercular, fungal, or bacterial infections are less frequent. Given the substantial imaging overlap between toxoplasmosis and PCNS, diagnosis of toxoplasmosis is usually confirmed by the radiological improvement after 1 week of anti-toxoplasma therapy. Should the lesions be unchanged or progressive, the diagnosis has to be reconsidered and the therapeutic strategy reevaluated. In any case, final diagnosis is given by brain biopsy, which is reserved only for patients who have failed 2–4 weeks of empirical therapy.

In most challenging cases, the use of advanced MRI technique is justified. In toxoplasma lesions, the internal cavity shows no restricted diffusivity; perfusion indices are reduced; spectroscopy reveals lipid and lactate peaks (Fig. 20.7).

As regards the nuclear medicine field, thallium-201 brain SPECT is very useful in the differentiation between toxoplasmosis and PCNS, because only in the last case a marked uptake can be observed.

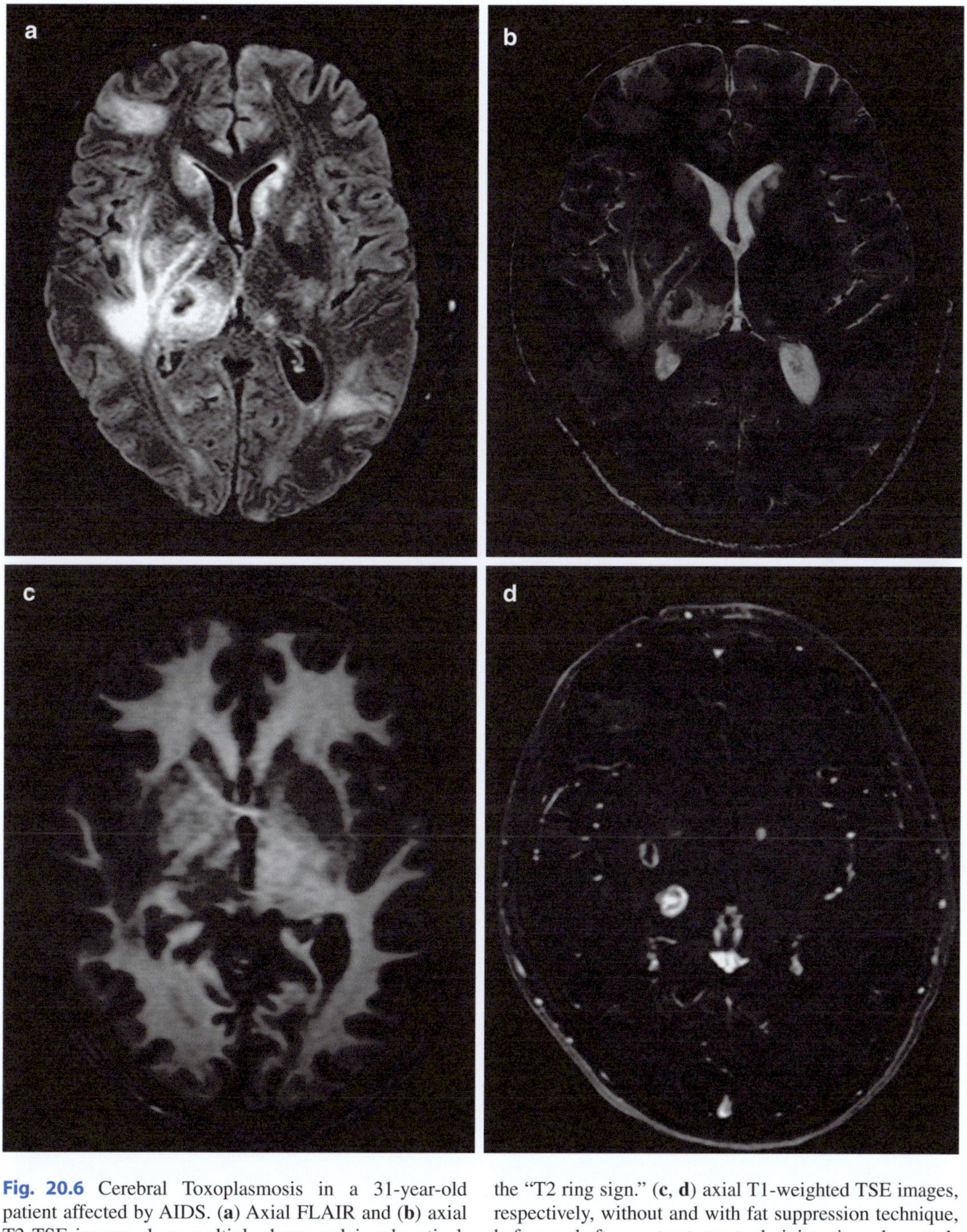


**Fig. 20.6** Cerebral Toxoplasmosis in a 31-year-old patient affected by AIDS. (**a**) Axial FLAIR and (**b**) axial T2 TSE images show multiple deep nuclei, subcortical, and deep white matter lesions surrounded by edema. Note the "T2 ring sign." (**c**, **d**) axial T1-weighted TSE images, respectively, without and with fat suppression technique, before and after contrast agent administration, show multiple ring-enhancing lesions of different size

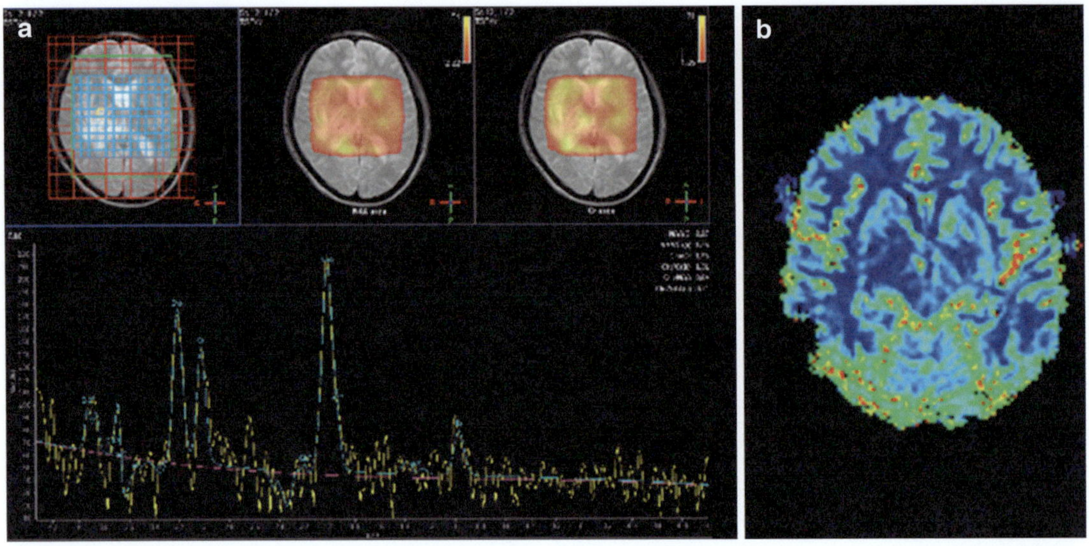

**Fig. 20.7** Same case as in Fig. 20.6. (**a**) 3 T multi-voxel long-echo time (TE = 144 ms) water-suppressed *1H*-MRS spectrum reveals lipid and lactate peaks in the internal cavity of the lesions. (**b**) 3 T dynamic susceptibility contrast-enhanced cerebral blood volume color map shows low CBV values in the lesions

## 20.5 Summary

CNS infectious diseases are often life-threatening conditions for which a prompt diagnosis is required in order to establish effective antimicrobial therapy as early as possible. Even if CSF analysis, biopsy analysis, and laboratory analyses remain the gold standard, MRI plays a crucial role in order to rule out conditions of emergency, to generate diagnostic hypotheses, to identify the site of infection, and to exclude and monitor possible complications. 3 T MRI allows shorter acquisition time for a given resolution and/or higher resolution for a given acquisition time with respect to 1.5 T. Furthermore, several advantages derive from performing advanced MRI techniques at 3 T with respect to 1.5 T. This is noteworthy if you consider that advanced MRI techniques can support conventional MRI in most challenging cases. In support of this statement, in our series, we observed that the diagnostic accuracy in the differential diagnosis between benign and malignant ring enhancing lesions (GBMs, metastases, and abscesses) significantly improves when ADC values measured in the internal cavity of the lesions are combined with other advanced technique-derived parameters.

## References


1. Tomar V, Yadav A, Rathore RK, Verma S, Awasthi R, Bharadwaj V, Ojha BK, Prasad KN, Gupta RK (2011) Apparent diffusion coefficient with higher b-value correlates better with viable cell count quantified from the cavity of brain abscess. AJNR Am J Neuroradiol 32(11):2120–2125
2. McIntyre PB, O'Brien KL, Greenwood B, van de Beek D (2012) Effect of vaccines on bacterial meningitis worldwide. Lancet 380(9854):1703–1711. doi:10.1016/S0140-6736(12)61187-8 . Review. PubMed PMID: 23141619
3. Adriani KS, Brouwer MC, van de Beek D (2015) Risk factors for community-acquired bacterial meningitis in adults. Neth J Med 73(2):53–60 . PubMed PMID: 25753069
4. Pons-Salort M, Parker EP, Grassly NC (2015) The epidemiology of non-polio enteroviruses: recent advances and outstanding questions. Curr Opin Infect Dis 28(5):479–487
5. Zunt JR, Baldwin KJ (2012) Chronic and subacute meningitis. Continuum (Minneap Minn) 18(6 Infectious Disease):1290–1318 . Review
6. Hauser SL, Josephson SA, English JD, Engstrom JW (2006) Harrison's neurology in clinical medicine. McGraw-Hill, New York, p 692
7. Hazany S, Go JL, Law M (2014) Magnetic resonance imaging of infectious meningitis and ventriculitis in adults. Top Magn Reson Imaging 23(5):315–325
8. Hughes DC, Raghavan A, Mordekar SR, Griffiths PD, Connolly DJ (2010) Role of imaging in the diagnosis of acute bacterial meningitis and its complications. Postgrad Med J 86(1018):478–485

9. Lin WC, Chen PC, Wang HC, Tsai NW, Chou KH, Chen HL, Su YJ, Lin CP, Li SH, Chang WN, Lu CH (2014) Diffusion tensor imaging study of white matter damage in chronic meningitis. PLoS One 9(6):e98210
10. Xu XX, Li B, Yang HF, Du Y, Li Y, Wang WX et al (2014) Can diffusion-weighted imaging be used to differentiate brain abscess from other ring-enhancing brain lesions? A meta-analysis. Clin Radiol 69(9): 909–915
11. Hartmann M, Jansen O, Heiland S, Sommer C, Münkel K, Sartor K (2001) Restricted diffusion within ring enhancement is not pathognomonic for brain abscess. AJNR Am J Neuroradiol 22: 1738–1742
12. Tung GA, Evangelista P, Rogg JM, Duncan JA 3rd (2001) Diffusion-weighted MR imaging of rim-enhancing brain masses: is markedly decreased water diffusion specific for brain abscess? AJR Am J Roentgenol 177(3):709–712
13. Nath K, Agarwal M, Ramola M, Husain M, Prasad KN, Rathore RK et al (2009) Role of diffusion tensor imaging metrics and in vivo proton magnetic resonance spectroscopy in the differential diagnosis of cystic intracranial mass lesions. Magn Reson Imaging 30:198–206
14. Reiche W, Schuchardt V, Hagen T, Il'yasov KA, Billmann P, Weber J (2010) Differential diagnosis of intracranial ring enhancing cystic mass lesions–role of diffusion-weighted imaging (DWI) and diffusion-tensor imaging (DTI). Clin Neurol Neurosurg 112(3):218–225
15. Garg M, Gupta RK, Husain M, Chawla S, Chawla J, Kumar R et al (2004) Brain abscesses: etiologic categorization with in vivo proton MR spectroscopy. Radiology 230:519–527 , 200
16. Erdogan C, Hakyemez B, Yildirim N, Parlak M (2005) Brain abscess and cystic brain tumor: discrimination with dynamic susceptibility contrast perfusion-weighted MRI. J Comput Assist Tomogr 29:663–667
17. Hakyemez B, Erdogan C, Bolca N, Yildirim N, Gokalp G, Parlak M (2006) Evaluation of different cerebral mass lesions by perfusion-weighted MR imaging. J Magn Reson Imaging 24:817–824
18. Masamed R, Meleis A, Lee EW, Hathout GM (2009) Cerebral toxoplasmosis: case review and description of a new imaging sign. Clin Radiol 64(5):560–563

# Use of fMRI Activation Paradigms: A Presurgical Tool for Mapping Brain Function

21

Daniela Cevolani, Raffaele Agati, and Marco Leonardi

Until not many years ago, the only reliable ways of mapping of brain eloquent areas were invasive methods, such as intraoperative cortical stimulation and somatosensory-evoked potentials. Invasive methods are accurate but time-consuming during the surgical procedure, often reducing the mapping analysis to "just sufficient" knowledge to enable the surgeon to proceed [53].

Obviously, the goal of neurosurgery is to maximize resection while preserving important brain functions. With this aim, it is important to provide the surgeon with all the available information to identify the eloquent cortex preoperatively; it is a well-known phenomenon that many tumours and their surrounding oedema cause a significant mass effect, which may markedly distort the cortical anatomy and make classical anatomical landmarks useless.

The presurgical use of functional magnetic resonance imaging (fMRI) paradigms enables the neurosurgeon to be given a complete mapping of brain eloquent areas before surgery, thus making the surgeon aware of the actual situation. Consequently, the surgeon may plan the surgery and decide the strategy of approach preoperatively, including the question of whether to operate or not [23].

The fMRI technique has a high spatial and temporal resolution, a non-invasive character, and is safe (the source of the signal is endogenous, and MRI has no known risks), thus also allowing the patient follow-up. It enables a correct definition of the relationships between, for instance, a tumour and the adjacent eloquent cortex. It is noteworthy that, sometimes, the intraoperative mapping by direct cortical stimulation is unsuccessful, especially when testing higher cognitive functions such as language, which requires the patient to be awake and not sedated as during the surgery [25]. In these cases, fMRI information becomes not only an invaluable help but also avoids the chance of a "surprise" during the surgical procedure [4].

Finally, fMRI can detect functional cortical reorganization and plasticity, namely, the displacement of brain function from one location to another [24, 42]. This phenomenon has clear-cut implications for the surgical management of the patient.

In this paper, we focus our attention on the phenomena at the root of eloquent brain maps, the description of some activation paradigms, their main presurgical application and some new approaches to fMRI.

D. Cevolani (✉)
Department of Specialized Diagnostics and Experimental Health, Department of Neuroradiology, Bellaria Hospital University of Bologna, Bologna, Italy
e-mail: daniela.cevolani@unibo.it

R. Agati • M. Leonardi
Department of Neuroradiology, Bellaria Hospital University of Bologna, Bologna, Italy
e-mail: raffaele.agati@ausl.bo.it; marco.leonardi@centauro.it



T. Scarabino et al. (eds.), *High Field Brain MRI*, DOI 10.1007/978-3-319-44174-0_21

## 21.1 The BOLD Phenomenon

Mapping eloquent areas by MRI is based on the blood oxygenation level-dependent (BOLD) contrast phenomenon. This is due to the paramagnetic properties of deoxyhaemoglobin. When a pool of neurons passes from a rest state to an activation state, the increased discharge of spikes induces a rise in regional oxygen consumption rate. This event brings two main effects: a regional increase in the absolute number of deoxyhaemoglobin molecules and a local vasodilation, due to the flow autoregulatory mechanism, which is characteristic of the brain circulation. The increase in blood regional flow largely overwhelms the amount of oxygen extracted by the activated neurons and leads to a relative decrease of deoxyhaemoglobin concentration. The resulting net effect is a local rise in oxyhaemoglobin and a local drop in deoxyhaemoglobin. The drop in paramagnetic deoxyhaemoglobin leads to an increased signal intensity in T2*- and T2-weighted images. The mapping of eloquent areas, then, is achieved by acquiring T2*- or T2-weighted images consecutively, while the subject is performing the task or is at rest. Finally, the difference between the performing condition and the resting condition is calculated [26].

## 21.2 3 T Versus 1.5 T

In the past 10–15 years, 1.5 T systems have been the most commonly used field strength in everyday clinical use. The advances in technology and the increased availability of higher fields have opened the door to a variety of exciting improvements in clinical and research application of MRI. In particular, 3 T systems have continued to gain wide acceptance as one of the main field strengths used for clinical and research studies [35]. The reasons for this acceptance are many. One of the main advantages of high-field imaging is the improvement of the signal-to-noise ratio (SNR). It has been shown [35] that the signal is expected to increase by a factor of 4 at 3 T, with respect to 1.5 T. Unfortunately, the noise also increases by a factor of 2. As a consequence, there is a twofold improvement in SNR, which may have profound clinical implications. (1) *Shortening of data acquisition times*. It is possible to decrease the total data acquisition times by a factor of 4 at 3 T, while maintaining a SNR comparable to that obtained at 1.5 T. This time reduction shortens the overall exam length and could minimize patient motion artefacts. (2) *Improving spatial resolution*, while keeping acquisition times similar to 1.5 T. Spatial resolution improves differently according to the acquisition approach used. Therefore, depending on the structures in exam and the imaging sequences used, it is possible to improve SNR to optimize the visualization of relevant details of interest.

Another effect observed with high-field imaging is an *increasing susceptibility*. fMRI is probably one of the best examples of converting artefacts into useful physiological information [35]. Signal changes due to BOLD effects are directly proportional to the magnetic field strength. The higher the field strength, the more sensitive the sequence will be to BOLD effects. Assuming the changes in the deoxyhaemoglobin concentration remain identical, the percentage signal changes are expected to increase twofold at 3 T when compared with that obtained from 1.5 T. However, since the absolute signal changes are small (~10 % with a 3 T system), appropriate task paradigms must be planned.

## 21.3 The "Ideal" Paradigm

Before starting any routine clinical application of fMRI on patients, it is useful to perform a survey of the literature in the search for the "ideal" paradigm. In our opinion, a reliable paradigm should have the following characteristics: (1) The activation induced should be *specific*. Specificity refers to the ability to localize a function: a high-specific paradigm should have a high localizing power, i.e. the ability to select and discover all and only the areas appertaining to that function considered. This way, evoked eloquent areas are defined unambiguously as to anatomical location and extent. (2) The activation induced should be *reproducible*: evoked eloquent areas have to remain unchanged as to location and extent, through different trials, made in the same and/or in different sessions, thus allowing patient follow-up. (3) The paradigm should be *easy* to learn by patients having different social and cultural backgrounds. If a patient does not understand clearly what to do or what will happen, he or she obviously will not perform the paradigm correctly, and the result will be a suboptimal activation. (4) The paradigm should be *short-lasting*. The length of time of a paradigm should enable the patient to maintain a high attention level all through the trial; otherwise, again a suboptimal activation will result. Unfortunately, an optimal duration is only a compromise between the time spent by the patient in the magnet and the need to acquire enough data for statistically significant mapping. Usually, an fMRI session includes more than one paradigm and lasts for almost an hour.

**A Few Words on Sensitivity** Sensitivity is the ability to detect low signals and/or to respond to small physical amounts or differences. As we have just seen ("3 T vs 1.5 T") and will see soon ("experimental design"), sensitivity does not depend only on the biological phenomena at the base of the BOLD contrast effect, but also on the characteristics of acquiring equipment (magnetic field strength, kind of sequence acquired, artefacts, etc.), as well as on the experimental design applied. Unfortunately, sensitivity and specificity are often in inverse relation. As a consequence, caution is needed in comparing results obtained by using different equipment and experimental designs.

It is useful, after the choice from the literature of the paradigms having the above characteristics, to select from them those producing the widest activation areas, with the aim, in a presurgical perspective, to spare as much eloquent tissue as possible. The result of such an operation is to obtain a set of paradigms, which, on the whole, constitute an adequate tool with which to explore the main eloquent cortical areas (cf. [9, 41] for review). After this, a safe strategy to set up the system is to implement and apply all paradigms to healthy volunteers before proceeding with the routine clinical application on patients. Finally, each patient has to receive a personalized set of paradigms, which are selected on the basis of the specific location and extent of the existing pathology.

## 21.4 Stimulating Apparatus

Usually, there is the need with some tools to apply a proper stimulation. For instance, we used goggles, earphones and a push-button panel (ten push buttons), to monitor patient response (Visual Stim XGA Digital Stereo Commander XG, Resonance Technology).

Stimuli could be administrated in different ways, but a careful procedure is to perform this step by software as automatically as possible. For instance, we use the Stim2 and Presentation software and a dedicated PC. The same PC synchronizes the beginning of stimulation to the beginning of acquisition using a radiofrequency pulse.

## 21.5 Experimental Design

The main limitation within fMRI experimental design planning arises from the fact that the signal changes being measured are very small. Thus, fMRI can be used only for determining *relative* signal intensity changes within a single image session [38]. There are two main methods of planning an fMRI experimental design: block design and event-related design.

A typical *block design* consists of two alternating situations: the "activation condition" and the "resting condition", which often have the same duration. Each condition is considered as a mean static value across the whole period. The principles of BOLD data processing are based on the subtraction of the rest from the active periods; thus the rest behaves as a baseline with respect to activation. The resulting difference between the two signals is the specific activation effect we are dealing with. It follows that the rest condition is very important, as much as the active condition, the more important the smaller the eloquent area to be revealed. Finally, the rest condition is not always the absence of anything, but may also consist of another task, which may differ in the different paradigms.

An *event-related design* considers the time course of the event and not a time-integrated averaging procedure. Each trial is considered separately, as being time locked to the beginning of the stimulus, and signal changes are explored in relation to the onset of the event generated by the trial. Event-related signal averaging requires the repetition of trials and the alignment of the data to a reference point, such that repeated time-locked epochs of data can be recorded and subsequently averaged together. In this way, event-related design can explore the temporal shape of the event and discover if there is a temporal evolution, e.g. if a transient signal change is followed by a sustained signal change (in a block paradigm the transient and sustained signal changes would not be resolved, because activity is mediated over each condition) [13].

With respect to event-related design, block design, besides being simpler, has a higher power in signal detection, i.e. has a higher sensitivity, due to the intrinsic characteristics of the method (to find significant differences between means). So a block design seems a more convenient way to perform presurgical fMRI paradigms [36].

## 21.6 Data Processing

Once data have been acquired, they need to be *preprocessed*. The purpose of this procedure is to remove various kinds of artefacts in order to maximize the sensitivity for later statistical analysis.

After reconstructing row data into images, looking like brain slices, *slice-timing correction* occurs. Actually, each slice is acquired at slightly different times, but further analysis needs to adjust the data so that it appears that all voxels within one volume have been acquired at exactly the same time. *Motion correction* follows: by using rotation and translation, each volume is transformed to be aligned with all the others [56]. Often but not always, a *spatial blurring* of each volume is taken into account, with the aim of reducing noise without significantly affecting the activation signal. Afterwards, overall intensity level is adjusted so that all volumes have the same mean intensity (*intensity normalization)* [51]. The final step is the filtering of each time series of voxels by linear or non-linear tools, in order to reduce low- and high-frequency noise. Now data are ready for statistical data processing [52].

A detailed description of statistical analysis is beyond the purpose of this paper, so only a few general points will be described and single subject data only are referred to. Statistical analysis is carried out to determine which voxels are activated by the stimulation. Various possible methods may be used to compute the significance level of these activated voxels. The principle is a model-based method (e.g. [15]), where an expected response is generated and compared with the data. Commonly, each time series of voxels is analysed independently (*univariate analysis*), in a *general linear model (GLM)*. To get the best fit of the model to the data, the "stimulus function", which is often a sharp on/off waveform, is smoothed, delayed and converted into the haemodynamic response function (HRF) [58]. Once the model fits the data, an estimate of the *goodness of fit* is found, expressed as a parameter estimate (the estimated $\beta$ value), which is converted, dividing it by the standard error, into the $t$ value. Proper standard statistical transformations convert the $t$ value into $P$ (probability) or $Z$ statistics, which contain the same statistical information: how significant the data are [57]. An important issue concerning these methods is the arbitrary establishment of the statistical threshold, above which the activity is significant, and below which data are rejected. If the significant ($P$) threshold is applied to every voxel in the brain, the huge amount of resulting voxels makes the number of false positives too high to be accepted; in this case a Bonferroni's correction is used (the significance level at each voxel is divided by the number of voxels, to correct the number of comparisons to be made). Otherwise, one may take into account clusters of activated voxels before estimating the significance. This

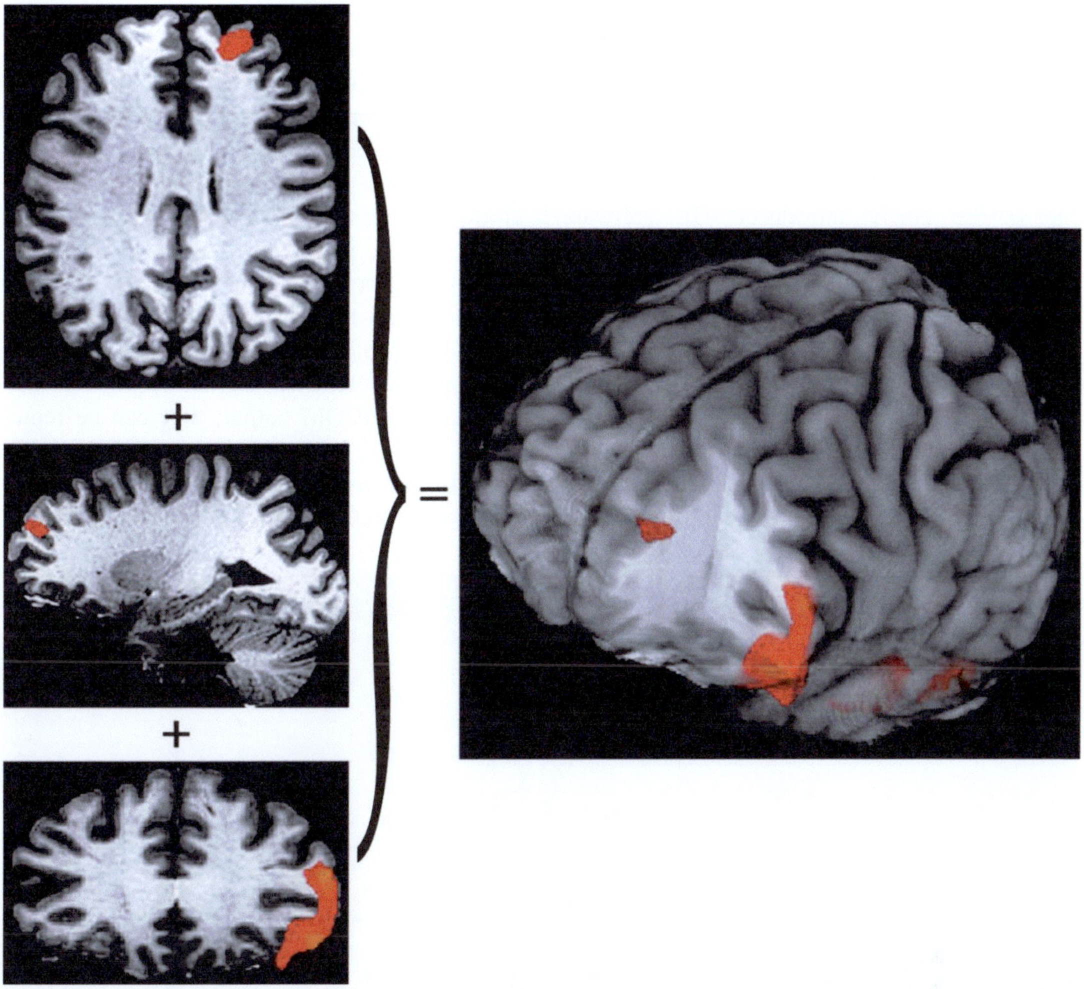

**Fig. 21.1** An example of 3D reconstruction. Activation maps are superimposed on the high-quality volumetric acquisition, giving a better opportunity to localize eloquent areas. MPR projections are also shown

method is more sensitive to activation but more arbitrary. Whatever the choice, the resulting output is a statistical map, which indicates those points where the brain has activated in response to the stimulus.

The above analysis concerns the low-resolution fMRI series, acquired during the performance of the task. An fMRI experiment typically includes also a single high-quality structural series, useful to better localize anatomically the task-related regions of increased signal. This isovolumetric morphological series needs in turn to be preprocessed [51], segmented [32] and coregistered with fMRI series, which, at last, are superimposed on the volumetric acquisition. In this way, activation areas may be viewed in the context of a good quality brain image (Fig. 21.1).

## 21.7 Software

The most commonly used packages are SPM and Brain Voyager; both import DICOM data, perform 2D and 3D statistical analysis and process single- or multi-subject data. Brain Voyager also has a real-time utility, Turbo Brain Voyager. There is no need to describe this well-known software in detail, suffice it to say that, at the beginning, fMRI was used only for research purposes and the software was targeted at this goal. With the increasing diffusion of this technique and its clinical application, manufacturers of magnetic equipment entered the market and began the production of new software. An example is the newly introduced GE software, *BrainWave*, which cannot process multi-subject data but is very convenient and has many advantages, so that we chose it as the software for fMRI analysis in the routine clinic. The package consists of two parts: real time and post-acquisition. *Real time* allows visualization of statistical t-maps during the acquisition; as the acquisition proceeds, statistical activation maps are processed and superimposed in real time on the fMRI series just acquired. This way, it is possible to monitor the situation and the activating effects from the very beginning of the acquisition. The *post-acquisition* package performs an in-depth analysis (similarly to Brain Voyager) but in a semiautomatic way; it may run in the background, during successive acquisitions or exams, and produces, in the final steps, two outputs: 3D-coloured activation maps and the so-called BIP maps, in which the activated areas, bounded by a white contour, are superimposed on the 3D structural isovolumetric sagittal acquisition. BIP maps are a DICOM output; they can be represented, in turn, in the three planes of the space (MPR) and, sent to the neuronavigator, are inestimable value to the neurosurgeon (Fig. 21.2).

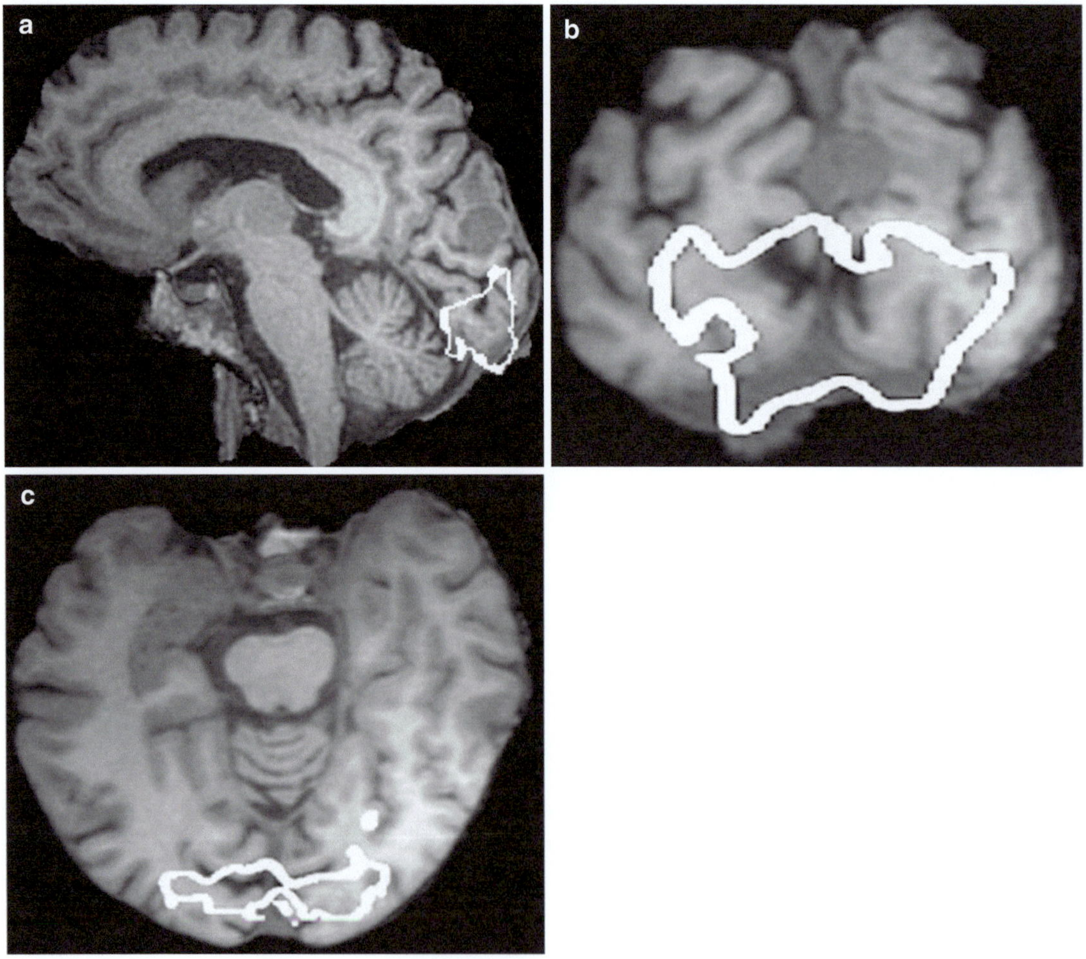


**Fig. 21.2** An example of BIP maps. The activated areas in the occipital lobe are bordered by a white line, leaving the inner area transparent, to better define the anatomical structures involved (Modified from Leonardi et al. [33], with permission)

## 21.8 Paradigms

### 21.8.1 Motor Paradigms

Motor and sensory paradigms were the the first to be implemented [46], both because of the ease with which they can be performed in the scanner with no additional equipment and their easy validation by preoperative and intraoperative cortical monitoring. The good correlation between cortical monitoring and fMRI results made fMRI motor tasks the method of choice for the presurgical evaluation of patients.

There are many motor tasks described in the literature. Owing to the cortical distortion of the sensorimotor homunculus, the wider areas of fingers, hands, tongue and lips are the most frequently explored to produce the highest BOLD signal. Furthermore, hands/fingers and lips/tongue are very important anatomical effectors, involved, respectively, in day-to-day manual activities and speaking. As a consequence, hand and lip movements are the most often used tasks to explore the activity of the primary motor cortex. When the lesion is located near the convexity of the brain, movements of the foot are also used.

As regards the hand movements, there is a wide spectrum of paradigms ranging from the simple opening and closing of the hand or squeezing a sponge to the more complex sequential tapping of fingers in predetermined fixed order or repetitive opposition of the thumb and each of the remaining fingers. Simple and complex hand motor tasks bring about different cortical activation patterns.

Simple hand movements activate only the contralateral primary motor cortex, the superior part of the precentral gyrus, in an area called the "precentral knob", otherwise named inverted Ω, which may also be divided by a sulcus in the middle and in that case is called horizontal ε [60, 61]. Complex hand movements activate not only the contralateral primary motor cortex, but also the ipsilateral motor cortex, the supplementary motor area, the premotor and the somatosensory cortex bilaterally [55]. There are different fundamental reasons for the primary sensory cortex activation. From the anatomical point of view, cytoarchitectonics show that pyramidal cells can be found either in the pre- or postcentral gyrus and motor fibres in the pyramidal tract originate not only from primary motor areas (MsI), but also from primary sensitive areas (SmI). According to classical neurophysiology, it is possible to elicit motor responses by electrically stimulating the precentral gyrus, as well as the postcentral gyrus, with a partial overlapping of the homunculi of cortical motor and sensory representation. Finally, both sensory proprioceptive and exteroceptive afferents can be activated by positional changes during the performance of motor tasks.

When the motor task is complex, there is also an asymmetry in lateralization, as regards the dominant hemisphere. In right-handed subjects, finger movements of the right hand substantially activate the dominant (left) hemisphere with almost no activation in the nondominant (right) hemisphere [29]. In left-handed subjects, the activation pattern may show a high degree of variability, but often both left- and right-hand movements produce activations comparable between dominant and nondominant hemispheres [50]. Obviously, all these differences must be taken into account in analysing an activation pattern.

Figure 21.3 shows an example of eloquent areas evoked by the repetitive sequential opposition of the thumb and each of the remaining fingers of the right hand.

### 21.8.2 Sensory Paradigms

Sensory paradigms are used less often than motor paradigms but have the advantage of being a passive task, which may also be performed on uncooperative patients (anaesthetized, unconscious, neurologically impaired, disabled, aged, babies, etc.). In this last case, they could be the only way to identify the sensorimotor cortex for surgical planning.

The most common way to perform a sensory paradigm is by tactile stimulation of the skin of the hand or, less frequently, of the foot or face. Simple plastic toothbrushes, blunt nails, air puffs and even the examiner's fingertips may accomplish this kind of stimulation.

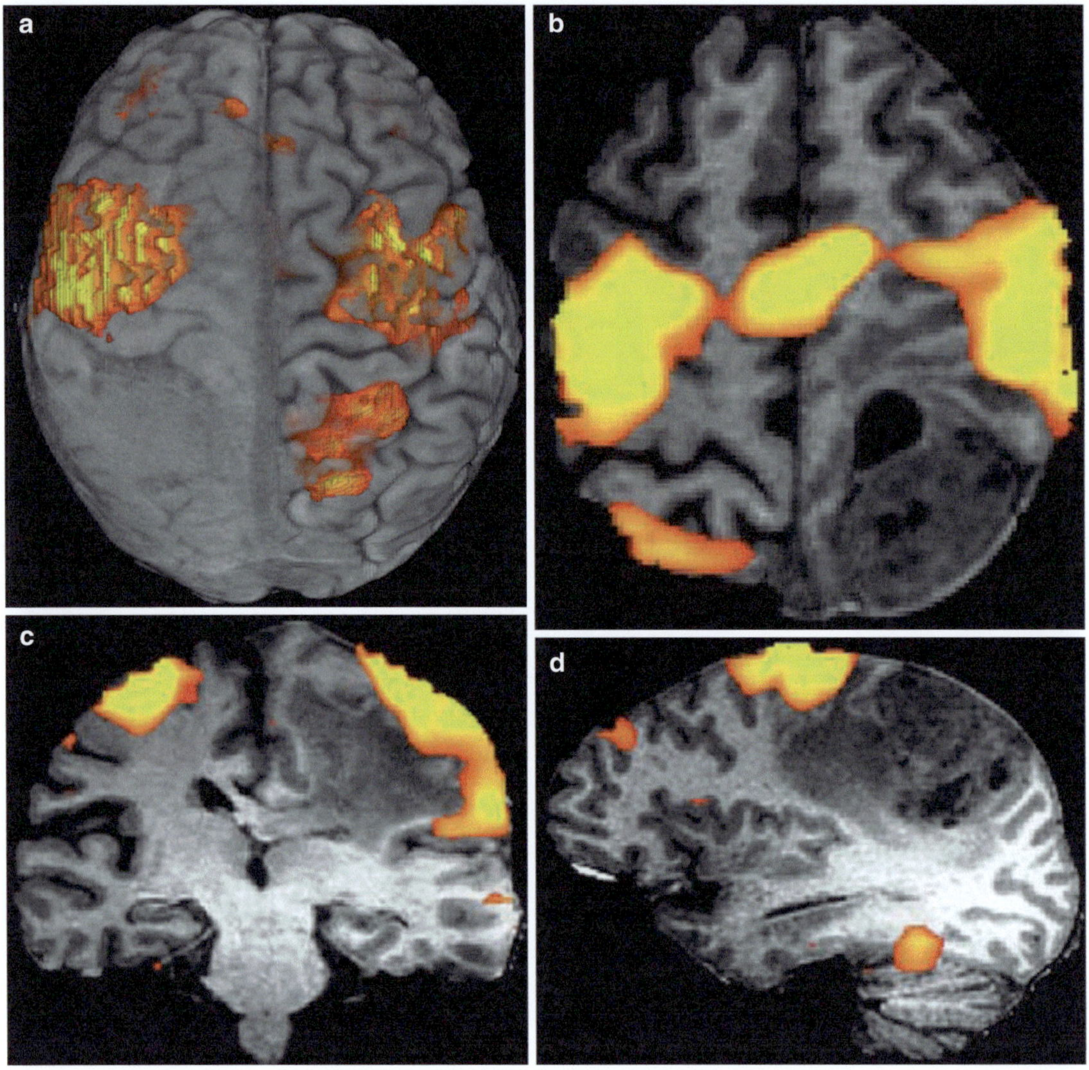


**Fig. 21.3** An example of motion paradigm (repetitive sequential opposition of the thumb and each of the remaining fingers of the right hand). Note that activated areas are adjacent to the lesion (a meningioma). The patient underwent surgery with no sequelae

Results show eloquent areas in both the postcentral and the precentral gyri [42]. The situation is similar to that which we have seen in motor paradigms: there is an anatomical cytoarchitectonic reason (i.e. the presence of granular cells not only in SmI but also in MsI) together with numerous connections through corticocortical or thalamocortical relays [59]; moreover, a direct cortical stimulation of the motor cortex in humans evokes sensory experiences [6]. The concept of a narrow, discrete, pre-Rolandic motor cortex separated from post-Rolandic sensory strip, although pervasive, has been challenged by evidence of a broad overlapping sensorimotor cortex [54].

## 21.8.3 Visual Paradigms

Before the introduction of fMRI, the most common way to obtain functional information about important anatomical visual areas, such as the fibre system of the optic radiations, the lateral geniculate nucleus and the striate/extrastriate cortices, was by perimetric examination of the visual field. This technique, however, provides only a subjective determination, at each point, of the functional variation in time and lacks direct anatomical information. Conventional neuroradiological imaging, on the other hand, simply outlines lesion location and its gross extent, but it is often difficult to establish if the presence of oedema or structural alterations of local anatomy imply neuronal death. A better understanding of the function-structure correlation of striate organization has been provided by functional PET imaging studies, but the associated radiation exposure and the limited availability of PET units have restricted its application for routine evaluation of patients with visual field defects to those described in a few clinical reports [30].

The enhanced spatial and temporal resolution of non-invasive fMRI, together with its safety and availability, has provided new and valuable information in understanding the organization and functional properties of visual areas in the human cortex. For instance, fMRI has been a precious method in confirming cortical retinotopy and quantitatively defining cortical extension of the central foveal vision [30, 48], results that, otherwise, could only have been obtained in an invasive manner. fMRI imaging can detect objective visual field deficits, caused by lesions not only producing destruction of the primary visual cortex, but also interrupting visual pathways and creating a lack of sensory input, without destroying neurons in the occipital cortex [30].

Visual stimulation may be delivered in plenty of modes: frequently used stimuli are flashing of white or coloured lights at certain frequencies or alternating checkerboards, stripes or bands. Stimuli may be presented by a video screen or by goggles. This last device is often preferred, because it allows different kinds of stimulations (e.g. monocular, different mixes of hemifields, quadrants) and allowed us to explore cortical visual retinotopy. Moreover, it provides a better concentration for the patient, who cannot see anywhere but into the goggles. The resting condition is frequently characterized by a black screen with a fixation point in the centre. We implemented visual paradigms in our department by using goggles and alternating (500 ms period) black and red vertical bands (Fig. 21.4).

### 21.8.4 Language and Lateralization Paradigms

Since the classical works of Wernicke and Broca, the location and definition of brain language areas have been a goal and a challenge for researchers. Language areas have traditionally ascribed to two discrete regions: Wernicke's area, which is responsible for the receptive aspects of language (comprehension), and Broca's area, which controls the expressive aspects of language (production). The former is located in the left posterior temporal lobe and the latter in the left inferior frontal lobe, anterior to the central fissure; both are interconnected by the arcuate fasciculus that allows information exchange between the two.

Language areas are usually located in only one hemisphere, more frequently the left, but lateralization may not remain constant: translocation of single Wernicke's [42] or single Broca's [24] areas to the contralateral hemisphere has been demonstrated in right-handed patients, when, for instance, a slowly growing tumour allows brain plasticity mechanisms to come into play.

Owing to the complexity of language-related functions, the exact location of these functional areas is somewhat variable and cannot be predicted on the basis of anatomy alone. Of course these areas are of great importance to the private and social life of the patient, and sparing them is essential when a surgical approach is required.

Before the arrival of PET and fMRI and for approximately half of the previous century, the Wada test represented the "gold standard" and the task routinely used to assess the language-dominant hemisphere. Briefly, the Wada test requires the catheterization of both the internal carotid arteries and the successive injection, for each side, of amobarbital (125 mg), followed by

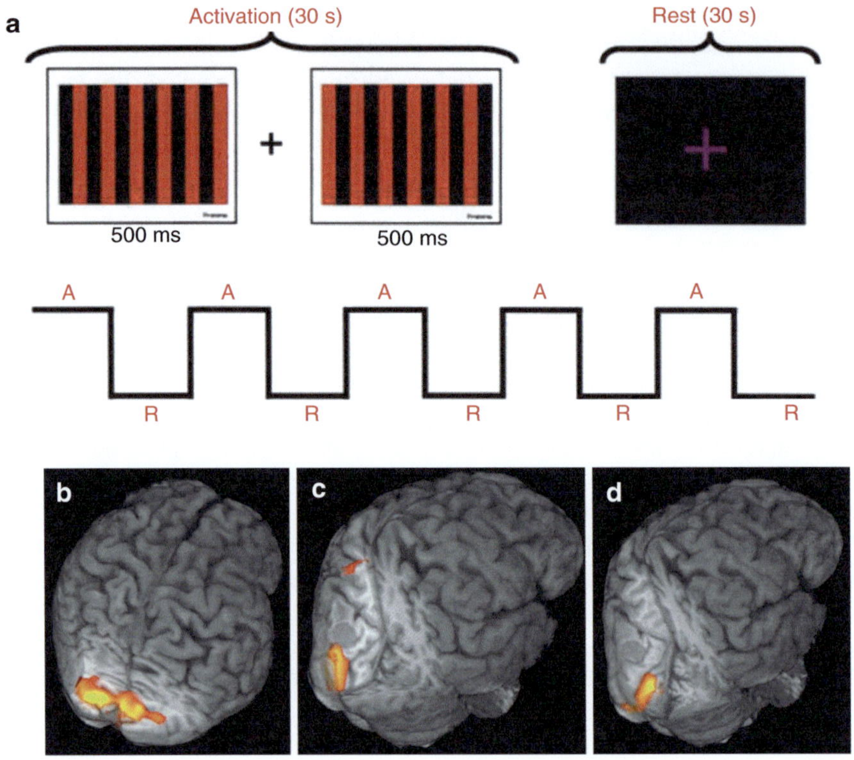


**Fig. 21.4** An example of visual paradigm. (**a**) Stimulation (alternating *black* and *red vertical bars* with a period of 500 ms) and rest alternate every 30 s. Stimulation may involve full visual fields bilaterally (**b**) or superior/inferior right quadrants (**c**, **d**, respectively). Cortical retinotopy is respected. Note the small meningioma on the left hemisphere (Modified from Leonardi et al. [33], with permission)

hemispheric anaesthetization, to exclude one hemisphere at a time; the final step is the study of the awake hemisphere to establish persistence or disruption of language functions. Of note, the Wada test is possible only when there are no vascular abnormalities allowing arterial crossflow between the two hemispheres.

The advent of fMRI has changed the approach to language exploration. As one can easily infer, the Wada test has many disadvantages with respect to fMRI: invasiveness, higher risk, higher cost and very short amounts of time (5–10 min) available to explore the awake hemisphere. fMRI, in addition to being non-invasive and cheaper, is not affected by underlying supply patterns; can be easily repeated, if necessary, without additional risk; and affords the examiner sufficient time to test a range of cortical functions. Moreover, owing to the fact that the entire brain is examined simultaneously, results are not confounded by difficulties in reproducing test conditions separately for each hemisphere, as in the Wada test. As a consequence, several studies have compared fMRI to the Wada test and have shown a significant correlation between results from both modalities in most cases. fMRI studies typically identify more language regions than direct electrocortical stimulation mapping and the Wada test, suggesting that fMRI not only identifies areas that are critical for language processing but also areas that participate in a less critical manner in networks that sustain language function. The result is a wider availability of information.

Plenty of paradigms have been used in the literature (cf. [7] for an exhaustive review) to define lateralization and locate language areas. On the whole, language paradigms may be classified into two main categories: the ones exploring receptive language and the ones exploring expressive language.

**Receptive Language Paradigms** This kind of task explores the comprehension aspect of language and elicits eloquent areas corresponding to Wernicke's areas proper (the posterior part of the superior temporal gyrus, posterior BA22) and the surroundings (the anterior-superior and middle temporal gyri, anterior BA22, the mid-superior temporal sulcus, midportion of BA21 and BA22), with the adjacent angular (BA39) and supramarginal (BA40) gyri, in the dominant hemisphere.

Receptive language paradigms are mainly divided into *reading comprehension* (visual input) and *auditory comprehension* (auditory input). The most common reading comprehension task consists of reading stories, in which each paragraph is presented at a fixed interval of time, according to the reader's speed. The most common auditory comprehension task consists of listening to stories. The latter is a passive task, which, like sensory paradigms, can also be performed on uncooperative patients.

When visual input is used, one has to consider brain activation induced by visual input, in addition. This activation does not concern the primary visual cortex only but also the ventral extrastriate inferior temporal/occipital regions, involved in transferring the modulated inputs to Wernicke's area. Otherwise, when auditory input is used, this will produce an auditory response in the adjacent auditory cortices of the superior temporal gyri. To isolate Wernicke's area and delete visual/auditory responses, other visual/auditory stimuli (e.g. uppercase/lowercase letters or backward text, respectively) may be used in the contrasting control task. However, this is not the case for presurgical purposes, because auditory/visual areas also have to be spared from the surgery.

Figure 21.5 shows an example of receptive language paradigm (listening to a reading).

**Expressive Language Paradigms** This kind of task explores the production aspect of language and elicits eloquent areas corresponding to Broca's area proper (the pars opercularis, BA44, and the posterior portion of the pars triangularis, posterior BA45, of the inferior frontal gyrus), plus the precentral gyrus of the insula, in the dominant hemisphere.

Most of the numerous existing paradigms can be classified into two main categories: *verbal fluency* and *semantic decision*. The main difference between the two is that semantic decision tasks do not only explore language production only but also some working memory functions; the result is the activation of other areas in addition to expressive language ones (see below).

*Verbal fluency tasks* rely on the ability to produce words in different ways. Worth noting is that the patient is requested to generate words covertly (inner speech), to avoid possible artefacts caused by movements of the lips, tongue and head in active word generation. When the task is of the phonological kind, the patient is visually or verbally cued with a letter of the alphabet at the beginning of each task period and asked to think of as many words as possible that begin with that letter. Of course, the letters change in each task period. When the task is of the semantic kind, the patient is visually or verbally cued with a certain category (e.g. animals, flowers) at the beginning of each task period and asked to think of as many words as possible that belong to that category. During the rest condition, the patient may repeat a single word (e.g. "bla", "bla", "bla") or may think of nothing. Receptive language areas are activated by both paradigms, but the phonological task gives a more clear-cut activation than the semantic one [44].

A verbal fluency task, which is very well used and reliable in disclosing lateralization, is verb generation from words. A sequence of words is aurally or visually presented to the patient, who has to think of a verb corresponding to each word (e.g. piano → to play), whereas the rest condition consists of silence. In addition to Broca's area, other eloquent areas may be activated in the dominant hemisphere: the pars orbitalis of the inferior frontal gyrus, BA47; the middle frontal gyrus, BA46 and 9; and the prefrontal and posterior temporal cortices.

*Semantic Decision Tasks* In this kind of task, a couple of words are sequentially presented to the

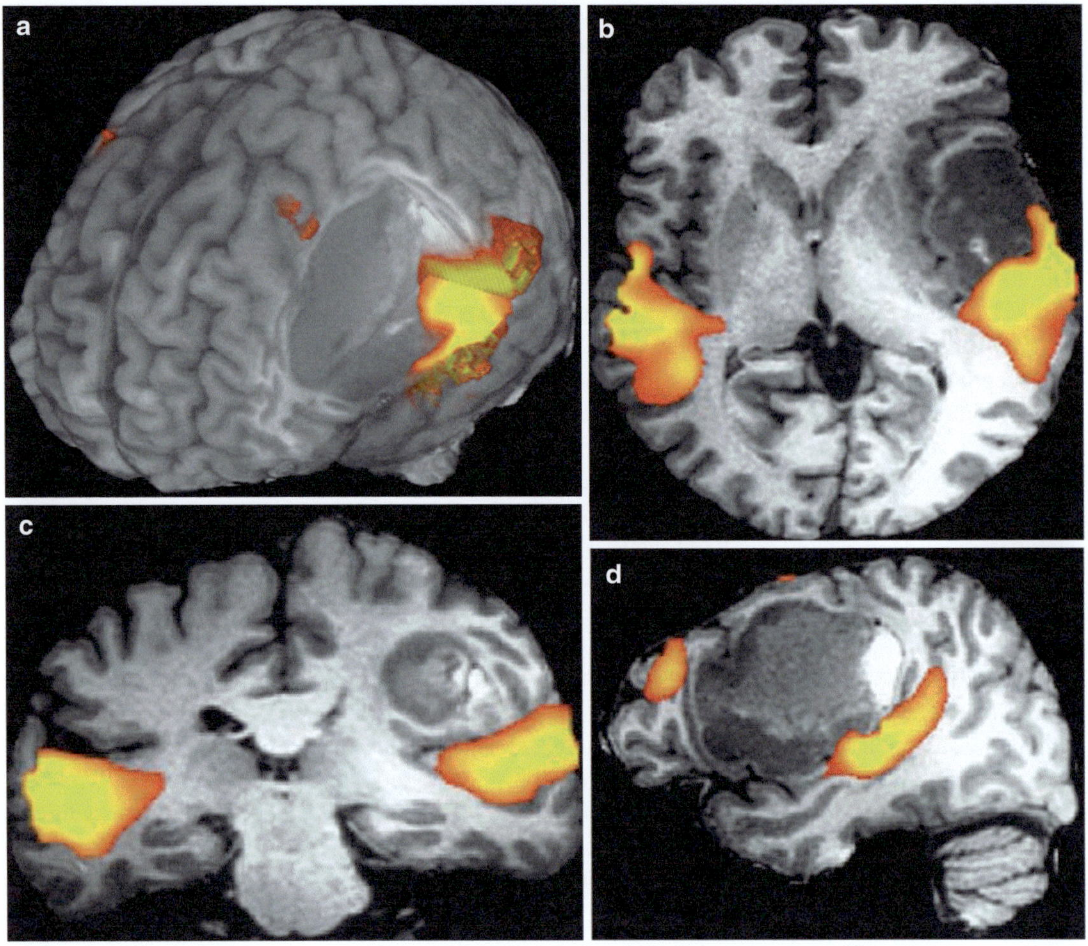


**Fig. 21.5** An example of receptive language paradigm (listening to a reading). Note that the activated areas are very adjacent to the lesion (glioma) and intermingled with it. The patient underwent surgery and had postsurgical deficits (aphasia)

patient, who has to decide if the couple appertain to a certain semantic category stated previously (e.g. synonyms vs antonyms, abstract vs concrete, living vs nonliving). Rest conditions differ according to whether the task is given aurally or visually. In the first case, couples of tones are presented, and the patient has to decide if they are identical or not. In the second case, couples of letter are shown, and the patient has to decide if they are written in uppercase or in lowercase. As already mentioned, these tasks activate other areas, besides Broca's area, and these are the middle and the inferior temporal gyri, fusiform and parahippocampal gyri, the cingulate cortex (BA32) and the superior frontal region (BA8) in the dominant hemisphere.

Figure 21.6 shows an example of an expressive language paradigm (words → verbs).

## 21.9 Presurgical Applications of fMRI

### 21.9.1 fMRI and Brain Tumours

Certainly, fMRI takes pride of place in the presurgical evaluation of brain tumours. As stated in the introduction, fMRI is of inestimable value in locating eloquent areas when normal relationships between anatomy and function are lost (e.g. when a mass effect distorts the anatomical land-

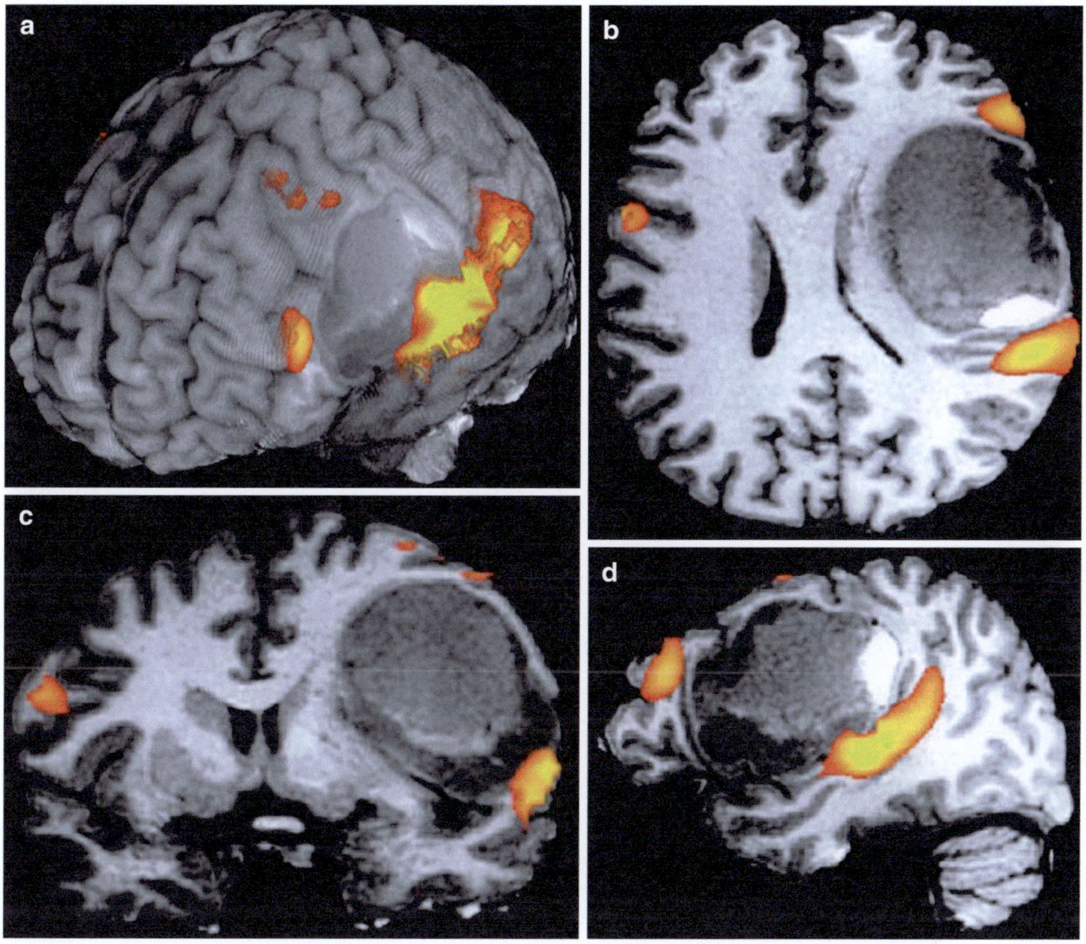


**Fig. 21.6** An example of expressive language paradigm (words→verbs). Note that the activated areas are again very adjacent to the lesion (glioma) and intermingled with it. The same patient as Fig. 21.5

marks or when functional areas may be relocated to other areas in the brain). However, in some situations, fMRI activation in and around tumours must be interpreted with caution.

Schreiber et al. [47] found that fMRI activation is reduced near glial tumours, but is usually not affected by non-glial tumours. They suggested that this phenomenon might be explained by the fact that glial tumours grow in a more infiltrative manner and thus alter the cellular architecture, whereas non-glial tumours show more delineation from normal tissue, leaving the cellular architecture intact.

Primary brain tumours, especially low-grade tumours, have been shown to have functional tissue preserved within the lesion itself. Negative findings may represent language cortex working but having an activity level below the sensitivity of the technique and thus not being detected. Moreover, it is known, from both angiographic and MR studies, that tumour vasculature in malignant gliomas loses the ability to autoregulate. If the brain's ability to autoregulate the flow of blood is lost in brain tissue, which is still functioning, then this area may not respond to increased neural activity by a corresponding increase in blood flow [25]. Another reason adduced by the same authors is the mass effect. Venous structures are normally under low pressure and are easily compressible. The increased tumour mass effect compresses the venules and larger veins, thereby speeding the egress of deoxyhaemoglobin-laden blood from the area of activation. This leads to a decrease in the relative concentration of deoxyhaemoglobin in the area of activation, which in turn results in an effective decrease in the difference in concentration of deoxyhaemoglobin between the resting and active states. This would lead to a decreased ability of fMRI to detect changes between the resting and active states [25].

However, intraoperative cortical mapping confirmed most of the fMRI findings and showed that the possible limitations of technique concerned only some selected cases and did not impede the successful identification of the eloquent cortex in the vast majority of patients of this kind.

### 21.9.2 fMRI and Epilepsy

Another important field of fMRI application is the presurgical evaluation of patients with refractory epilepsy. It is well known that about 90 % of well-selected patients become seizure-free after surgical treatment [17]. As far as the surgical outcome is concerned, fMRI becomes an important tool for selecting and better characterizing these patients.

fMRI in fact plays a significant role not only in defining the lateralization of language functions but also in localizing the specific language areas. As to this last point, it has been shown that patients with epilepsy tend to have more "bilateral" activation: they reveal a significantly higher recruitment of contralateral homologous language areas, compared to the normal controls. Moreover, the earlier the onset of dominant temporal lobe seizure foci, the more widespread and atypical the distribution of language areas; expressive and receptive language skills can also dissociate in people with brain lesions occurring early in life [2]. In this context, fMRI becomes an invaluable help in mapping clinically relevant language functions in the epilepsy surgery population.

Another advantage of fMRI use is the possibility of defining the seizure spatially and temporally. Krings et al. [31] performed fMRI on a patient, who happened to experience a simple partial seizure; the seizure was associated with changes in MR signal in different regions, showing the spatiotemporal course of spreading. fMRI data correlated with EEG-determined seizure foci. Hence, it is possible to use fMRI not only to detect the cortical location of activations associated with the seizure but also to define the epileptogenic focus in the originally activated area. The recent development of EEG-triggered fMRI allows interpretable electroencephalographic data to be recorded during MRI scanning. In this way, it is possible to combine the spatial resolution of MRI with the temporal resolution of electrophysiology in the seizure localization. EEG-linked fMRI acquisition is a promising technique in the field of epilepsy.

### 21.9.3 fMRI and AVM

The presurgical evaluation of arteriovenous malformations (AVMs) is another interesting and controversial application of fMRI. They are the most common of cerebrovascular malformations and consist of a coiled mass of arteries and veins, without an intervening capillary network, lying in a bed formed by displacement rather than invasion of normal brain tissue. Functionally, they are direct arteriovenous communications causing a shunt of blood from the arterial to the venous side. The high flow volume shunted through an AVM fistula appears as "voids" within the structure in morphological MR images and may induce a decrease in cerebral perfusion pressure in the downhill artery [37].

The surgical importance of AVMs is related to their high probability of bleeding and giving epileptic crisis. In such situations, the localization of eloquent cortices near AVMs becomes important not only presurgically but also during possible embolization procedures, because, when there is doubt that an AVM is close to eloquent tissue, particular care must be exercised to avoid devascularizing these functional areas.

The debate about the use of fMRI in AVMs revolves around the peculiar haemodynamics of this pathology. AVMs produce high-velocity, low-resistance blood flow and induce feeding artery hypotension and draining vein hypertension, with a potential net reduction in cerebral perfusion pressure in neighbouring territories. Chronic hypotension does not necessarily result in loss of neuronal function in brain tissues surrounding AVMs, but haemodynamic perturbations may reduce or impede the BOLD signal in adjacent eloquent cortex, obscuring activation where neuronal function may be present.

More specifically, there is a possible disagreement with respect to the presence or absence of significant activation within and around the nidus. The nidus represents the area, interposed between the distal segments of feeding arteries and the emerging proximal segments of draining veins, where arteriovenous shunting occurs. As revealed by histopathological findings, the nidus excludes intervening brain, whereas feeding and draining vessels are separated by brain parenchyma. Therefore, shunted blood within the nidus should not take part in metabolic changes occurring during neuronal activity, including oxygen consumption. Considering that the origin of the fMRI signal is the BOLD phenomenon, activation should not be measurable within the nidus of an AVM. The conflicting results in the literature may derive from the morphological difficulty in distinguishing the exact border of the nidus from the adjacent complex and variably dilated vessels on MR images. Intervening brain between distal feeding and proximal draining vessels could be mistaken for intranidal activation [1].

The above haemodynamic problems occur when there are severe flow anomalies; yet many patients have only moderate or any flow alterations at all. In these cases, a high correlation has been shown between fMRI mapping and electrocortical stimulation mapping [43].

Finally, Cannestra et al. propose the subdivision of MAVs into three groups on the basis of fMRI results. In group I (minimal risk), AVM and eloquent areas are disjoined by at least one gyrus free from activation; in group II (high risk) AVM and eloquent areas are intimately associated; in group III (indeterminate risk) AVM and eloquent areas are adjacent to each other. Group I patients may undergo direct surgical excision of the AVMs solely on the basis of fMRI maps. Group II patients are considered inoperable and are referred for radiosurgery. In group III patients, eloquent areas are too close to the AVMs (less than 1 cm) to allow estimation of risk; these patients are considered candidates for intraoperative electrocortical stimulation [8].

### 21.9.4 fMRI and Other Pathologies

fMRI is rapidly moving into the clinical setting, including being used for traumas, vascular diseases, inflammations, multiple sclerosis, Alzheimer disease, developmental disorders, learning disabilities and many other conditions.

One good example is the presurgical evaluation of a hydrocephalus case, which had a temporo-occipital cyst as an EEG documented source of epilepsy. The surgical question was the removal of the temporo-occipital cyst, in a patient with nearly normal full visual fields. fMRI revealed the existence of an eloquent area medial to the cyst, a result that documented a functional reorganization of the visual cortex. This way of presurgically defining visual cortex plasticity called for a conservative resection of the temporo-occipital region, with sparing of the medial aspect of the cyst [14].

### 21.9.5 fMRI and Presurgical Risk

The presurgical evaluation of patients with cerebral lesions involves the evaluation of the risk of postsurgery sequelae. Of course it is imperative for the patients to know the kind of deficit they are going to meet, as well as the probability this deficit will actually occur. In other words, the methodological approach to the risk assessment should be qualitative and quantitative. The qualitative aspect examines which function is at risk of being damaged and refers to the location of eloquent areas concerning that function (e.g. motor cortex for motion, Wernicke's and Broca's areas for language, etc.). The quantitative aspect is far more difficult to evaluate. Many studies have investigated this problem (cf. [53] for review), and the resultant quantitative best parameter to evaluate this risk is the distance between eloquent areas and lesions. The outcome of such a kind of analysis gives the following resulting values: when the distance lesion-eloquent areas exceeded 2 cm, surgical resection was considered safe, and no sequelae occurred in patients. As the distance decreased, the risk of deficits increased: when the value was between 1 and 2 cm, 33 % of patients showed postoperative deficits. Finally, when the distance was less than 1 cm, 50 % of patients experienced postoperative sequelae. Similar results were obtained by Haglund et al. [22] some years previously. These authors, by intraoperative cortical stimulation, showed no sequelae for distances over 2 cm, 17 % sequelae for distances between 0.7 and 1 cm, and 43 % sequelae for distances under 0.7 cm. Many authors (cf. [53] for review) also compared fMRI mapping of eloquent areas with results obtained by direct cortical mapping, and a good spatial correlation between the two methods was shown.

These results indicate a reliability of fMRI not only in defining the anatomical locations of an explored function but also in determining the presurgical risk. In this way, the patients are given reliable information on possible postoperative loss of function, making them clearly and fully aware at the moment of informed consent, and, at the same time, it is possible to set up a process of proper presurgical planning.

### 21.9.6 Our Experience

We received our 3 T GE Signa Excite MRI system in February 2004, but our experience with fMRI dates only from October 2004, when we received the stimulating apparatus. From October 2004 to June 2005, we performed fMRI on 27 patients with the following pathologies: 15 tumours, 4 AVMs, 4 cavernous angiomas, 2 dysplasias, 1 Parkinson's disease and 1 aphasia. Of these patients, 12 did not undergo surgery, 2 because of nonsurgical pathologies (aphasia and Parkinson) and the other 5 because fMRI showed eloquent areas strictly adjacent to the lesions. The remaining 15 patients underwent surgery. Again, of these, 7 did not show activation areas adjacent to the lesions and had no postsurgical sequelae (cf., e.g. Fig. 19.3), whereas the last 8 had eloquent cortices adjacent to the lesions. Of these, 3 % experienced postsurgical sequelae (1 serious deficit and 2 moderate deficits; cf., e.g. Figs. 21.5 and 21.6). The above percentage values are in good agreement with the previously described values of presurgical risk (cf. 33 % in [53]).

## 21.10 Some New Approaches to fMRI

### 21.10.1 The "Resting State Functional Connectivity"

In 1995, Bharat B. Biswal and colleagues [3] were studying brain activity in healthy subjects "instructed to refrain from any cognitive, language or motor tasks": they noted some slow seemingly spontaneous oscillations, having the intensities of BOLD signal and frequencies lower than 0.1 Hz, which was distinct from cardiac and respiratory activity (by a Fourier analysis). The authors also identified primary sensorimotor areas in the same subject group, by a bilateral hand movement block paradigm, and observed that the described spontaneous slow oscillations in the right-hand sensorimotor area were *temporally correlated* to the corresponding spontaneous slow oscillations in the left-hand sensorimotor area. Since such temporally correlated BOLD activities were far away (on the other hemisphere) from one another and not induced by any motor paradigm, the authors concluded that this temporal "correlation of low frequency fluctuations … is a manifestation of functional connectivity of the brain". Moreover, because BOLD oscillations occurred during a rest condition (resting state, RS), this "functional connectivity of the brain" was named as *resting state functional connectivity*.

### 21.10.2 The "Default Mode" Brain Function

Since the 1990s, many papers have been published on functional activation by using both PET (positron emission tomography) and fMRI: these works contributed to discover and explain many features of brain functions. However, many authors noticed that, during the ON phases of block paradigms, some brain areas showed reduced activities below the baseline (called deactivations) in areas seemingly different from the specifically activated ones. On the other hand, during the OFF phases of block paradigms, many of the ON phase-deactivated areas showed increased activities. Such a ON/OFF behaviour was also called *task-induced deactivation/activation*, respectively.

The physiological interpretation of these phenomena is due to Marcus E. Raichle and co-workers [45, 49], who studied a group of healthy subjects both while they "rested quietly but awake, with eyes closed" and "again while they passively viewed a visual fixation cross" with eyes open, in a PET scanner. During the eyes-closed condition, they observed many spontaneously activated areas and, among them, are precuneus (PreCu), posterior cingulate cortex (PCC), lateral parietal cortex (LPC) and medial prefrontal cortex (MPFC). When the subjects opened their eyes, a task-induced deactivation occurred in the aforesaid structures. These deactivations were not correlated to the specific kind of task (task-independent), and the same aforesaid structures were the more deactivated the higher the attentive/cognitive task demand. The authors hypothesized that this tonic activity of the spontaneously activated areas during eyes-closed rest represented a sort of baseline activity of the brain and called it the *default mode* brain function.

### 21.10.3 The "Default Mode Network"

Few years later, Michael D. Greicius and co-workers [18] succeeded in defining the connectivity of the brain structures involved in the default mode brain function. They asked themselves three questions: (1) "Does such a resting-state network exist in the human brain?" (2) "Is it modulated during simple sensory processing?" (3) "How is it modulated during cognitive processing?" To answer these questions, they performed three kinds of fMRI scans: (1) an eyes-closed resting state condition, (2) a simple passive visual block paradigm (a black and white checkerboard pattern appearing in normal and reverse way), and (3) a two-back working memory block task. The first task confirmed the previously demonstrated resting state activated areas, with particular regard to PCC/PreCu, ventral ACC (vACC) and MPFC; the second task showed no task-dependent deactivated area, whereas the third memory task showed both a task-related activity decrease in PCC, vACC, MPFC and left inferior parietal cortex (IPC), and a task-related activity increase in both left and right ventrolateral prefrontal cortex (VLPFC) and right dorsolateral prefrontal cortex (DLPFC). The authors converted deactivated and activated areas in regions of interest (ROI) and statistically inferred their connections by an analysis of the oscillation coherence (direct correlation for deactivated ROIs and inverse correlation for activated ROIs). This way, they defined the following correlations: (1) RS condition, PCC showed significant connectivity with vACC/MPFC, orbitofrontal cortex (OFC), bilateral IPC, left DLPFC, left inferolateral temporal cortex (ITC) and left parahippocampal gyrus (PHG); vACC showed significant connectivity with PCC, MPFC/OFC, nucleus accumbens and hypothalamus/midbrain. (2) Visual task: PCC and vACC connectivity patterns were virtually identical to RS condition. (3) Memory task: both VLPFC and DLPFC were inversely correlated with PCC only.

Since deactivated areas during memory task matched default mode activated areas during resting state, and these last ones showed an important connectivity, the authors defined this network of connections as the *Default Mode Network* (DMN) (Fig. 21.7). While tasks with important cognitive demands inhibit the DMN, DMN is not inhibited by simpler tasks (Fig. 21.8).

The described results suggest the existence of an inhibitory interaction between DMN areas (active at rest) and task-activated areas. The study of conditions producing DMN deactivation allows us to infer what cognitive processes DMN supports or not. For instance, the lack of deactivation in simple passive visual tasks shows that

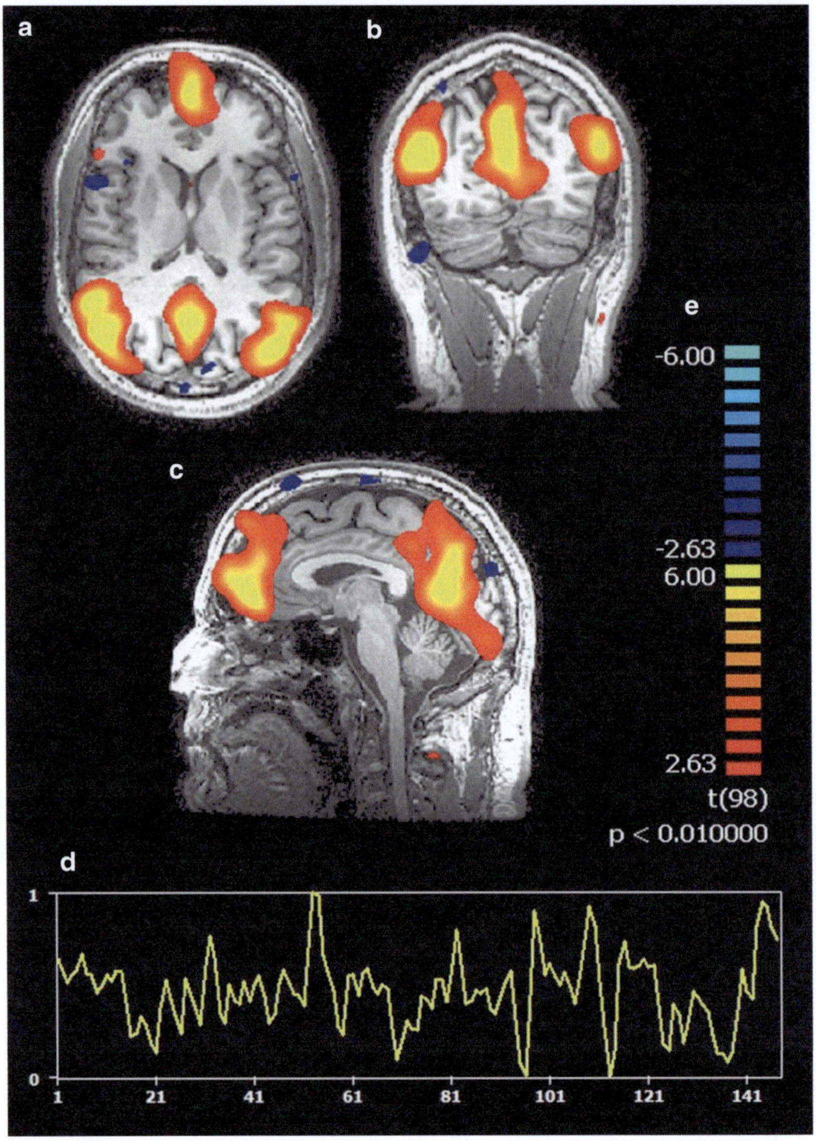


**Fig. 21.7** An example of default mode network. Eloquent areas were obtained by ICA analysis (see text). (**a**) Axial, (**b**) coronal and (**c**) sagittal brain views. (**d**) Time course of the ICA selected component, (**e**) colour scale. The activation pattern showed was obtained in a healthy volunteer lying relaxed in a supine position, with his eyes closed and not thinking about anything. No stimulation paradigm was applied. Note some spontaneously activated areas in PCC/PreCu, ACC/MPFC and lateral temporoparietal cortex

DMN is different from the network involved in the EEG alpha rhythm block when eyes pass from close to open condition.

### 21.10.4 Some Methodological Issues

In block paradigms, the mean of OFF conditions is subtracted from the mean of ON conditions: the noise of the two conditions subtract each other, and the resulting BOLD signal is relatively clean. In RS acquisitions, otherwise, more attention should be taken to the signal quality. Acquired sequences need to be properly filtered to delete cardiac and respiratory oscillations as well as other possible drifts.

There are several methods of analysis, but the most commonly used are mainly two: ROI-based analysis and independent component analysis (ICA).

The ROI-based analysis has been the first to be employed and is still the most used. ROIs are defined a priori (and named *seed regions*), according to anatomical or functional criteria.

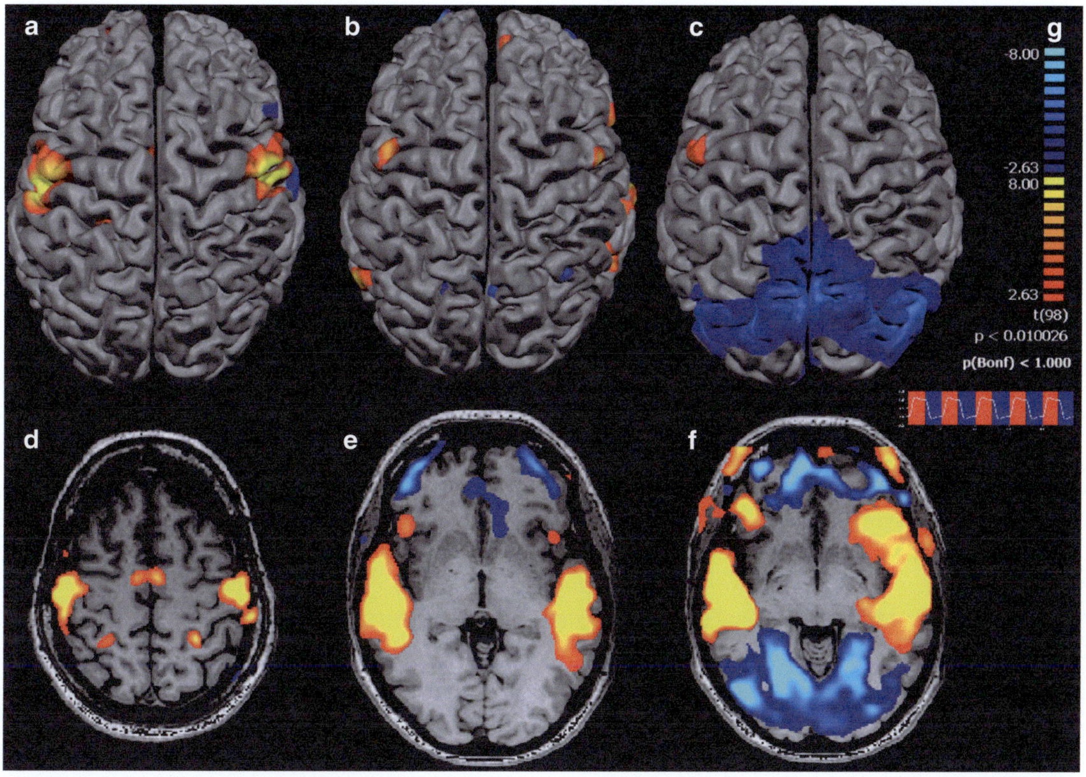


**Fig. 21.8** An example of DMN deactivation. (**a–c**) Surface 3D maps, (**d–f**) axial 2D maps, (**g**) colour scale and reference time course of the block paradigms. In this example, a healthy volunteer performed the following block paradigms. (**a**, **d**) Active motion of his lips: note the bilateral eloquent areas in the corresponding lip motor areas of the precentral gyrus. (**b**, **e**) Passive text listening: note the bilateral temporal eloquent areas in (**d**) and no deactivated area in (**e**). (**c**, **f**) Silent words-verbs generation: note the important deactivations in wide areas corresponding to bilateral PreCu/lateral temporoparietal cortex and MPFC (axial only). (**c/f**) Task requires much higher cognitive/attentive demands compared to (**a/d**) and (**b/e**) tasks

After the setting of a threshold, the next step is to average the BOLD ROI time courses at each point, thus cancelling out extraneous noise. The mean time course is then correlated to the BOLD time courses of all the other regions of the brain, resulting in a functional connectivity map, which provides information about with which regions the seed region is functionally connected and to what extent. This method has some advantages: it is simple to perform, and results may be easily explained; however, the disadvantages are it needs an a priori ROI choice, and the concurrent study of multiple systems is not possible, making it difficult to examine functional connection pattern on a whole brain scale.

The ICA analysis [39] is a mathematical-statistical multivariate method, which assumes that fMRI data set consists of a mix of independent signals from a number of spatially distributed sources, and decomposes the data into several independent components. By this technique, the many independent components are statistically decomposed in many spatial maps (each associate with a single time course), and the results are the spatial distribution of distinct functional connectivity networks. Some advantages of this technique are it is automatic; there is no need of a priori ROI, i.e. it does not require initial assumptions about network locations; and ICA is capable to discern activations which could not be predicted in advance of the experiment and allows the simultaneous study of multiple systems. However, ICA has the disadvantage of requiring a priori specification of the number of components. Some software may automatically estimate such a number, but, in practice, the number of components are often estimated by the user. Finally, ICA requires an important a posteriori selection of valid components (e.g. some resulting noise maps can be excluded).

### 21.10.5 Clinical Uses

The most important advantage, in the use of RS, is to allow the BOLD analysis in non-collaborating patients. Moreover, some studies [21] have shown the surprising persistence of DMN during a light sedation (the so-called conscious sedation), initially performed by midazolam and now achieved by propofol. In this kind of sedation, patients do not need any respiratory assistance and are sufficiently conscious to answer to vocal calls or to light tactile stimulations but are, at the same time, sedated enough to be completely relaxed and to show retrograde amnesia, after the procedure. Conscious sedation is usually used in some moderately invasive procedures such as gastroscopy or bronchoscopy.

In the last decade, the study of resting state connectivity extended to various pathologies, including both neurological and psychiatric diseases. In this chapter, a brief overview will be done to show the main clinical uses where some encouraging results have already been obtained.

#### 21.10.5.1 Alzheimer Disease (AD)

This pathology was the first clinical application of RS connectivity examined. In 2002, Li et al. [34] studied patients both at an advanced stage and with only slight cognitive deficits with respect to a control group. Results showed an important and significant connectivity change in both hippocampi (HIPP), in the case of full-blown pathology; otherwise, in the case of mild pathology, patients showed a significant connectivity decrease only: Moreover, the more the pathology progression, the more the decrease of connectivity.

Two years later, Greicius and co-workers [19] studied HIPP connectivity in AD with respect to controls and showed no DMN connectivity in PCC/PreCu: this result at last explained the PCC hypometabolism usually found in these patient's PET.

#### 21.10.5.2 Schizophrenia

This is a complex pathology, having many different symptomatological subtypes. Some of the several morphological changes involve PreCu grey matter, corpus callosum genu and anterior commissure white matter. Studies [16, 27, 28] on the DMN connectivity in these patients have shown an increase of DMN connectivity (even if with some discordant results), with respect to the control groups. Particularly, the increased connectivity occurred in MPFC and PreCu: these areas are very close to zones, where anatomical changes were shown. Once more, connectivity changes went hand in hand with the seriousness of the pathology.

#### 21.10.5.3 Disorders of Consciousness (DOC)

A critical problem, in this pathology, is that the clinical evaluation of these patients is based mainly on patient behaviour. This way, the diagnosis may result inaccurate in a percentage even reaching the 40 % of cases. Damages to nervous structures may be very variable (according to the damages in motor, sensory, visual pathways, etc.). In these patients, fMRI may successfully use block paradigms with a passive stimulation (e.g. acoustic stimulation): this kind of stimulation has revealed very useful to show activations in areas classically considered as the functional correlate of language associative areas (Wernicke's and Broca's areas).

Connectivity analysis, however, finds its pivotal role in these non-cooperating patients. There are some studies (e.g. [5]) showing the DMN (PCC/PreCu) preservation in DOC but with a reduced connectivity compared to controls. In case of cerebral death, otherwise, DMN is no more present.

#### 21.10.5.4 Other Applications

Many other applications are appearing in literature. For instance, the connectivity analysis was studied in autism (e.g. [10]), depression (e.g. [20]), temporal lobe epilepsy [62], amyotrophic lateral sclerosis [40], paediatrics [11, 12] and in the presurgical location of eloquent areas [63].

**Conclusions**

fMRI has proved to be a reliable, safe, reproducible method with which to presurgically define eloquent areas. This technique gives us the opportunity to know in advance the actual situation of a lesion so that the surgeons may plan their approach strategy. This technique also allows the establishment of a presurgical evaluation of risk and enables the patient to be fully aware at the moment of informed consent. Despite the increase in its clinical applications, fMRI is still underused in the clinical field and should be performed almost routinely before surgery. Finally, also the application of the new described functional approaches may reveal as a new added value, useful to better define eloquent areas and presurgical risk.

## References


1. Alkadhi H, Kollias SS, Crelier GR et al (2000) Plasticity of the human motor cortex in patients with arteriovenous malformations: a functional MR imaging study. AJNR 21:1423–1433
2. Baxendale S (2002) The role of functional MRI in the presurgical investigation of temporal lobe epilepsy patients: a clinical perspective and review. J Clin Exp Neuropsychol 24:664–676
3. Biswal B, Yetkin FZ, Haughton VM et al (1995) Functional connectivity in the motor cortex of resting human brain using echo-planar MRI. Magn Reson Med 34:537–541
4. Bogomolny DL, Petrovich NM, Hou BL et al (2004) Functional MRI in the brain tumor patients. Top Magn Reson Imaging 14:325–335
5. Boly M, Tshibanda L, Vanhaudenhuyse A et al (2009) Functional connectivity in the default network during resting state is preserved in a vegetative but not in a brain dead patient. Hum Brain Mapp 30:2393–2400
6. Bumgartner C, Barth DS, Levesque MF et al (1992) Human hand and lip sensimotor cortex as studied on electrocorticography. Electroencephalogr Clin Neurophysiol 84:115–126
7. Cabeza R, Nyberg L (2000) Imaging cognition II: an empirical review of 275 PET anf FMRI studies. J Cogn Neurosci 12:1–47
8. Cannestra AF, Pouratian N, Forage J et al (2004) Functional magnetic resonance imaging and optical imaging for dominant-hemisphere perisylvian arterovenous malformations. Neurosurgery 55:804–814
9. Cevolani D, Agati R, Albini Riccioli L et al (2004) Pre-surgical use of functional paradigms in brain fMRI mapping: our initial 3 T experience. Rivista di Neuroradiologia 17:836–848
10. Cherkassky VL, Kana RK, Keller TA, Just MA (2006) Functional connectivity in a baseline resting-state network in autism. Neuroreport 17:1687–1690
11. de Bie HM, Boersma M, Adriaanse S et al (2012) Resting-state networks in awake five- to eight-year old children. Hum Brain Mapp 33:1189–1201
12. Degnan AJ, Wisnowski JL, Choi S et al (2015) Altered structural and functional connectivity in late preterm preadolescence: an anatomic seed-based study of resting state networks related to the posteromedial and lateral parietal cortex. PLoS One 10:e0130686
13. Donaldson DI, Buckner RL (2004) Effective paradigm design. In: Jezzard P, Matthews PM, Smith SM (eds) Functional MRI. an introduction to methods. Oxford University Press, New York/Oxford
14. Fried I, Nenov VI, Ojermann SG et al (1995) Functional MR and PET imaging of rolandic and visual cortices for neurosurgical planning. J Neurosurg 83:854–861
15. Friston K, Holmes A, Poline J-B et al (1995) Analysis of fMRI time series revisited. Neuroimage 2:45–53
16. Garrity AG, Pearlson GD, McKiernan K et al (2007) Aberrant "default mode" functional connectivity in schizophrenia. Am J Psychiatry 164:450–457
17. Golby AJ, Poldrack RA, Illes J et al (2002) Memory lateralization in medial temporal lobe epilepsy assessed by functional MRI. Epilepsia 43:855–863
18. Greicius MD, Krasnow B, Reiss AL et al (2003) Functional connectivity in the resting brain: a network analysis of the default mode hypothesis. Proc Natl Acad Sci U S A 100:253–258
19. Greicius MD, Srivastava G, Reiss AL, Menon V (2004) Default mode network activity distinguishes Alzheimer's disease from healthy aging: evidence from functional MRI. Proc Natl Acad Sci U S A 101:4637–4642
20. Greicius MD, Flores BH, Menon V et al (2007) Resting-state functional connectivity in major depression: abnormally increased contributions from subgenual cingulate cortex and thalamus. Biol Psychiatry 62:429–437
21. Greicius MD, Kiviniemi V, Tervonen O et al (2008) Persistent default-mode network connectivity during light sedation. Hum Brain Mapp 29:839–847
22. Haglund MM, Berger MS, Mitchel S et al (1994) Cortical localization of temporal lobe language sites in patients with gliomas. Neurosurgery 34:567–576

23. Sunaert S (2006) Presurgical planning for tumor resectioning. J Magn Reson Imaging 23:887–905
24. Holodny AI, Schulder M, Ybasco A et al (2002) Translocation of Broca's area to the contralateral hemisphere as the result of the growth of a left inferior frontal glioma. J Comput Assist Tomogr 26:941–943
25. Holodny AI, Schulder M, Liu WC et al (2000) The effect of brain tumors on BOLD functional MR imaging activation in the adjacent cortex: implications for image-guided neurosurgery. AJNR 21:1415–1422
26. Hu X, Norris D (2004) Advances in high-field magnetic resonance imaging. Annu Rev Biomed Eng 6:157–184
27. Hulshoff Pol HE, Schnack HG, Mandl RC et al (2001) Focal gray matter density changes in schizophrenia. Arch Gen Psychiatry 58:1118–11251
28. Hulshoff Pol HE, Schnack HG, Mandl RC et al (2004) Focal white matter density changes in schizophrenia: reduced interhemispheric connectivity. Neuroimage 21:27–35
29. Kim SG, Ashe J, Hendrich K et al (1993) Functional magnetic resonance imaging of motor cortex: hemispheric asymmetry and handedness. Science 261:615–617
30. Kollias SS, Landau K, Khan N et al (1998) Functional evaluation using magnetic resonance imaging of the visual cortex in patients with retrochiasmatic lesions. J Neurosurg 89:780–790
31. Krings T, Topper R, Reinges MH et al (2000) Hemodynamic changes in simple partial epilepsy: a functional fMRI study. Neurology 54:524–527
32. Lemieux L, Hammers A, Mackinnon T et al (2003) Automatic segmentation of the brain and intracranial cerebrospinal fluid in T1-weighted volume MRI scans of the head, and Its application to serial cerebral and intracranial volumetry. Magn Reson Med 49:872–884
33. Leonardi M, Agati R, Cevolani D et al (2004) Potential impact of advanced 3 Tesla diagnostics in the management of patients with brain tumours. Rivista di Neuroradiologia 17:849–881
34. Li SJ, Li Z, Wu G et al (2002) Alzheimer disease: evaluation of a functional MR imaging index as a marker. Radiology 225:253–259
35. Lin W, An H, Chen Y et al (2003) Practical consideration for 3 T imaging. Magn Reson Imaging Clin N Am 11:615–639
36. Liu TT, Frank LR, Wong EC et al (2001) Detection power, estimation efficiency, and predictability in event-related fMRI. Neuroimage 13:759–773
37. Mast H, Mohr JP, Osipov A et al (1995) Steal is an unestablished mechanism for the clinical presentation of cerebral arteriovenous malformations. Stroke 26:1215–1220
38. Matthews PM (2004) An introduction to functional magnetic resonance in the brain. In: Jezzard P, Matthews PM, Smith SM (eds) Functional MRI. an introduction to methods. Oxford University Press, New York/Oxford
39. McKeown MJ, Makeig S, Brown GG et al (1998) Analysis of FMRI data by blind separation into independent spatial components. Hum Brain Mapp 6:160–188
40. Mohammadi B, Kollewe K, Samii A et al (2009) Changes of resting state brain networks in amyotrophic lateral sclerosis. Exp Neurol 217:147–153
41. Moritz C, Haughton V (2003) Functional MR imaging: paradigms for clinical preoperative mapping. Magn Reson Imaging Clin N Am 11:529–542
42. Petrovich NM, Holodny AI, Brennan CW et al (2004) Isolated translocation of Wernicke's area to the right hemisphere in a 62-year-man with a temporo-parietal glioma. AJNR 25:130–133
43. Pouratian N, Bookheimer SY, Rex DE et al (2000) Utility of preoperative functional magnetic resonance imaging for identifying language cortices in patients with vascular malformations. J Neurosurg 97:21–32
44. Pujol J, Vendrell P, Deus J et al (1996) Frontal lobe activation during word generation studied by functional MRI. Acta Neurol Scand 93:403–410
45. Raichle ME, Macleod AM, Snyder AZ et al (2001) A default mode of brain function. Proc Natl Acad Sci U S A 98:676–682
46. Rao SM, Binder JR, Hammeke TA et al (1995) Somatotopic mapping of the human primary motor cortex with functional magnetic resonance imaging. Neurology 45:919–924
47. Schreiber A, Hubbe U, Ziyeh S et al (2000) The influence of gliomas and non-glial space occupying lesions on blood-oxygen-level-dependent contrast enhancement. AJNR 21:1055–1063
48. Sereno MI, Dale AM, Reppas JB et al (1995) Borders of multiple visual areas in humans, revealed by functional magnetic resonance imaging. Science 268:889–893
49. Shulman GL, Fiez JA, Corbetta M et al (2007) Common blood flow changes across visual tasks: II.: decreases in cerebral cortex. J Cogn Neurosci 9:648–663
50. Singh LN, Higano S, Takahashi S et al (1998) Comparison of ipsilateral activation between right- and left-handers: a functional MR imaging study. Neuroreport 9:1861–1186
51. Sled JG, Zijdenbos AP, Evans AC (1998) A nonparametric method for automatic correction of intensity nonuniformity in MRI data. IEEE Trans Med Imaging 17:87–97
52. Smith SM (2004) Overview of fMRI analysis. In: Jezzard P, Matthews PM, Smith SM (eds) Functional MRI. An introduction to methods. Oxford University Press, New York/Oxford
53. Sunaert S, Yousry TA (2001) Clinical applications of functional magnetic resonance imaging. Neuroimaging Clin N Am 11:221–236
54. Uematsu S, Lesser RP, Gordon B (1992) Localization of sensimotor cortex: the influence of Sherrington and Cushing on the modern concept. Neurosurgery 30:904–913

55. Wexler BE, Fulbright RK, Lacadie CM et al (1997) An fMRI study of the human cortical motor system response to increasing functional demands. Magn Reson Imaging 15:385–396
56. Woods RP, Grafton ST, Holmes CJ et al (1998) Automated image registration: I. General methods and intrasubject, intramodality validation. J Comput Assist Tomogr 22:139–152
57. Worsley KJ, Marrett S, Neelin P et al (1996) A unified statistical approach for determining significant signals in images of cerebral activation. Hum Brain Mapp 4:58–73
58. Worsley KJ, Friston KJ (1995) Analysis of fMRI time series revisited – again. Neuroimage 2:173–181
59. Yetkin FZ, Mueller WM, Hammeke TA et al (1995) Functional magnetic resonance imaging mapping of the sensimotor cortex with tactile stimulation. Neurosurgery 36:921–925
60. Yoursy I, Naidich TP, Yoursy TA (2001) Functional magnetic resonance imaging. Factors modulating the cortical activation pattern of the motor system. Neuroimaging Clin N Am 11:195–202
61. Yoursy TA, Schmid UD, Alkadhi H et al (1997) Localization of the motor hand area to a knob on the precentral gyrus. Brain 120:141–157
62. Zhang Z, Lu G, Zhong Y et al (2009) Impaired attention network in temporal lobe epilepsy: a resting fMRI study. Neurosci Lett 458:97–101
63. Zhang D, Johnston JM, Fox MD et al (2009) Preoperative sensorimotor mapping in brain tumor patients using spontaneous fluctuations in neuronal activity imaged with functional magnetic resonance imaging: initial experience. Neurosurgery 65: 226–236

# 3.0 T fMRI in Psychiatry

# 22

Linda Antonella Antonucci, Alessandro Bertolino, and Giuseppe Blasi

## 22.1 Introduction

Neuroimaging techniques are giving an outstanding contribution to the understanding of the pathophysiology of major psychiatric disorders. Differently from other fields of medicine, the brain cannot be directly investigated in vivo with invasive procedures. Furthermore, diagnosis in psychiatry is still syndromal and based on a constellation of symptoms without known biological correlates to date. In this context, noninvasive imaging techniques including functional magnetic resonance imaging (fMRI) are crucial tools in order to shape functional aspects of the brain likely at the basis of emergent phenomena characterizing the clinical presentation of psychiatric disorders.

Importantly, major psychiatric disorders are heritable, and it is likely that their risk is mainly explained by multiple genes, each adding a small effect [113, 129]. Therefore, it is crucial to link genes effects to phenotypes key for brain disorders in order to shed light on causative pathophysiological chains. Indeed, fMRI correlates are at a shorter biological distance from genes products compared to clinical symptoms, which should increase the likelihood to disambiguate the relationship between specific genetic configurations and specific fMRI phenotypes. This is actually one of the assumptions of the Research Domain Criteria (RDoC) approach, which integrates genetic, imaging, and behavioral information in order to better characterize the biology of psychiatric disorders [72]. In this line of reasoning, fMRI is considered an important tool in order to characterize so-called intermediate phenotypes [64], i.e., quantitative, heritable traits that co-segregate with a psychiatric disorder and are tightly related to the molecular genetics of the disease [7]. Intermediate phenotypes allow to build a tight link between genes and their biological and measurable effects related to a psychiatric disorder. In other words, by identifying intermediate phenotypes, it is more likely that we could understand more about how genetic susceptibility for a psychiatric disorder affects brain function.

L.A. Antonucci
Group of Psychiatric Neuroscience, Department of Basic Medical Sciences, Neuroscience and Sense Organs, University of Bari "Aldo Moro", 70100 Bari, Italy

Department of Education Science, Psychology and Communication Science, University of Bari "Aldo Moro", Bari, Italy

A. Bertolino
Group of Psychiatric Neuroscience, Department of Basic Medical Sciences, Neuroscience and Sense Organs, University of Bari "Aldo Moro", 70100 Bari, Italy

G. Blasi (✉)
Group of Psychiatric Neuroscience, Department of Basic Medical Sciences, Neuroscience and Sense Organs, University of Bari "Aldo Moro", 70100 Bari, Italy

Unit of Psychiatry, Azienda Ospedaliero-Universitaria Consorziale Policlinico, Bari, Italy
e-mail: blasi.seppe@gmail.com


T. Scarabino et al. (eds.), *High Field Brain MRI*, DOI 10.1007/978-3-319-44174-0_22

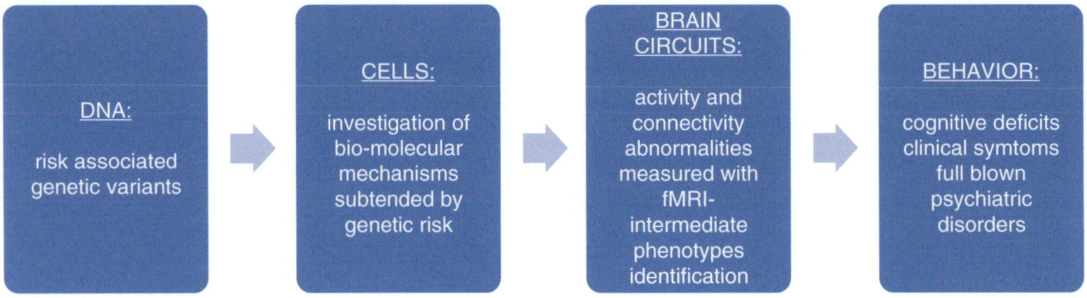


**Fig. 22.1** The path from genes to behavior. fMRI phenotypes are closer to genes effect compared to behavioral correlates

The main features of intermediate phenotypes are that (1) they are present also in healthy relatives of patients suffering from the disorder [63], (2) they are strongly involved in one or some biological pathogenic mechanisms of the disease [37], and (3) they have good psychometric properties and are measurable with sufficient validity and reproducibility. In this regard, high-field fMRI is particularly relevant for the identification of intermediate phenotypes because it deeply characterizes brain activity with high reproducibility and spatial resolution, such that it may capture even subtle genetic effects of relevance to brain disorders (Fig. 22.1).

In this chapter, we will first focus on how high-field fMRI is helping in revealing pathophysiological aspects of a prototypical brain disorder, i.e., schizophrenia. In particular, we will first describe key concepts related to this brain disorder and to its genetics. Then, we will describe intermediate phenotypes for schizophrenia as identified with fMRI. Furthermore, we will focus on studies addressing the relationship between such intermediate phenotypes and genetic variations of relevance to schizophrenia. Finally, we will highlight recent applications of high-field functional neuroimaging as a tool for delineating trajectories of risk for this brain disorder using the intermediate phenotype approach.

## 22.2 Schizophrenia: Key Concepts

Schizophrenia has a lifetime prevalence of approximately 0.3–0.7 % (Diagnostic and Statistical Manual of Mental Disorders, version V (DSM V) [3]) and is considered the most severe and disabling mental disorder for several reasons. First, schizophrenia symptoms including delusions, hallucinations, and flattened affect lead to a significant decline in personal and social functioning of the patients [136]. Moreover, it is characterized by a chronic course with frequent relapses [59], and the rehabilitation of patients suffering from this disorder is hard because of the frequent insufficient response to the pharmacological treatment, which often fails in improving personal and social functioning of patients.

Heritability plays a crucial role in schizophrenia: about 80 % of the susceptibility for this disorder is explained by genetic factors [94]. Nonetheless, the likely complex, heterogeneous, and non-Mendelian genetic architecture [69] of schizophrenia makes it extremely difficult to discover causative genes. There is not a single gene explaining genetic risk for schizophrenia [12]. In this regard, genome-wide association studies (GWAS) using very large sample sizes suggest that risk for this brain disorder is associated with several genetic variants, each with a small effect [113]. In particular, the Schizophrenia Working Group of the Psychiatric Genomics Consortium analyzed genome-wide data from more than 36,000 patients with schizophrenia as well as more than 113,000 healthy subjects and identified 108 genetic loci associated with diagnosis for this brain disorder [113]. These results are giving an outstanding contribution and impulse to further studies investigating the biological pathways implicated in mechanisms of risk for this devastating disease, which are not fully understood to date. Importantly, gene-environment interactions may be relevant in increasing such risk [12, 36]. This scenario, together with the uncertainty and variability of the clinical phenotype [12], makes it crucial for the investigation of intermediate phenotypes characterized by fMRI in order to link small and complex gene effects to measurable biological correlates, such that new light could be shed on key pathophysiological aspects of schizophrenia.

### 22.2.1 Schizophrenia and fMRI Intermediate Phenotypes

A starting point of fMRI studies in schizophrenia is that patients exhibit deficits while performing tasks eliciting high-order cognitive functions as working memory and attention [47, 77, 145]. Moreover, evidence revealed that such cognitive deficits are also present in their unaffected siblings [47, 137]. On this basis, past research devoted to the investigating of neurobiological correlates of these cognitive impairments identified abnormal activation of the dorsolateral prefrontal cortex (DLPFC) as a reliable and robust intermediate phenotype for schizophrenia (Bertolino and Blasi in Pancheri, [11]). Indeed, this brain region is key for working memory [62] and attentional control [17] processing. More in detail, a large body of literature suggested decreased prefrontal activation in patients with schizophrenia when compared to healthy controls during working memory (hypofrontality) [6, 103, 104, 112]. On the other hand, further studies proposed a more elaborated interpretation of the relationship between schizophrenia and dorsolateral prefrontal abnormalities, positing that prefrontal capacity in patients with schizophrenia reaches saturation at a lower level of working memory demand when patients are compared to normal controls [13, 32, 91, 118, 130, 132]. Thus, patients may have greater DLPFC activity than controls at low working memory demands because of the need to recruit a large amount of prefrontal resources. At a greater load of working memory, patients may have lower DLPFC response, because of the failure of performing the task when the load is too high for their working memory capacity [91].

Similarly, studies focusing on attentional control and selective attention suggest a decrease in activation in patients with schizophrenia in DLPFC [6, 22, 34, 35, 78, 80, 87, 107, 108, 119, 149] and in cingulate cortex [17, 18]. On the other hand, there is evidence of hyperfrontality in patients with schizophrenia when compared to controls while performing attentional control tasks [78, 92, 148]. Again, an earlier saturation of capacity also during attentional processing may reconcile these apparently discrepant findings [22]. Apart of these interpretations, these studies testify the strong involvement of DLPFC in the pathophysiology of schizophrenia, suggesting that abnormalities in functional activation during both working memory and attentional control tasks are core features of this disorder.

As stated above, one of the key features of intermediate phenotypes is that they must be present also in healthy relatives of patients suffering from the disease. In this line of reasoning, further studies have investigated whether healthy siblings of patients with schizophrenia share with their affected relatives patterns of functional abnormalities during brain processing. For example, Callicott et al. [30] demonstrated that, despite the absence of significant behavioral differences between groups, siblings had greater DLPFC activation than normal controls while performing the N-Back task, suggesting that siblings require the engagement of a greater amount of neuronal resources compared to controls in order to perform the working memory task at the same level of proficiency. This pattern is similar to those found in several previous studies ([24, 29, 45, 67, 78, 90]; Manoach et al. 1999; [92, 122, 126, 134, 148]) and consistent with the model of decreased prefrontal capacity during cognition in schizophrenia described above [91].

Recent studies on schizophrenia have also focused on another key brain function, i.e., the processing of reward. This is a form of action-outcome learning about an organized behavior that is performed in order to obtain a positive experience [154]. Indeed, previous models have posited that reward processing may play a key role in the pathophysiology of schizophrenia [61], possibly because of the inability of patients in integrating feedback over extended learning.

In this context, several fMRI studies have demonstrated abnormal lower activation of the ventral striatum in patients with schizophrenia during reward anticipation compared to healthy controls, as well as a negative correlation between such striatal response and negative symptoms scores [41, 50, 75, 76, 97, 124, 156]. Consistent with a role of the neural network subtending reward in the pathophysiology of schizophrenia, a recent study using a multivariate approach [84] found that diagnosis of schizophrenia is predicted by the activation pattern of several key nodes of the reward system (frontal, temporal, and midbrain regions) (93 % accuracy rate). Activation in ventral striatum was associated with 88 % accuracy rate in the prediction analysis. Moreover, activity of ventral striatum also predicted negative symptoms scores. These results suggest that investigation of the brain network subserving reward processing is a promising target for the identification of novel neurobiological markers of schizophrenia. Accordingly, few recent studies comparing the brain activation of normal controls and relatives of patients with schizophrenia revealed that relatives have the same pattern of reduced ventral striatum activation characterizing patients [44, 66] and that such ventral striatal activation negatively correlates with subclinical negative symptoms [44].

Overall, these findings suggest that region-specific fMRI activity during different brain processes is crucially associated with schizophrenia. In particular, DLPFC fMRI response during high-order cognitive processing is consistently altered in patients as well as in their healthy siblings. Consistent findings have also highlighted the putative relevance of ventral striatal activity during reward processing for schizophrenia. This evidence strongly suggests that these fMRI correlates could be useful intermediate phenotypes for this brain disorder.

A growing body of evidence obtained using high-field MRI is also highlighting the crucial relevance for schizophrenia of anomalies in functional connectivity between key regions for working memory and attention. In this context, evidence indicated lower cortical (prefrontal) and subcortical (especially thalamic) connectivity during cognitive processing in patients with schizophrenia and in subjects with genetic liability for this disorder [42, 105, 140, 141, 155], although evidence of increased prefrontal connectivity has also been found [152]. Moreover, other studies have revealed that connectivity abnormalities related to schizophrenia are also present in regions not directly participating to cognitive processing, such as nodes of the default mode network (DMN) [109, 127], which is composed of a set of brain areas including the medial prefrontal cortex (mPFC), the posterior cingulate cortex, the inferior parietal lobule, the precuneus, and the medial temporal lobe [117]. This network has been implicated in self-reference [68] and introspection [110]. In particular, abnormalities in DMN connectivity have been found in both patients with schizophrenia and people at genetic risk for the disease, even if patterns of anomalies are not always consistent [38, 58, 82, 99, 101, 116, 133, 152, 155]. A recent study [5] investigated with Independent Component Analysis the relationship between genetic risk for schizophrenia and connectivity strength in both DMN and nodes of cognition during attentional control using the Variable Attentional Control (VAC) task [18] in patients with schizophrenia, unaffected siblings of patients, and normal controls. Results revealed that patients with schizophrenia and healthy siblings, compared to healthy controls, had attenuated connectivity strength in left thalamus within an attentional control network (Fig. 22.2) as well as greater connectivity in right medial prefrontal cortex (PFC) within the DMN.

These results are in line with studies demonstrating the key role of the thalamus in cognition [71, 139, 163] as well as with those indicating its abnormal activation in patients with schizophrenia and in their healthy siblings during cognitive processing (Braus et al. 2002; [70, 88, 90]; Salgado-Pineda et al. 2004). Furthermore, they are also consistent with the hypothesis that connectivity dysfunctions are a core feature of schizophrenia, especially in the thalamic-prefrontal network [4, 102, 123, 150], such that they could be considered a reliable intermediate phenotype for schizophrenia.

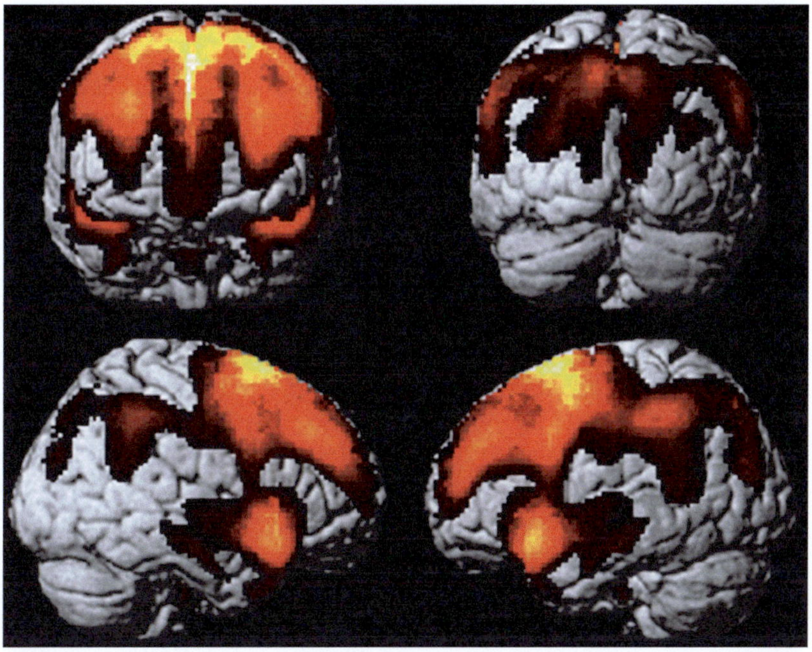

**Fig. 22.2** Render depicting an independent component of brain functional connectivity correlated with attentional control processing, as found in Antonucci et al. [5]

## 22.3 The Relationship Between fMRI Intermediate Phenotypes and Genetics of Schizophrenia

It is crucial to link intermediate phenotypes with biological pathogenic mechanisms of the disease. Shaping this relationship is relevant in order to shed light on the effects of such mechanisms on the physiology of the brain, as well as to unveil how pharmacological treatments modulating specific biological targets affect system-level phenotypes key for brain disorders. With respect to schizophrenia, a large body of evidence suggests that risk for this brain disorder is predicted by multiple genetic variants [113], that dopamine plays a key role in its pathophysiology ([14, 16, 26, 33, 65]; Weinberger 1987), and that genetic variability of an important determinant of dopamine signaling as the D2 dopamine receptor (DRD2) is associated with diagnosis of schizophrenia [113]. Importantly, D2 is target of all the antipsychotics to date and modulates prefrontal cognition (Seamans 2004 [121]). Its relevance in psychotic disorders is further testified by evidence of increased D2 density in striatum in patients [85]. Furthermore, both clinical and cognitive symptoms in patients with schizophrenia may be associated with abnormalities in D2 signaling [46, 81, 144]. Thus, it is crucial to investigate the relationship between genetic variations affecting D2 signaling and intermediate phenotypes as identified with high-field fMRI in order to add knowledge to the relationship between genes effect and brain correlates of relevance to schizophrenia.

In this regard, it is important to note that there are two alternatively spliced isoforms of the D2 receptor [138]: the D2 long (D2L) isoform is primarily postsynaptic, while the D2 short (D2S) isoform is mainly presynaptic and acts as an autoreceptor. Previous evidence has indicated that an intronic DRD2 single-nucleotide polymorphism (SNP) (rs1076560) affects the D2S/D2L ratio in both prefrontal and striatal regions, with GG subjects having higher D2S density than subjects carrying the T allele [162]. Importantly, this SNP also predicts in healthy subjects behavioral performance as well as cortical and subcortical activity during working memory and attention, with subjects homozygous for the guanine (G) allele being more efficient than subjects carrying the timine (T) allele (i.e., GG subjects exhibited lower prefrontal and striatal activation and greater performance during working memory when compared to T carriers). Other findings indicate that this genetic variant interacts with diagnosis of schizophrenia in modulating cognitive and neurobiological phenotypes. In particular, Bertolino et al. [15] replicated the association of rs1076560 with D2S/D2L ratio of expression in healthy subjects and found similar results in patients with schizophrenia. Furthermore, they reported an interaction between genotype and diagnosis on prefrontal activity and behavior during working memory. In particular, T carrier healthy subjects had lower working memory performance in the face of greater prefronto-striatal activation when compared to healthy GG subjects. Differently, patients carrying the T allele had lower working memory accuracy but also lower prefronto-striatal activity relative to GG patients. The authors interpreted these results on the basis of a differential dopamine level in patients with schizophrenia and healthy subjects, such that suboptimal prefrontal processing during working memory might be differentially elicited in this group of individuals. Apart of possible interpretations, overall these findings strongly suggest a key relevance of functional variation in the D2 receptor gene in the modulation of crucial system-level phenotypes of schizophrenia, as measured with high-field fMRI.

D2 signaling is transducted in the neuron by different signaling pathways, which allow D2 related molecular adjustments possibly relevant for pathophysiological aspects of schizophrenia. In one of these molecular cascades, D2 receptors interact with the serine/threonine kinase AKT1, which phosphorylates to inhibit the protein kinase glycogen synthase kinase (GSK-3β) in a cAMP-independent pathway [51]. In particular, D2 stimulation by dopamine inhibits AKT1 through dephosphorylation [8, 9]. This mechanism in turn modulates activity of another serine/threonine kinase, GSK-3β, which has beta-catenin as a crucial substrate involved in gene expression [19, 20, 51]. Importantly, both AKT1 and GSK-3β have been involved in schizophrenia. For example, AKT1 levels in peripheral lymphocytes and in the prefrontal cortex are reduced in schizophrenia patients [49]. Furthermore, the AKT1 coding gene (14q32.32) has been associated with diagnosis of schizophrenia [73, 98, 120, 131, 135]. Moreover, imaging genetic results revealed that the A allele of a synonymous SNP in the gene coding for AKT1 (rs1130233, G>A) has been associated with less efficient prefrontal activity during working memory. With regard to GSK-3β, evidence indicated lower phosphorylation of this kinase in postmortem prefrontal cortex of patients with schizophrenia [2, 49] as well as genetic association of GSK-3β with diagnosis [86, 128]. Other studies have also indicated that GSK-3β genetic variation affects temporal lobe volumes in schizophrenia patients [10]. Moreover, a recent fMRI study [19] tested the association of a polymorphism (rs12630592) in GSK-3β coding gene with prefrontal activity during cognitive processing and prefrontal cortical thickness in healthy humans. Results demonstrated that the TT genotype for rs12630592 was associated with attenuated fMRI prefrontal activity during working memory and attentional control processing. Furthermore, TT genotype was associated with reduced prefrontal cortical thickness and with diagnosis of schizophrenia.

Given the complex genetic architecture of schizophrenia, other studies have also tested if the interaction between genetic variants relevant to D2 signaling affect brain phenotypes crucially associated with this brain disorder. In this context, a recent study [20] investigated the interaction between DRD2 rs1076560 and AKT1 rs1130233 on multilevel correlates in healthy subjects and patients with schizophrenia. Results indicated that the interaction between the T allele of DRD2 rs1076560 and the A allele of AKT1 rs1130233 was associated with reduced AKT1 levels, reduced GSK-3β phosphorylation and altered cingulate cortex activation during attentional control. Furthermore, in a sample of patients with schizophrenia, the authors found that the interaction between the two alleles was associated with better response after 8 weeks of treatment with a second-generation antipsychotic. Moreover, Blasi et al. [21] investigated the interaction between functional genetic variations in genes coding for D2 (rs1076560) and 5HT2A (rs6314) [19] coding genes, whose signaling likely converges on common molecular pathways [43]. Here [21] the authors demonstrated that healthy subjects carrying the T allele for both genetic variants have greater prefrontal activity during working memory and attentional control tasks, as well as lower behavioral accuracy during N-Back. Furthermore, patients carrying the T allele for both DRD2 rs1076560 and HTR2A rs6314 had lower clinical improvements after antipsychotic treatment, relative to the other genotypic groups. Other results add evidence to the complex interaction between genetic variants in modulating intermediate phenotypes for schizophrenia. In particular, Tan et al. [131] found an epistatic interaction between *AKT1* rs1130233 and *COMT* rs4680, a functional polymorphism located in the gene coding for the cathecol-O-methyltransferase, which acts as the main enzyme for the catabolism of dopamine in prefrontal cortex. Specifically, healthy individuals carrying both the *AKT1* rs1130233 A allele (associated with decreased AKT1 expression) and the *COMT* rs4680 valine allele – which increases COMT activity compared to the met allele [39], possibly lowering synaptic dopamine tone – had lower prefrontal efficiency relative to all other *AKT1-COMT* genotypic configurations while performing a working memory task during fMRI.

Altogether, these results highlight the relevance of high-field fMRI in elucidating how functional genetic variation of relevance for schizophrenia affects brain phenotypes crucially associated with this brain disorder. Furthermore, they are consistent with the notion that the genetic architecture of schizophrenia is heterogeneous and more likely associated with interactive mechanisms among several genetic variants. Therefore, the investigation of association between single genetic variants and brain intermediate phenotypes of schizophrenia would probably have only a limited amount of information on the pathophysiological mechanisms of the disease. Accordingly, recent advances in this field are starting to address the relationship between polygenic effects of multiple genetic variants and brain intermediate phenotypes. For example, Walton et al. [142] derived a polygenic risk score, based on more than 600 genetic variants associated with schizophrenia in a separate discovery sample, and demonstrated that increased polygenic risk for schizophrenia predicted DLPFC inefficiency during a working memory task, coherently with other reports [143, 151]. These results strengthen the notion that a polygenic approach is able to detect complex patterns of schizophrenia-related neural dysfunctions, which is in line with the complex genetic architecture underlying the disease. Consistent with this notion, novel and intriguing methodological concepts are arising, which are pushing this field of research toward the investigation of the relationship between genetic networks and brain functional activity. This approach integrates to the analysis of a large amount of genetic and molecular information in order to identify biological ensembles implicated in brain disorders [57]. Using this perspective, Richiardi et al. [111] report findings suggesting that physiological resting state brain functional connectivity is linked with the coordinated activity of several genes possibly modulating ion channels and synaptic function. A logical following step of this investigation will be the study of the relationship between gene networks and intermediate phenotypes of relevance to schizophrenia.

## 22.4 fMRI as a Prevention Tool: The At-Risk Mental State for Psychosis and Brain Functional Imaging-Associated Features

High-field fMRI allows the detection of intermediate phenotypes for schizophrenia as well as the investigation of their association with individual genetic variability of relevance for this brain disorder. However, if risk for schizophrenia is genetically mediated and affects neurodevelopmental mechanisms [147], it is likely that schizophrenia-specific brain functional features are present before the clinical onset of the disorder. Extending knowledge on brain functional anomalies during the period of life preceding full-blown schizophrenia would be useful for clinical research and practice in order to early identify people at risk for the illness and might allow the implementation of prevention and/or intervention strategies targeting these individuals [159, 160].

In this regard, schizophrenia is often preceded at the clinical level by a "prodromal phase," defined as a critical period which could last from few days to around 5 years, characterized by a marked behavioral alteration and by a significant personal and social decline. Moreover, during the prodromal period, some psychotic-like symptoms may appear, which are usually different from those characterizing the acute phase of schizophrenia in terms of attenuated frequency, duration, and/or intensity. Because of this attenuated symptomatology, none of these symptoms could fall into any diagnostic category [159–161]. Current evidence has highlighted that some clinical variables could be predictive of the transition to psychosis. For example, high levels of unusual content of thoughts, high level of paranoid thoughts, low personal, occupational and social functioning, history of drug addiction, and exposure to stressful life events seem to increase risk for conversion to acute psychosis [74]. Previous studies have used specific criteria in order to identify the subclinical population of "at-risk mental state" (ARMS), i.e., individuals between 15 and 30 years [40] who suffer from attenuated psychotic symptoms but cannot be diagnosed with psychosis yet [161]. Meta-analytic [52, 53] and longitudinal studies [31, 83, 96, 160] on ARMS subjects suggest that the risk of transition to full-blown psychosis progressively increases during the subsequent 3 years after their first evaluation.

A wide body of literature demonstrated that cognitive deficits in the domains of working memory, attention, executive functioning, verbal fluency, and social cognition are present in at-risk subjects [52], in whom they could be considered as primary symptoms [23] and independent from drug treatment and course of the disease [48]. Previous literature suggests that they could be also considered as an index of functional outcome and response to treatment [79]. Specifically, results in literature demonstrated that people at risk who subsequently convert to psychosis, compared with those who do not convert, have more severe cognitive impairment in several cognitive domains [158], especially in verbal fluency and memory [60, 106]. However, the neural substrates of the cognitive deficits exhibited by ARMS subjects have not been fully investigated. Furthermore, results published in this context are often weak, also due to the small sample sizes used.

fMRI studies performed to date have indicated that the brain functional abnormalities found in ARMS subjects are qualitatively similar, but less severe, than those exhibited by subjects at their first episode of psychosis (FEP, [56]) and that ARMS have patterns of brain activation which are intermediate between those displayed by full-blown psychotic patients and normal controls [27, 95]. For example, Morey et al. [95] found that the behavioral performances of ARMS subjects during a cognitive control task were lower than those of normal controls, but greater than those of FEP and chronic schizophrenia patients. Furthermore, fMRI activity during the task revealed that ARMS subjects, when compared to normal controls, had lower BOLD response in the middle and the inferior frontal gyrus, while they had greater activation of these loci when compared to FEP and schizophrenia patients. Overall, these results suggest that both behavioral and imaging abnormalities are associated with the progression of the disease. Furthermore, they also suggest that brain functional anomalies predate the onset of the illness and are associated with vulnerability to psychosis, rather than with the diagnosis itself. On the other hand, other studies have indicated that ARMS subjects exhibit greater activation than normal controls in medial and inferior frontal regions [28, 54, 100]. Moreover, further work found patterns of both increased and decreased activation in ARMS subjects during cognitive processing in basal ganglia, precuneus, occipital, parietal, postcentral, and supramarginal gyrus compared to controls [1, 54, 55, 114, 157]. Also, other findings indicate that prefrontal, cingulate, and parietal cortex hypoactivation is associated with transition from ARM state to full psychosis [125, 153]. All together, these results suggest that ARMS are characterized by different brain functional anomalies compared to healthy controls and FEP on one hand. On the other hand, the lack of consistency of the results makes it difficult to clearly identify an unambiguous pathophysiological pattern characterizing ARMS.

An emerging approach for the characterization of potential markers of risk for psychosis is the analysis of brain functional networks. In this regard, Allen et al. [1] used dynamic causal modeling (DCM) techniques in order to investigate effective frontotemporal connectivity during a sentence completion task. Results of this study indicate an increase in activation of the cingulate cortex in ARMS subjects when compared to healthy controls. Furthermore, there was a relationship between cingulate activity and frontotemporal connectivity, such that the more the activity of cingulate cortex in ARMS, the more the frontotemporal connectivity was similar between these subjects and controls. These results could suggest that ARMS subjects need compensatory activation of the cingulate cortex in order to maintain optimal levels of frontotemporal connectivity, thus revealing connectivity anomalies associated with the prodromal phase of psychosis. Similarly, Lord et al. [89] used a graph theory approach to investigate patterns of abnormal connectivity in ARMS during a verbal fluency task. The anterior cingulate cortex (ACC) was the network hub of this analysis. Results revealed that ARMS and normal controls did not differ in terms of global connectivity and efficiency of networks. However, ACC was less involved in contributing to task relevant functional connections in high symptomatic compared to low symptomatic ARMS subjects and to normal controls, as suggested by the analysis of topological centrality. These results suggest that connectivity abnormalities predate the onset of full-blown psychosis and could be associated with psychosis risk. Furthermore, they also suggest that advanced neuroimaging techniques could have a predictive value in order to detect anomalies associated with the risk for psychosis. In this regard, the strong and groundbreaking clinical potential of high-field fMRI for the early identification of at risk individuals should be well explored in the next future.

**Conclusions**

All studies here reported support the notion that high-field fMRI is capable to detect neurobiological anomalies that are associated with schizophrenia, which has heterogeneous clinical correlates. Indeed, fMRI, more than behavioral and clinical tools, is providing brain phenotypes closer to the effect of the complex genetic architecture of this disease and, as such, is likely to characterize markers of its risk. These markers might in future provide clinical practice with useful information about potential predictors of psychosis, such that they might be used as targets for strategies of prevention in order to mitigate trajectories of development of schizophrenia. However, the heterogeneity of findings and the lack of robust longitudinal studies comparing individuals who subsequently develop psychosis with subjects who do not call for stronger efforts in order to shed more light on the brain correlates of schizophrenia and of risk for this brain disorder. Such efforts might also help in softening the social burden associated with this devastating brain illness, which is paradigmatic of the relevant impact of psychiatric diseases for the entire community.

## References

1. Allen P, Stephan KE, Mechelli A, Day F, Ward N, Dalton J, Williams SC, McGuire P (2010) Cingulate activity and fronto-temporal connectivity in people with prodromal signs of psychosis. NeuroImage 49:947–955
2. Amar S, Shaltiel G, Mann L, Shamir A, Dean B, Scarr E, Bersudsky Y, Belmaker RH, Agam G (2008) Possible involvement of post-dopamine D2 receptor signalling components in the pathophysiology of schizophrenia. Int J Neuropsychopharmacol 11:197–205
3. American Psychiatric Association (2013) Diagnostic and statistical manual of mental disorders, 5th edn. American Psychiatric Publishing, Arlington
4. Anticevic A, Cole MW, Repovs G, Murray JD, Brumbaugh MS, Winkler AM, Savic A, Krystal JH, Pearlson GD, Glahn DC (2014) Characterizing thalamo-cortical disturbances in schizophrenia and bipolar illness. Cereb Cortex 24:3116–3130

5. Antonucci LA, Taurisano P, Fazio L, Gelao B, Romano R, Quarto T, Porcelli A, Mancini M, Di Giorgio A, Caforio G, Pergola G, Popolizio T, Bertolino A, Blasi G (2016) Association of familial risk for schizophrenia with thalamic and medial prefrontal functional connectivity during attentional control. Schizophr Res 173:23–29
6. Barch DM, Carter CS, Braver TS, Sabb FW, MacDonald A 3rd, Noll DC, Cohen JD (2001) Selective deficits in prefrontal cortex function in medication-naive patients with schizophrenia. Arch Gen Psychiatry 58:280–288
7. Bearden CE, Freimer NB (2006) Endophenotypes for psychiatric disorders: ready for primetime? Trends Genet 22:306–313
8. Beaulieu JM, Sotnikova TD, Marion S, Lefkowitz RJ, Gainetdinov RR, Caron MG (2005) An Akt/beta-arrestin 2/PP2A signaling complex mediates dopaminergic neurotransmission and behavior. Cell 122:261–273
9. Beaulieu JM, Tirotta E, Sotnikova TD, Masri B, Salahpour A, Gainetdinov RR, Borrelli E, Caron MG (2007) Regulation of Akt signaling by D2 and D3 dopamine receptors in vivo. J Neurosci 27:881–885
10. Benedetti F, Poletti S, Radaelli D, Bernasconi A, Cavallaro R, Falini A, Lorenzi C, Pirovano A, Dallaspezia S, Locatelli C, Scotti G, Smeraldi E (2010) Temporal lobe grey matter volume in schizophrenia is associated with a genetic polymorphism influencing glycogen synthase kinase 3-beta activity. Genes Brain Behav 9:365–371
11. Bertolino A, Blasi G (2007) Fisiopatologia e alterazioni funzionali. In: Pancheri P (ed) Trattato italiano di psichiatria. La schizofrenia. Elsevier Masson.
12. Bertolino A, Blasi G (2009) The genetics of schizophrenia. Neuroscience 164:288–299
13. Bertolino A, Caforio G, Petruzzella V, Latorre V, Rubino V, Dimalta S, Torraco A, Blasi G, Quartesan R, Mattay VS, Callicott JH, Weinberger DR, Scarabino T (2006) Prefrontal dysfunction in schizophrenia controlling for COMT Val158Met genotype and working memory performance. Psychiatry Res 147:221–226
14. Bertolino A, Esposito G, Callicott JH, Mattay VS, Van Horn JD, Frank JA, Berman KF, Weinberger DR (2000) Specific relationship between prefrontal neuronal N-acetylaspartate and activation of the working memory cortical network in schizophrenia. Am J Psychiatry 157:26–33
15. Bertolino A, Fazio L, Caforio G, Blasi G, Rampino A, Romano R, Di Giorgio A, Taurisano P, Papp A, Pinsonneault J, Wang D, Nardini M, Popolizio T, Sadee W (2009) Functional variants of the dopamine receptor D2 gene modulate prefronto-striatal phenotypes in schizophrenia. Brain 132:417–425
16. Bertolino A, Knable MB, Saunders RC, Callicott JH, Kolachana B, Mattay VS, Bachevalier J, Frank JA, Egan M, Weinberger DR (1999) The relationship between dorsolateral prefrontal N-acetylaspartate measures and striatal dopamine activity in schizophrenia. Biol Psychiatry 45:660–667
17. Blasi G, Goldberg TE, Elvevag B, Rasetti R, Bertolino A, Cohen J, Alce G, Zoltick B, Weinberger DR, Mattay VS (2007) Differentiating allocation of resources and conflict detection within attentional control processing. Eur J Neurosci 25:594–602
18. Blasi G, Mattay VS, Bertolino A, Elvevag B, Callicott JH, Das S, Kolachana BS, Egan MF, Goldberg TE, Weinberger DR (2005) Effect of catechol-O-methyltransferase val158met genotype on attentional control. J Neurosci 25:5038–5045
19. Blasi G, Napolitano F, Ursini G, Di Giorgio A, Caforio G, Taurisano P, Fazio L, Gelao B, Attrotto MT, Colagiorgio L, Todarello G, Piva F, Papazacharias A, Masellis R, Mancini M, Porcelli A, Romano R, Rampino A, Quarto T, Giulietti M, Lipska BK, Kleinman JE, Popolizio T, Weinberger DR, Usiello A, Bertolino A (2013) Association of GSK-3beta genetic variation with GSK-3beta expression, prefrontal cortical thickness, prefrontal physiology, and schizophrenia. Am J Psychiatry 170:868–876
20. Blasi G, Napolitano F, Ursini G, Taurisano P, Romano R, Caforio G, Fazio L, Gelao B, Di Giorgio A, Iacovelli L, Sinibaldi L, Popolizio T, Usiello A, Bertolino A (2011) DRD2/AKT1 interaction on D2 c-AMP independent signaling, attentional processing, and response to olanzapine treatment in schizophrenia. Proc Natl Acad Sci U S A 108:1158–1163
21. Blasi G, Selvaggi P, Fazio L, Antonucci LA, Taurisano P, Masellis R, Romano R, Mancini M, Zhang F, Caforio G, Popolizio T, Apud J, Weinberger DR, Bertolino A (2015) Variation in dopamine D2 and serotonin 5-HT2A receptor genes is associated with working memory processing and response to treatment with antipsychotics. Neuropsychopharmacology 40:1600–1608
22. Blasi G, Taurisano P, Papazacharias A, Caforio G, Romano R, Lobianco L, Fazio L, Di Giorgio A, Latorre V, Sambataro F, Popolizio T, Nardini M, Mattay VS, Weinberger DR, Bertolino A (2010) Nonlinear response of the anterior cingulate and prefrontal cortex in schizophrenia as a function of variable attentional control. Cereb Cortex 20:837–845
23. Bora E, Yucel M, Pantelis C (2010) Neurocognitive markers of psychosis in bipolar disorder: a meta-analytic study. J Affect Disord 127:1–9
24. Brahmbhatt SB, Haut K, Csernansky JG, Barch DM (2006) Neural correlates of verbal and nonverbal working memory deficits in individuals with schizophrenia and their high-risk siblings. Schizophr Res 87:191–204
25. Braus DF, Weber-Fahr W, Tost H, Ruf, M, Henn FA (2002) Sensory information processing in neuroleptic-naive first-episode schizophrenic patients: a functional magnetic resonance imaging study. Arch. Gen. Psychiatry 59:696–701
26. Breier A, Su TP, Saunders R, Carson RE, Kolachana BS, de Bartolomeis A, Weinberger DR, Weisenfeld

N, Malhotra AK, Eckelman WC, Pickar D (1997) Schizophrenia is associated with elevated amphetamine-induced synaptic dopamine concentrations: evidence from a novel positron emission tomography method. Proc Natl Acad Sci U S A 94:2569–2574
27. Broome MR, Matthiasson P, Fusar-Poli P, Woolley JB, Johns LC, Tabraham P, Bramon E, Valmaggia L, Williams SC, Brammer MJ, Chitnis X, McGuire PK (2009) Neural correlates of executive function and working memory in the 'at-risk mental state'. Br J Psychiatry 194:25–33
28. Brune M, Ozgurdal S, Ansorge N, von Reventlow HG, Peters S, Nicolas V, Tegenthoff M, Juckel G, Lissek S (2011) An fMRI study of "theory of mind" in at-risk states of psychosis: comparison with manifest schizophrenia and healthy controls. NeuroImage 55:329–337
29. Callicott JH, Bertolino A, Mattay VS, Langheim FJ, Duyn J, Coppola R, Goldberg TE, Weinberger DR (2000) Physiological dysfunction of the dorsolateral prefrontal cortex in schizophrenia revisited. Cereb Cortex 10:1078–1092
30. Callicott JH, Egan MF, Mattay VS, Bertolino A, Bone AD, Verchinksi B, Weinberger DR (2003) Abnormal fMRI response of the dorsolateral prefrontal cortex in cognitively intact siblings of patients with schizophrenia. Am J Psychiatry 160:709–719
31. Cannon TD, Cadenhead K, Cornblatt B, Woods SW, Addington J, Walker E, Seidman LJ, Perkins D, Tsuang M, McGlashan T, Heinssen R (2008) Prediction of psychosis in youth at high clinical risk: a multisite longitudinal study in North America. Arch Gen Psychiatry 65:28–37
32. Cannon TD, Glahn DC, Kim J, Van Erp TG, Karlsgodt K, Cohen MS, Nuechterlein KH, Bava S, Shirinyan D (2005) Dorsolateral prefrontal cortex activity during maintenance and manipulation of information in working memory in patients with schizophrenia. Arch Gen Psychiatry 62:1071–1080
33. Carlsson A, Hansson LO, Waters N, Carlsson ML (1999) A glutamatergic deficiency model of schizophrenia. Br J Psychiatry 37:2–6
34. Carter CS, Perlstein W, Ganguli R, Brar J, Mintun M, Cohen JD (1998) Functional hypofrontality and working memory dysfunction in schizophrenia. Am J Psychiatry 155:1285–1287
35. Carter JD, Bizzell J, Kim C, Bellion C, Carpenter KL, Dichter G, Belger A (2010) Attention deficits in schizophrenia – preliminary evidence of dissociable transient and sustained deficits. Schizophr Res 122:104–112
36. Caspi A, Sugden K, Moffitt TE, Taylor A, Craig IW, Harrington H, McClay J, Mill J, Martin J, Braithwaite A, Poulton R (2003) Influence of life stress on depression: moderation by a polymorphism in the 5-HTT gene. Science 301:386–389
37. Castellanos FX, Tannock R (2002) Neuroscience of attention-deficit/hyperactivity disorder: the search for endophenotypes. Nature reviews. Neuroscience 3:617–628
38. Chang X, Shen H, Wang L, Liu Z, Xin W, Hu D, Miao D (2014) Altered default mode and fronto-parietal network subsystems in patients with schizophrenia and their unaffected siblings. Brain Res 1562:87–99
39. Chen J, Lipska BK, Halim N, Ma QD, Matsumoto M, Melhem S, Kolachana BS, Hyde TM, Herman MM, Apud J, Egan MF, Kleinman JE, Weinberger DR (2004) Functional analysis of genetic variation in catechol-O-methyltransferase (COMT): effects on mRNA, protein, and enzyme activity in postmortem human brain. Am J Hum Genet 75:807–821
40. Cocchi A, Meneghelli A (2012) Rischio ad esordio psicotico: una sfida che continua. Manuale d'intervento precoce. Edi-ermes
41. Da Silva Alves F, Bakker G, Schmitz N, Abeling N, Hasler G, van der Meer J, Nederveen A, de Haan L, Linszen D, van Amelsvoort T (2013) Dopaminergic modulation of the reward system in schizophrenia: a placebo-controlled dopamine depletion fMRI study. Eur Neuropsychopharmacol 23:1577–1586
42. Dauvermann MR, Whalley HC, Romaniuk L, Valton V, Owens DG, Johnstone EC, Lawrie SM, Moorhead TW (2013) The application of nonlinear Dynamic Causal Modelling for fMRI in subjects at high genetic risk of schizophrenia. NeuroImage 73:16–29
43. De Bartolomeis A, Buonaguro EF, Iasevoli F (2013) Serotonin-glutamate and serotonin-dopamine reciprocal interactions as putative molecular targets for novel antipsychotic treatments: from receptor heterodimers to postsynaptic scaffolding and effector proteins. Psychopharmacology 225:1–19
44. De Leeuw M, Kahn RS, Vink M (2015) Fronto-striatal dysfunction during reward processing in unaffected siblings of schizophrenia patients. Schizophr Bull 41:94–103
45. Delawalla Z, Csernansky JG, Barch DM (2008) Prefrontal cortex function in nonpsychotic siblings of individuals with schizophrenia. Biol Psychiatry 63:490–497
46. Durstewitz D, Seamans JK (2008) The dual-state theory of prefrontal cortex dopamine function with relevance to catechol-o-methyltransferase genotypes and schizophrenia. Biol Psychiatry 64:739–749
47. Egan MF, Goldberg TE, Gscheidle T, Weirich M, Rawlings R, Hyde TM, Bigelow L, Weinberger DR (2001) Relative risk for cognitive impairments in siblings of patients with schizophrenia. Biol Psychiatry 50:98–107
48. Elvevag B, Weickert T, Wechsler M, Coppola R, Weinberger DR, Goldberg TE (2002) An investigation of the integrity of semantic boundaries in schizophrenia. Schizophr Res 53:187–198
49. Emamian ES, Hall D, Birnbaum MJ, Karayiorgou M, Gogos JA (2004) Convergent evidence for impaired AKT1-GSK3beta signaling in schizophrenia. Nat Genet 36:131–137

50. Esslinger C, Englisch S, Inta D, Rausch F, Schirmbeck F, Mier D, Kirsch P, Meyer-Lindenberg A, Zink M (2012) Ventral striatal activation during attribution of stimulus saliency and reward anticipation is correlated in unmedicated first episode schizophrenia patients. Schizophr Res 140:114–121
51. Freyberg Z, Ferrando SJ, Javitch JA (2010) Roles of the Akt/GSK-3 and Wnt signaling pathways in schizophrenia and antipsychotic drug action. Am J Psychiatry 167:388–396
52. Fusar-Poli P, Bonoldi I, Yung AR, Borgwardt S, Kempton MJ, Valmaggia L, Barale F, Caverzasi E, McGuire P (2012) Predicting psychosis: meta-analysis of transition outcomes in individuals at high clinical risk. Arch Gen Psychiatry 69:220–229
53. Fusar-Poli P, Borgwardt S, Bechdolf A, Addington J, Riecher-Rossler A, Schultze-Lutter F, Keshavan M, Wood S, Ruhrmann S, Seidman LJ, Valmaggia L, Cannon T, Velthorst E, De Haan L, Cornblatt B, Bonoldi I, Birchwood M, McGlashan T, Carpenter W, McGorry P, Klosterkotter J, McGuire P, Yung A (2013) The psychosis high-risk state: a comprehensive state-of-the-art review. JAMA Psychiatry 70:107–120
54. Fusar-Poli P, Broome MR, Matthiasson P, Woolley JB, Mechelli A, Johns LC, Tabraham P, Bramon E, Valmaggia L, Williams SC, McGuire P (2011) Prefrontal function at presentation directly related to clinical outcome in people at ultrahigh risk of psychosis. Schizophr Bull 37:189–198
55. Fusar-Poli P, Howes OD, Allen P, Broome M, Valli I, Asselin MC, Grasby PM, McGuire PK (2010) Abnormal frontostriatal interactions in people with prodromal signs of psychosis: a multimodal imaging study. Arch Gen Psychiatry 67:683–691
56. Fusar-Poli P, Perez J, Broome M, Borgwardt S, Placentino A, Caverzasi E, Cortesi M, Veggiotti P, Politi P, Barale F, McGuire P (2007) Neurofunctional correlates of vulnerability to psychosis: a systematic review and meta-analysis. Neurosci Biobehav Rev 31:465–484
57. Gaiteri C, Ding Y, French B, Tseng GC, Sibille E (2014) Beyond modules and hubs: the potential of gene coexpression networks for investigating molecular mechanisms of complex brain disorders. Genes Brain Behav 13:13–24
58. Garrity AG, Pearlson GD, McKiernan K, Lloyd D, Kiehl KA, Calhoun VD (2007) Aberrant "default mode" functional connectivity in schizophrenia. Am J Psychiatry 164:450–457
59. Geller V, Gorzaltsan I, Shleifer T, Belmaker RH, Bersudsky Y (2005) Clotiapine compared with chlorpromazine in chronic schizophrenia. Schizophr Res 80:343–347
60. Giuliano AJ, Li H, Mesholam-Gately RI, Sorenson SM, Woodberry KA, Seidman LJ (2012) Neurocognition in the psychosis risk syndrome: a quantitative and qualitative review. Curr Pharm Des 18:399–415
61. Gold JM, Waltz JA, Prentice KJ, Morris SE, Heerey EA (2008) Reward processing in schizophrenia: a deficit in the representation of value. Schizophr Bull 34:835–847
62. Goldberg TE, Torrey EF, Gold JM, Bigelow LB, Ragland RD, Taylor E, Weinberger DR (1995) Genetic risk of neuropsychological impairment in schizophrenia: a study of monozygotic twins discordant and concordant for the disorder. Schizophr Res 17:77–84
63. Gottesman II, Gould TD (2003) The endophenotype concept in psychiatry: etymology and strategic intentions. Am J Psychiatry 160:636–645
64. Gottesman II, Shields J (1971) Schizophrenia: geneticism and environmentalism. Hum Hered 21:517–522
65. Grace AA (1993) Cortical regulation of subcortical dopamine systems and its possible relevance to schizophrenia. J Neural Transm Gen Sect 91:111–134
66. Grimm O, Heinz A, Walter H, Kirsch P, Erk S, Haddad L, Plichta MM, Romanczuk-Seiferth N, Pohland L, Mohnke S, Muhleisen TW, Mattheisen M, Witt SH, Schafer A, Cichon S, Nothen M, Rietschel M, Tost H, Meyer-Lindenberg A (2014) Striatal response to reward anticipation: evidence for a systems-level intermediate phenotype for schizophrenia. JAMA Psychiatry 71:531–539
67. Gur RE, Turetsky BI, Loughead J, Snyder W, Kohler C, Elliott M, Pratiwadi R, Ragland JD, Bilker WB, Siegel SJ, Kanes SJ, Arnold SE, Gur RC (2007) Visual attention circuitry in schizophrenia investigated with oddball event-related functional magnetic resonance imaging. Am J Psychiatry 164:442–449
68. Gusnard DA, Akbudak E, Shulman GL, Raichle ME (2001) Medial prefrontal cortex and self-referential mental activity: relation to a default mode of brain function. Proc Natl Acad Sci U S A 98:4259–4264
69. Harrison PJ, Weinberger DR (2005) Schizophrenia genes, gene expression, and neuropathology: on the matter of their convergence. Mol Psychiatry 10:40–68 ; image 45
70. Hazlett EA, Buchsbaum MS, Zhang J, Newmark RE, Glanton CF, Zelmanova Y, Haznedar MM, Chu KW, Nenadic I, Kemether EM, Tang CY, New AS, Siever LJ (2008) Frontal-striatal-thalamic mediodorsal nucleus dysfunction in schizophrenia-spectrum patients during sensorimotor gating. NeuroImage 42:1164–1177
71. Hulme OJ, Whiteley L, Shipp S (2010) Spatially distributed encoding of covert attentional shifts in human thalamus. J Neurophysiol 104:3644–3656
72. Insel T, Cuthbert B, Garvey M, Heinssen R, Pine DS, Quinn K, Sanislow C, Wang P (2010) Research Domain Criteria (RDoC): toward a new classification framework for research on mental disorders. Am J Psychiatry 167:748–751
73. Ikeda M, Iwata N, Suzuki T, Kitajima T, Yamanouchi Y, Kinoshita Y, Inada T, Ozaki N (2004) Association of AKT1 with schizophrenia confirmed in a Japanese population. Biol Psychiatry 56:698–700

74. Johnstone EC, Ebmeier KP, Miller P, Owens DG, Lawrie SM (2005) Predicting schizophrenia: findings from the Edinburgh High-Risk Study. Br J Psychiatry 186:18–25
75. Juckel G, Schlagenhauf F, Koslowski M, Filonov D, Wustenberg T, Villringer A, Knutson B, Kienast T, Gallinat J, Wrase J, Heinz A (2006a) Dysfunction of ventral striatal reward prediction in schizophrenic patients treated with typical, not atypical, neuroleptics. Psychopharmacology 187:222–228
76. Juckel G, Schlagenhauf F, Koslowski M, Wustenberg T, Villringer A, Knutson B, Wrase J, Heinz A (2006b) Dysfunction of ventral striatal reward prediction in schizophrenia. NeuroImage 29:409–416
77. Kahn RS, Keefe RS (2013) Schizophrenia is a cognitive illness: time for a change in focus. JAMA Psychiatry 70:1107–1112
78. Karch S, Leicht G, Giegling I, Lutz J, Kunz J, Buselmeier M, Hey P, Sporl A, Jager L, Meindl T, Pogarell O, Moller HJ, Hegerl U, Rujescu D, Mulert C (2009) Inefficient neural activity in patients with schizophrenia and nonpsychotic relatives of schizophrenic patients: evidence from a working memory task. J Psychiatr Res 43:1185–1194
79. Keefe RS, Eesley CE, Poe MP (2005) Defining a cognitive function decrement in schizophrenia. Biol Psychiatry 57:688–691
80. Kerns JG, Cohen JD, MacDonald AW 3rd, Johnson MK, Stenger VA, Aizenstein H, Carter CS (2005) Decreased conflict- and error-related activity in the anterior cingulate cortex in subjects with schizophrenia. Am J Psychiatry 162:1833–1839
81. Kellendonk C, Simpson EH, Polan HJ, Malleret G, Vronskaya S, Winiger V, Moore H, Kandel ER (2006) Transient and selective overexpression of dopamine D2 receptors in the striatum causes persistent abnormalities in prefrontal cortex functioning. Neuron 49:603–615
82. Khadka S, Meda SA, Stevens MC, Glahn DC, Calhoun VD, Sweeney JA, Tamminga CA, Keshavan MS, O'Neil K, Schretlen D, Pearlson GD (2013) Is aberrant functional connectivity a psychosis endophenotype? A resting state functional magnetic resonance imaging study. Biol Psychiatry 74:458–466
83. Klosterkotter J, Hellmich M, Steinmeyer EM, Schultze-Lutter F (2001) Diagnosing schizophrenia in the initial prodromal phase. Arch Gen Psychiatry 58:158–164
84. Koch SP, Hagele C, Haynes JD, Heinz A, Schlagenhauf F, Sterzer P (2015) Diagnostic classification of schizophrenia patients on the basis of regional reward-related FMRI signal patterns. PLoS One 10:e0119089
85. Laruelle M (1998) Imaging dopamine transmission in schizophrenia. A review and meta-analysis. Q J Nucl Med 42:211–221
86. Li M, Mo Y, Luo XJ, Xiao X, Shi L, Peng YM, Qi XB, Liu XY, Yin LD, Diao HB, Su B (2011) Genetic association and identification of a functional SNP at GSK3beta for schizophrenia susceptibility. Schizophr Res 133:165–171
87. Liddle PF, Laurens KR, Kiehl KA, Ngan ET (2006) Abnormal function of the brain system supporting motivated attention in medicated patients with schizophrenia: an fMRI study. Psychol Med 36:1097–1108
88. Liemburg EJ, Dlabac-De Lange JJ, Bais L, Knegtering H, van Osch MJ, Renken RJ, Aleman A (2015) Neural correlates of planning performance in patients with schizophrenia–relationship with apathy. Schizophr Res 161:367–375
89. Lord LD, Allen P, Expert P, Howes O, Lambiotte R, McGuire P, Bose SK, Hyde S, Turkheimer FE (2011) Characterization of the anterior cingulate's role in the at-risk mental state using graph theory. NeuroImage 56:1531–1539
90. MacDonald AW 3rd, Thermenos HW, Barch DM, Seidman LJ (2009) Imaging genetic liability to schizophrenia: systematic review of FMRI studies of patients' nonpsychotic relatives. Schizophr Bull 35:1142–1162
91. Manoach DS (2003) Prefrontal cortex dysfunction during working memory performance in schizophrenia: reconciling discrepant findings. Schizophr Res 60:285–298
92. Manoach DS, Gollub RL, Benson ES, Searl MM, Goff DC, Halpern E, Saper CB, Rauch SL (2000) Schizophrenic subjects show aberrant fMRI activation of dorsolateral prefrontal cortex and basal ganglia during working memory performance. Biol Psychiatry 48:99–109
93. Manoach DS, Press DZ, Thangaraj V, Searl MM, Goff DC, Halpern E, Saper CB, Warach S (1999) Schizophrenic subjects activate dorsolateral prefrontal cortex during a working memory task, as measured by fMRI. Biol Psychiatry 45:1128–1137
94. McGuffin P, Gottesman II (1999) Risk factors for schizophrenia. N Engl J Med 341:370–371
95. Morey RA, Inan S, Mitchell TV, Perkins DO, Lieberman JA, Belger A (2005) Imaging frontostriatal function in ultra-high-risk, early, and chronic schizophrenia during executive processing. Arch Gen Psychiatry 62:254–262
96. Nelson B, Thompson A, Yung AR (2013) Not all first-episode psychosis is the same: preliminary evidence of greater basic self-disturbance in schizophrenia spectrum cases. Early Interv Psychiatry 7:200–204
97. Nielsen MO, Rostrup E, Wulff S, Bak N, Lublin H, Kapur S, Glenthoj B (2012) Alterations of the brain reward system in antipsychotic naive schizophrenia patients. Biol Psychiatry 71:898–905
98. Norton N, Williams HJ, Dwyer S, Carroll L, Peirce T, Moskvina V, Segurado R, Nikolov I, Williams NM, Ikeda M, Iwata N, Owen MJ, O'Donovan MC (2007) Association analysis of AKT1 and schizophrenia in a UK case control sample. Schizophr Res 93:58–65
99. Orliac F, Naveau M, Joliot M, Delcroix N, Razafimandimby A, Brazo P, Dollfus S, Delamillieure

P (2013) Links among resting-state default-mode network, salience network, and symptomatology in schizophrenia. Schizophr Res 148:74–80
100. Pauly K, Seiferth NY, Kellermann T, Ruhrmann S, Daumann B, Backes V, Klosterkotter J, Shah NJ, Schneider F, Kircher TT, Habel U (2010) The interaction of working memory and emotion in persons clinically at risk for psychosis: an fMRI pilot study. Schizophr Res 120:167–176
101. Peeters SC, van Bronswijk S, van de Ven V, Gronenschild EH, Goebel R, van Os J, Marcelis M (2015) Cognitive correlates of frontoparietal network connectivity 'at rest' in individuals with differential risk for psychotic disorder. Eur Neuropsychopharmacol 25:1922–1932
102. Pergola G, Suchan B (2013) Associative learning beyond the medial temporal lobe: many actors on the memory stage. Front Behav Neurosci 7:162
103. Perlstein WM, Carter CS, Noll DC, Cohen JD (2001) Relation of prefrontal cortex dysfunction to working memory and symptoms in schizophrenia. Am J Psychiatry 158:1105–1113
104. Perlstein WM, Dixit NK, Carter CS, Noll DC, Cohen JD (2003) Prefrontal cortex dysfunction mediates deficits in working memory and prepotent responding in schizophrenia. Biol Psychiatry 53:25–38
105. Pettersson-Yeo W, Allen P, Benetti S, McGuire P, Mechelli A (2011) Dysconnectivity in schizophrenia: where are we now? Neurosci Biobehav Rev 35:1110–1124
106. Pflueger MO, Gschwandtner U, Stieglitz RD, Riecher-Rossler A (2007) Neuropsychological deficits in individuals with an at risk mental state for psychosis – working memory as a potential trait marker. Schizophr Res 97:14–24
107. Polli FE, Barton JJ, Thakkar KN, Greve DN, Goff DC, Rauch SL, Manoach DS (2008) Reduced error-related activation in two anterior cingulate circuits is related to impaired performance in schizophrenia. Brain 131:971–986
108. Quintana J, Wong T, Ortiz-Portillo E, Marder SR, Mazziotta JC (2004) Anterior cingulate dysfunction during choice anticipation in schizophrenia. Psychiatry Res 132:117–130
109. Raichle ME, MacLeod AM, Snyder AZ, Powers WJ, Gusnard DA, Shulman GL (2001) A default mode of brain function. Proc Natl Acad Sci U S A 98:676–682
110. Reiman EM, Caselli RJ (1999) Alzheimer's disease. Maturitas 31:185–200
111. Richiardi J, Altmann A, Milazzo AC, Chang C, Chakravarty MM, Banaschewski T, Barker GJ, Bokde AL, Bromberg U, Buchel C, Conrod P, Fauth-Buhler M, Flor H, Frouin V, Gallinat J, Garavan H, Gowland P, Heinz A, Lemaitre H, Mann KF, Martinot JL, Nees F, Paus T, Pausova Z, Rietschel M, Robbins TW, Smolka MN, Spanagel R, Strohle A, Schumann G, Hawrylycz M, Poline JB, Greicius MD (2015) BRAIN NETWORKS. Correlated gene expression supports synchronous activity in brain networks. Science 348:1241–1244
112. Riehemann S, Volz HP, Stutzer P, Smesny S, Gaser C, Sauer H (2001) Hypofrontality in neuroleptic-naive schizophrenic patients during the Wisconsin Card Sorting Test – a fMRI study. Eur Arch Psychiatry Clin Neurosci 251:66–71
113. Ripke S, Neale BM, Corvin A, Walters JT, Farh K, Holmans PA, Lee P, Schizophrenia Working Group of the Psychiatric GenomicsConsortium et al (2014) Biological insights from 108 schizophrenia-associated genetic loci. Nature 511:421–427
114. Sabb FW, van Erp TG, Hardt ME, Dapretto M, Caplan R, Cannon TD, Bearden CE (2010) Language network dysfunction as a predictor of outcome in youth at clinical high risk for psychosis. Schizophr Res 116:173–183
115. Salgado-Pineda P, Junque C, Vendrell P, Baeza I, Bargallo N, Falcon C, Bernardo M (2004) Decreased cerebral activation during CPT performance: structural and functional deficits in schizophrenic patients. NeuroImage 21:840–847
116. Sambataro F, Blasi G, Fazio L, Caforio G, Taurisano P, Romano R, Di Giorgio A, Gelao B, Lo Bianco L, Papazacharias A, Popolizio T, Nardini M, Bertolino A (2010) Treatment with olanzapine is associated with modulation of the default mode network in patients with Schizophrenia. Neuropsychopharmacology 35:904–912
117. Sambataro F, Fazio L, Taurisano P, Gelao B, Porcelli A, Mancini M, Sinibaldi L, Ursini G, Masellis R, Caforio G, Di Giorgio A, Niccoli-Asabella A, Popolizio T, Blasi G, Bertolino A (2013) DRD2 genotype-based variation of default mode network activity and of its relationship with striatal DAT binding. Schizophr Bull 39:206–216
118. Schlosser R, Gesierich T, Kaufmann B, Vucurevic G, Hunsche S, Gawehn J, Stoeter P (2003) Altered effective connectivity during working memory performance in schizophrenia: a study with fMRI and structural equation modeling. NeuroImage 19:751–763
119. Schneider F, Habel U, Reske M, Kellermann T, Stocker T, Shah NJ, Zilles K, Braus DF, Schmitt A, Schlosser R, Wagner M, Frommann I, Kircher T, Rapp A, Meisenzahl E, Ufer S, Ruhrmann S, Thienel R, Sauer H, Henn FA, Gaebel W (2007) Neural correlates of working memory dysfunction in first-episode schizophrenia patients: an fMRI multi-center study. Schizophr Res 89:198–210
120. Schwab SG, Hoefgen B, Hanses C, Hassenbach MB, Albus M, Lerer B, Trixler M, Maier W, Wildenauer DB (2005) Further evidence for association of variants in the AKT1 gene with schizophrenia in a sample of European sib-pair families. Biol Psychiatry 58:446–450
121. Seamans JK, Yang CR (2004) The principal features and mechanisms of dopamine modulation in the prefrontal cortex. Prog Neurobiol 74:1–58
122. Seidman LJ, Thermenos HW, Poldrack RA, Peace NK, Koch JK, Faraone SV, Tsuang MT (2006) Altered brain activation in dorsolateral prefrontal cortex in adolescents and young adults at genetic

risk for schizophrenia: an fMRI study of working memory. Schizophr Res 85:58–72
123. Sherman SM, Guillery RW (2006) Exploring the thalamus and its role in cortical function. MIT Press, Cambridge, MA
124. Simon JJ, Cordeiro SA, Weber MA, Friederich HC, Wolf RC, Weisbrod M, Kaiser S (2015) Reward system dysfunction as a neural substrate of symptom expression across the general population and patients with schizophrenia. Schizophr Bull 41:1370–1378
125. Smieskova R, Fusar-Poli P, Allen P, Bendfeldt K, Stieglitz RD, Drewe J, Radue EW, McGuire PK, Riecher-Rossler A, Borgwardt SJ (2010) Neuroimaging predictors of transition to psychosis–a systematic review and meta-analysis. Neurosci Biobehav Rev 34:1207–1222
126. Smieskova R, Marmy J, Schmidt A, Bendfeldt K, Riecher-Rssler A, Walter M, Lang UE, Borgwardt S (2013) Do subjects at clinical high risk for psychosis differ from those with a genetic high risk?–A systematic review of structural and functional brain abnormalities. Curr Med Chem 20:467–481
127. Smith SM, Miller KL, Moeller S, Xu J, Auerbach EJ, Woolrich MW, Beckmann CF, Jenkinson M, Andersson J, Glasser MF, Van Essen DC, Feinberg DA, Yacoub ES, Ugurbil K (2012) Temporally-independent functional modes of spontaneous brain activity. Proc Natl Acad Sci U S A 109: 3131–3136
128. Souza RP, Romano-Silva MA, Lieberman JA, Meltzer HY, Wong AH, Kennedy JL (2008) Association study of GSK3 gene polymorphisms with schizophrenia and clozapine response. Psychopharmacology 200:177–186
129. Sullivan PF (2012) Puzzling over schizophrenia: schizophrenia as a pathway disease. Nat Med 18:210–211
130. Tan HY, Choo WC, Fones CS, Chee MW (2005) fMRI study of maintenance and manipulation processes within working memory in first-episode schizophrenia. Am J Psychiatry 162:1849–1858
131. Tan HY, Nicodemus KK, Chen Q, Li Z, Brooke JK, Honea R, Kolachana BS, Straub RE, Meyer-Lindenberg A, Sei Y, Mattay VS, Callicott JH, Weinberger DR (2008) Genetic variation in AKT1 is linked to dopamine-associated prefrontal cortical structure and function in humans. J Clin Invest 118:2200–2208
132. Tan HY, Sust S, Buckholtz JW, Mattay VS, Meyer-Lindenberg A, Egan MF, Weinberger DR, Callicott JH (2006) Dysfunctional prefrontal regional specialization and compensation in schizophrenia. Am J Psychiatry 163:1969–1977
133. Tang J, Liao Y, Song M, Gao JH, Zhou B, Tan C, Liu T, Tang Y, Chen J, Chen X (2013) Aberrant default mode functional connectivity in early onset schizophrenia. PLoS One 8:e71061
134. Thermenos HW, Seidman LJ, Breiter H, Goldstein JM, Goodman JM, Poldrack R, Faraone SV, Tsuang MT (2004) Functional magnetic resonance imaging during auditory verbal working memory in nonpsychotic relatives of persons with schizophrenia: a pilot study. Biol Psychiatry 55:490–500
135. Thiselton DL, Vladimirov VI, Kuo PH, McClay J, Wormley B, Fanous A, O'Neill FA, Walsh D, Van den Oord EJ, Kendler KS, Riley BP (2008) AKT1 is associated with schizophrenia across multiple symptom dimensions in the Irish study of high density schizophrenia families. Biol Psychiatry 63: 449–457
136. Tohen M, Strakowski SM, Zarate C Jr, Hennen J, Stoll AL, Suppes T, Faedda GL, Cohen BM, Gebre-Medhin P, Baldessarini RJ (2000) The McLean-Harvard first-episode project: 6-month symptomatic and functional outcome in affective and nonaffective psychosis. Biol Psychiatry 48:467–476
137. Toulopoulou T, Goldberg TE, Mesa IR, Picchioni M, Rijsdijk F, Stahl D, Cherny SS, Sham P, Faraone SV, Tsuang M, Weinberger DR, Seidman LJ, Murray RM (2010) Impaired intellect and memory: a missing link between genetic risk and schizophrenia? Arch Gen Psychiatry 67:905–913
138. Usiello A, Baik JH, Rouge-Pont F, Picetti R, Dierich A, LeMeur M, Piazza PV, Borrelli E (2000) Distinct functions of the two isoforms of dopamine D2 receptors. Nature 408:199–203
139. Van der Werf YD, Scheltens P, Lindeboom J, Witter MP, Uylings HB, Jolles J (2003) Deficits of memory, executive functioning and attention following infarction in the thalamus; a study of 22 cases with localised lesions. Neuropsychologia 41: 1330–1344
140. Wagner G, De la Cruz F, Schachtzabel C, Gullmar D, Schultz CC, Schlosser RG, Bar KJ, Koch K (2015) Structural and functional dysconnectivity of the fronto-thalamic system in schizophrenia: a DCM-DTI study. Cortex 66:35–45
141. Wagner G, Koch K, Schachtzabel C, Schultz CC, Gaser C, Reichenbach JR, Sauer H, Bar KJ, Schlosser RG (2013) Structural basis of the fronto-thalamic dysconnectivity in schizophrenia: a combined DCM-VBM study. NeuroImage Clin 3:95–105
142. Walton E, Geisler D, Lee PH, Hass J, Turner JA, Liu J, Sponheim SR, White T, Wassink TH, Roessner V, Gollub RL, Calhoun VD, Ehrlich S (2014) Prefrontal inefficiency is associated with polygenic risk for schizophrenia. Schizophr Bull 40:1263–1271
143. Walton E, Turner J, Gollub RL, Manoach DS, Yendiki A, Ho BC, Sponheim SR, Calhoun VD, Ehrlich S (2013) Cumulative genetic risk and prefrontal activity in patients with schizophrenia. Schizophr Bull 39:703–711
144. Wang M, Vijayraghavan S, Goldman-Rakic PS (2004) Selective D2 receptor actions on the functional circuitry of working memory. Science 303:853–856
145. Weickert TW, Goldberg TE, Gold JM, Bigelow LB, Egan MF, Weinberger DR (2000) Cognitive impairments in patients with schizophrenia displaying preserved and compromised intellect. Arch Gen Psychiatry 57:907–913

146. Weinberger DR (1987) Implications of normal brain development for the pathogenesis of schizophrenia. Arch Gen Psychiatry 44:660–669
147. Weinberger DR, Egan MF, Bertolino A, Callicott JH, Mattay VS, Lipska BK, Berman KF, Goldberg TE (2001) Prefrontal neurons and the genetics of schizophrenia. Biol Psychiatry 50:825–844
148. Weiss EM, Golaszewski S, Mottaghy FM, Hofer A, Hausmann A, Kemmler G, Kremser C, Brinkhoff C, Felber SR, Fleischhacker WW (2003) Brain activation patterns during a selective attention test-a functional MRI study in healthy volunteers and patients with schizophrenia. Psychiatry Res 123:1–15
149. Weiss EM, Siedentopf C, Golaszewski S, Mottaghy FM, Hofer A, Kremser C, Felber S, Fleischhacker WW (2007) Brain activation patterns during a selective attention test–a functional MRI study in healthy volunteers and unmedicated patients during an acute episode of schizophrenia. Psychiatry Res 154:31–40
150. Welsh RC, Chen AC, Taylor SF (2010) Low-frequency BOLD fluctuations demonstrate altered thalamocortical connectivity in schizophrenia. Schizophr Bull 36:713–722
151. Whalley HC, Hall L, Romaniuk L, Macdonald A, Lawrie SM, Sussmann JE, McIntosh AM (2015) Impact of cross-disorder polygenic risk on frontal brain activation with specific effect of schizophrenia risk. Schizophr Res 161:484–489
152. Whalley HC, Simonotto E, Marshall I, Owens DG, Goddard NH, Johnstone EC, Lawrie SM (2005) Functional disconnectivity in subjects at high genetic risk of schizophrenia. Brain 128:2097–2108
153. Whalley HC, Simonotto E, Moorhead W, McIntosh A, Marshall I, Ebmeier KP, Owens DG, Goddard NH, Johnstone EC, Lawrie SM (2006) Functional imaging as a predictor of schizophrenia. Biol Psychiatry 60:454–462
154. White NM (2011). Reward: What Is It? How Can It Be Inferred from Behavior? Chapter 3 In: Gottfried JA. Neurobiology of sensation and reward. CRC Press/Taylor & Francis, Boca Raton
155. Whitfield-Gabrieli S, Thermenos HW, Milanovic S, Tsuang MT, Faraone SV, McCarley RW, Shenton ME, Green AI, Nieto-Castanon A, LaViolette P, Wojcik J, Gabrieli JD, Seidman LJ (2009) Hyperactivity and hyperconnectivity of the default network in schizophrenia and in first-degree relatives of persons with schizophrenia. Proc Natl Acad Sci U S A 106:1279–1284
156. Wolf DH, Satterthwaite TD, Kantrowitz JJ, Katchmar N, Vandekar L, Elliott MA, Ruparel K (2014) Amotivation in schizophrenia: integrated assessment with behavioral, clinical, and imaging measures. Schizophr Bull 40:1328–1337
157. Wood SJ, Reniers RL, Heinze K (2013) Neuroimaging findings in the at-risk mental state: a review of recent literature. Can J Psychiatry 58:13–18
158. Woodberry KA, Giuliano AJ, Seidman LJ (2008) Premorbid IQ in schizophrenia: a meta-analytic review. Am J Psychiatry 165:579–587
159. Yung AR, McGorry PD (1996) The prodromal phase of first-episode psychosis: past and current conceptualizations. Schizophr Bull 22:353–370
160. Yung AR, Phillips LJ, Yuen HP, Francey SM, McFarlane CA, Hallgren M, McGorry PD (2003) Psychosis prediction: 12-month follow up of a high-risk ("prodromal") group. Schizophr Res 60:21–32
161. Yung AR, Yuen HP, McGorry PD, Phillips LJ, Kelly D, Dell'Olio M, Francey SM, Cosgrave EM, Killackey E, Stanford C, Godfrey K, Buckby J (2005) Mapping the onset of psychosis: the comprehensive assessment of at-risk mental states. Austr N Z J Psychiatry 39:964–971
162. Zhang Y, Bertolino A, Fazio L, Blasi G, Rampino A, Romano R, Lee ML, Xiao T, Papp A, Wang D, Sadee W (2007) Polymorphisms in human dopamine D2 receptor gene affect gene expression, splicing, and neuronal activity during working memory. Proc Natl Acad Sci U S A 104:20552–20557
163. Zikopoulos B, Barbas H (2012) Pathways for emotions and attention converge on the thalamic reticular nucleus in primates. J Neurosci 32:5338–5350

# 7 T MR: From Basic Research to Human Applications

# 23

Laura Biagi, Mirco Cosottini, and Michela Tosetti

The recent ultra-high field magnetic resonance (UHF MR, ≥7 T) scanners are demonstrating incredible potential, especially in the analysis of cerebral tissues. The technological achievements and the principles associated with the use of 7 T MRI systems are now being turned to applications on human, increasing both physiological and physiopathological knowledge as prelude to future clinical applications.

## 23.1 Ultra-High Field (UHF) MR

From the early days of magnetic resonance imaging, great interest was shown in obtaining ever stronger static magnetic fields since, according to the principles of NMR, all physical quantities are functions of the magnetic field applied $B_0$. It was therefore not by chance that in 1981, the same year in which the first clinical MR scanner was introduced to the biomedical market, Lauterbur and Budinger attempted to build the first superconductor magnet with a magnetic field of 6 T, the strongest magnetic field ever created at that time for human applications. Neither the time nor technology was right for such an undertaking; however, it is not difficult to see how in the 30-years history of magnetic resonance and its applications in medicine, there was an inexorable and very rapid increase in the strength of the static magnetic fields used in the medical context with 0.3–0.5 T systems seen in the early 1980s, 1–1.5 T in the early 1990s and the 3 T introduced between the late 1990s and the early 2000s. The same period also saw the development of revolutionary technologies in terms of image acquisition such as phased array systems and parallel imaging techniques. The power of these new approaches allowed the promises of ultra-high field MR (≥7 T magnetic field, ultra-high field, UHF), which had been predicted 20 years before, to be made possible, and led to the development of suitable tools for resolving many hypothetical and real problems which had been encountered in terms of the quality of images and safety.

In the late 1990s, 3 T systems were introduced to clinical practice. In the same period, in 1998, the first 8 T system for human applications was installed in Ohio State University, followed in 1999 by the installation of a 7 T scanner in the Magnetic Resonance Research Center of the

Translated in part with permission from: L. Biagi, M. Cosottini, M. Tosetti, "La risonanza magnetica a 7 T: dalla ricerca di base alle applicazioni sull'uomo", Il Nuovo Saggiatore (Bulletin of the Italian Physical Society), vol 30 (2014) pp. 34–48, ©SIF 2014.

L. Biagi • M. Tosetti (✉)
IRCCS Stella Maris Founation, Pisa, Italy

Foundationa Research Imago 7, Pisa, Italy
e-mail: michela.tosetti@inpe.unipi.it

M. Cosottini
Foundationa Research Imago 7, Pisa, Italy

University of Pisa, Pisa, Italy



T. Scarabino et al. (eds.), *High Field Brain MRI*, DOI 10.1007/978-3-319-44174-0_23

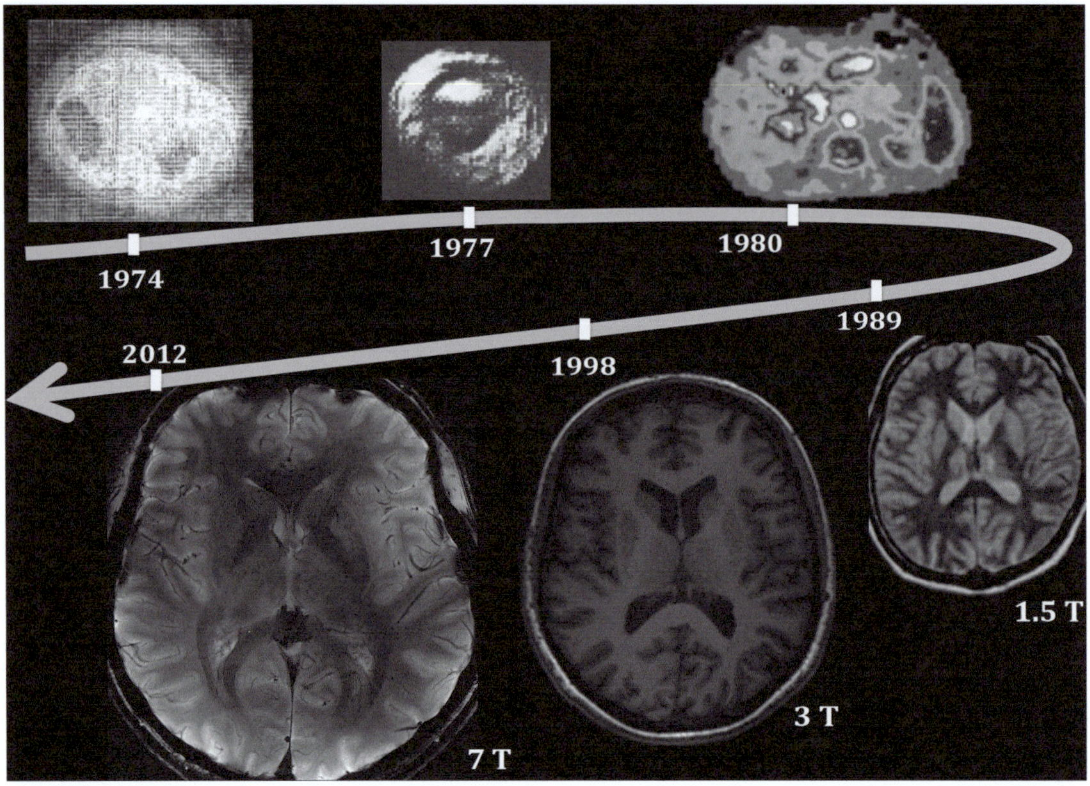


**Fig. 23.1** The evolution of MR images over time. In 1974, the first image of a small animal was obtained by Lauterbur using a technique called zeugmatography at that time. The Mansfield's group obtained the first human anatomical image in vivo, an axial cross section of a finger (1977). On 28 August 1980 in Aberdeen, the first clinical image of a cross section of the abdomen was obtained. In the late 1980s, the use of 1.5 T magnetic resonance began to spread around the world followed in the late 1990s by 3 T systems. In the 21st century the MR image acquired at 7 T has an in-plane resolution of 192 μm *in plane*

University of Minnesota. Both these systems were for experimental purposes only and were assembled with great effort and dedication by research laboratories using components made on-site.

The incredible results obtained opened the road to the main manufacturers at that time, Siemens, General Electric and Philips, to develop ultra-high field magnetic resonance (UHF MR) technologies, which led to the first Siemens 7 T system being installed in Massachusetts General Hospital in Boston and, in rapid succession, a General Electric scanner at the Bethesda National Institute of Health (NIH). Today, around the world, there are more than 60 systems with ≥7 T magnetic fields installed and dedicated to the development and use in experimental protocols for human clinical research.

In retrospect, given the history of the discoveries in MR, the progress made towards the use of UHF technology would appear no less than logical (Fig. 23.1).

The trend forward high magnetic fields derives from the quite low sensitivity of MRI. This originates from the small difference in the population of two consecutive Zeeman energy levels caused by the difference in energy of these levels. The slight excess of spin in the fundamental state generates a small polarisation, which depends on the temperature and the magnetic field applied, and it is only from this small fraction of sample that the whole absorption signal is detected in correspondence with the radio frequency associated with the nuclear transition. One direct method for increasing the low sensitivity was identified as increasing the static magnetic field $B_0$. In more detail, the MR signal increases in quadratic mode with the strength of the static magnetic field, while the associated noise demonstrates linear dependence. Therefore, the use of MR 7 T equipment allows a significant increase in the signal-to-noise ratio (SNR) in comparison with lower fields. For example, an image obtained with a clinical 1.5 T or even a 3 T system has a spatial resolution limit of about 1 cubic millimetre, while the combination of the benefits of ultra-high field can lead to a resolution of some hundredths of microns with similar signal-to-noise ratio. The significant increase in SNR produces a great improvement of all the imaging parameters and can be used not only in terms of spatial resolution but also in terms of sensitivity to modifications of the composition of the tissue or in terms of temporal resolution for dynamic phenomena or in terms of spectral resolution of signals. In addition, many other benefits could come out from the potential of new sources of mechanisms of contrast. Particularly in the brain, but also generally in the human body, there are potential sources of signal which cannot be fully explored using standard magnetic fields, because of low SNR, poor spatial resolution and/or their scarcity. It is the case of myelin, iron or metabolites which contain nuclei that differ from hydrogen ($^{13}C$, $^{23}Na$, $^{31}P$) that can be in principle detected by MR. These further signal sources can be extremely useful for providing additional and complementary information about molecular structure and/or the physiological, metabolic and functional dynamics of physiopathological processes. Moreover, the improvement in SNR and consequently in the intrinsic sensitivity of MR experiment can make possible the study of spontaneous distribution of nuclei different from proton that are normally found within structures of biological interest. For the same reason, it becomes possible to explore the distribution and the metabolic dynamics of molecular probes that are artificially enriched with stable isotopes that are visible in MR.

Increasing the magnetic field however causes some physical and instrumental problems that must be considered and fully investigated so that the potential of an ultra-high field MR system can be fully exploited. The major issues are related to the signal losses associated with the effects of magnetic susceptibility and inhomogeneities of the static magnetic field $B_0$, to the increase of chemical shift artefacts and to the variations in the relaxation times $T_1$ and $T_2$, which completely change the semeiotics of the images and the strategies of signal acquisition.

Moreover, the wavelength and dielectric effects of the radio frequency (RF) signal produce an uneven excitation and can cause an inhomogeneous distribution of radio frequency energy deposition on tissues. At 7 T, the resonance frequency for hydrogen is 298 MHz. Raising the operating frequency leads to the so-called wavelength effect: the radio frequency wavelength becomes comparable with the dimensions of the sample being investigated (limbs, brain and trunk) which per se brings stationary wavelength effects to the whole sample. The experiment becomes more complicated due to the dielectric properties of the sample irradiated by the radio frequency that further decreases the radiation wavelength (e.g. at 7 T, the wavelength in anatomical tissue with a high concentration of water is about 12 cm). This effect shows up as inconsistencies in the RF field transmitted ($B_1$) distribution, which is known as dielectric resonance. This generates peculiar artefacts in images that present hypo- and hyperintense zones caused by the presence of peaks and dips in the RF magnetic field $B_1$ and as a consequence generates locally different flip angles. The inhomogeneities in the $B_1$ magnetic field inevitably translate into inhomogeneous depositing of energy on the patient and give rise to possible "hot spots" of energy deposited. Specific absorption rate (SAR) is the parameter that measures this energy and forms the basis for both national and international patient safety standards. Commercial UHF MR systems monitor this parameter and use acquisition thresholds to do not exceed the abovementioned standards. However, given the uneven distribution of the transmitted fields and the possible presence of "hot spots", new methods for assessing variations in local magnetic field are mandatory. These may involve the simulation of electromagnetic fields and experimental measures [1], as well as the development of sensors for the real-time monitoring of SAR specifically for each individual patient (Fig. 23.2).

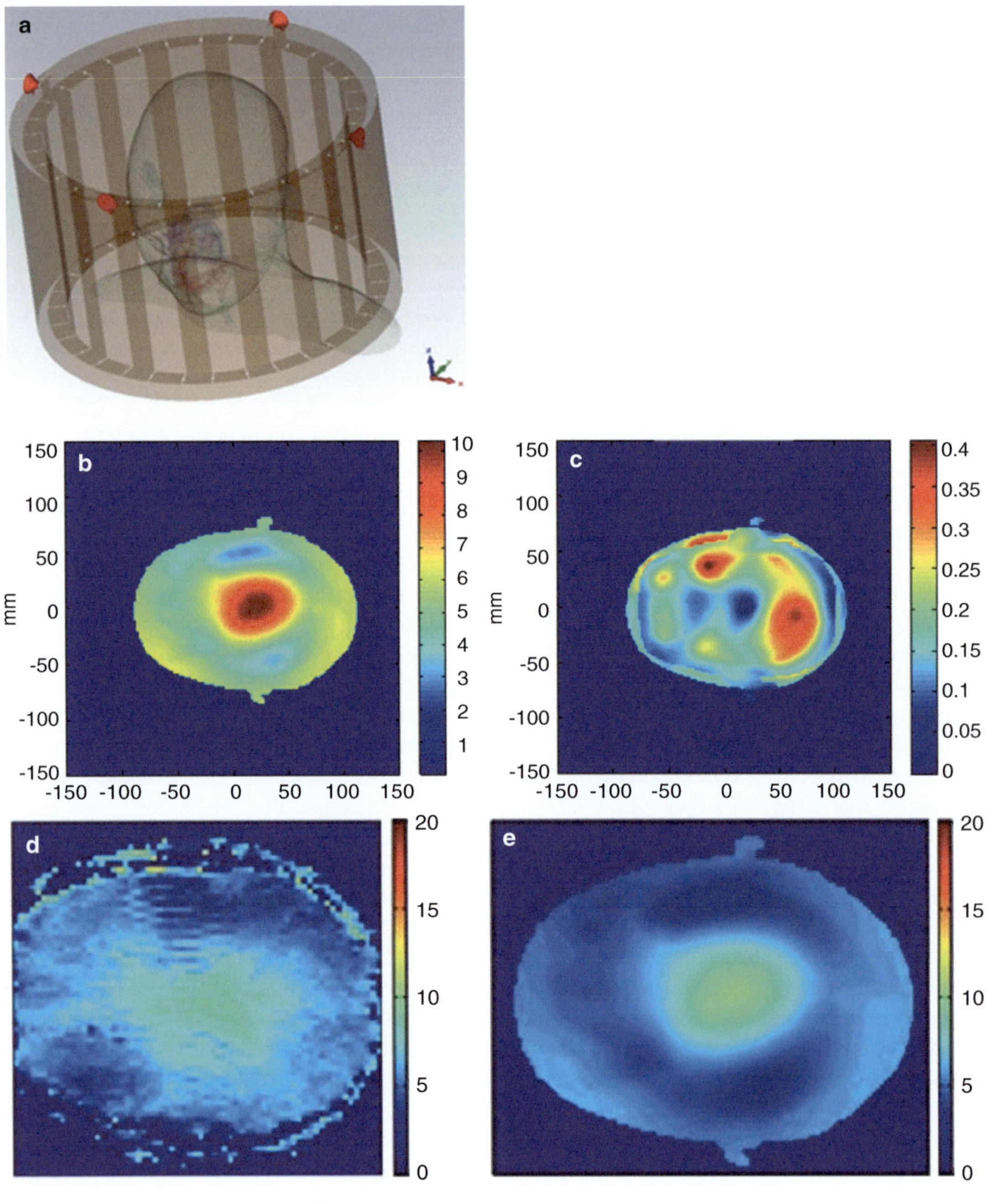


**Fig. 23.2** The use of UHF MR in human needs a very careful safety assessment. In this context, calculating the specific absorption rate (SAR) becomes vitally important. SAR is a measure of the rate at which energy is absorbed by the tissue when exposed to radio frequency (RF) magnetic field per unit of mass. At ultra-high field, the distribution of the SAR within a patient becomes very uneven; this lack of uniformity is associated with the high-radio frequency (RF) output of the coil (298 MHz at 7 T). The calculation of RF fields and SAR is usually performed using full-wave electromagnetic simulators. In our case, we used the CST MW suite to simulate the volume transmitter in quadrature loading it with anatomical models of the human body (Hugo, Virtual Family, Virtual Classroom). In all the models, the voxel discretization has a resolution of 1 $mm^3$, whereas the dielectric properties of tissue are taken from literature. Figure (**a**) shows Ella's head (female Virtual Family model) within the volume transmitter in quadrature. Figures (**b**) and (**c**) show the map of B1+ (magnitude, in [μT]) and the SAR [W/kg] on the axial section passing through the eyes. Lastly, simply to validate the simulator, Figures (**d**) and (**e**) show the map of B1+ measured on a volunteer with characteristics similar to Ella [μT] and the appropriately scaled map of Ella [μT], respectively [11]

In recent years, huge technological progress has been made in attempting to resolve the problem of inhomogeneities in the excitation and in the receiving of RF signals in terms of both hardware and software. Rewriting the pulse sequence for UHF to enable the use of less sensitive sequences and eliminate errors in the flip angles applied to prevent sequence "refocusing" has proved extremely difficult. As the use of multichannel coils for signal receiving revolutionised MRI by allowing increased SNR and reduction of acquisition times, the introduction of parallel transmission opened new scenarios for UHF, creating a fundamental turning point in the use of UHF. Parallel transmission uses and controls a multichannel array system for the signal transmission, adjusting independently phase and amplitude of signals sent to each channel, with the aim of producing uniform excitation inside the sample. This led to what is now known as "RF shimming" (radio frequency calibration). Recently, parallel transmission systems allow to manage the different channels of signal transmission not only by adjusting the phases and amplitudes of signals but also by sending completely independent signals to single channels, increasing the spatial selectivity of the RF pulses. Thanks to this technological advance, it is possible to compensate specific $B_1$ inhomogeneities induced by specific geometry and dielectric properties of each single human body exanimated. Corrections of $B_1$ are therefore "customised" and allow the quality of imaging to be improved while at the same time minimising the depositing of energy for each patient with his or her specific characteristics (gender, age, dimensions such as weight and height, muscle mass and the presence of physiopathological signs).

As described above, some physical key UHF MR phenomena are not favourable for the application of 7 T in a clinical context such as inhomogeneities in B1 and the corresponding distribution of SAR. Moreover, the shortening of the RF wavelength used at UHF can interfere more strongly with metal objects increasing the heating effect. For this reason, the presence of implanted metal objects remains the main cause of exclusion from UHF MR exams.

With knowledge of above-mentioned limits and the significant results expected from awareness of the physical phenomena of UHF MR, the encouraging results of experimental studies carried out on patients suffering from diseases of the central nervous system have recently started to arrive.

## 23.2 Applications of UHF MR

From its first introduction into clinical practice in the 1980s, MRI has become a key tool for studying the anatomy and function of the central nervous system (CNS). At present, 7 T scanners around the world are used only for experimental purposes, and most of these experiments involve improving both hardware and software of the systems, in order to overcome the technological limitations intrinsic in the ultra-high field.

Studies about the applications to diseases of the CNS are still limited and are aimed to assess the diagnostic-clinical benefits of UHF with respect to clinical scanner, as well as to investigate safety aspects of application of UHF in humans (Fig. 23.3).

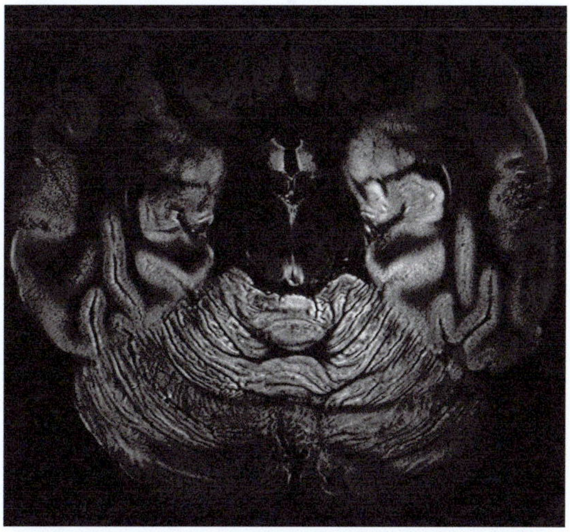

**Fig. 23.3** Ex vivo 7 T cerebellum. Ex vivo imaging of the cerebellum at 7 T: a gross specimen from a human cadaver was fixed in a 10 % aqueous solution of formaldehyde, placed in a perfluoropolyether suspension and imaged with an IR sequence. The image resolution was about 100 microns and allows the appreciation of extremely fine details of the human anatomy such the cerebellar folia

The physical phenomena of UHF MR regulate the diagnostic possibilities obtainable with these scanners in a counteracting manner and provide benefits in some cases and disadvantages in others. The limited diffusion of UHF, the high costs involved and the presence of artefacts in the images limit its use in experimental studies, but at the same time push the development of new signal treatment methods and technological development. The possibility of obtaining new contrasts acts as a stimulus for the development of a new imaging semeiotics of the CNS in both healthy and unhealthy subjects. This is a true challenge for future clinical applications.

In effect, with increase of the applied magnetic field, relaxation times vary, particularly lengthening T1 while shortening T2 and T2*. In some applications, such variations can be beneficial, e.g. an increase in T1 which favours the saturation of stationary spins or a decrease in T2 which provides faster sequences. On the other hand, as relaxation times do not change uniformly in different parts of the CNS, contrasts between different structures can vary. Based on new signal treatment methods, new signal semiotics must be redefined and new imaging techniques can be discovered [2, 3].

An increase in SNR allows spatial resolution (in the order of hundredths of micron) able to provide anatomical imaging never seen in vivo. The phenomena of magnetic susceptibility have pros and cons for the clinical application of UHF. On the one hand, they allow greater sensitivity in detecting paramagnetic and diamagnetic substances such as haemosiderin in micro-haemorrhages, calcium in tumoural calcifications and iron in degenerated portions of the CNS, while on the other hand, they increase distortions in anatomical images and decrease diagnostic quality. Greater sensitivity to the effects of magnetic susceptibility however allows new types of contrast to be obtained (susceptibility-weighted imaging, phase mapping, susceptibility mapping) (Fig. 23.4) which allow to distinguish anatomical components with different susceptibilities within an anatomical structure such as the laminar aspect of the cerebral cortex.

At the same time, the increased sensitivity to deoxyhaemoglobin in the veins causes greater sensitivity to the blood oxygenation level-dependent (BOLD) effect. This effect exploits the magnetic properties of the blood and of haemoglobin in particular, as an endogenous source of contrast, and forms the basis of the classical detection techniques of cortical activation. The functional magnetic resonance imaging (fMRI) technique is considered as one of the main applications that benefits from the use of UHF, thanks to the two simultaneous advantages of increased SNR and increased sensitivity to the BOLD effect. The improvement of both these factors can be exploited to study cerebral function with greater spatial resolution and greater sensitivity. It has been demonstrated that an increase in the spatial resolution of UHF fMRI can allow the definition of the functional architecture of the cerebral cortex at columnar level. In addition, the increase in the sensitivity of fMRI at 7 T allows to obtain statistically significant functional maps of cerebral activation not only in group of subjects but also for individual patients and individual events, opening new perspectives in the use of fMRI for clinical purposes.

The increase in the static magnetic field produces also an increase of the phenomenon of chemical shift, which can be also a negative effect, by worsening the chemical shift artefact typical of the fluid-fat interface. However, the increase of chemical shift forms the basis of a better spectral resolution of the frequency signal obtainable with UHF MR spectroscopy. The applicability of proton spectroscopy in a medical context is limited by the low concentration of most of the cerebral metabolites of interest compared with the quantity of water present in the tissue (over 50 mM). As the SNR and chemical shift are proportional to the strength of the static magnetic field, 7 T MR systems allow the quantification of about 13 brain metabolites, and thanks to spectral editing techniques, the direct detection

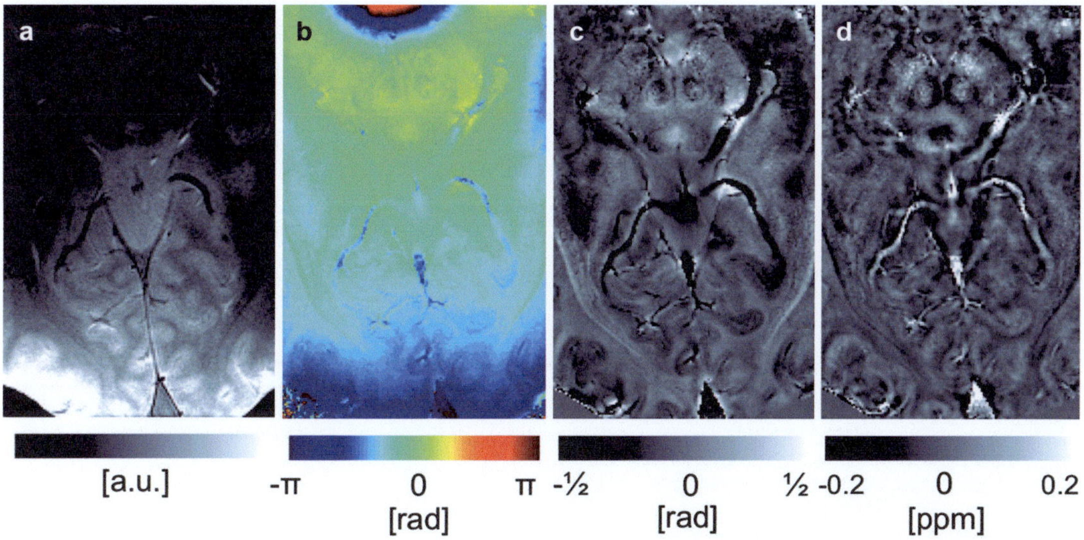


**Fig. 23.4** From the acquisition of signal (real and imaginary component), the phase can be extracted, and therefore information can be obtained regarding the physical measurements associated with the static magnetic field which affect the precession frequency. In other words, it is possible to obtain a map of the magnetic susceptibility of the tissue being examined. The latter physical property has proven to be a new and powerful endogenic contrast agent that can detect significant tissue characteristics in clinical practice. Susceptibility is in fact directly proportional to the presence of iron and inversely proportional to myelin density – two key parameters in the study of neurodegenerative diseases for example. The extraction of susceptibility maps is performed starting from the signal (**a**) and the reconstruction of phase images (**b**) which are processed in order to isolate the contributions of phase from the large-scale ones caused by inhomogeneities of the static magnetic field. From these maps of local phase variations (**c**), frequency variation maps and therefore quantitative magnetic susceptibility maps QSM (**d**) can be reconstructed and applied in clinical protocol [12]

of important neurotransmitters such as glutamate in few minutes (Fig. 23.5 MRS).

Thanks to an increase in the sensitivity of spectral resolution, the introduction of UHF systems also opens new horizons for the study of other nuclei such as $^{31}P$, and significant results have also been obtained with $^{13}C$, $^{23}Na$ and $^{17}O$, which are key elements in the study of cerebral metabolism and metabolism energy balance.

7 T scanning offers huge benefits when investigating structures and ultrastructures in vivo in human as in the field of neurometabolic studies and of cortical activation, improving our knowledge about anatomy and normal physiology in vivo. It is also for this reason that part of the research carried out at the UHF MR centres is aimed at fine-tuning sequences, identifying new contrast and optimising acquisition protocols on healthy volunteers. Moreover, the use of UHF offers a great potential for improving the characterisation of a wide spectrum of diseases of the CNS such as multiple sclerosis, neurodegenerative diseases, cerebral neoplasms and epilepsy.

The evaluation of multiple sclerosis at UHF allows to better clarify the underlying inflammatory process. In particular, the high resolution combined with the sensitivity to susceptibility of UHF allows to reveal the development of plaques along the perivenular white matter as a marker of MS in the differential diagnosis with other demyelinating disorders. Moreover, susceptibility-weighted imaging seems to detect paramagnetic rims at the lesion edge reflecting the expanding inflammatory phenomena of acute MS plaques [4].

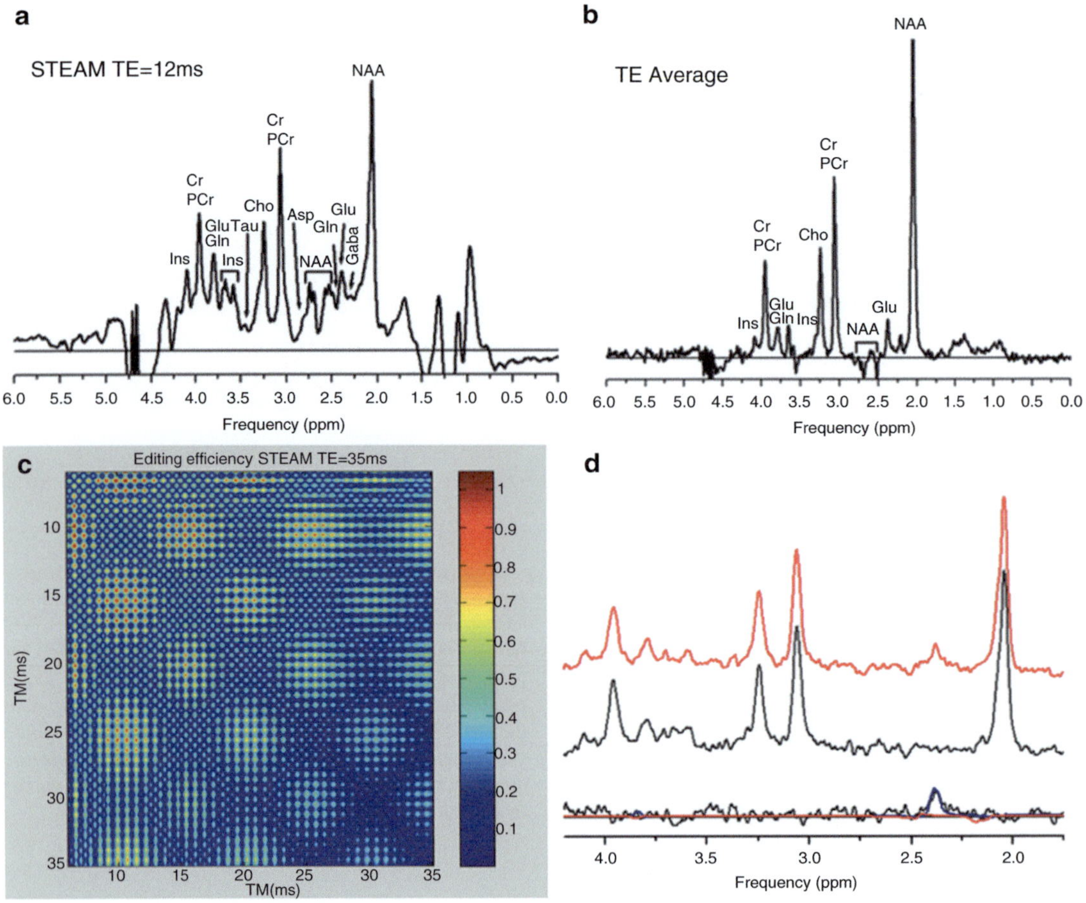


**Fig. 23.5** MR spectroscopy in vivo. Thanks to the use of UHF systems, and the subsequent increases in SNR and spectral resolution, signals from a larger number of cerebral metabolites can be detected and separated than with clinical magnetic fields. (a) Example of standard acquisition with stimulated echo acquisition mode (STEAM) short echo time sequence for detecting the greatest number of metabolites. (b) The technique of spectral simplification, which allows the detection of metabolites of interest by eliminating the spectral components of multiplets. (c) The simulation of the quantum evolution of spins for optimising acquisition parameters (TE, TM) to detect particularly weak signals and/or signals that are spectrally overlapped with others (STEAM-MiTis, *mixing time subtraction* technique). The STEAM-MiTis technique is optimised for detecting glutamate, an important neurotransmitter involved in numerous pathological processes [13]

As regards neurodegenerative diseases, most of the attention is focused on Alzheimer-type dementia, Parkinson's disease and, to a smaller extent, amyotrophic lateral sclerosis.

The studies on Alzheimer's are aimed at evaluating hippocampal formations at high resolution (Fig. 23.6) to measure substructures of the Ammon's horn such as the reticular or lacunosum moleculare layer sites of the initial phase of the neurodegenerative process. In comparison with normal subjects, these studies also regard hippocampal morphology in patients with mild cognitive impairment. Thanks to the combination of high resolution and sequences that are sensitive to magnetic susceptibility, other studies are dedicated to detecting amyloid plaques that are the pathological substrate of the disease. Such consistent results in ex vivo animal experiments are however a matter of debate when applied to humans in vivo.

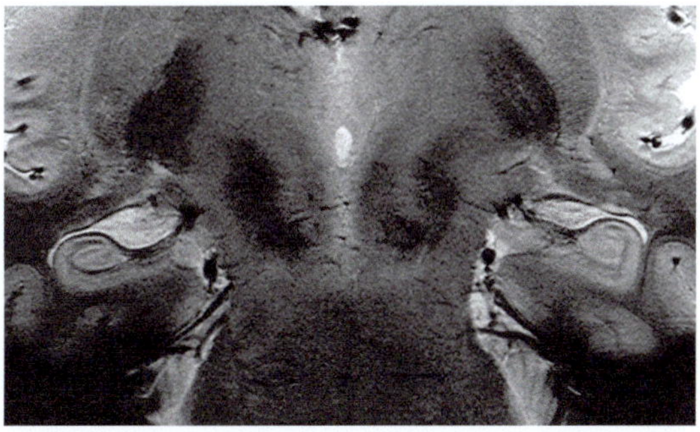

**Fig. 23.6** Images acquired with the MR 7 T system with very high spatial resolution (200 µm *in plane*) by using a gradient-recalled echo (GRE) sequence targeted on the hippocampus regions. This portion of the brain plays an important role in long-term memory and in spatial navigation. Simultaneous research into high spatial resolution and contrast in the hippocampus is aimed at measuring fine substructures of the Ammon's horn such as the reticular layers and incomplete molecular sites and locations of the initial phase of the neurodegenerative process of Alzheimer's disease

In Parkinson's disease, UHF MR has shown its additional value compared with clinical MR systems at conventional field strength, using targeted sequences sensitive to susceptibility. For the first time in vivo, UHF MR has allowed the identification of components of the substantia nigra including that responsible for the disease [5]. The disappearance of the pars compacta of the substantia nigra, containing the nigrosome, demonstrates its degeneration, which is the pathological counterpart of dopaminergic deficit. Moreover, UHF MRI allows identifying patients in the initial phase of Parkinson's disease with great diagnostic accuracy. These radiological signs are not specific of Parkinson's disease but constitute a hallmark of nigrostriatal degeneration common to other forms of atypical parkinsonisms. In addition, the possibility of obtaining quantitative maps of magnetic susceptibility will also provide more information about the pathogenesis of the neurodegeneration seen in Parkinson's disease.

In amyotrophic lateral sclerosis, high-resolution UHF imaging of the motor cortex has revealed an unusual accumulation of iron in the deeper layers of the cortex corresponding with what can be detected by an anatomopathological examination. This accumulation would seem to correspond with the severity of the disability [6]. In the field of motor neuron diseases, however, there are great expectations for high-resolution imaging of the spinal cord. This is currently under study to resolve hardware problems associated with the receiving of MR signals in an anatomically complex region and to increase the sensitivity of MRI in identifying the ultrastructure of the spinal cord.

In the evaluation of cerebral neoplasia, conventional MR, proton spectroscopy and advanced techniques such as diffusion and perfusion are currently the techniques used for neoplasia grading and for defining the bioptic target. The new contrasts that can be obtained with UHF (intratumoural susceptibility signals) seem to provide additional elements that are indicative of greater aggressiveness such as the presence of micro-haemorrhages or venographic studies, which, thanks to the sensitivity of the UHF for deoxyhaemoglobin, have become an index of oxygen consumption. Specific patterns of neoplasia in differential diagnostics with radionecrosis or expansive lesions of another nature have not yet been studied, but there are great hopes for the demarcation of neoplastic tissue, which remains a challenge unresolved at conventional fields. Moreover, a great expectancy is about the differential diagnosis and grading of gliomas. Sodium MR imaging greatly improved at 7 T for the increased SNR. Sodium signal has been shown to increase in brain tumours, and it seems to be a probe of tissue viability able to differentiate low- and high-grade gliomas [7]. 1H-MR spectroscopy provides a benefit for measuring metabolic markers of tumours for the increased spectral resolution and metabolite sensitivity compared with conventional magnetic field strength.

In epilepsy, the introduction of UHF allows to identify more epileptogenic lesions than those detectable with lower magnetic field strength, so that the number of patients with secondary focal epilepsy increases, reducing the incidence of patients with cryptogenic focal epilepsy. 7 T MR shows structural and biochemical abnormalities in greater detail to delineate seizure foci and probably could contribute to the surgical planning and to the improvement of patients outcome [8, 9].

Lastly, for all the experimental protocols on humans, many studies have been carried out about safety and tolerability of 7 T MR, providing encouraging results regarding the absence of significant side effects. Only annoying sensations have been reported, such as vertigo result, the most frequent at high magnetic fields [10].

Based on the laws of physics which govern it, UHF magnetic resonance has created great expectations and hopes for the creation of new semeiotics of many diseases of both the CNS in the first instance and in the future of many other regions of the body, e.g. the musculoskeletal system. In recent years, there have been numerous efforts made to provide 7 T scanners with coils and sequences for application on human to thus gain greater physiological and physiopathological knowledge as a prelude to future clinical applications. Many problems have been resolved but many others still remain to be fixed, before the full potential of UHF could be exploited at all. Only through continuous research, multidisciplinary synergy and the comparison of expertise from different sectors (physics, chemistry, engineering and medicine), the effective diagnostic progress of UHF in comparison with conventional fields can be demonstrated in different diseases, a fundamental step for putting UHF MR at the service of medicine.

## References


1. Tiberi G, Fontana N, Costagli M, Stara R, Biagi L, Symms MR, Monorchio A, Retico A, Cosottini M, Tosetti M (2015) Investigation of maximum local specific absorption rate in 7T magnetic resonance with respect to load size by use of electromagnetic simulations. Bioelectromagnetics 36(5):358–366
2. Costagli M, Kelley DA, Symms MR, Biagi L, Stara R, Maggioni E, Tiberi G, Barba C, Guerrini R, Cosottini M, Tosetti M (2014) Tissue Border Enhancement by inversion recovery MRI at 7.0. Neuroradiology 56(7):517–523
3. Costagli M, Symms MR, Angeli L, Kelley DAC, Biagi L, Farnetani A, Rua C, Donatelli G, Tiberi G, Tosetti M, Cosottini M (2016) Assessment of Silent T1-weighted head imaging at 7 T. Eur Radiol 26(6):1879–1888
4. Absinta M, Sati P, Gaitán MI, Maggi P, Cortese IC, Filippi M, Reich DS (2013) Seven-tesla phase imaging of acute multiple sclerosis lesions: A new window into the inflammatory process. Ann Neurol 74(5):669–678
5. Cosottini M, Frosini D, Pesaresi I, Costagli M, Biagi L, Ceravolo R, Bonuccelli U, Tosetti M (2014) MR imaging of the substantia nigra at 7 T enables diagnosis of Parkinson disease. Radiology 271(3):831–838
6. Cosottini M, Donatelli G, Costagli M, Caldarazzo Ienco E, Frosini D, Pesaresi I, Biagi L, Siciliano G, Tosetti M (2016) High-resolution 7 T MR imaging of the motor cortex in amyotrophic lateral sclerosis. Am J Neuroradiol 37(3):455–461
7. Biller A, Badde S, Nagel A, Neumann JO, Wick W, Hertenstein A, Bendszus M, Sahm F, Benkhedah N, Kleesiek J (2016) Improved brain tumor classification by sodium MR imaging: prediction of IDH mutation status and tumor progression. AJNR Am J Neuroradiol 37(1):66–73. doi:10.3174/ajnr.A4493
8. De Ciantis A, Barba C, Tassi L, Cosottini M, Tosetti M, Costagli M, Bramerio M, Bartolini E, Biagi L, Cossu M, Pelliccia V, Symms MR, Guerrini R (2016 Mar) 7 T MRI in focal epilepsy with unrevealing conventional field strength imaging. Epilepsia 57(3):445–454. doi:10.1111/epi.13313
9. De Ciantis A, Barkovich AJ, Cosottini M, Barba C, Montanaro D, Costagli M, Tosetti M, Biagi L, Dobyns WB, Guerrini R (2015) Ultra-high-field MR imaging in polymicrogyria and epilepsy. Am J Neuroradiol 36(2):309–316
10. Cosottini M, Frosini D, Biagi L, Pesaresi I, Costagli M, Tiberi G, Symms M, Tosetti M (2014) Short-term side-effects of brain MR examination at 7 T: A single-centre experience. Eur Radiol 24(8):1923–1928
11. Tiberi G, Costagli M, Biagi L, Ciantis AD, Fontana N, Stara R, Symms MR, Cosottini M, Guerrini R, Tosetti M (2016) SAR prediction in adults and children by combining measured B1+ maps and simulations at 7.0 Tesla. J Magn Reson Imaging. doi:10.1002/jmri.25241
12. Costagli M, Donatelli G, Biagi L, Caldarazzo Ienco E, Siciliano G, Tosetti M, Cosottini M (2016) Magnetic susceptibility in the deep layers of the primary motor cortex in Amyotrophic Lateral Sclerosis. Neuroimage. doi:10.1016/j.nicl.2016.04.011
13. Toncelli A, Noeske R, Cosottini M, Costagli M, Domenici V, Tiberi G, Tosetti M (2015) STEAM-MiTiS: An MR spectroscopy method for the detection of scalar-coupled metabolites and its application to glutamate at 7 T. Magn Reson Med 74(6):1515–1522

## Further Reading

Robert W, Brown, Y-C, Cheng N, Haacke EM, Thompson MR, Venkatesan R (2014) Magnetic Resonance Imaging: Physical Principles and Sequence Design, 2nd Edition Wiley-Blackwell

Hennig J, Speck O (2012) High-field MR imaging. Springer Science & Business Media

Pierre-Marie R, Lawrence B (eds) (2007) Ultra high field magnetic resonance imaging. Series: Biological magnetic resonance, vol 26. Springer Science & Business Media

# Index




T. Scarabino et al. (eds.), *High Field Brain MRI*, DOI 10.1007/978-3-319-44174-0

MIX
Papier aus verantwortungsvollen Quellen
Paper from responsible sources
FSC® C105338

If you have any concerns about our products,
you can contact us on
**ProductSafety@springernature.com**

In case Publisher is established outside the EU,
the EU authorized representative is:
**Springer Nature Customer Service Center GmbH**
**Europaplatz 3, 69115 Heidelberg, Germany**

Printed by Libri Plureos GmbH
in Hamburg, Germany